UNDERSTANDING HEALTHCARE FINANCIAL MANAGEMENT

Third Edition

Louis C. Gapenski

Understanding Healthcare Financial Management

Third Edition

Including Student Learning Diskette

AUPHA Press, Washington, D.C.

Health Administration Press, Chicago, Illinois

05   04   03   02   5   4   3   2

The paper used in this publication meets the minimum requirements of American National Standards for Information Sciences—Permanence of Paper for Printed Library Materials, ANSI Z39.48–1984. ⊗™

Library of Congress Cataloging-in-Publication Data

Gapenski, Louis C.
    Understanding healthcare financial management / Louis C. Gapenski. — 3rd ed.
        p.   cm.
    "AUPHA/HAP."
    Includes bibliographical references and index.
    ISBN 1-56793-144-8 (alk. paper)
    1. Health facilities—Business management.   2. Health facilities—United States—Business management.   3. Medical care—United States—Finance.
    4. Health services administration—Economic aspects—United States.
    I. Association of University Programs in Health Administration.   II Title.
    RA971.3.G37   2000
    362.1'068'1—dc21   00-061341
                                                                    CIP

Health Administration Press
A division of the Foundation
  of the American College of
  Healthcare Executives
1 North Franklin Street, Suite 1700
Chicago, IL 60606-3491
(312) 424-2800

Association of University Programs
  in Health Administration
730 11th St., NW
4th Floor
Washington, DC 2001
(202) 638-1448

CONTENTS

PART V Capital Allocation

PART VI Financial Analysis and Forecasting

PART VII Other Topics

PREFACE

After years of teaching corporate finance and writing related textbooks and casebooks, I began teaching the healthcare financial management course in the University of Florida's Graduate Program in Health and Hospital Administration. The first thing that struck me was that no textbook was available that truly focused on healthcare financial management. To me, financial management primarily involves analysis and decision making, yet the textbooks available at the time mostly covered accounting and institutional detail, with only a very limited number of pages devoted to financial management.

Thus, I set about creating a textbook that emphasized (1) financial management rather than accounting and (2) analysis and decision making rather than institutional detail. In creating this textbook, I set out to do two things. First, I adopted a very broad definition of the health services industry that included medical practices, managed care organizations, nursing homes, and home health care providers, in addition to hospitals. Today, more and more health services administration students are electing careers outside of the hospital industry, and it is important that a textbook on healthcare financial management presents a broad range of provider settings. Second, I identified the environmental factors that are unique to the health services industry and hence make healthcare financial management different from corporate finance. Then, I made sure that these factors played an important role in the textbook discussions.

Concept of the Textbook

My goals in writing the first edition were to create a textbook that provided health services administration students with (1) an operational knowledge of financial management theory and concepts; (2) the opportunity to apply these ideas to "real-world" healthcare business settings; and (3) the opportunity to use spreadsheet analyses to help make better financial decisions. Additionally, I wanted to create a textbook that could be used as a reference during residencies and after graduation. Finally, I wanted a textbook that students would find "user friendly," meaning one that they would enjoy reading and could learn from on their own. If students don't find a textbook interesting, understandable, and useful, they won't read it!

This third edition of the textbook continues to meet those goals. It begins with basic concepts about both the health services industry and financial management. The textbook then progresses to show how financial management theory and concepts can be applied to healthcare businesses to help managers make better financial decisions, where "better" is defined as promoting the financial well-being of the organization.

Intended Market and Use

The textbook is targeted for the healthcare financial management course required in graduate programs in health services administration. Students typically have some background in basic business topics such as financial and managerial accounting, probability and statistics, spreadsheet analysis, and perhaps even corporate finance. However, the textbook contains a great deal of background information in these areas, and it can be used in programs where students have not had prior exposure to business topics. The textbook is useful also to healthcare professionals, including both those holding general management positions and those working as members of financial staffs.

Alternative Course Formats

There is no single best approach to teaching a healthcare financial management course—the optimal approach varies with students' backgrounds, instructors' interests, class contact hours, and the role of the course in the overall curriculum. Because these factors change, most instructors vary their approaches over time. Still, it may be useful to adopters to learn how the textbook has been used at the University of Florida.

In the Florida program, students first take introductory corporate finance and accounting courses in the College of Business. Thus, the healthcare financial management course is the second, and typically last, finance course in the curriculum. The second financial management course in any curriculum generally is taught either as a theoretically based lecture course, as a pragmatically based pure case course, or as a blend of theory and practice where lectures are combined with some cases. Over time, I have used all three approaches, but the one that I have found best is a blend of theory and practice—lecturing occasionally, but also using a large number of cases to provide insights into the complex financial decisions faced by practicing healthcare managers.

Understanding Healthcare Financial Management provides both the theory and concepts behind financial decision making in the health services industry and the "nuts and bolts" tools required to implement the theory and concepts. Students learn the theory and concepts of healthcare financial management from the textbook and lectures, and then implement the material by working cases. In the first two editions, the cases were contained in the textbook. However, the editorial and production burden of having both textbook and casebook in a single edition created constraints that became too confining. The publisher and I agreed that the optimal solution to this problem was to separate the cases from the textbook, which we have done beginning with this edition. I will have much more to say about this decision later in the preface.

I cover most of the textbook, along with 12 cases (one per week, after some introductory material), in a one-semester course; but I acknowledge that some depth is sacrificed to obtain this breadth. However, our students are studying to be general managers, not financial staff specialists, and hence I am willing to sacrifice depth to expose students to a large range of topics. The course runs fast and furious, but this tends to keep students, and instructors, on their toes and in high gear.

Although the textbook is designed for use in the second course in financial management, a great deal of introductory material has been included. In spite of the fact that the Florida students have already had one course in corporate finance, I have found that many of them still do not have a good grasp of the basic fundamentals of financial management. Thus, they appreciate the fact that *Understanding Healthcare Financial Management* reviews basic concepts in addition to presenting new material. After all, repetition is the key to learning.

Because the textbook contains so much introductory material, it is also suitable for use in courses in which students have not had an introductory finance course, including two-course sequences. In this situation, I would tend to go slower to give students more time to digest the material, and the lectures would be more extensive to ensure that students really know the fundamentals before working the cases, which would be fewer in number. In a two-course sequence, instructors could easily supplement the textbook with outside readings and/or additional cases.

Changes in the Third Edition

Since the second edition of the textbook was published, I have used the text-book several times in courses I have taught and have received many comments from users at other universities. Furthermore, Health Administration Press has solicited and received a number of thoughtful reviews. The reaction of students, other professors, and the market in general has been overwhelmingly positive—every comment indicates that the basic concept of the textbook is sound. Even so, nothing is perfect, and the health services industry is evolving at a dizzying pace. These circumstances have led to a number of changes to the textbook; the most important of which are listed below:

- The most significant change for users of *Understanding Healthcare Financial Management* is the removal of the cases and the creation of a separate casebook. The new casebook is described in a later section.

- The textbook now includes a *Student Learning Diskette*, which is discussed in a later section.
- I updated and clarified all aspects of textbook discussion and references. Particular care was taken to include the most recent reimbursement changes and to update the real-world examples.
- New sections have been added that deal with the complications that arise in small businesses, especially medical practices. Many physicians are enrolling in health services administration programs, and hence the financial management of medical practices merits more discussion. Even students who choose careers with large providers, such as hospitals, should be aware of the financial management challenges facing small businesses.
- A separate chapter that deals with security valuation, market efficiency, and debt refunding was created. Although much of the material in the new chapter had been included in the second edition—in the debt financing and equity financing chapters—placing it in a separate chapter consolidates the material so that it can be presented in a more logical manner, as well as allow for somewhat greater coverage in the debt and equity financing chapters.
- A new chapter was added titled "Distributions to Owners: Bonuses, Dividends, and Repurchases." Although many students continue to seek careers with not-for-profit providers, an increasing proportion are going to work at investor-owned businesses, where return to owners is an important consideration in the financial management decision process. In adddition, this material is highly relevant to medical practices.
- A new chapter was added that deals with financial risk management. It is important that students, and practicing managers, recognize the financial risks facing healthcare providers as well as the tools that are available to help deal with those risks.
- The chapter on lease financing was moved into the Capital Acquisition section. Leasing is clearly an alternative form of financing, and hence part of capital acquisition.
- Each chapter now begins with a set of learning objectives, which allow students to gain a perspective of the chapter contents before they start reading.
- A short list of key web site references has been placed at the end of most chapters. Students need to get an idea of the types and extent of information available on the World Wide Web, and these references provide a start.

The Student Learning Diskette

The textbook now contains a *Student Learning Diskette*, which has two major sections. The first, and most important, section contains spreadsheet files for most chapters that illustrate some of the textbook calculations, as well as additional calculations that are relevant to the chapter material. The purpose of this section of the diskette is twofold. First, students can learn the material better because they can more easily visualize how various input factors influence a model or calculation. For example, the spreadsheet model for capital budgeting allows students to change input values and immediately see the effect on profitability. Second, the spreadsheets permit students to learn the mechanics of spreadsheet analysis in a less-challenging context than the cases because the models on the *Student Learning Diskette* are not part of a graded assignment. Text sections that have accompanying calculations on the diskette are identified by a diskette logo placed next to the heading.

The second section of the diskette contains a Word file with the web site addresses that are listed at the end of each chapter in the textbook. Thus, to go to any of the web sites suggested in the textbook, students can access this file and merely click on the address rather than enter it from scratch.

The Casebook

Healthcare finance can be a fascinating, exciting subject, yet students often regard it as either too theoretical or too mechanical. The fact is good financial decision making requires both sound quantitative analysis and a great deal of insight and judgment. The best way to get this point across to students, and to demonstrate the inherent richness of the subject matter, is to relate classroom work to real-world decision making. When this is done, students must not only grapple with the theory and concepts, but, more importantly, with how they are applied in practice.

Of course, the most realistic application of healthcare finance occurs within health services organizations, and there is no substitute for "on-the-job" experience. The next best thing, and the only real option for the classroom, is to use cases to simulate, to the extent possible, the environment in which finance decisions are actually made. Cases provide students with the opportunity to bridge the gap between learning concepts in a lecture setting and actually applying them on the job. By using cases, students can be better prepared to deal with the multitude of problems that arise in the practice of healthcare financial management. Thus, previous editions of *Understanding Healthcare Finance* contained cases in lieu of questions and problems. By placing these cases in a separate book, *Cases in Healthcare Finance*, we have been able to provide a more complete set of cases as well as expand the material in the textbook.

Cases in Healthcare Finance contains 26 cases that focus on the practice of healthcare finance within provider organizations. In general, each case addresses a single financial issue, such as a capital investment decision; but the uncertainty of the input data, along with the presence of relevant nonfinancial factors, make each case interesting and challenging. The case settings include a wide variety of provider organizations, including integrated delivery systems and managed care organizations. In addition to cases that focus purely on financial decisions, the casebook contains six mini-cases on ethics. The mini-cases are not quantitative in nature, but rather are designed to promote discussion about a finance situation that has potential ethical implications.

In general, cases may be classified as *directed* or *nondirected*. Directed cases include a specific set of questions that students must answer to complete the case, while nondirected cases (as I use the term) contain general guidance to point students in the right direction. Most of the cases in the casebook are nondirected. The primary advantage of nondirected cases is that they closely resemble how real-world managers confront financial decision making because they require students to develop their own solution approach. The disadvantage is that students who stray from the key issues of the case often do not obtain full value from their effort.

I have found that students with more advanced finance skills gain the most from nondirected cases, while students that have had less finance exposure gain most from directed cases. The *Instructor's Manual* for the casebook contains a set of case questions that can be used to convert each nondirected case to a directed case. Thus, instructors have the option of using the nondirected cases in either way, depending on the experience of the students, the objectives of the course, and the extent to which cases will be used.

Spreadsheet analysis has become extremely important in all aspects of healthcare finance. Students must be given the opportunity to develop computer skills and be allowed, or required, to use spreadsheet programs to assist in case analyses. If students have not previously learned about spreadsheets, they must be exposed to them because "functional literacy" in any area of management today means at least some knowledge of spreadsheet modeling. Furthermore, spreadsheet models can reduce the amount of "busywork" required to perform the required calculations, and hence leave students with more time to focus on financial management issues.

Because of these factors, I developed well-structured, user-friendly spreadsheet models for those cases where models would help to create a more efficient analysis. Most of the cases could, of course, be done with a calculator; but the spreadsheet models are far more efficient, and hence big time savers, especially when conducting risk assessment using techniques such as sensitivity and scenario analyses. In addition, spreadsheet models allow students to easily create graphics and other computer output that enhance the quality of both the analyses and any required presentations.

The student versions of the case models are complete in the sense that no modeling is required to obtain a base case solution. However, zeros have been entered for all input data, and hence students must identify and then enter the appropriate input values. When this is done, the model automatically calculates the base case solution. However, the models do not contain risk analyses or other extensions such as graphics, so students must modify the models as necessary to make them most useful in completing the cases. The student versions of the case models are distributed with the casebook, so when students buy the casebook they also receive the student version case models.

The instructor versions of the case models are similar to the student versions, except that the input values are intact. Thus, instructors can view the base case solution without entering any data. In addition, some instructor version models have additional modeling, such as risk analyses, included. The instructor versions of the case models are distributed with the *Instructor's Manual* to the casebook.

Using the Textbook and Casebook Together

Health Administration Press is keenly aware of the increasing financial burden that students face as course materials escalate in both quantity and price. Thus, when both the textbook and casebook are adopted for a single course, the publisher will give a discount on the joint purchase. For more information, call the Health Administration Press marketing department at (312) 424-9470 or e-mail *khumbert@ache.com*.

Acknowledgments

This book reflects the efforts of many people. First, I would like to thank the following individuals, who reviewed previous editions of the textbook and provided many valuable comments and suggestions for improving it:

Doug Conrad	University of Washington
Tom Getzen	Temple University
Mike McCue	Virginia Commonwealth University
Dean Smith	University of Michigan
Jack Wheeler	University of Michigan

Special thanks are due to Barbara Langland-Orban and Christy Harris Lemak, who coauthored Chapter 1; and to Mike McCue and Jack Wheeler, who coauthored some sections.

Colleagues, students, and staff at the University of Florida provided inspirational support, as well as more tangible support, during the development and class testing of each edition of the textbook. And last, but certainly not least, I would like to thank the Health Administration Press staff, who was instrumental in ensuring the quality and usefulness of the textbook.

Errors in the Textbook

In spite of the significant effort that has been expended on this edition, it is safe to say that some errors exist. In an attempt to create the most error-free and useful textbook possible, I strongly encourage both instructors and students to write me at the address below with comments and suggestions for improving the textbook. I welcome and value your input!

Conclusion

Good financial management is vital to the economic well-being of the health services industry. Because of its importance, financial management theory and concepts should be thoroughly understood; but this is easier said than done. I hope that *Understanding Healthcare Financial Management* will help you better appreciate the financial management problems faced by the health services industry today, and that it will provide guidance on how best to solve them.

Louis C. Gapenski, PhD
Box 100195
Health Science Center
University of Florida
Gainesville, Florida 32610-0195

THE HEALTHCARE ENVIRONMENT

INTRODUCTION*

Learning Objectives

After studying this chapter, readers should be able to:

- Explain the difference between accounting and financial management.
- Discuss the role of financial management in health services organizations.
- Briefly outline the organization of the book.
- Describe in general terms the composition of the health services industry, its manpower requirements, and how healthcare is financed in the United States.
- Discuss the major trends in the healthcare environment and how these trends influence the provision of health services.

Introduction

The study of healthcare financial management is both fascinating and rewarding. It is fascinating because so many of the concepts involved have implications for both professional and personal behavior. It is rewarding because, rightly or wrongly, the healthcare environment today, and into the foreseeable future, is forcing managers to place an increasing emphasis on financial implications when making operating decisions.

First and foremost, financial management is a *decision science*. Whereas accounting provides decision makers with a rational means by which to budget for and measure a business's financial performance, financial management provides the theory, concepts, and tools necessary to make better decisions. Thus, the primary purpose of this text is to help health services administrators and students become better decision makers. The text is designed primarily for general managers rather than for financial management specialists, although such specialists—especially those with accounting rather than finance backgrounds or those who are moving into the health services industry from other industries—will also find the text useful.

The major difference between this text and corporate finance texts is that this text focuses on factors that are unique to the health services industry. For example, the provision of health services is dominated by *not-for-profit* organizations—both private and governmental—which are inherently

---

*This chapter was coauthored by Barbara Langland-Orban of the University of South Florida and Christy Harris Lemak of the University of Florida.

different from *investor-owned* businesses.[1] Also, the majority of payments for services made to healthcare providers are not made by the consumers of the service, but rather by some *third-party payer* (for example, a commercial insurance company or a government program). Indeed, even the purchase of health insurance is dominated by employers rather than by the individuals who will receive the services. Throughout this text, we emphasize ways in which the unique features of the health services industry affect financial management decisions.

Although this text contains some theory, and a great number of financial management concepts, its primary emphasis is on how managers can apply the theory and concepts; thus, it does not contain the traditional end-of-chapter questions and problems. Rather, the text is designed to be used with the casebook *Cases in Healthcare Finance*, which contains cases that are based on "real-life" decisions faced by practicing healthcare managers. The cases are designed to enable students to apply the skills learned in this text's chapters in a realistic context, where judgment is just as critical to good decision making as numerical analysis. Furthermore, the cases are semidirected, which means that although students receive some guidance, they must formulate their own approach to the analyses just as real-world decision makers must do.[2]

Also, personal computers are changing the way managers think about structuring and performing financial analyses. Managers, and students, must recognize that computers are capable of providing answers to questions that were not even asked a few years ago. Thus, both this text and the casebook are oriented toward using spreadsheets to help make better decisions. This text has an accompanying diskette with spreadsheet models that illustrate the key concepts presented in many of the chapters. The casebook has a diskette with spreadsheet models that make the quantitative portion of the case analyses both easier to do and more complete.

Note, however, that it is impossible to create a text that includes everything that a manager needs to know about healthcare financial management. Indeed, it would be foolish even to try because the industry is so vast and is changing so rapidly that many of the details needed to become completely knowledgeable in the field can only be learned through contemporary experience. Thus, we do not expect readers to fully understand every nuance of every financial management theory and concept that pertains to the industry, nor do we expect readers to become experts in quantitative analysis. Nevertheless, this text will provide the competencies required to enable readers to (1) judge the validity of analyses performed by others, usually financial staff specialists or consultants; and (2) incorporate sound financial management theory and concepts in their own managerial and personal decision making.

The Role of Financial Management in the Health Services Industry

Until the 1960s, *financial management* in all industries was generally viewed as descriptive in nature, with its primary role being to secure the financing needed to meet a business's operating objectives. A business's marketing, or planning, department would project demand for the firm's goods or services; operating personnel would estimate the assets needed to meet the projected demand; and the finance department would raise the money needed to purchase the required plant, equipment, and supplies. The study of financial management concentrated on business securities and the markets in which they are sold, and on how businesses could interact with the financial markets to raise capital. Consequently, financial management textbooks of that era were almost totally descriptive in nature.

Today, financial management plays a much larger role in the overall management of a business. Now, the primary role of financial management is to plan for, acquire, and utilize funds (capital) to maximize the efficiency and value of the enterprise. Because of this role, financial management is known also as *capital finance*. The specific goals of financial management depend on the nature of the business, so we must postpone that discussion until Chapter 2. In general, financial management and accounting are separate functions, although the accounting function is often carried out under the direction of the organization's *chief financial officer (CFO)*, and hence falls under the overall category of "finance."

In general, the financial management function includes the following activities:

- **Evaluation and planning.** First and foremost, financial management involves evaluating the financial effectiveness of current operations and planning for the future.
- **Long-term investment decisions**. Although more important to senior management, managers at all levels must be concerned with the capital investment decision process. Such decisions, which focus on the acquisition of new plant and equipment (i.e., fixed assets), are the primary means by which businesses implement strategic plans, and hence they play a key role in a business's financial future.
- **Financing decisions.** All organizations must raise funds to buy the assets necessary to support operations. Such decisions involve the choice between internal and external funds, the use of debt versus equity capital, and the use of long-term versus short-term debt. Although senior managers typically make financing decisions, these decisions have ramifications for managers at all levels.
- **Working capital management.** An organization's current, or short-term, assets, such as cash, marketable securities, receivables, and inventories,

must be properly managed both to ensure operational effectiveness and to reduce costs. Generally, managers at all levels are involved, to some extent, in short-term asset management, which is often called working capital management.

- **Contract management.** In today's healthcare environment, health services organizations must negotiate, sign, and monitor contracts with managed care organizations and third-party payers. The financial staff typically has primary responsibility for these tasks, but managers at all levels are involved in these activities and must be aware of their effect on operating decisions.
- **Financial risk management.** Many financial transactions that take place to support the operations of a business can, themselves, increase a business's risk. Thus, an important financial management activity is to control financial risk.

In times of high profitability and abundant financial resources, the finance function tends to decline in importance. Thus, when most healthcare providers were reimbursed on the basis of costs incurred, the role of finance was minimal. At that time, the most critical finance function was cost accounting because it was more important to account for costs than it was to control them. Today, however, healthcare providers are facing an increasingly hostile environment, and any business that ignores the finance function runs the risk of financial deterioration, which ultimately could lead to bankruptcy and closure.

In recent years, providers have been redesigning their finance functions to recognize the changes that have been occurring in the health services industry. For the most part, the practice of finance had been driven by the Medicare program, which demanded that providers (primarily hospitals) churn out a multitude of reports both to comply with regulations and to maximize Medicare revenues. Third-party reimbursement complexities meant that a large amount of time had to be spent on cumbersome accounting, billing, and collection procedures. Thus, instead of focusing on value-adding activities, most finance work focused on bureaucratic functions. Today, to be of maximum value to the enterprise, the finance function must support cost-containment efforts, managed care and other payer contract negotiations, joint venture decisions, and integrated delivery system participation. In essence, finance must help lead organizations into the future, rather than merely record what has happened in the past.

In this text, the emphasis is on financial management, but there are no unimportant functions in health services organizations. Managers must understand a multitude of functions such as marketing, accounting, and human resource management in addition to financial management. Still, all business decisions have financial implications, so all managers—whether in operations, marketing, personnel, or facilities—must know enough about financial management to incorporate financial implications in decisions made within their own specialized areas. Thus, all managers must understand the theory and principles of financial management because this knowledge will make them even more effective at their own specialized work.

1. What is the role of financial management in today's health services organizations?
2. How has this role changed over time?

Self-Test Questions

Organization of the Text

Lewis Carroll wrote in *Alice in Wonderland*: "Any road will do if you don't know where you are going." With that caution in mind, we have carefully identified our destination—the readers of this text need to learn financial management theories, concepts, and tools that are most important to managers in the health services industry. The organization of this text paves the road to our destination.

Part I contains fundamental background materials on the healthcare environment on which the remainder of the text builds. Chapter 1 introduces the text, while Chapters 2 and 3 provide additional insights into the uniqueness of the health services industry. Healthcare financial management cannot be studied in a vacuum because financial decisions are profoundly influenced by the economic and social environment of the industry in which they are made.

Part II contains two concepts fundamental to virtually all financial management decisions. Chapter 4 discusses time value analysis, which provides techniques for valuing cash flows that are expected to occur in the future, and Chapter 5 presents financial risk and required return, which are two of the cornerstones of financial decision making.

Part III turns to the capital acquisition process. Businesses need capital, or funds, to purchase assets. Chapters 6 and 7 provide descriptive information about the two primary types of financing—debt and equity—and the markets in which they are traded. In Chapter 8, we discuss security valuation and bond refunding decisions, along with the concept of market efficiency. Finally, Chapter 9 explores lease financing, which is gaining popularity as an alternative to traditional financing sources.

Part IV sets forth the framework for analyzing the appropriate mix of financing and for assessing its cost to the business. In essence, businesses use the particular mix of debt and equity financing that maximizes the value of the firm or, alternatively, minimizes the business's overall cost of funds. In turn, the cost of funds raised sets the business's cost of capital, which is the return that investment opportunities must provide if they are to be financially acceptable.

In Chapters 12 and 13 (Part V), we consider the vital subject of long-term investment decisions, or *capital budgeting*. Because major capital projects take years to plan and execute, and because these decisions generally are not easily reversed and will affect operations for many years, their impact on a business's financial condition is profound.

Part VI focuses on financial analysis and forecasting. It is important for healthcare managers to be able to assess the current financial condition of the business. Even more important, managers must be able to monitor and control current operations, and to assess ways in which alternative courses of action will affect the business's future financial condition. The tools used to analyze a business's financial and operating strengths and weaknesses, as well as to forecast future financial condition, are discussed here.

Finally, in Part VII, we examine some other topics of relevance to healthcare financial management. Chapter 16, with its emphasis on working capital, examines current, ongoing operations, as opposed to long-term, strategic decisions. Chapter 17, which is of relevance only within for-profit businesses, focuses on the means by which such businesses provide profit distributions to owners. In Chapter 18, we focus on business valuation, mergers, and acquisitions, which are areas of current importance as healthcare businesses combine to help position themselves to better cope with the ever-changing healthcare environment. Chapter 19 focuses on capitation and risk sharing. The trend toward a more integrated delivery of health services is creating new challenges for managers, and some of the unique issues associated with integration are covered in this chapter. Finally, Chapter 20 provides information on financial risk management, especially on the techniques used to reduce or limit the riskiness inherent in financial transactions.

Self-Test Question

1. Briefly, explain the organization of the text.

Healthcare Expenditures

The healthcare sector in the United States is a diverse collection of industries that involve, either directly or indirectly, the provision of *healthcare services*. The major players in the sector are (1) the *providers* of health services, such as medical (physician) practices, hospitals, and nursing homes; (2) the *suppliers* of drugs and equipment, such as the pharmaceutical firms and medical equipment manufacturers; (3) the *traditional third-party payers*, including both government programs and commercial insurers; (4) *managed care organizations*, such as health maintenance and preferred provider organizations; and (5) a diverse collection of other entities, ranging from consulting firms to educational institutions to government and private research agencies. This text generally focuses on providers because they are the unique element of the healthcare sector, but one must never forget that the sector includes firms such as General Electric, which makes, markets, and leases medical diagnostic equipment, along with lightbulbs, appliances, and jet engines.

The healthcare sector is the second largest business sector in the United States (only the real estate sector is larger). As shown in Table 1.1, with total spending estimated at over $1.3 trillion in 2000, the sector consumed about 14 percent of the nation's gross domestic product. As measured by percentage of GNP, the resources devoted to healthcare in the United States have more than tripled since 1950.

Although it is impossible to effectively pinpoint the causes of rapidly escalating healthcare expenditures in the United States, the reasons most often cited include the following:

- The rapid advance in the use of technology, including biotech, genetic, and pharmaceutical technology, to diagnose and treat disease coupled with the high cost of new technology;
- The aging of the population;
- Society's view of the value of life, and the resultant belief that good health is worth any price (It has been said that Americans are the only people on earth who believe that death is optional.);
- The fact that the third-party-payer system removes the economic responsibility from the consumers of healthcare goods and services;
- The high cost of malpractice insurance;
- Operational and administrative inefficiencies, including duplication of

TABLE 1.1 Historical and Estimated National Health Expenditures, 1950–2008

Calendar Year	Total (in Billions)	Per Capita	Percentage of GDP
1950	$ 12.7	$ 82	4.4%
1960	26.9	141	5.1
1970	73.2	341	7.1
1980	247.3	1,052	8.9
1990	699.4	2,689	12.2
1993	898.5	3,350	13.7
1995	993.7	3,638	13.7
1997	1,092.4	3,927	13.5
1999*	1,228.5	4,340	13.9
2000*	1,316.2	4,611	14.3
2001*	1,403.6	4,877	14.6
2002*	1,495.5	5,155	14.9
2003*	1,590.4	5,439	15.2
2004*	1,690.4	5,737	15.4
2005*	1,799.5	6,061	15.6
2006*	1,917.3	6,409	15.8
2007*	2,043.1	6,708	16.0
2008*	2,176.6	7,170	16.2

*Estimated.
Source: Health Care Financing Administration (HCFA) online statistics and data. 2000. www.hcfa.gov.

services, excess capacity, and inefficiencies in billing and payment mechanisms;
• The willingness of the federal government to fund healthcare expenditures through its Medicare and Medicaid programs; and
• The high cost of physician education.

Table 1.2 provides a breakdown of direct expenditures for healthcare goods and services. Hospitals capture the largest percentage of the healthcare dollar, while physicians are the next largest beneficiary of healthcare expenditures. However, hospitals have been losing their share of the healthcare dollar in recent years while physicians have been gaining. It is interesting to note that nursing home care now consumes over 8 percent of healthcare expenditures, whereas nursing home care was almost nonexistent 40 years ago. Because hospitals and physicians combined receive over half of all healthcare expenditures, cost-containment efforts were first directed toward these two providers. However, in recent years, we have witnessed dramatic growth rates in payments for nursing home care, home health care, and pharmaceuticals. Thus, the most recent cost-containment efforts have focused on these areas.

Self-Test Questions

1. What has been the trend in healthcare expenditures over the past several decades?
2. How is the healthcare dollar split among the providers of goods and services and what are the trends?

Healthcare Financing Sources and Trends

Funding for healthcare goods and services is provided by private as well as by federal, state, and local government sources. Although total spending by all sources has increased, the percentage of total expenditures covered by private

TABLE 1.2
Estimated Health Expenditures by Type of Good or Service, 2000

Healthcare Expenditure	Percentage of Total
Hospital care	36.9%
Physician services	22.6
Prescription drugs	10.0
Nursing home care	8.1
Other professional services	6.8
Dental services	5.3
Medical products and equipment	4.1
Home health care	3.1
Other health services	3.1
Total	100.0%

Source: Health Care Financing Administration (HCFA) online statistics and data. 2000. www.hcfa.gov.

sources decreased, the percentage from the federal government increased, and the percentage from state and local governments remained roughly constant from the years 1950 to 2000. The trend of increasing participation by the federal government is a direct result of the Medicare and Medicaid programs.

In 2000, private sources covered 55.4 percent of all expenditures for healthcare goods and services, the federal government paid for 31.9 percent, and state and local governments covered 12.7 percent. Table 1.3 summarizes the sources of national healthcare expenditures.

Numerous factors led to the development and growth of health insurance programs, particularly as health services became more expensive and the provision of charity care became less practical. In this section, we provide a brief overview of the *third-party-payer system*. Because reimbursement is an essential element of healthcare financial management, we will discuss this subject in much more detail in Chapter 3.

During the 1920s, the science of medicine advanced and hospital care became more expensive. By the decade's end, the country faced the Great Depression. As a result, the financial condition of hospitals began to erode and the need for insurance protection became evident. Hospitals, through the American Hospital Association, encouraged the development of hospital insurance plans, primarily Blue Cross plans. (Blue Shield plans provide insurance for physician care.) Private health insurance grew rapidly after World War II, increasing both the proportion of the population with insurance and the scope of coverage. In 1966, the Medicare and Medicaid programs—the two largest government programs that finance healthcare services—were initiated to provide coverage to the elderly and poor.

Medicare is a federal insurance program designed primarily to cover healthcare services for people 65 years and older. In 2000, about 40 million individuals were enrolled in Medicare. Medicare has two parts, and each part has its own federal trust fund originally established to ensure that adequate funds are available. The health insurance portion—Part A—pays for inpatient hospital care, posthospital skilled nursing care, home healthcare, and hospice

Source	Percentage of Total Funding
Private health insurance	34.5%
Medicare	19.2
Out-of-pocket payments	17.4
Medicaid	15.2
Other government programs	10.2
Other private sources	3.5
Total	100.0%

TABLE 1.3
Estimated Healthcare Financing Sources, 2000

Source: Health Care Financing Administration (HCFA) online statistics and data. 2000. www.hcfa.gov.

care. The supplementary medical insurance portion—Part B—covers physician, hospital outpatient, and selected other services. Although Medicare is currently funded at adequate levels by payroll taxes and by Part B charges to enrollees, the rapid aging of the population together with healthcare costs that are increasing faster than general inflation have caused concern over the future viability of the program. Thus, many recent changes that attempt to moderate the growth in expenditures have occurred in the Medicare program.

Medicaid is funded jointly by federal and state governments. The federal government establishes the minimum requirements for eligibility and specifies the services that must be provided, and the states are allowed to design the scope of their programs within these guidelines. States receive roughly one dollar from the federal government for each dollar they contribute to the program. This creates an incentive for the states, especially the more affluent ones, to expand Medicaid coverage because they have to bear only half the costs. In 2000, over 30 million people received some type of Medicaid benefit; the majority of these benefits were provided to the aged, blind, and disabled.

Private health insurance is offered by state and local *Blue Cross/Blue Shield* organizations, which are either not-for-profit or for-profit corporations established for the sole purpose of providing health insurance, and by *commercial insurers*, such as Aetna and Prudential, which are investor-owned insurance companies that typically offer a complete line of insurance services. Private health insurance varies widely in terms of hospital and physician benefits, depth of major medical coverage, and protection against large out-of-pocket expenses.

Traditional health insurance, or *indemnity plans*, typically use *deductibles* and *copayments* to curtail the demand for health services. Such out-of-pocket payments require beneficiaries to share some level of expense, thus avoiding first-dollar coverage. Despite the use of these financial incentives, indemnity plans, which provide almost unlimited access to services with relatively small out-of-pocket costs, encourage consumers to seek additional or higher-quality healthcare services, and thus place considerable pressure on overall costs.

Managed care organizations, which reflect the current movement to control healthcare spending, strive to combine providers and insurers into a single entity. One type of managed care organization is the *health maintenance organization (HMO)*. HMOs are based on the premise that the current fee-for-service system creates perverse incentives that reward providers for treating patients' illnesses while offering few or no incentives for providing prevention and rehabilitation services. By combining the financing and delivery of comprehensive healthcare services into a single system, HMOs, at least theoretically, have as strong an incentive to prevent illnesses as to treat illnesses.

Because of the many different types of organizational structures, ownership, and financial incentives provided, HMOs vary widely in cost and quality. HMOs use a variety of methods to control costs. These methods include limiting patients to particular providers, including "gatekeeper" physicians who must authorize any specialized or referral services; utilization review to ensure that services rendered are appropriate and needed; discounted rate schedules for providers; and payment methods that transfer some risk to providers. In general, services are not covered if beneficiaries bypass their gatekeeper physician or use non-HMO providers.

The federal Health Maintenance Act of 1973 encouraged the development of HMOs and created a great deal of interest in the concept by providing federal funds for HMO-operating grants and loans. In addition, the Act requires larger employers that offer healthcare benefits to their employees to include a federally qualified HMO as one of the healthcare alternatives, if one is available, in addition to traditional insurance plans.

Another type of managed care plan, the *preferred provider organization (PPO)*, evolved during the early 1980s. PPOs are a hybrid of HMOs and traditional healthcare insurance. They use many of the cost-saving strategies developed by HMOs such as specific provider panels, utilization review, and reduced rate schedules for providers. However, PPOs do not mandate that beneficiaries use specific providers, although financial incentives are created that encourage members to use those providers with which the PPO has discounted-fee contracts (i.e., the PPO panel). Unlike HMOs, PPOs do not require beneficiaries to use preselected gatekeeper physicians who serve as the initial contact and authorize all services received. PPOs are less likely than HMOs to provide preventive services, and they do not assume any responsibility for quality assurance because enrollees are not constrained to use only the PPO panel of providers.

HMOs and PPOs grew rapidly in numbers and size during the 1980s and 1990s. Furthermore, hybrids of HMOs and PPOs continue to develop, such as *exclusive provider organizations*, which are PPO-like plans that require members to use only participating providers but do not designate a specific gatekeeper, and *point of service (POS) plans*, in which enrollees may choose either to obtain services from within the HMO or to bear higher out-of-pocket costs to obtain services from providers outside the HMO. Managed care plans now dominate employer-provided health insurance, covering over 80 percent of all individuals with such insurance compared to less than 30 percent only ten years ago.

In an effort to achieve the potential cost savings of managed care plans, conventional health insurers have started to apply managed care strategies to their own plans. Such plans, which are called *managed fee-for-service plans*, are using preadmission certification, utilization review, and second surgical opinions to control inappropriate utilization. Although the distinctions between managed care and conventional plans were once quite apparent, considerable overlap now exists in the strategies and incentives employed. Thus, the term "managed care" now describes a continuum of plans, which can vary significantly in their approaches to providing combined insurance and healthcare services. The common feature in managed care programs and plans is that the insurer has some mechanism by which it controls, or at least influences, patients' utilization of healthcare services.

Of course, managed care has its critics. The biggest problem facing the industry is the criticism that managed care is more about limiting costs than providing care. The media has jumped on the bandwagon by highlighting case after case where patients have suffered because a managed care plan has denied or delayed treatment. The problem, of course, is that it is difficult to find the balance between too much and too little when healthcare services are concerned. A fee-for-service system without constraints pushes costs out of control, while a managed care system that is overly managed can reduce care too much. For managed care to work, the industry has to focus on reducing costs by improving quality of care rather than by just reducing the amount of care provided.

In addition to costs that grow, on average, at twice the general rate of inflation, another problem facing the U.S. healthcare system is the fact that at any one time about 45 million Americans are without any type of insurance. This lack of healthcare insurance effectively denies these Americans complete access to services, even though a large percentage of national expenditures are devoted to those services. Although the health system appears well funded, at least when compared with other industrialized nations, it clearly does not meet the complete healthcare needs of the entire population.

Regardless of the details of the future of the healthcare system, healthcare managers undoubtedly will be facing more and more pressure from both government and private payers to offer quality services at the lowest possible costs. This means that the financial consequences of actions will become more and more important to the decision-making process, and that managers will have to become more and more sophisticated in their financial management skills.

Self-Test Questions

1. What are the major sources of financing for healthcare services?
2. Describe the recent trends in healthcare financing.
3. What are the implications of these trends for healthcare managers?

Delivery Settings and Trends

Healthcare services are provided in numerous settings including hospitals, ambulatory care facilities, long-term care facilities, and even at home. Prior to the 1980s, most health services organizations were freestanding and not formally linked with other organizations. Those that were linked tended to be part of horizontally integrated systems that control a single type of healthcare facility, such as hospitals or nursing homes. Recently, however, many health services organizations have diversified and become vertically integrated either through direct ownership or through contractual arrangements.

Hospitals

Hospitals provide diagnostic and therapeutic services to individuals who require more than several hours of care, although most hospitals are actively engaged in ambulatory services as well. To ensure a minimum standard of safety and quality, hospitals must be licensed by the state and undergo inspections for compliance with state regulations. In addition, most hospitals are accredited by the *Joint Commission on Accreditation of Healthcare Organizations (JCAHO)*. JCAHO accreditation is a voluntary process that is intended to promote high standards of care. Although the cost to achieve and maintain compliance with standards can be substantial, accreditation provides eligibility for participation in the Medicare program; hence, most general acute care hospitals seek accreditation.

Recent environmental and operational changes have created significant challenges for hospital managers. For example, hospitals are experiencing decreasing admission rates and shorter average lengths of stay, resulting in excess capacity. At the same time, hospitals have been pressured to give discounts to managed care plans, to limit the growth in patient charges, and to assume greater risk in their contracts with third-party payers. These trends are illustrated in Table 1.4, which contains selected hospital statistics for 1979, 1989, and 1998. As can be seen, the number of hospitals and beds is declining, and increasing cost-containment pressures are likely to accelerate the trend toward fewer, more efficient hospitals.

Hospitals differ in function, length of patient stay, size, and ownership. These factors affect the type and quantity of fixed assets, programs, and management requirements, and often determine the type and level of reimbursement available. Hospitals are classified as either general acute care facilities or specialty facilities. Function not only dictates the type of patients who will be treated, but also the source of patients, capital intensity required— the amount of fixed assets such as buildings and equipment, staff mix, and reimbursement structure.

General acute care hospitals provide general medical and surgical services and selected acute specialty services. General acute care hospitals are

Measure	1979	1989	1998
Number of hospitals	5,842	5,455	5,015
Total number of beds	984,000	933,000	839,988
Average number of beds per hospital	168	171	167
Average length of stay (days)	7.6	7.2	6.0
Average occupancy rate	73.9%	65.5%	62.4%
Profit margin	5.6%	3.7%	5.5%

TABLE 1.4
Selected General Acute Care Hospital Operating Measures

Source: *AHA Hospital Statistics*, 2000 and previous years.

short-stay facilities, and account for the majority of hospitals. *Specialty hospitals*, such as psychiatric, children's, women's, rehabilitation, and cancer, limit admission of patients to specific ages, sexes, illnesses, or conditions. The number of psychiatric and rehabilitation hospitals has grown significantly in the past decade because of the increased needs created by substance abuse, as well as increased government reimbursement for such services.

Hospitals vary in size from fewer than 25 beds to more than 1,000 beds; general acute care hospitals tend to be larger than specialty hospitals. Small hospitals, those with fewer than 100 beds, tend to be located in rural areas. Many rural hospitals have experienced financial difficulties in recent years because they have less ability than larger hospitals to lower costs in response to ever-tighter reimbursement rates. Most of the largest hospitals are academic health centers or teaching hospitals, which offer a wide range of services including tertiary services.

Hospitals are classified by ownership as private not-for-profit, investor owned, and governmental.[3] *Governmental hospitals*, which make up 25 percent of all hospitals, are broken down into federal and public (nonfederal) entities. *Federal hospitals*, such as those run by the military services or the Department of Veterans Affairs, serve special purposes. *Public hospitals* are funded wholly or in part by a city, county, tax district, or state. In general, federal and public hospitals provide substantial services to indigent patients. In recent years, many public hospitals have converted to other ownership categories—primarily private, not-for-profit—because the financial burdens placed on local governments has limited the amount of public funds available for hospital care. In addition, the inability of bureaucratic organizations to respond quickly to changes in the healthcare-operating environment contributed to many conversions.

Private not-for-profit hospitals are nongovernment entities organized for the sole purpose of providing inpatient healthcare services. Because of the charitable origins of U.S. hospitals and a tradition of community service, roughly 80 percent of all private hospitals (60 percent of all hospitals) are not-for-profit entities. In return for serving a charitable purpose, these hospitals receive numerous benefits including exemption from federal and state income taxes, exemption from property and sales taxes, eligibility to receive tax-deductible charitable contributions, favorable postal rates, favorable tax-exempt financing, and tax-favored annuities for employees.

The remaining 20 percent of private hospitals (15 percent of all hospitals) are *investor owned*. This means that they have shareholders that benefit directly from any profits generated by the hospital and that they do not share the charitable mission of not-for-profit hospitals. Historically, most investor-owned hospitals have been owned by physicians, but now most are owned by large corporations such as HCA–The Healthcare Company (formerly Columbia/HCA Healthcare) and Tenet Healthcare, each of which owns over a hundred hospitals. Unlike not-for-profit hospitals, investor-owned hospitals pay taxes and forgo the other benefits of not-for-profit status. Despite the expressed differences in mission between investor-owned and not-for-profit hospitals, not-for-profit hospitals are now being forced to place greater emphasis on the financial implications of operating decisions than in the past. This trend has raised concerns in some quarters that many not-for-profit hospitals are now failing to meet their charitable mission. As this perception grows, some people are now arguing that these hospitals should lose some, if not all, of the benefits associated with their not-for-profit status.

Hospitals are labor-intensive because of their duty to provide continuous nursing supervision to patients, in addition to the other services they provide through professional and semiprofessional staffs. Physicians petition for privileges to practice in hospitals. While they admit and provide care to hospitalized patients, physicians, for the most part, are not hospital employees, and hence are not directly accountable to hospital management. However, physicians retain a major responsibility for determining which hospital services will be provided to patients, so physicians play a critical role in determining a hospital's costs and revenues, and hence its financial condition.

Ambulatory (Outpatient) Care

Ambulatory care, also known as *outpatient care*, encompasses services provided to noninstitutionalized patients. Traditional outpatient settings include medical (physician) practices, hospital outpatient departments, and emergency rooms. In addition, the 1980s and early 1990s witnessed substantial growth in nontraditional ambulatory care settings such as home health care, ambulatory surgery centers, urgent care centers, diagnostic imaging centers, rehabilitation/sports medicine centers, and clinical laboratories. In general, the new settings offer patients increased amenities and convenience compared to hospital-based services and, in many situations, provide services at a lower cost than hospitals. For example, urgent care and ambulatory surgery centers are typically less expensive than their hospital counterparts because hospitals have higher overhead costs.

Many factors have contributed to the expansion of ambulatory services, but technology has been a leading factor. Often, patients who once required hospitalization because of the complexity, intensity, invasiveness, or risk associated with certain procedures can now be treated in outpatient settings. In addition, third-party payers have encouraged providers to expand their outpatient services through mandatory authorization for inpatient services and by payment mechanisms that provide incentives to perform services on an outpatient basis. Finally, fewer entry barriers to developing outpatient services relative to institutional care exist. Ordinarily, ambulatory facilities are less costly, less often subject to licensure and certificate-of-need regulations (exceptions are hospital outpatient units and ambulatory surgery centers), and generally are not accredited. (Licensure and certificate-of-need regulation are discussed in detail in a later section.)

As outpatient care consumes an increasing portion of the healthcare dollar, and efforts to control outpatient spending are enhanced, the traditional role of the ambulatory care manager is changing. Ambulatory care managers have typically met the needs of physician owners, specifically assuring adequate billing, collections, staffing, scheduling, and patient relations, while physicians have tended to make the more important business decisions. However, reimbursement changes, including a new Medicare prospective payment system and increased managed care affiliations, are requiring a higher level of management expertise. Increasing competition as well as the increasing complexity of the environment are forcing managers of ambulatory care facilities to become more sophisticated in making business decisions, including financial management decisions.

Long-Term Care

Long-term care entails healthcare services, as well as some personal services, provided to individuals who lack some degree of functional ability. It usually covers an extended period of time and includes both inpatient and outpatient services, many of which focus on mental health, rehabilitation, and nursing home care. Although the greatest use is among the elderly, long-term care services are used by individuals of all ages.

Long-term care is concerned with levels of independent functioning, specifically activities of daily living such as eating, bathing, and locomotion. Individuals become candidates for long-term care when they become too mentally or physically incapacitated to perform tasks necessary to their environment, and when their family members are unable to provide the services needed. Long-term care is a hybrid of health services and social services, and *nursing homes* are a major source of such care.

Three levels of nursing home care exist: (1) skilled nursing facilities, (2) intermediate care facilities, and (3) residential care facilities. *Skilled nursing facilities (SNFs)* provide the level of care closest to hospital care. Services must be under the supervision of a physician and must include 24-hour daily nursing care. *Intermediate care facilities (ICFs)* are intended for individuals who do not require hospital or SNF care, but whose mental or physical conditions require daily continuity of one or more medical services. *Residential care* facilities are sheltered environments that do not provide professional healthcare services, and thus for which most insurance programs, including Medicare and Medicaid, do not provide coverage.

It is interesting to note that the dominant payer for nursing home services, by far, is Medicaid. In the United States, most of the patients in nursing homes, at least those that stay for more than a year or two, exhaust their life savings and are forced to turn to the government to fund the care.[4] Nursing homes, with almost 20,000 facilities, are more abundant than hospitals and are also smaller, with average bed size of about 100 beds, compared with about 170 beds for hospitals. Nursing homes have a high 92 percent occupancy rate and an average patient length of stay is 2.9 years. Nursing homes are licensed by states, and nursing home administrators are licensed as well. Although the Joint Commission accredits nursing homes, only a small percentage participate because accreditation is not required for reimbursement, and the standards to achieve accreditation are much higher than licensure requirements.

The long-term care industry has experienced tremendous growth in the past three decades. Long-term care accounted for only 1 percent of healthcare expenditures in 1960, but by 2000, it accounted for over 8 percent. Further demand increases are anticipated, as the percentage of the U.S. population 65 and older increases from less than 16 percent in 2000 to a forecasted 20 percent in 2030. The elderly are disproportionately high users of healthcare services and are major users of long-term care.

Although long-term care is often perceived as nursing home care, many new services are developing to meet society's needs in less-institutional surroundings such as adult day care, life care centers, and hospice programs. These services tend to offer a higher quality of life, although they are not necessarily less expensive than institutional care. Home health care, provided for an extended time period, can be an alternative to nursing home care for many patients, but it is not as readily available as nursing home care in many rural areas. Furthermore, third-party payers, especially Medicare, have sent mixed signals about their willingness to adequately pay for home health care. In fact, many home health care businesses have been forced to close in the last few years as a result of a new, and less generous, Medicare payment system.

Integrated Delivery Systems

Many healthcare experts have extolled the benefits of providing hospital care, ambulatory care, long-term care, and business support services through a single entity usually called an *integrated delivery system*. The proposed benefits of such systems include the following:

- Patients are kept in the corporate network of services (*patient capture*).
- Providers have access to managerial and functional specialists (for example, reimbursement and marketing professionals).
- Information systems that track all aspects of patient care, as well as insurance and other data, can be developed more easily, and the costs to develop them are shared.
- Linked organizations have better access to capital.
- The ability to recruit and retain management and professional staff is enhanced.
- Integrated delivery systems are able to offer insurers a complete package of services ("one-stop shopping").
- By offering all services, integrated delivery systems are better able to plan for and deliver a full range of healthcare services to meet the needs of a defined population, including chronic disease management and health

status improvement programs. Many of these population-based efforts are not typically offered by stand-alone providers.

- Incentives that encourage all providers in the system to work together for the common good of the system can be created, which has the potential to both improve quality and control costs.

Although integrated delivery systems can be structured in many different ways, the defining characteristic of such systems is that the organization has the ability to assume full clinical responsibility for the healthcare needs of a defined population. Because of current state laws, which typically mandate that the insurance function can be assumed only by licensed insurers, integrated delivery systems typically contract with managed care plans. Sometimes, the managed care plan is owned by the integrated delivery system itself, but often the managed care plan is separately owned. In contracts with managed care plans, the integrated delivery system often receives a fixed payment per plan member, and hence assumes both the financial and clinical risks associated with providing healthcare services.

To be an effective competitor, integrated delivery systems must minimize the provision of unnecessary services because additional services create added costs but do not necessarily result in additional revenues. Thus, the objective of integrated delivery systems is to provide all needed services to its member-population in the lowest cost setting. To achieve this goal, integrated delivery systems invest heavily in primary care services, especially prevention, early intervention, and wellness programs. The primary care gatekeeper concept is frequently used to control utilization and, hence, costs. While hospitals continue to be centers of technology, integrated delivery systems have the incentive to shift patients toward lower-cost settings. Thus, clinical integration among the various providers and components of care is essential to achieving quality, cost efficiency, and patient satisfaction.

One of the most common types of integrated delivery system is the *physician-hospital organization (PHO)*, which is a separate organization formed by a hospital and a physician group to provide contracted healthcare services to managed care plans and, when permitted, directly to employers. The PHO must provide utilization and quality management, physician credentialing, claims processing, marketing, and revenue distribution for the system. Another common type is the *management service organization (MSO)*, which is a hospital-based organization that provides physician billing and medical group management services. Some of the larger integrated systems are a combination of PHOs, MSOs, and managed care organizations, which can provide all clinical services as well as the insurance function. Most of these large systems were developed by hospitals, but others were started by health plans or by large physician group practices.

In spite of the hypothesized benefits of vertical integration, executives of healthcare systems have found it more difficult than they originally thought to manage large, diverse enterprises. This difficulty has been especially true when hospitals or health systems have acquired medical (physician) practices. Many of the gains predicted were not realized, and hence many of the acquisitions have unraveled. In fact, as many integrated delivery systems are breaking up as are currently being formed. It appears that the benefits ascribed to such systems are more difficult to realize than had been anticipated. It is not clear today whether or not large vertically integrated health systems are better suited for success than are smaller, more-focused organizations. Only time will tell.

1. What are some different types of hospitals, and what trends are occurring **Self-Test** in the hospital industry? **Questions**
2. What trends are occurring in outpatient and long-term care?
3. What is an integrated delivery system?
4. Do you think that integrated delivery systems will be more or less prevalent in the future? Explain your answer.

Health Services Manpower

About 8 million individuals are employed in the health services industry, and of its full-time equivalents (FTEs), 4 million are employed in hospitals and 1.5 million are employed in long-term care facilities. The health services industry is not only labor intensive, its labor force has also moved toward extreme specialization. For example, large hospitals have over 300 different types of job descriptions, and that number is growing. Furthermore, many health services jobs require professional and paramedical staff who are licensed, registered, or certified.

Specialization of professionals creates a number of problem areas for managers. First, specialization reduces continuity of patient care. As providers deliver a more narrow scope of services, a greater number of providers must be involved in the overall management of an individual patient. In this environment, continuity of services can be achieved only at the cost of additional resources to coordinate services. Second, specialists demand higher incomes, and hence higher levels of reimbursement than generalists, which increases costs. Such cost increases are especially burdensome when specialists provide routine care along with specialized care.

When one thinks about health services professionals, the first profession that comes to mind is the *physician*. Because of a perceived shortage of physicians during the 1960s and 1970s, federal assistance programs encouraged growth in the number of medical schools, as well as the number of students enrolled in existing schools. Thus, the number of physicians per 100,000 population increased from 168 in 1970 to almost 350 in 2000. Today, most of the growth incentives have been eliminated, partly as a result of the forecasts that the United States currently has, or will soon have, a surplus of physicians. Although a national surplus is not readily apparent, primarily because of growth in specialization and increased opportunities in primary care, many communities are "over-doctored."

Physicians primarily control the quantity and mix of healthcare services utilized, and thus their role in healthcare expenditures receives much attention from health policymakers. It has been estimated that about 70 percent of all healthcare costs for services result directly from physician decisions. In addition, it has been argued that physicians even have some ability to create demand for health services.[5] Optimizing physician numbers, mix, distribution, and practice patterns are key factors in controlling healthcare costs.

Many types of nonphysician professionals also provide direct health services to patients. Some of them, such as dentists, podiatrists, psychologists, and chiropractors, are independent *health professionals* who do not practice under physician supervision. Numerous other *paramedical personnel*, such as pharmacists, dieticians, and physician assistants, are educated in universities. Depending on the profession, paramedical personnel are either licensed by the state or registered or certified by a professional association. Their roles are narrower in focus than those of physicians, independent health professionals, or nurses. The diversity of healthcare professionals and restrictions on their scope of practice make cost-control strategies that attempt to utilize personnel across service areas impractical in many healthcare settings.

Nurses comprise the largest professional group in healthcare services. Active registered nurses total about 1.7 million, with hospitals as their dominant employer. Unlike medical schools, the numbers of nursing schools and graduates have decreased since 1980. The decline in nursing education, together with the growing demand for healthcare services, resulted in nursing shortages in some geographic areas, especially in hospitals and nursing homes. However, this shortage has been somewhat offset in recent years by the reduction in demand for hospital services. The nursing profession is confronting many problems, including low levels of work satisfaction, similar to that of other professional occupations. Satisfaction studies indicate that nurses perceive the need for more autonomy, higher salaries, and greater professional respect.

One dominant problem that must be overcome before the profession can enhance its image is the variety of educational programs that produce different skill levels needed to obtain licensure. About 42 percent of hospital nurses have associate degrees in nursing, 32 percent have nursing diplomas, 23 percent have baccalaureate degrees in nursing, and 3 percent have master's degrees in nursing. The current system of licensure recognizes only one skill level, although nursing education produces professionals with very different levels of technical and professional expertise. With only one licensure level, nursing salaries are rarely adjusted to recognize the educational and skill differences among nurses.

Technicians and *technologists*, such as radiology technicians and medical technologists, are usually trained in community colleges or hospital-based programs, although some baccalaureate programs exist for these paramedical personnel. Such personnel are essential to the provision of many types of healthcare service, although their scope of responsibility is quite narrow. Facilities often face problems in retaining technicians and technologists because the profession's focused education and training generally limit advancement opportunities.

A major factor that contributes to increasing healthcare costs is growing labor expenses. Labor costs now represent almost half of hospitals' total costs, and, in general, labor costs are rising more rapidly than nonlabor costs. Tight labor markets, minimum wage laws, the growth of unionization, and the "catching-up" process explain much of the increase in healthcare labor costs that has taken place. Historically, health services employees have been underpaid compared to workers in other industries, and thus wage increases in excess of inflation have been necessary to achieve wage parity. Despite the prolonged upward trend in real wages, an equilibrium has not yet been reached and wage inflation continues to be a major factor in increasing healthcare costs.[6]

1. What types of professionals work in the health services industry?
2. Which healthcare professional has the greatest impact on healthcare utilization and, hence, costs?

Self-Test Questions

Environmental Changes: Technology, Demographics, and the Internet

Changing technology, including the Internet, and demographics alter the need for the delivery of healthcare services, and both factors ultimately affect healthcare costs. The advancement and proliferation of technology is a controversial area in health services because cost/benefit assessments are difficult to perform and unnecessary duplication of expensive technologies is readily apparent. The rapid development of technology and the Internet, as well as demographic changes, create opportunities and challenges for both providers and payers.

Technology

Technologies include drugs, equipment, devices, procedures, and application of specialized knowledge. New technologies are developed with the goal of improving patients' health, but their impact is often to shift delivery sites, stimulate reorganization of systems, and escalate costs.

Rapid and far-reaching technological improvements in diagnosing and treating patients have occurred in the healthcare sector. Such developments have resulted in improved patient care and outcomes, alternatives to invasive procedures, and enhanced patient comfort and convenience. Sophisticated diagnostic imaging devices, such as magnetic resonance imaging and digital subtraction angiography, provide examples of how technology can improve patient care. These technologies use enhanced computer capabilities to generate clinical information that was previously unavailable from diagnostic equipment. In addition, new drugs, devices, gene therapies, and surgical knowledge are facilitating highly complicated procedures, such as organ or tissue transplants and artificial implant surgeries, as well as offering treatments to diseases that heretofore had been untreatable.

Surgery is also experiencing rapid technological change. Less-invasive procedures are being developed including arthroscopic, endoscopic, percutaneous, laser, microsurgery, cryosurgery, and lithotripsy techniques. Such recently developed techniques are improving patient outcomes, reducing complication rates, and reducing risk of adverse outcomes. In addition, some techniques, such as balloon angioplasty, provide therapeutic interventions coincident with relatively noninvasive diagnostic equipment. Less-invasive technologies also enhance patient satisfaction by reducing discomfort and recovery time.

Patient convenience is also improved by substituting ambulatory care for institutional care. New diagnostic imaging devices and less-invasive surgical procedures permit more patients to be managed as outpatients. Also, improvements in anesthetics have permitted more procedures to be safely performed on an outpatient basis. In addition, new developments in clinical laboratory equipment allow an increased number of tests to be accurately performed in physicians' offices, so fewer patients must be referred to outside laboratories, while the development of mobile diagnostic and therapeutic units offers patients access to specialized services in more convenient locations. Finally, patient care has been improved by the development of comprehensive centers organized to manage particular diagnoses. For example, comprehensive cancer centers provide highly coordinated multidisciplinary services to patients, enhance communication among specialists, and improve patient education and information. Although cancer care is experiencing only incremental improvements in therapy (surgery, radiation therapy, and chemotherapy), the art of providing cancer care is being advanced in such centers and survival rates are gradually improving.

Important new pharmaceuticals are discovered each year, and such developments have facilitated major improvements in health outcomes. For example, cyclosporin has permitted the development of organ transplant programs, and drug "cocktails" have extended average longevity among patients with AIDS. In recent years, several of the largest pharmaceutical firms have each developed drugs that generate annual sales of more than a billion dollars, thus generating the profits necessary to further develop new drugs. Despite significant advances in drug therapy, much of the research and development among pharmaceutical manufacturers has produced drugs that contribute little to patient health because alternative medications already exist. Indeed, critics accuse pharmaceutical firms of price gouging because the industry's profit margin has averaged over 17 percent during the last five years, whereas the average for the S&P 500 firms has been about 10 percent. While generally praised for advances in drug therapies, rapidly increasing drug prices are becoming a problem for the entire healthcare system that will have to be addressed in the near future.

As noted in a previous section, technological advancements are responsible for at least some portion of recent healthcare cost increases. Some, such as imaging devices, require heavy capital investment, and many complement, rather than substitute for, existing services. Technological developments have also been criticized for creating an imperative for use, regardless of their expense or whether patient benefit is incremental or substantial. Providers generally perceive new technologies as providing greater prestige, and hence offering a competitive advantage. Thus, in the current competitive environment, providers are often compelled to purchase and use more expensive technologies to maintain a progressive up-to-date image. There appears to be nothing in the near term that will reverse this trend in technological development or minimize the impact of new technology on costs.

The Internet

The rapid development and use of the Internet is another important trend that is likely to make an impact on health services organizations over the coming decade. Internet applications may profoundly affect (1) how patients and other consumers access and use health information; (2) the exchanges of information and financial resources between providers, insurers, and other intermediaries on behalf of patients and enrollees; and (3) the ability of providers to access, analyze, and use clinical data in their everyday medical decision making. Some futurists suggest that the effects of the Internet on the structure and processes of the healthcare system will be tempered by privacy concerns and the resistance of physicians and other healthcare professionals to this new technology. Nonetheless, many of the key relationships among providers, insurers, and patients are likely to be dramatically influenced by the Internet as its full capabilities are explored and developed.

Demographics

Demographic changes have an impact on the demand for services and the type of services required. The most significant demographic change is the aging of the population. The number of elderly (individuals over 65) is expected to increase from 34.7 million in 2000 to 53.2 million in 2020 to 75.2 million in 2040. The "oldest old" (individuals over 85) are expected to jump from 4.3 million in 2000 to 6.5 million in 2020 to 13.6 million in 2040. The "graying of America" is a result of increased longevity coupled with the post–World War II baby boom. This trend is a major concern to policymakers because the elderly are disproportionate users of health services, and a majority of their care is funded through public sources.

Although many elderly people are independent and active, they are likely to experience multiple chronic conditions that may become disabling. The elderly are admitted to hospitals three times more often than the general population, and their average length of stay is over three days longer than the general average. In addition, the elderly visit their physicians more often than younger people, and they comprise the majority of residents in nursing homes. Providers are concerned about the growth in elderly population because public funding sources—Medicare and Medicaid—have not been increasing their reimbursement rates sufficiently to cover inflation; therefore, providers earn a smaller real return on elderly patients each year.

The aging population also creates funding concerns because the percentage of employed individuals, who pay most of the income tax and all social security taxes, will decrease as the elderly population increases. Reform is needed to ensure adequate delivery of healthcare services as the population ages. Suggestions for reform include increasing the age limits for Medicare eligibility, requiring beneficiaries to pay for a greater proportion of services provided, increasing the availability and coverage of long-term care insurance, increasing the incentives for prevention, and creating less-expensive and more-efficient delivery settings.

Self-Test Questions

1. What are the costs and benefits associated with the relentless drive for technological innovation in health care?
2. What demographic factors will have the largest impact on the delivery of healthcare services in the future?

Regulatory and Legal Issues

Entry into the health services industry is heavily regulated. Examples of such regulation include licensure, certificate of need, rate setting, and review programs. In addition, legal issues, specifically malpractice and antitrust, are prominent in discussions of healthcare cost control.

States require *licensure* of certain health services providers in an effort to protect the health, safety, and welfare of the public. Licensure regulations establish minimum standards that must be met to provide a service. Many types of providers are licensed, including whole facilities such as hospitals and nursing homes, as well as individuals such as physicians, dentists, and nurses. Facilities that are licensed must submit to periodic inspections and review activities. Such reviews have focused more on physical features and safety and less on patient care services and outcomes, although some progress is being made in outcomes research. Thus, licensure has not necessarily ensured that the public will receive quality services. Critics of licensure contend that it is designed to protect providers rather than consumers. For example, licensed paramedical professionals are required to work under the supervision of a physician or dentist, and thus it is impossible for the paramedical professions to compete with physicians or dentists. Despite the limitations of licensure, it is probably here to stay.

Certificate of need (CON) legislation was enacted by Congress in the early 1970s in an effort to control increasing healthcare costs. States were required to conduct healthcare planning, and a logical extension of this planning was to require providers to obtain approval based on community need for construction and renovation projects that either relate to specific services or exceed a defined cost threshold. This attempt to control capital expenditures by controlling expansion and preventing duplication of services lasted less than a decade before the Reagan administration began to downplay CON regulation and to promote cost controls through competition, although CON regulation still exists in about half the states.

Criticisms of CON regulation include the following: (1) It does not provide as much control over capital expenditures as originally envisioned; (2) it increases healthcare costs by forcing providers to incur the administrative costs associated with applying for a CON; and (3) it creates a territorial franchise for services that it covers. That is, CON regulation makes it difficult for new entities to enter markets, even though those new entities may be able to provide services more efficiently than entrenched providers.

In addition to CON regulation, *cost-containment programs* were enacted in many states at a time when most health services reimbursement was based on costs. By the late 1970s, nine states had mandatory cost-containment programs, and many other states had voluntary programs or programs that did not mandate compliance. The primary tool for cost-containment programs is the *rate review* system. Three types of systems have been used: (1) detailed budget reviews with approval or setting of rates; (2) formula methods, which use inflation formulas to set target rates; and (3) negotiated rates involving joint decision making between the provider and the rate setter. Some states that use rate review systems have reduced the rate of increase in healthcare costs below the national average, while others have failed. However, rate review, as a sole means of cost containment, has been criticized because it does not address the issue of demand for health services.

Health services are subject to many other forms of regulation. For example, pharmacy services are regulated by state and federal laws, and radiology services are highly regulated because of the handling and disposal of radioactive materials. The costs of complying with regulation are not trivial. The CEO of one 430-bed hospital estimated that the cost of dealing with regulatory agencies, including third-party payers, is about $8 million annually, requiring a staff of 140 full-time workers to handle the process.

In addition, both federal and state agencies are involved in the regulation of *mergers* and *acquisitions*. In essence, *antitrust laws* prohibit businesses from combining in any way that would unduly limit future competition. Antitrust regulation will be considered in more detail in Chapter 18 in our discussion of mergers and acquisitions.

Finally, *professional liability* is yet another legal concern for healthcare providers. Malpractice suits are the oldest forms of quality assurance in the U.S. healthcare system, and such suits now are used to an extreme extent. Many people believe that the United States is facing a malpractice insurance crisis. Total malpractice premiums, which have doubled in the last ten years, have been passed on to healthcare purchasers. Some specialists pay malpractice premiums of more than $100,000 per year, and each month U.S. courts manage approximately 20,000 new malpractice suits, with awards averaging $300,000 for cases that go to trial. Although providers have been successful in achieving some tort reforms, malpractice litigation continues to be perceived as inefficient because it diverts resources to lawyers and courts and creates disincentives for physicians to practice high-risk specialties and for hospitals to offer high-risk services.

A major problem with the existing malpractice system is the lack of uniformity in compensating victims and protecting providers. Medical malpractice not only affects healthcare costs in terms of malpractice insurance premiums; it also encourages the practice of defensive medicine, in which physicians overutilize diagnostic services in an effort to protect themselves. Although professional liability is the most visible legal concern in health services, the industry is subject to many other legal issues, including those typical of other industries such as general liability. Finally, healthcare providers are confronted with unique ethical issues such as the right to die or to prolong life, which are often resolved through the legal system.

Self-Test Question

1. What are some regulatory and legal issues facing healthcare providers today?

Key Concepts

This chapter introduced the health services industry, discussed the role of financial management, and introduced the concept and organization of the text. Here are its key concepts:

- Financial management is a *decision science*, so the primary objective of this text is to provide students and practicing healthcare managers with the theory, concepts, and tools necessary to make effective decisions. The text is structured to support this goal.
- The *primary role of financial management* is to plan for, acquire, and utilize funds to maximize the efficiency and value of the enterprise.
- Specific financial management functions include (1) *evaluation and planning*; (2) *long-term investment decisions*; (3) *financing decisions*; (4) *working capital management*, (5) *contract management*, and (6) *financial risk management*.
- The U.S. healthcare sector is a diverse collection of industries that are directly or indirectly involved in the provision of *healthcare services*.

- The major players in the healthcare sector are (1) the *providers* of healthcare services, such as hospitals and nursing homes; (2) the *suppliers* of drugs and equipment, such as pharmaceutical and medical equipment firms; (3) the *insurers*, including both governmental programs, such as Medicare, and private insurers; (4) *managed care plans*, such as health maintenance and preferred provider organizations; and (5) a diverse collection of other entities ranging from consulting firms to educational institutions to research agencies.
- Healthcare financing is provided by private and federal, state, and local government sources. Although total spending by all sources has increased, the percentage of total expenditures covered by private sources decreased from 1950 to 2000, while the percentage derived from the federal government has increased.
- Most of the reimbursement for healthcare providers occurs through the *third-party-payer system*, which includes (1) *private insurers* such as Blue Cross/Blue Shield and Prudential, (2) *public insurance plans* such as Medicare and Medicaid, and (3) *managed care plans* such as health maintenance organizations (HMOs) and preferred provider organizations (PPOs).
- Healthcare services are provided in numerous settings, including *hospitals, ambulatory care* facilities, *long-term care* facilities, in the home, and in *integrated delivery systems.*
- The health services industry is not only *labor intensive*, its labor force is also extremely specialized. For example, large hospitals have over 300 different types of jobs, and that number is growing. Furthermore, many of its employees are professional and paramedical staffs who are licensed, registered, or certified.
- *Changing technology,* the *Internet,* and *demographics* alter the needs and delivery of health services and ultimately affect healthcare costs.
- Entry into the health services industry has been heavily regulated. Examples of regulation include *licensure, certificate of need,* and *rate setting and review* programs.
- Legal issues, such as *malpractice* and *antitrust,* are prominent in discussions about controlling healthcare costs.

This chapter introduces the book and the healthcare sector. In the next two chapters, more detailed information about health services organizations is presented.

Selected References

For more information on the healthcare industry, see

        Barton, Phoebe Lindsey. 1998. *Understanding the U.S. Health Services System.* Chicago: Health Administration Press.

Long, Michael J. 1998. *Health and Healthcare in the United States.* Chicago: Health Administration Press.

For the latest information on events that effect the health services industry, see

Medical Benefits, published semimonthly by Kelly Communications, Inc., Charlottesville, Virginia.

Modern Healthcare, published weekly by Crain Communications, Inc., Chicago.

For some ideas on where the health services industry is headed, see

Morrison, Ian. 1999. *Health Care in the New Millennium.* New York: Joseph Wiley & Sons.

Goldsmith, Jeff. 2000. "How Will the Internet Change Our Health System." *Health Affairs* (January/February): 148–156.

Nauert, Roger C. 2000. "The New Millennium: Health Care Evolution in the 21st Century." *Journal of Health Care Finance* (Spring): 1–14.

Selected Web Sites

One of the best ways to learn more about the healthcare sector is to go to the web sites of the major professional and industry organizations.

See the American Hospital Association web site at *www.aha.org*.

See the American Medical Association web site at *www.ama-assn.org*.

See the American Association of Health Plans web site at *www.aahp.org*.

For U.S. demographic information, see the online version of the Statistical Abstract of the United States at *www.census.gov/statab/www/*.

The National Center for Health Statistics has a web site that provides a great deal of information about the health status of the U.S. population. The index to the site can be found at *www.cdc.gov/nchs*.

Notes

1. Not-for-profit organizations are also called *nonprofit*, but the former designation is becoming dominant within the health services industry. Also, investor-owned businesses are sometimes called *proprietary*, or *for-profit*. We will discuss the differences in these forms of ownership in detail in Chapter 2.

2. There is a set of questions for each case in the Instructor's Manual to the casebook. Instructors who want to provide more guidance to students than given in the case itself can distribute these questions to their students.

3. Here, we briefly discuss hospital ownership. We will have much more to say about the impact of ownership on financial management goals in Chapter 2.

4. The cost to stay in a nursing home varies widely, but the average cost is over $3,000 per month. At roughly $40,000 a year, it does not take long for most people to exhaust their savings. Also, about one in five people in the United States will eventually require nursing home care. Considering all of these facts, it is not surprising that many elderly individuals with substantial savings are setting up trusts or other legal devices to try to protect their wealth from being spent on nursing home care. Additionally, long-term care insurance is beginning to

become more widely available, but thus far has not achieved the same widespread acceptance as other forms of health insurance.

5. For example, a recent study by the Florida Health Care Cost Containment Board found that clinical laboratories owned by doctors performed almost twice as many tests per patient as similar laboratories with no physician investors. The average charge in a physician-owned lab was $43 per patient, as compared with $20 per patient in other labs. Such findings have prompted Congress to set limits on physician ownership and referrals.

6. *Real* wages are wages that are adjusted for inflation effects. Thus, for real wages to grow, the growth rate in wages must exceed inflation. In recent years, wages to healthcare workers, on average, have grown at about twice the inflation rate.

BUSINESS ORGANIZATION, OWNERSHIP, GOALS, AND TAXES

Learning Objectives

After studying this chapter, readers should be able to:

- Describe the basic forms of business organization along with their advantages and disadvantages.
- Discuss the two basic types of ownership and explain why ownership type is so important in the healthcare sector.
- Explain how the goals of investor-owned and not-for-profit businesses differ.
- Describe, in general terms, the tax laws that apply both to individuals and to healthcare businesses.

Introduction

In this chapter, we discuss four important, and interrelated, topics. Unlike most industries, which tend to be dominated by one form of business organization and ownership, businesses in the healthcare sector have diverse ownership and organizational structures. For example, health services are provided by both investor-owned and not-for-profit businesses that are organized as proprietorships, partnerships, corporations, joint ventures, and loose alliances. The diverse forms of organization and ownership create an industry in which the participants can have significantly different goals and tax structures. Because financial management decisions are greatly influenced by the goals and ownership of the organization, and the resulting tax consequences, it is necessary for managers to have a good understanding of the similarities and differences in ownership and organization that occur within health services businesses.

Alternative Forms of Business Organization

Throughout the text, the focus is on business finance—that is, the practice of financial management within business organizations. There are three primary forms of *business organization*: (1) proprietorship, (2) partnership, and (3) corporation. Because most healthcare managers work for corporations and because not-for-profit businesses are organized as corporations, this form of organization is emphasized. However, many individual physician practices are organized as proprietorships, and partnerships are common in group practices and joint ventures. Healthcare managers must, therefore, be familiar with all forms of business organization.

Proprietorship

A *proprietorship*, sometimes called a *sole proprietorship*, is a business owned by one individual. Going into business as a proprietor is easy—the owner merely begins business operations. However, most cities require even the smallest businesses to be licensed, and state licensure is required for most healthcare professionals.

The proprietorship form of organization is easily and inexpensively formed, is subject to few governmental regulations, and pays no corporate income taxes. All earnings of the business, whether reinvested in the business or withdrawn by the owner, are taxed as personal income to the proprietor. In general, a sole proprietorship will pay lower total taxes than a comparable, taxable corporation because corporate profits are taxed twice—once at the corporate level and once by stockholders at the personal level when profits are distributed as dividends or when capital gains are realized.

Partnership

A *partnership* is formed when two or more individuals associate to conduct a nonincorporated business. Partnerships may operate under different degrees of formality, ranging from informal, verbal understandings to formal agreements filed with the state in which the partnership does business. Like a proprietorship, the major advantage of the partnership form of organization is its low cost and ease of formation. In addition, the tax treatment of a partnership is similar to that of a proprietorship; the partnership's earnings are allocated to the partners and taxed as personal income regardless of whether the earnings are actually paid out to the partners or retained in the business.[1]

Proprietorships and partnerships have three important limitations:

1. It typically is difficult for owners to sell, or transfer, their interest in the business.
2. The owners have unlimited personal liability for the debts of the business, which can result in losses greater than the amount invested in the business. In a proprietorship, unlimited liability means that the owner is personally responsible for the debts of the business. In a partnership, it means that if any partner is unable to meet his or her pro rata obligation in the event of bankruptcy, the remaining partners are responsible for the unsatisfied claims and must draw on their personal assets if necessary.
3. The life of the business is limited to the life of the owners.

These three disadvantages—difficulty in transferring ownership, unlimited liability, and impermanence of the business—lead to the fourth, and perhaps the most important, disadvantage from a finance perspective: It is difficult for proprietors and partners to attract substantial amounts of capital. This difficulty is not a particular problem for a slow-growing business or when the owners are very wealthy, but for most businesses, it becomes a real handicap if the business needs to expand rapidly to take advantage of market opportunities. For this reason, proprietorships and most partnerships are restricted primarily to small businesses.[2] However, almost all businesses start out as sole proprietorships or partnerships, and then ultimately convert to the corporate form of organization.

Corporation

A *corporation* is a legal entity that is separate and distinct from its owners and managers. Although corporations can be either investor-owned or not-for-profit, this section mostly focuses on investor-owned corporations. The unique features of not-for-profit corporations will be discussed in later sections. The creation of a separate business entity gives the corporation three main advantages:

1. A corporation has unlimited life and can continue in existence after its original owners and managers have died or left the firm.
2. It is easy to transfer ownership in a corporation because ownership is divided into shares of stock that can be easily sold.
3. Owners of a corporation have limited liability.

To illustrate limited liability, suppose that one person made an investment of $10,000 in a partnership that subsequently went bankrupt, and owed $100,000. Because the partners are liable for the debts of the partnership, that partner could be assessed for a share of the partnership's debt in addition to the initial $10,000 contribution. In fact, if the other partners were unable to pay their shares of the indebtedness, one partner would be held liable for the entire $100,000. However, if the $10,000 had been invested in a corporation that went bankrupt, the potential loss for the investor would be limited to the $10,000 investment. (However, in the case of small, financially weak corporations, the limited liability feature of ownership is often fictitious because bankers and other lenders will require personal guarantees from the stockholders.) With these three factors—unlimited life, ease of ownership transfer, and limited liability—corporations can more easily raise money in the financial markets than sole proprietorships or partnerships can.[3]

The corporate form of organization has two primary disadvantages. First, corporate earnings of taxable entities are subject to double taxation— once at the corporate level and once at the personal level when dividends are paid to stockholders or capital gains are realized. Second, setting up a corporation, and then filing the required periodic state and federal reports, is more costly and time consuming than what is required to establish a proprietorship or partnership.

Although a proprietorship or partnership can begin operations without much legal paperwork, setting up a corporation requires that the founders, or their attorney, prepare a charter and a set of bylaws. Today, attorneys have standard forms for charters and bylaws on their computers, so they can set up a "no-frills" corporation with much less work than what would have been required in the past. However, setting up a corporation remains relatively difficult when compared to a proprietorship or partnership, and still more difficult if the corporation has nonstandard features.

The *charter* includes the name of the corporation, its proposed activities, the amount of stock to be issued (if investor-owned), and the number and names of the initial set of directors. The charter is filed with the appropriate official of the state in which the business will be incorporated, and, when approved, the corporation is officially in existence.[4] After the corporation has been officially formed, it must file quarterly and annual financial and tax reports with state and federal agencies.

The *bylaws* are a set of rules drawn up by the founders to provide guidance for the governing and internal management of the corporation. Bylaws include information about how directors are to be elected; whether the existing shareholders have the first right to buy any new shares that the firm issues; and the procedures for changing the charter or bylaws.

The value of any investor-owned business, other than a very small one, generally will be maximized if it is organized as a corporation for the following three reasons:

1. Limited liability reduces the risks borne by equity investors (the owners); with all else the same, the lower the risk, the higher the value of the investment.
2. A business's value is dependent on growth opportunities, which in turn are dependent on the business's ability to attract capital. Because corporations can obtain capital more easily than other forms of business can, they are better able to take advantage of growth opportunities.
3. The value of any investment depends on its *liquidity*, which means the ease at which the investment can be sold for a fair price. Because an equity investment in a corporation is much more liquid than a similar investment in a proprietorship or partnership, the corporate form of organization creates more value for its owners.

Hybrid Forms of Organization

Although the three basic forms of organization—proprietorship, partnership, and corporation—dominate the overall business scene, several hybrid forms of organization also are used by businesses. Some of these forms are found in the health services industry.

Several specialized types of partnerships have characteristics somewhat different than a standard form of partnership. First, limiting some of the partners' liabilities is possible by establishing a *limited partnership*, wherein certain partners are designated *general partners* and others *limited partners*. The limited partners, like the owners of a corporation, are liable only for the amount of their investment in the partnership, while the general partners have unlimited liability. However, the limited partners typically have no control, which rests solely with the general partners. Limited partnerships are quite common in real estate and mineral investments; they are not as common in the health services industry, however, because in this setting it is difficult to find one partner that is willing to accept all of the business's risk and a second partner that is willing to relinquish control.

The *limited liability partnership (LLP)* is a relatively new type of partnership that is available in many states. In a limited liability partnership, the general partners have joint liability for all actions of the partnership, including personal injuries and indebtedness. However, all partners enjoy limited liability regarding professional malpractice because partners are only liable for their own individual malpractice actions, not those of the other partners. In spite of limited malpractice liability, the partners are jointly liable for the partnership's debts. Menomonee Falls Ambulatory Surgery Center in Wisconsin is an example of a LLP.

The *limited liability company (LLC)* is another new type of business organization. It has some characteristics of both a partnership and a corporation. The owners of a LLC are called *members*, and they are taxed as if they are partners in a partnership. However, a member's liability is like that of a stockholder of a corporation because liability is limited to the member's initial contribution in the business. Personal assets are only at risk if the member assumes specific liability, such as by signing a personal loan guarantee. Both the LLP and LLC are new and complex forms of organizations, so setting them up can be time consuming and costly. Charter Behavioral Health Systems, the nation's largest behavioral health system, is an example of a LLC.

The *professional corporation (PC)*, which is called a *professional association (PA)* in some states, is a form of organization that is common among physicians and other individual and group practice healthcare professionals. All 50 states have statutes that prescribe the requirements for such corporations, which provide the usual benefits of incorporation, but do not relieve the participants of professional liability. Indeed, the primary motivation behind the professional corporation, which is a relatively old business form compared to the LLP and LLC, was to provide a way for professionals to incorporate, yet still be held liable for professional malpractice.

PCs have tight restrictions, however. First, one or more owners must be licensed in the profession of the PC. Second, PCs are taxed as corporations; they cannot be designated as an S corporation for tax purposes (see the following paragraph). The Atlanta Cardiology Group, comprising 20 physicians who provide a full range of cardiac services at multiple sites, typifies a PC.

For tax purposes, standard for-profit corporations are called *C corporations*. If certain requirements are met, either one or a few individuals can incorporate, but, for tax purposes only, elect to be treated as if the business were a proprietorship or partnership. Such corporations, which differ only in how the owners are taxed, are called *S corporations*. Although S corporations are similar to LLPs and LLCs regarding taxes, LLPs and LLCs provide more flexibility and benefits to owners. Many businesses, especially group practices, are, therefore, converting to the newer forms.

Self-Test Questions

1. What are the three major forms of business organization, and how do they differ?
2. What are some different types of partnerships?
3. What are some different types of corporations?

Alternative Forms of Ownership

Unlike other sectors in the economy, not-for-profit corporations play a major role in the healthcare sector, especially among providers. For example, only 20 percent of non-governmental hospitals are investor-owned; the remaining 80 percent are not-for-profit. Furthermore, not-for-profit ownership is common in the nursing home, home health care, and managed care industries.

Investor-Owned Corporations

As discussed in the previous section, for-profit businesses can be organized in a variety of ways. However, because of their size, corporations are by far the largest employers of healthcare professionals. When the average person thinks of a corporation, he or she probably thinks of an *investor-owned*, or *for-profit*, *corporation*. Virtually all large businesses (e.g., Ford, Microsoft, IBM, and General Electric) are investor-owned corporations.

Investors become owners of such businesses by buying shares of *common stock* in the firm. Investors may buy common stock when it is first sold by the firm. Such sales are called *primary market transactions*. In a primary market transaction, the funds raised from the sale generally go to the corporation.[5] After the shares have been initially sold by the corporation, they are traded in the *secondary market*. These sales may take place on *exchanges* such as the New York Stock Exchange (NYSE) and the American Stock Exchange (AMEX). They may also take place in the *over-the-counter (OTC) market*, which is composed of a large number of dealer/brokers connected by a sophisticated electronic trading system. When shares are bought and sold in the secondary market, the corporations whose stocks are traded receive no funds from the trades—corporations receive funds only when shares are first sold to investors.

Investor-owned corporations may be either publicly held or privately held. The shares of *publicly held* firms are owned by a large number of investors and are widely traded. For example, HCA, which currently (2000) owns and operates about 200 hospitals and has over 550 million shares outstanding, is owned by some 50,000 individual and institutional stockholders. Another example is Beverly Enterprises, which owns and operates over 600 nursing homes and has over 100 million shares outstanding owned by about 8,000 stockholders. Drug manufacturers such as Merck and Pfizer; and medical equipment manufacturers such as St. Jude Medical, which makes heart valves; and U.S. Surgical, which makes surgical stapling instruments; are all publicly held corporations.

Conversely, the shares of *privately held,* also called *closely held,* firms are owned by just a handful of investors and are not publicly traded. In general, the managers of privately held firms are major stockholders. In regards to ownership and control, therefore, privately held firms are more similar to partnerships than to publicly held firms. Often, the privately held corporation is a transitional form of organization that exists for a short time between a proprietorship or partnership and a publicly owned corporation in which the motivation to go public is driven by capital needs. Community Health Systems, a Tennessee firm that owns or manages over 35 hospitals in 14 states, is an example of a closely held firm in the health services industry.

The *stockholders,* also called *shareholders,* are the owners of investor-owned firms. As owners, they have three basic rights:

1. **The right of control.** Common stockholders have the right to vote for the corporation's board of directors, which oversees the management of the firm. Each year, a firm's stockholders receive a *proxy* ballot, which they use to vote for directors and to vote on other issues that are proposed by management or stockholders. In this way, stockholders exercise control. In the voting process, stockholders cast one vote for each common share held.

2. **A claim on the residual earnings of the firm.** A corporation sells products or services and realizes revenues from the sales. To produce these revenues, the corporation must incur expenses for materials, labor, insurance, debt capital, and so on. Any excess of revenues over expenses—the residual earnings—belong to the shareholders of the business. Often, a portion of these earnings are paid out in the form of *dividends,* which are merely cash payments to stockholders, or *stock repurchases,* in which the firm buys back shares held by stockholders. However, management typically elects to reinvest some, or all, of the residual earnings in the business, which presumably will produce even higher payouts to stockholders in the future.

3. **A claim on liquidation proceeds.** In the event of bankruptcy and liquidation, shareholders are entitled to any proceeds that remain after all other claimants have been satisfied.

In summary, there are three key features of investor-owned corporations. First, the owners (the stockholders) of the business are well defined, and exercise control of the firm by voting for directors. Second, the residual earnings of the business belong to the owners, so management is responsible only to the stockholders for the profitability of the firm. Finally, investor-owned corporations are subject to taxation at the local, state, and federal levels.

Not-for-Profit Corporations

If an organization meets a set of stringent requirements, it can qualify for incorporation as a *tax-exempt*, or *not-for-profit, corporation*. Tax-exempt corporations are sometimes called *nonprofit corporations*. Because nonprofit **businesses** (as opposed to pure charities) need profits to sustain operations, and because it is hard to explain why nonprofit corporations should earn profits, the term "not-for-profit" is more descriptive of such health services corporations.

Tax-exempt status is granted to businesses that meet the tax definition of a charitable corporation, as defined by Internal Revenue Service (IRS) Tax Code Section 501(c)(3) or (4). Hence, such corporations are also known as *501(c)(3) or (4) corporations*. The tax code defines a charitable organization as, "any corporation, community chest, fund, or foundation that is organized and operated exclusively for religious, charitable, scientific, public safety, literary, or educational purposes." Because the promotion of health is commonly considered a charitable activity, a corporation that provides healthcare services can qualify for tax-exempt status, provided that it meets other requirements.[6]

In addition to the charitable purpose, a not-for-profit corporation must be organized and operated so that it operates exclusively for the public, rather than private, interest. Thus, no profits can be used for private gain and no political activity can be conducted. Also, if the corporation is liquidated or if sold to an investor-owned firm, the proceeds from the liquidation or sale must be used for a charitable purpose. Because individuals cannot benefit from the profits of not-for-profit corporations, such organizations cannot pay dividends. However, prohibition of private gain from profits does not prevent parties of not-for-profit corporations, such as managers and physicians, from benefiting through salaries, perquisites, contracts, and so on.

Not-for-profit corporations differ significantly from investor-owned corporations. Because not-for-profit firms have no shareholders, no single body of individuals has ownership rights to the firm's residual earnings, or exercises control of the firm. Rather, control is exercised by a *board of trustees*, which is not constrained by outside oversight. Also, not-for-profit corporations are generally exempt from taxation, including both property and income taxes, and have the right to issue tax-exempt debt (municipal bonds). Finally, individual contributions to not-for-profit organizations can be deducted from taxable income by the donor, so not-for-profit firms have access to tax-subsidized contribution capital. (The tax benefits enjoyed by not-for-profit corporations are reviewed in a later section on tax laws.)

The financial problems facing most federal, state, and local governments have caused politicians to take a closer look at the tax subsidies provided to not-for-profit hospitals. For example, several bills that require hospitals to meet minimum standards of care to the indigent to retain tax-exempt status have been introduced in Congress. Also, officials in several states have been fighting to restrict or strip tax exemptions to hospitals, or to specify mandatory levels of charity care. For example, Texas has established minimum requirements for charity care, which in effect hold not-for-profit hospitals accountable to the public for the tax exemptions they receive. The Texas law specifies four tests, and each hospital must meet at least one of them. The test that most hospitals use to comply with the law requires that at least 4 percent of net patient service revenue be spent on charity care.

Finally, money-starved municipalities in several states have attacked the property tax exemption of not-for-profit hospitals that have "neglected" their charitable missions. For example, tax assessors are fighting to remove property tax exemptions from not-for-profit hospitals in several Pennsylvania cities after a recent appellate court ruling supported the Erie school district's authority to tax a local hospital that had strayed too far from its charitable purpose. According to one estimate, if all not-for-profit hospitals had to pay taxes comparable to their investor-owned counterparts, local, state, and federal governments would garner an additional $3.5 billion in tax revenues. This estimate explains why tax authorities in some jurisdictions are pursuing not-for-profit hospitals as a source of revenue.

The inherent differences between investor-owned and not-for-profit organizations have profound implications for many elements of healthcare financial management, including organizational goals, financing decisions (i.e., the choice between debt and equity financing and the specific types of securities issued), and capital investment decisions. How ownership affects the application of healthcare financial management theory and concepts will be addressed throughout the book.

1. What are the major differences between investor-owned and not-for-profit corporations? **Self-Test Questions**
2. What pressures recently have been placed on not-for-profit hospitals to ensure that they meet their charitable mission?

Organizational Structures

Whether investor-owned or not-for-profit, the number of ways of organizing a health services organization is almost unlimited. At the most basic level, a healthcare provider can be a single entity with one operating unit. In this situation, all of the financial management decisions for the organization are made by a single set of managers. Alternatively, corporations can be set up with separate operating divisions or as holding companies with wholly or partially owned subsidiary corporations, in which different management layers have different financial management responsibilities.

Holding Companies

Today, many organizations, both investor-owned and not-for-profit, have adopted *holding company* structures to take advantage of economies of scale, or scope, in operations and financing or to gain favorable legal or tax treatment. Holding companies date from 1889, when New Jersey became the first state to pass a law permitting corporations to be formed for the sole purpose of owning the stocks of other firms. Many of the advantages and disadvantages of holding companies are identical to those inherent in a large firm with several divisions. Whether a firm is organized on a divisional basis or as a holding company with several subsidiary corporations does not affect the basic reasons for conducting large-scale, multiproduct or multiservice, multifacility operations. However, the holding company structure has some distinct advantages and disadvantages over the divisional structure.

There are several advantages of holding companies.

- **Control with fractional ownership.** A holding company may buy 5, 10, or 50 percent of the stock of another corporation. Such fractional ownership may be sufficient in giving the acquiring firm effective working control, or at least substantial influence, over the operations of the firm in which it has acquired stock ownership. Working control is often considered to entail more than 25 percent of the common stock, but it can be as low as 10 percent if the stock is widely held.
- **Isolation of risks.** Because the various operating firms in a holding company system are separate legal entities, the obligations of one unit are separate from those of the other units. Therefore, catastrophic losses incurred by one unit of the system are not transferable into claims against the other units. This separation can be especially beneficial when the operating units carry the potential for large losses from malpractice or other liability lawsuits. Note, though, that the parent firm often voluntarily steps in to aid a subsidiary with large losses, either to protect the good name of the firm or to protect its investment in the subsidiary.
- **Separation of for-profit and not-for-profit subsidiaries.** Holding company organization facilitates expansion into both tax-exempt and taxable activities well beyond patient care. However, a tax-exempt holding company must ensure that all transactions with the taxable subsidiaries are conducted at arm's length, otherwise the tax-exempt status of the parent holding company could be challenged. Investor-owned multihospital systems are organized similarly, except that all of the entities are taxable, for-profit organizations.

Holding companies have the following disadvantages.

- **Partial multiple taxation.** Investor-owned holding companies that own at least 80 percent of a subsidiary's common stock can file a consolidated return for federal income tax purposes. In effect, the holding company and the subsidiary are treated as a single entity, with all of the revenues and costs aggregated. However, when less than 80 percent of the stock is owned, the only way that the subsidiary can transfer funds to the holding company is by paying dividends, and such dividends face partial multiple taxation. For example, holding companies that own over 20 percent but less than 80 percent of the stock of another corporation must pay tax on 20 percent of the dividends received (80 percent are nontaxable), and companies that own less than 20 percent must pay tax on 30 percent of the dividends (70 percent are nontaxable). Because the subsidiary must pay taxes on the earnings prior to making the dividend payment, the funds transferred to the parent are taxed twice.
- **Ease of forced divestiture.** In the event of antitrust action, it is relatively easy for a holding company to relinquish ownership in a subsidiary by selling the stock to another party. This transfer is considered a disadvantage because it increases the likelihood that government agencies will demand divestiture if antitrust concerns arise.

Multihospital Systems

Multihospital systems, including both tax-exempt and for-profit organizations, have grown much faster than freestanding hospitals over the past 30 years. Several advantages of multihospital systems have been hypothesized including the following:

- Better access to capital markets, which results in lower capital costs;
- Elimination of duplicated services, which increases the volume of services at the remaining sites and results in lower unit costs and increased quality;
- Economies of scale;
- Access to specialized managerial skills within the system;
- Ability to recruit and retain better personnel because of superior training programs, advancement opportunities, and transfer opportunities; and
- Increased political power to deal with governmental issues such as property taxes, certificates of need, and government reimbursement systems.

In recent years, the largest systems have tended to shed some hospitals, although there continues to be some consolidation within local markets. It appears that hospital systems have more economies of scale within local markets than they do regionally or nationally.

Corporate Alliances

Corporate alliances potentially can provide some of the benefits of multi-institutional systems without requiring common ownership. Perhaps the least binding alliances are industry trade groups, which tend to operate at both state and national levels. To illustrate the concept, note that the American Hospital Association and its state organizations—for example, the Florida Hospital Association—constitute one major hospital trade association. Also, the American Association of Equipment Lessors is the trade group for firms that lease equipment to the health services industry.

Other types of alliances can be more binding, but provide more benefits to their members. For example, several hospital alliances exist primarily to provide purchasing clout for their members. One of the largest of such alliances is VHA (formerly Voluntary Hospitals of America), which is a for-profit firm whose shareholders are the member hospitals, all not-for-profit institutions, and their physicians. VHA's firms and subsidiaries provide members and affiliates with management services in such areas as procurement, data management, marketing, and even capital acquisition. VHA's members and affiliates retain local control and autonomy, yet gain many of the advantages of a large system.

In addition to alliances among similar organizations, alliances are also being formed among dissimilar providers to offer a more complete range of services. Such vertical alliances are discussed in the next section.

Integrated Delivery Systems

In recent years, the most dynamic changes in organizational structures in health services have centered on the *integrated delivery system*.[7] In the 1970s, horizontal integration, such as the combining of hospitals, was the dominant trend in organization evolution. In the 1980s and well into the 1990s, the dominant organizational movement was toward vertically integrated systems. In an integrated delivery system, a single organization, or a closely aligned group of organizations, offers a broad range of patient care and support services operated in a unified manner. The range of services offered by an integrated delivery system may focus on a particular area, such as long-term care or mental health, or, more commonly, it may offer a full range of subacute, acute, and postacute services.

An integrated delivery system may have a single owner, or it may have multiple owners joined together by contracts and agreements. The driving force behind these systems is the motivation to offer a full line of coordinated services, and hence to increase the overall effectiveness and lower the overall cost of the services provided. Cost reduction is obtained by providing only necessary services and ensuring that the services are provided at the most cost-effective clinical level. Integrated delivery systems may be formed by managed care plans or even directly by employers, but more often they are formed by providers to facilitate contracting with plans or employers.

Perhaps the key feature of integrated delivery systems is that, to be successful, the primary focus must be the clinical effectiveness and profitability of the system as a whole, as opposed to each individual element. This requires a much higher level of administrative and clinical integration than is seen in most organizations and, more importantly, it requires that managers of the individual elements of the system place their own interests second to that of the overall system. Although it would appear that single-owner systems would have advantages over systems that are contractually created, such advantages, if they do exist, have proven to be difficult to realize in practice.

1. What are the advantages and disadvantages of the holding company form of organization?
2. What is the difference between horizontal and vertical integration?
3. What are integrated delivery systems, how are they created, and what is the driving force behind them?

Self-Test Questions

Organizational Goals

Financial decisions are not made in a vacuum, but with an objective in mind. Financial management goals within an organization clearly must be consistent with and in support of the overall goals of the business. Thus, by discussing organizational goals, a framework for financial decision making within health services organizations is provided.

In a proprietorship, partnership, or small privately owned corporation, the owners of the business generally are also its managers. In theory, the business can be operated for the exclusive benefit of the owners. If the owners want to work very hard to maximize wealth, they can. On the other hand, if every Wednesday is devoted to golf, no one is hurt by such actions. (Of course, the business still has to cater to its customers or else it will not survive.) It is in large public-owned corporations, in which owners and managers are separate parties, that organizational goals become most important.

Large, Investor-Owned Corporations

From a financial management perspective, the primary goal of investor-owned corporations is generally assumed to be *shareholder wealth maximization*, which translates to stock price maximization. Investor-owned corporations do, of course, have other goals. Managers, who make the actual decisions, are interested in their own personal welfare, in their employees' welfare, and in the good of the community and of society at large. Still, the goal of stock price maximization is a reasonable operating objective upon which to build financial decision rules.

The primary obstacle to shareholder wealth maximization as the goal of investor-owned corporations is the *agency problem*. An agency problem exists when one or more individuals (the *principals*) hire another individual or group of individuals (the *agents*) to perform a service on their behalf, and then delegate a decision-making authority to those agents. Within a health-care financial management framework, the agency problem exists between stockholders and managers, and between debtholders and stockholders. (The stockholder/manager problem is reviewed in this chapter, but the review of the debtholder/stockholder problem is deferred until Chapter 6.)

The agency problem between stockholders and managers occurs because the managers of large, investor-owned corporations hold only a very small proportion of the firm's stock, so they benefit very little from stock price increases. On the other hand, managers benefit substantially from actions often detrimental to shareholders' wealth such as increasing the size of the firm to justify higher salaries and more fringe benefits; awarding themselves generous retirement plans; and spending too much on office space, personal staff, and travel. Clearly, many situations can arise in which managers are motivated to take actions that are in their best interests, rather than in the best interests of stockholders.

However, shareholders recognize the agency problem and counter it by creating incentives for managers to act in shareholders' interests. Additionally, other factors are at work to keep managers focused on shareholder wealth maximization. Here are some of the factors that mitigate the agency problem:

- **The creation of managerial incentives.** More and more firms are creating *incentive compensation plans* that tie managers' compensation to the firm's performance. One tool often used is *stock options*, which allows managers to purchase stock at some time in the future at a given price. Because the options are valuable only if the stock price climbs above the *exercise price* (the price that the managers must pay to buy the stock), managers are motivated to take actions to increase stock price. However, because a firm's stock price is a function both of the actions taken by managers and the general state of the economy, a firm's managers could be doing a superlative job for shareholders and the options still prove to be worthless. To overcome the inherent shortcoming of stock options, many firms today now use *performance shares* as the managerial incentive. Performance shares are given to managers on the basis of the firm's performance as indicated by objective measures such as earnings per share, return on equity, and so on. In addition to getting more shares when targets are met, the value of the shares is enhanced if the firm's stock price rises. Finally, many businesses now are using the concept of *economic value added (EVA)* to structure managerial compensation. (EVA is discussed in some detail in Chapter 14.) All incentive compensation plans—stock options, performance shares, profit-based bonuses, and so forth—are designed with two purposes in mind. First, they offer managers incentives to act on those factors under their control in a way that will contribute to stock price maximization. Second, the existence of such plans helps firms attract and retain top-quality managers.[8]
- **The threat of firing.** Until the 1980s, the probability of a large firm's management being ousted by its stockholders was so remote that it posed

little threat. This situation existed because ownership of most firms was so widely held, and management's control over the proxy (voting) mechanism was so strong, that it was almost impossible for dissident stockholders to fire a firm's managers. Today, however, about 50 percent of the stock of an average large corporation is held by large institutions, such as pension funds and mutual funds, rather than by individual investors. These institutional money managers have the clout, if they choose to use it, to exercise considerable influence over a firm's managers and, if necessary, to remove the current management team by voting them off the board.

- **The threat of takeover.** *Hostile takeovers*, in which a firm is bought against its management's wishes, are most likely to occur when a firm's stock is undervalued relative to its potential because of poor management. In a hostile takeover, a potential acquirer makes a direct appeal to the shareholders of the target firm to *tender*, or sell, their shares at some stated price. If 51 percent of the shareholders agree to tender their shares, the acquirer gains control. When a hostile takeover occurs, the managers of the acquired firm often lose their jobs, and any managers permitted to stay on generally lose the autonomy they had prior to the acquisition. Thus, managers have a strong incentive to take actions to maximize stock price. In the words of the president of a major drug manufacturer, "If you want to keep control, don't let your company's stock sell at a bargain price."

In summary, it is clear that managers of investor-owned firms can have motivations that are inconsistent with shareholder wealth maximization. Still, sufficient mechanisms are at work to force managers to view shareholder wealth maximization as an important, if not primary, goal. Thus, shareholder wealth maximization is a reasonable goal for financial management decision making within investor-owned firms.

Not-for-Profit Corporations

Because not-for-profit corporations do not have shareholders, shareholder wealth maximization is not an appropriate goal for such organizations. Not-for-profit firms consist of a number of classes of *stakeholders* who are directly affected by the organization. Stakeholders include all parties that have an interest, usually of a financial nature, in the organization. For example, a not-for-profit hospital's stakeholders include the board of trustees, managers, employees, physicians, creditors, suppliers, patients, and even potential patients, which may include the entire community. An investor-owned hospital has the same set of stakeholders, plus one additional class—stockholders. While managers of investor-owned firms have to please only one class of stakeholders—the shareholders—to keep their jobs, managers of not-for-profit firms face a different situation. They have to try to please all of the organization's stakeholders because no single, well-defined group exercises control.

Many people argue that managers of not-for-profit firms do not have to please anyone at all because they tend to dominate the board of trustees who are supposed to exercise oversight. Others argue that managers of not-for-profit firms have to please all of the firm's stakeholders to a greater or lesser extent because all are necessary to the successful performance of the business. Of course, even managers of investor-owned firms should not attempt to enhance shareholder wealth by treating any of their firm's other stakeholders unfairly because such actions ultimately will be detrimental to shareholders.

Typically, the goal of not-for-profit firms is stated in terms of a mission. An example is the current mission statement of Bayside Memorial Hospital, a 450-bed, not-for-profit, acute care hospital:

> "Bayside Memorial Hospital, along with its medical staff, is a recognized, innovative healthcare leader dedicated to meeting the needs of the community. We strive to be the best comprehensive healthcare provider through our commitment to excellence."

Although this mission statement provides Bayside's managers and employees with a framework for developing specific goals and objectives, it does not provide much insight into the goal of the hospital's finance function. For Bayside to accomplish its mission, its managers have identified five financial goals:

1. The hospital must maintain its financial viability.
2. The hospital must generate sufficient profits to continue to provide the current range of healthcare services to the community. This goal means that current buildings and equipment must be replaced as they become obsolete.
3. The hospital must generate sufficient profits to invest in new medical technologies and services as they are developed and needed.
4. The hospital should not rely on its philanthropy program or government grants to fund its operations and growth, although it will aggressively seek such funding.
5. The hospital will strive to provide services to the community as inexpensively as possible, given the above financial requirements.

In effect, Bayside's managers are saying that to achieve the hospital's commitment to excellence as contained in its mission statement, the hospital must remain financially strong and profitable. Financially weak organizations cannot continue to accomplish their stated missions over the long run. What is interesting is that Bayside's five financial goals are probably not much different from the finance goals of Jefferson Regional Medical Center (JRMC), a for-profit competitor. Of course, JRMC has to worry about providing a return to its shareholders, and it receives only a very small amount of contributions and grants. However, to maximize shareholder wealth, JRMC also must retain its financial viability and have the financial resources necessary to offer new services and technologies. Furthermore, competition in the market for hospital services will not permit JRMC to charge appreciably more for services than its not-for-profit competitors.

1. What is the difference in goals between investor-owned and not-for-profit **Self-Test** firms? **Questions**
2. What is the agency problem, and how does it apply to investor-owned firms?
3. What factors tend to reduce the agency problem?

Tax Laws

The value of any financial asset—such as a share of stock issued by HCA or a municipal bond issued by the Alachua County Healthcare Financing Authority on behalf of Shands HealthCare, as well as the value of many real assets such as a MRI machine, medical office building, or hospital—depends on the stream of usable cash flows that the asset is expected to produce. Because taxes reduce the cash flows that are usable to the business, financial management analyses must include the impact of local, state, and federal taxes. Local and state tax laws vary widely, so we will not attempt to cover them in this text. Rather, we will focus on the federal income tax system because these taxes dominate the taxation of business income. Then, in our examples, we will typically increase the tax rate to approximate the effects of state and local taxes.

Tax laws can be changed by Congress, and major changes have occurred every three to four years, on average, since 1913 when the federal tax system was initiated. Furthermore, certain aspects of the Tax Code are tied to inflation, so changes automatically occur each year based on the previous year's inflation rate. Therefore, although this section will give you an understanding of the basic nature of our federal tax system, **it is not intended to be a guide for actual use**. Tax laws are so complicated that many law schools offer a master's degree in taxation, and many of the lawyers who hold this degree also are CPAs. Managers and investors should and do, therefore, rely on tax experts rather than trust their own limited knowledge. Still, it is important to know the basic elements of the tax system as a starting point for discussions with tax specialists. In a field complicated enough to warrant such detailed study, we can cover only the highlights.

Current (2000) federal income tax rates on personal income go up to 39.6 percent, and when state and local income taxes are added, the marginal rate can approach or even exceed 50 percent. Business income is also taxed heavily. The income from partnerships and proprietorships is reported by the individual owners as personal income and, consequently, is taxed at rates going up to 50 percent. Corporate income, in addition to state and local income taxes, is taxed by the federal government at marginal rates as high as 38 percent. Because of the magnitude of the tax bite, taxes play an important role in most financial management decisions made by individuals and by for-profit organizations.

Individual (Personal) Income Taxes

Individuals pay personal taxes on wages and salaries; on investment income such as dividends, interest, and profits from the sale of securities; and on the profits of sole proprietorships, partnerships, and S corporations. For tax purposes, investors received two types of income: (1) ordinary and (2) capital gains. *Ordinary income* includes wages and salaries, dividends, and interest income. *Capital gains*, which are taxed at different rates from ordinary income, arise when the investor sells a capital asset for a profit.

Taxes on Wages and Salaries

Federal income taxes on ordinary income are *progressive*; that is, the higher one's income, the larger the *marginal tax rate*, which is the rate applied to the last dollar of earnings. Marginal rates on ordinary income begin at 15 percent, then rise to 28, 31, and 36 percent, and finally top out at 39.6 percent. Because the levels of income for each bracket are adjusted for inflation annually, and because the brackets are different for single individuals and married couples who file a joint return, we will not provide a complete discussion here. However, to help put things in perspective, it takes a taxable income of roughly $275,000 to be in the highest (39.6 percent) bracket, so most people belong in the lower brackets.

Taxes on Dividend and Interest Income

Individuals can receive *dividend income* on stocks that they own and *interest income* on savings accounts, certificates of deposit, bonds, and the like. Such income from securities, like wages and salaries, is taxed as ordinary income, and hence is taxed at federal rates that go up to 39.6 percent, in addition to applicable state and local income taxes. Because investor-owned corporations pay dividends out of earnings that have already been taxed, there is double taxation on corporate income.

Note, however, that under federal tax laws, interest on most state and local government bonds, called *municipals* or "*munis*," is not subject to federal income taxes. Such bonds include those issued by municipal healthcare authorities on behalf of not-for-profit healthcare providers. Thus, investors get to keep all of the interest received from municipal bonds, but only a proportion of the interest received from bonds issued by the federal government or by corporations. This means that a lower interest rate muni bond could provide the same or higher after-tax return as a higher yielding corporate or Treasury bond. For example, consider an individual in the 39.6 percent federal tax bracket who could buy a taxable corporate bond that pays a 10 percent interest rate. What rate would a similar-risk muni bond have to offer to make the investor indifferent between the muni and the corporate? Here is a way to think about this problem:

After-tax rate on corporate bond = Pre-tax rate − Yield lost to taxes

$$= \text{Pre-tax rate} - (\text{Pre-tax rate} \times \text{Tax rate})$$

$$= \text{Pre-tax rate} \times (1 - \text{T})$$

$$= 10\% \times (1 - 0.396) = 10\% \times 0.604 = 6.04\%.$$

Here, T is the investor's marginal tax rate. Thus, the investor would be indifferent between a corporate bond with a 10 percent interest rate and a municipal bond with a 6.04 percent rate.

If the investor wants to know what yield on a taxable bond is equivalent to, say, a 7.0 percent interest rate on a muni bond, then he or she would follow this procedure:

$$\text{Equivalent rate on taxable bond} = \frac{\text{Rate on municipal bond}}{1 - \text{T}}$$

$$= \frac{7.0\%}{1 - 0.396} = \frac{7.0\%}{0.604} = 11.59\%.$$

The exemption of municipal bonds from federal taxes stems from the separation of power between the federal government and state and local governments, and its primary effect is to allow state and local governments, and not-for-profit healthcare providers, to borrow at lower interest rates than otherwise would be possible.

Capital Gains Income

Assets such as stocks, bonds, real estate, and plant and equipment (land, buildings, x-ray machines, and the like) are defined as *capital assets*. If an individual buys a capital asset and later sells it at a profit—that is, if the individual sells it for more than the purchase price—the profit is called a *capital gain*. If the individual sells it for less than the purchase price, the loss is called a *capital loss*. An asset sold within one year of the time it was purchased produces a *short-term capital gain or loss*, whereas an asset held for more than one year produces a *long-term capital gain or loss*. To illustrate the concept, consider that if you buy 100 shares of Beverly Enterprises, a nursing home business, for $10 per share and sell the stock later for $15 per share, you will make a capital gain of 100 × ($15 − $10) = 100 × $5 = $500. However, if you sell the stock for $5 per share, you will incur a capital loss of $500. If you held the stock for one year or less, the gain or loss is short term; otherwise, it is a long-term gain or loss. Note that if you sell the stock for $10 a share, you will make neither a capital gain nor a loss; you will simply get your $1,000 back and no taxes are due on the transaction.

Short-term capital gains are taxed as ordinary income at the same rates as wages, interest, and dividends. However, long-term capital gains are taxed at lower rates than ordinary income. If an individual is in the 28 percent, or higher, tax bracket, long-term capital gains are taxed at 20 percent. If in the lowest (15 percent) tax bracket, the long-term capital gains tax rate is only 10 percent. To illustrate the effect of this tax benefit on long-term capital gains, consider an investor in the top 39.6 percent tax bracket who makes a $500 long-term capital gain on the sale of her Beverly Enterprises stock. If the $500 were ordinary income, she would have to pay federal income taxes of 0.396 × $500 = $198. However, as a long-term capital gain, the tax would be only 0.20 × $500 = $100, for a savings of $98 in taxes. There are many nuances to capital gains taxes, especially regarding how losses can affect taxes. However, our purpose here is merely to introduce the concept.

The purpose of the reduced tax rate on long-term capital gains is to encourage individuals to invest in those assets that contribute to economic growth. The effect of capital gains taxes is to encourage the owners of both large and small healthcare businesses to favor reinvestment of earnings in the business rather than the payment of bonuses or dividends. Ultimately, owners will receive the value of the reinvested earnings in the form of lower-taxed capital gains.

Corporate Income Taxes

The corporate tax structure, shown in Table 2.1, has marginal rates as high as 38 percent, which brings the average rate up to 35 percent. To illustrate this concept, consider the following example. If Midwest Home Health Services, an investor-owned home healthcare business headquartered in Chicago, had $80,000 of taxable income, its federal income tax bill would be $15,450:

$$\text{Corporate taxes} = \$13,750 + [0.34 \times (\$80,000 - \$75,000)]$$
$$= \$13,750 + (0.34 \times \$5,000)$$
$$= \$13,750 + \$1,700 = \$15,450.$$

Midwest's marginal tax rate would be 34 percent, but its average tax rate would be $15,450/$80,000 = 19.3%. Note that the average federal corporate income tax rate is progressive to $18,333,333 of income, but is constant thereafter.

Unrelated Business Income   Even though tax-exempt holding companies can be created with both tax-exempt and taxable subsidiaries, it is also possible for tax-exempt corporations to have taxable income, which is usually referred to as *unrelated business income (UBI)*. UBI is created when a tax-exempt corporation has income from a trade or business that (1) is not substantially related to the charitable goal of the organization and (2) is carried on with the frequency and regularity of comparable for-profit commercial businesses.

As an example of UBI, consider Bayside Memorial Hospital's pharmacy sales. In addition to its services to the hospital's patients, the not-for-profit hospital's pharmacy has a second location, adjacent to the parking garage, that sells drugs and supplies to the general public. In general, the IRS views the

TABLE 2.1
Corporate Tax
Rates for 2000

Taxable Income	Tax	Average Tax Rate at Top of Bracket
Up to $50,000	15% of taxable income	15.0%
$50,000–$75,000	$7,500 + 25% of excess over $50,000	18.3
$75,000–$100,000	$13,750 + 34% of excess over $75,000	22.3
$100,000–$335,000	$22,250 + 39% of excess over $100,000	34.0
$335,000–$10,000,000	$113,900 + 34% of excess over $335,000	34.0
$10,000,000–$15,000,000	$3,400,000 + 35% of excess over $10,000,000	34.3
$15,000,000–$18,333,333	$5,150,000 + 38% of excess over $15,000,000	35.0
Over $18,333,333	$6,416,667 + 35% of excess over $18,333,333	35.0

charitable purpose of a hospital as providing healthcare services to its patients, so the income from Bayside's sale of drugs and supplies to nonpatients, which is done on a regular basis, is taxable. The fact that the profits from the sales are used for charitable purposes is immaterial. Note, however, that if the trade or business engaged in by a not-for-profit entity (1) is run by volunteers, (2) is run for the convenience of employees, or (3) involves the sale of merchandise contributed to the organization, then the income generated remains tax exempt. Thus, the profits on Bayside's sale of drugs and supplies to its employees, as well as the profits on the sale of items in its gift shop run by volunteer "pink ladies," is exempt from taxation.

UBI tax returns must be filed annually with the IRS by not-for-profit organizations if the gross income from unrelated business activity exceeds $1,000. In determining taxable income, expenses related to UBI income production are deducted from gross income. Then, taxes are calculated as if the income were earned by a taxable corporation.

Interest and Dividend Income Received by an Investor-Owned Corporation

Interest income received by a taxable corporation is taxed as ordinary income at the regular tax rates contained in Table 2.1. However, a portion of the dividends received by one corporation from another is excluded from taxable income. As we mentioned earlier in our discussion of holding companies, the size of the dividend exclusion actually depends on the degree of ownership. In general, we will assume that corporations that receive dividends have only nominal ownership in the dividend-paying corporations, so 30 percent of the dividends received are taxable. The purpose of the dividend exclusion is to lessen the impact of triple taxation. Triple taxation occurs when the earnings of Firm A are taxed; then dividends are paid to Firm B, which must pay partial taxes on the income; and then Firm B pays out dividends to Individual C, who must pay personal taxes on the income.

To illustrate the effect of the dividend exclusion, consider the following example. A corporation that earns $500,000 and pays a 34 percent marginal tax rate would have an *effective tax rate* of only $0.30 \times 0.34 = 0.102 = 10.2\%$ on its dividend income. If this firm had $10,000 in pre-tax dividend income, its after-tax dividend income would be $8,980:

$$\text{After-tax income} = \text{Pre-tax income} - \text{Taxes}$$

$$= \text{Pre-tax income} - (\text{Pre-tax income} \times \text{Effective tax rate})$$

$$= \text{Pre-tax income} \times (1 - \text{Effective tax rate})$$

$$= \$10,000 \times [1 - (0.30 \times 0.34)]$$

$$= \$10,000 \times (1 - 0.102) = \$10,000 \times 0.898 = \$8,980.$$

If a taxable corporation has surplus funds that can be temporarily invested in securities, the tax laws favor investment in stocks, which pay dividends, rather than in bonds, which pay interest. For example, suppose Midwest Home Health Services has $100,000 to invest temporarily, and it could buy either bonds that paid interest of $8,000 per year or preferred stock that paid dividends of $7,000 per year. Because Midwest is in the 34 percent tax bracket, its tax on the interest if it bought the bonds would be $0.34 \times \$8,000 = \$2,720$, and its after-tax income would be $\$8,000 - \$2,720 = \$5,280$. If it bought the preferred stock, its tax would be $0.34 \times (0.30 \times \$7,000) = \$714$, and its after-tax income would be $6,286. Other factors might lead Midwest to invest in the bonds, or in other securities, but the tax laws certainly favor stock investments when the investor is a corporation. (See Chapter 16 for a discussion of both short-term and long-term securities investments by healthcare businesses.)

Interest and Dividend Income Received by a Not-for-Profit Corporation

Interest and dividend income received from securities purchased by not-for-profit corporations with **temporary surplus cash** is not taxable. However, note that not-for-profit firms are prohibited from issuing tax-exempt bonds for the sole purpose of reinvesting the proceeds in other securities, although such firms can temporarily invest the proceeds from a tax-exempt issue in taxable securities while waiting for the planned expenditures to occur. If not-for-profit firms could engage in such *tax arbitrage* operations, they could, in theory, generate an unlimited amount of income by issuing tax-exempt bonds for the sole purpose of raising funds to invest in higher-yielding securities that are taxable to most investors. For example, a not-for-profit firm might sell tax-exempt bonds with an interest rate of 5 percent and use the proceeds to invest in U.S. Treasury bonds that yield 6 percent.

A firm's assets can be financed either with debt or equity capital. If it uses debt financing, it must pay interest on that debt, whereas if an investor-owned firm uses equity financing, normally it will pay dividends to its stockholders. The interest paid by a taxable corporation is deducted from the corporation's operating income to obtain its taxable income, but dividends are not deductible. Put another way, dividends are paid from after-tax income. Therefore, Midwest Home Health Services, which is in the 34 percent tax bracket, needs only $1 of pre-tax earnings to pay $1 of interest expense, but it needs $1.52 of pre-tax earnings to pay $1 in dividends:

Interest and Dividends Paid by an Investor-Owned Corporation

$$\text{Dollars of pre-tax income required} = \frac{\$1}{1 - \text{Tax rate}}$$

$$= \frac{\$1}{0.66} = \$1.52.$$

The fact that interest is a tax-deductible expense, while dividends are not, has a profound impact on the way taxable businesses are financed—the U.S. tax system favors debt financing over equity financing. This point will be discussed in detail in Chapter 11.

At one time, corporate long-term capital gains were taxed at lower rates than ordinary income. However, under current law, corporate capital gains are taxed at the same rate as operating income.

Corporate Capital Gains

Corporate operating losses that occur in any year can be used to offset taxable income in other years. Such losses can be carried back to each of the preceding three years and forward for the next 15 years. For example, an operating loss by Midwest Home Health Services in 2000 would be applied first to 1997. If Midwest had taxable income in 1997, and hence paid taxes, the loss would be used to reduce 1997's taxable income, so the firm would receive a refund on taxes paid for 1997. If the 2000 loss exceeded the taxable income for 1997, the remainder would be applied to reduce taxable income for 1998, then 1999. If Midwest had losses in the previous three years, the cumulative losses, including the loss for 2000, would be carried forward to 2001, then 2002, and so on—up to year 2015. Note that losses that are carried back provide immediate tax benefits, but the tax benefits of losses that are carried forward are delayed until some time in the future. The tax benefits of losses that cannot be used to offset taxable income in 15 years or less are lost to the firm. The purpose of this provision in the tax laws is to avoid penalizing corporations whose incomes fluctuate substantially from year to year.

Corporate Loss Carry-Back and Carry-Forward

As we mentioned earlier, if a corporation owns 80 percent or more of another corporation's stock, it can aggregate income and expenses and file a single

Consolidated Tax Returns

consolidated tax return. Thus, the losses of one firm can be used to offset the profits of another. No business wants to incur losses (it can go broke losing $1 to save 34 cents in taxes), but tax offsets do make it more feasible for large multicompany businesses to undertake risky new ventures that might suffer start-up losses.

Self-Test Questions

1. Briefly, explain the individual (personal) and corporate income tax systems.
2. What are capital gains and losses, and how are they differentiated from ordinary income?
3. What is unrelated business income?
4. How do federal income taxes treat dividends received by corporations as compared to dividends received by individuals? Why is this distinction made?
5. With regards to investor-owned businesses, do tax laws favor financing by debt or by equity? Explain your answer.

Depreciation

Suppose Northside Family Practice buys a x-ray machine for $100,000 and uses it for ten years, after which time the machine becomes obsolete. The cost of the services provided by the machine must include a charge for the cost of the machine; this charge is called *depreciation*. Because depreciation reduces profit (net income) as calculated by accountants, the higher a business's depreciation charge, the lower its reported profit. However, depreciation is a noncash charge—it is an allocation of previous cash expenditures—so higher depreciation expense does not actually reduce cash flow. In fact, for taxable businesses, higher depreciation increases cash flow because the greater a business's depreciation expense in any year, the lower its tax bill.

To see more clearly how depreciation expense affects cash flow, consider Table 2.2. Here, we examine the impact of depreciation on two investor-owned hospitals that are alike in all regards except for the amount of depreciation expense each hospital has. Hospital A, with $100,000 of depreciation expense, has $200,000 of taxable income, pays $80,000 in taxes, and has $120,000 of after-tax income. Hospital B, with $200,000 of depreciation expense, has only $100,000 of taxable income, pays $40,000 in taxes, and has an after-tax income of $60,000.

However, depreciation is a noncash expense, whereas we assume that all other entries in Table 2.2 represent actual cash flows. To determine each hospital's cash flow, depreciation must be added back to after-tax income. When this is done, Hospital B, with the larger depreciation expense, has the larger cash flow. In fact, Hospital B's cash flow is larger by $260,000 − $220,000 = $40,000, which represents the tax savings, or *tax shield*, on its additional $100,000 in depreciation expense:

	Hospital A	Hospital B
Revenue	$1,000,000	$1,000,000
Costs except depreciation	700,000	700,000
Depreciation	100,000	200,000
Taxable income	$ 200,000	$ 100,000
Federal plus state taxes (assumed to be 40%)	80,000	40,000
After-tax income	$ 120,000	$ 60,000
Add back depreciation	100,000	200,000
Net cash flow	$ 220,000	$ 260,000

TABLE 2.2
The Effect of Depreciation on Cash Flow

$$\text{Tax shield} = \text{Tax rate} \times \text{Depreciation expense}$$

$$= 0.40 \times \$100,000 = \$40,000.$$

Because a business's financial condition depends on the actual amount of cash that it earns, as opposed to some arbitrarily determined accounting profit, owners and managers should be more concerned with cash flow than reported profit. Note that if the hospitals in Table 2.2 were **not-for-profit hospitals**, taxes would be zero for both hospitals, and both hospitals would have $300,000 in net cash flow. However, Hospital A would report $200,000 in earnings, while Hospital B would report only $100,000 in earnings.

For-profit businesses generally calculate depreciation one way for tax returns and another way when reporting income on their financial statements. For *tax depreciation*, businesses must follow the depreciation guidelines laid down by tax laws, but for other purposes, businesses usually use *accounting*, or *book*, *depreciation* guidelines.

To determine **book depreciation**, the most common method is the *straight-line* method. To apply the straight-line method, (1) start with the *capitalized cost* of the asset (generally price plus shipping plus installation); then (2) subtract the asset's *salvage value*, which, for book purposes, is the estimated value of the asset at the end of its useful life; and, finally, (3) divide the net amount by the asset's useful life. For example, consider Northside's x-ray machine that costs $100,000 and has a ten-year useful life. Furthermore, assume that it costs $10,000 to deliver and install the machine, and that its estimated salvage value after ten years of use is $5,000. In this case, the capitalized cost, or *basis*, of the machine is $100,000 + $10,000 = $110,000, and the annual depreciation expense is ($110,000 − $5,000)/10 = $10,500. Thus, the depreciation expense reported on Northside's income statement would include a $10,500 charge for "wear and tear" on the x-ray machine. The name "straight line" comes from the fact that the annual depreciation under this method is constant; the *book value* of the asset, which is the cost minus the accumulated depreciation to date, declines evenly (follows a straight line) over time.

For **tax purposes**, depreciation is calculated according to the *Modified Accelerated Cost Recovery System (MACRS)*. MACRS actually spells out two procedures for calculating tax depreciation: (1) The *standard (accelerated) method*, which is faster than the straight-line method because it allows businesses to depreciate assets on an accelerated basis; and (2) an *alternative straight-line method*, which is optional for some assets, but mandatory for others. Because taxable businesses want to gain the tax shields from depreciation as quickly as possible, they will normally use the standard (accelerated) MACRS method when it is allowed.

The calculation of MACRS deprecation uses three components: (1) The depreciable basis of the asset, which is the total amount to be depreciated; (2) a recovery period that defines the length of time over which the asset is depreciated; and (3) a set of allowance percentages for each recovery period that, when multiplied by the basis, gives each year's depreciation expense.

Depreciable Basis

The *depreciable basis* is a critical element of the depreciation calculation because each year's recovery allowance depends jointly on the asset's depreciable basis and its recovery period. The depreciable basis under MACRS generally is equal to the purchase price of the asset plus any transportation and installation costs. Unlike the calculation of book depreciation, the basis for MACRS depreciation is **not** adjusted for salvage value regardless of whether the standard accelerated or alternate straight-line method is used.

MACRS Recovery Periods

Table 2.3 describes the general types of property that fit into each *recovery period*. Property in the 27.5- and 39-year classes (real estate) must be depreciated using the alternate straight-line method, but 3-, 5-, 7-, and 10-year property (personal property) can be depreciated either by the accelerated method or by the alternate straight-line method.

MACRS Recovery Allowances

Once the property is placed in the correct recovery period, the yearly recovery allowance, or depreciation expense, is determined by multiplying the asset's depreciable basis by the appropriate recovery percentage shown in Table 2.4. The specific calculation is discussed in the following sections.

Under MACRS, the assumption is generally made that an asset is placed in service in the middle of the first year. Thus, for three-year recovery period property, depreciation begins in the middle of the year the asset is placed in service and ends three years later. The effect of the *half-year convention* is to extend the recovery period out one more year, so three-year property is

TABLE 2.3
MACRS
Recovery
Periods

Period	Type of Property
3–year	Tractor units and certain equipment used in research
5–year	Automobiles, trucks, computers, and certain special manufacturing tools
7–year	Most equipment, office furniture, and fixtures
10–year	Certain longer-lived types of equipment
27.5–year	Residential rental property such as apartment buildings
39–year	All nonresidential property such as commercial and industrial buildings

Note: Land cannot be depreciated.

TABLE 2.4
MACRS
Recovery
Allowances

Ownership Year	Recovery Period			
	3-Year	5-Year	7-Year	10-Year
1	33%	20%	14%	10%
2	45	32	25	18
3	15	19	17	14
4	7	12	13	12
5		11	9	9
6		6	9	7
7			9	7
8			4	7
9				7
10				6
11				3
	100%	100%	100%	100%

Note: The tax tables carry the recovery allowances out to two decimal places, but for ease of illustration, we will use the rounded allowances shown in this table throughout this text.

depreciated over four calendar years, five-year property is depreciated over six calendar years, and so on. This convention is incorporated in the values listed in Table 2.4.

MACRS Depreciation Illustration

Assume that the $100,000 x-ray machine is purchased by Northside Family Practice and placed in service in 2000. Furthermore, assume that Northside paid another $10,000 to ship and install the machine, and that the machine falls into the MACRS five-year class. Because salvage value does not play a part in tax depreciation, and because delivery and installation charges are included (are capitalized) in the basis rather than expensed in the year incurred, the machine's depreciable basis is $110,000.

Each year's recovery allowance (tax depreciation expense) is determined by multiplying the depreciable basis by the applicable recovery percentage. Thus, the depreciation expense for 2000 is $0.20 \times \$110,000 = \$22,000$, and for 2001 it is $0.32 \times \$110,000 = \$35,200$. Similarly, the depreciation expense is $20,900 for 2002, $13,200 for 2003, $12,100 for 2004, and $6,600 for 2005. The total depreciation expense over the six-year recovery period is $110,000, which equals the depreciable basis of the x-ray machine. Note that the depreciation expense reported for tax purposes each year is different from the book depreciation reported on Northside's income statement that we calculated earlier.

The *book value* of a depreciable asset at any point in time is its depreciable basis minus the depreciation accumulated to date. Thus, at the end of 2000, the x-ray machine's tax book value is $\$110,000 - \$22,000 = \$88,000$; at the end of 2001, the machine's tax book value is $\$110,000 - \$22,000 - \$35,200 = \$52,800$ (or $\$88,000 - \$35,200 = \$52,800$); and so on. Again, note that the book value for accounting purposes is different from the book value for tax purposes.

According to the IRS, the value of a depreciable asset at any point in time is its tax book value. If a business sells an asset for more than its tax book value, the implication is that the firm took too much depreciation, and the IRS will want to recover the excess tax benefit. Similarly, if an asset is sold for less than its book value, the implication is that the firm did not take sufficient depreciation, and it can take additional depreciation upon the sale of the asset. For example, suppose Northside sells the x-ray machine in early 2002 for $60,000. Because the machine's tax book value is $52,800 at the time, $\$60,000 - \$52,800 = \$7,200$ is added to the Northside's operating income and taxed. Conversely, if Northside received only $40,000 for the machine, it would be able to deduct $\$52,800 - \$40,000 = \$12,800$ from taxable income, and hence reduce its taxes in 2002.

Self-Test Questions

1. Briefly, describe the MACRS tax depreciation system.
2. What is the effect of the sale of a depreciable asset on the firm's taxes?

Key Concepts

This chapter presented some background information on business organization, ownership, goals, and taxes. Here are its key concepts:

- The three main forms of business organization are the *sole proprietorship*, the *partnership*, and the *corporation*.
- Although each form of organization has its own unique advantages and disadvantages, most large organizations, and all not-for-profit entities, are organized as *corporations*.
- *Investor-owned corporations* have *shareholders* who are the owners of the firm. Shareholders exercise control through the *proxy* process, in which

they elect the firm's board of directors and vote on matters of major consequence to the firm. As owners, the shareholders have a claim on the residual earnings of the firm. Investor-owned firms are fully taxable.

- Organizations that serve a charitable purpose that meet certain criteria can be organized as *not-for-profit corporations*. Rather than have a well-defined set of owners, such organizations have a large number of *stakeholders* who have an interest in the organization. Not-for-profit firms do not pay taxes, they can accept tax-deductible contributions and they can issue tax-exempt (municipal) debt.

- From a financial management perspective, the goal of investor-owned firms is *shareholder wealth maximization*, which translates to stock price maximization. For not-for-profit firms, a reasonable goal for financial management is to *ensure the organization can fulfill its mission*, which translates to *maintaining the organization's financial viability*.

- An *agency problem* is a potential conflict of interests that can arise between principals and agents. One type of agency problem that can arise in financial management is the conflict between the owners and managers of a for-profit corporation.

- The value of any income stream depends on the amount of *usable*, or *after-tax, income*. Thus, tax laws play an important role in financial management decisions.

- Separate tax laws apply to *personal* income and *corporate* income.

- Fixed assets are *depreciated* over time to reflect the decline in their values. Depreciation is a deductible, but noncash, expense. Thus, for a taxable entity, the higher its depreciation, the lower its taxes, and hence the higher its cash flow, with other things held constant.

- Current laws specify that the *Modified Accelerated Cost Recovery System (MACRS)* be used to depreciate assets for tax purposes.

Although the first two chapters provide a great deal of background information relevant to healthcare financial management, it is necessary to have a more thorough understanding of the reimbursement system. This important topic is covered in the next chapter.

Selected References

Blair, John D., Grant T. Savage, and Carlton J. Whitehead. 1989. "A Strategic Approach for Negotiating with Hospital Stakeholders." *Health Care Management Review* (Winter): 13–23.

Clement, Jan P., Dean G. Smith, and John R. C. Wheeler. 1994. "What Do We Want and What Do We Get from Not-for-Profit Hospitals?" *Hospital & Health Services Administration* (Summer): 159–178.

Fallon, Robert P. 1991. "Not-For-Profit≠No Profit: Profitability Planning in Not-For-Profit Organizations." *Health Care Management Review* (Summer): 47–59.

Fottler, Myron D., John D. Blair, Carlton J. Whitehead, Michael D. Laus, and Grant
  T. Savage. 1989. "Assessing Key Stakeholders: Who Matters to Hospitals and
  Why?" *Hospital & Health Services Administration* (Winter): 525–546.

Healthcare Financial Management. The July 1997 issue has several articles related
  to the tax sanctions imposed on not-for-profit corporations when transactions
  result in excess benefits to individuals.

Herzlinger, Regina E., and William S. Krasker. 1987. "Who Profits From Nonprofits"
  Harvard Business Review (January–February): 93–105.

McLean, Robert A. 1989. "Agency Costs and Complex Contracts in Health Care
  Organizations." *Health Care Management Review* (Winter): 65–71.

Nauert, Roger C., A. Beckwith Sanborn, II, Charles F. MacKelvie, and James L.
  Harvitt. 1988. "Hospitals Face Loss of Federal Tax-Exempt Status." *Healthcare Financial Management* (September): 48–60.

Pink, George H., and Peggy Leatt. 1991. "Are Managers Compensated for Hospital
  Financial Performance." *Health Care Management Review* (Summer): 37–45.

Umbdenstock, Richard J., Winifred M. Hageman, and Bruce Amundson. 1990. "The
  Five Critical Areas for Effective Governance of Not-for-Profit Hospitals."
  Hospital & Health Services Administration (Winter): 481–492.

Walker, C. Langford and L. Wade Humphreys. 1993. "Hospital Control and Decision
  Making: A Financial Perspective." *Healthcare Financial Management* (June):
  90–96.

Wolfson, Jay and Scott L. Hopes. 1994. "What Makes Tax-Exempt Hospitals Special?"
  Healthcare Financial Management (July): 57–60.

Selected Web Sites

There are a multitude of web sites that pertain to this chapter.

For more information on taxes, see the Tax Guide for Investors at *www.fairmark.com*.

To get some feel for the services offered by a corporate alliance, see the VHA site at
  www.vha.com.

Two of the largest integrated health systems in the United States are Kaiser Permanente
  and the Henry Ford Health System. To gain a better idea of what constitutes
  such systems, see *www.kaiserpermanente.org*; or *www.henryfordhealth.org*.

Notes

1. Note that a tax-exempt corporation, which is discussed later in this chapter,
   can be one partner of a partnership. In this situation, profits allocated to the
   tax-exempt partner are not taxed, but those allocated to taxable partners are
   subject to taxation.

2. Although most partnerships are small, there are some very large firms that are
   organized as partnerships or as hybrid organizations, which will be discussed in
   a later section. Examples include the major public accounting firms and many
   large law firms.

3. *Financial markets* bring together individuals and businesses that need money
   with other individuals and businesses that have excess funds to invest. In a

developed economy, such as in the United States, there are a great many financial markets. Some markets deal with debt capital while some deal with equity capital; some deal with short-term capital and others deal with long-term capital, and so on. How financial markets operate and their benefits to healthcare businesses will be discussed throughout the text.

4. Over 60 percent of corporations in the United States are chartered in Delaware, which over the years has provided a favorable governmental and legal environment for business activities. A firm does not have to be headquartered or even conduct business in its state of incorporation.

5. In rare situations, shares can be sold to the public for the first time by the corporation's original owners or by a foundation established by the owners, rather than directly by the firm. In such situations, the proceeds from the sale go to the original owners or foundation and not to the firm. Stock sales are discussed in more detail in Chapter 7.

6. An entire chapter could easily be filled with the details of obtaining and maintaining tax-exempt status, but our focus is on the impact of such status on financial management decision making.

7. For a more thorough discussion of integrated delivery systems, see Douglas A. Conrad and William L. Dowling, "Vertical Integration in Health Services: Theory and Managerial Implications," *Health Care Management Review*, Fall 1990.

8. Incentive compensation plans are also used by not-for-profit organizations. For more information, see the Winter 1989 issue of *Topics in Health Care Financing*, "Incentive Compensation"; and William O. Cleverley and Roger K. Harvey, "Economic Value Added—A Framework for Health Care Executive Compensation," *Hospital & Health Services Administration*, Summer 1993.

THE THIRD-PARTY-PAYER SYSTEM

Learning Objectives

After studying this chapter, readers should be able to:

- Describe the key features of insurance.
- Discuss, in general terms, the reimbursement methods used by third-party payers, and the incentives and risks that they create for providers.
- Describe the major types of third-party payers.
- Discuss the specific reimbursement methods used by Medicare.

Introduction

In general, businesses in the healthcare sector that do not provide products or services directly to patients have the same operating environment as businesses in any other industry. For example, Cincinnati Milicron, a machine tool manufacturer, and General Electric's Medical Equipment Division sell their products in roughly the same way. Cincinnati sells its machines directly to manufacturers that use the machines to produce other goods, and GE Medical sells its diagnostic equipment directly to hospitals, medical practices, and other organizations that use the equipment for diagnostic testing. The prices that the two firms charge for their products are set in the competitive marketplace, and it is relatively easy for buyers to distinguish among competing products. In general, the more expensive the product, the better the performance, where performance can be judged on the basis of a set of more or less objective measures. Thus, in some industries in the healthcare sector, and in most other industries, the consumer of the product or service (1) has a choice among many suppliers, (2) can distinguish the quality of competing goods or services, (3) makes a (presumably) rational decision regarding the purchase on the basis of quality and price, and (4) pays for the full cost of the purchase.

However, for the most part, the provision of healthcare services takes place in a unique way. First, often there are few providers of a particular service at hand. Next, it is very difficult, if not impossible, to judge the quality of competing goods or services. Then, the decision about which goods or services to purchase is usually not made by the consumer of those goods or services, but rather by a physician or some other clinician. Also, payment to the provider is not normally made by the user of the goods or services, but by a *third-party payer*. Finally, for most individuals, the purchase of health insurance from third-party payers is totally paid for or heavily subsidized by employers or government agencies, so patients are insulated from the costs of healthcare. This highly unusual marketplace for healthcare services has a profound effect on the supply of, and demand for, such services. We will leave most of the discussion concerning the market for healthcare services for economics courses, but, to get a better understanding of the unique payment mechanisms involved, we must examine the third-party-payment system in more detail. Thus, in this chapter, we discuss those elements of the payer system that directly affect financial management decisions.

Insurance Concepts

To begin our discussion, note that the third-party-payer system is really an insurance system with a wide variety of insurance "companies" that come in all types and sizes. Some are investor-owned, while others are not-for-profit or government sponsored. Furthermore, some "companies" require their policyholders, who may or may not be the beneficiaries of the insurance, to make the policy payments, while other "companies" collect partially or totally from society at large. Because insurance is the cornerstone of the third-party-payment system, an appreciation of the nature of insurance will help you better understand the marketplace for healthcare services.[1]

A Simple Illustration

To better understand insurance concepts, consider a simple example. Assume that no health insurance exists, and that you face only two medical outcomes in the coming year:

Outcome	Probability	Cost
Stay healthy	0.99	$ 0
Get sick	0.01	20,000
	1.00	

Furthermore, assume that every other individual faces the same medical outcomes, and hence "sees" the same odds and costs associated with healthcare. Then, what is your expected healthcare cost, E(Cost), for the coming year? To find the answer, we must multiply the cost of each outcome by its probability of occurrence, and then sum the products:

$$E(Cost) = (\text{Probability of Outcome 1} \times \text{Cost of Outcome 1})$$

$$+ (\text{Probability of Outcome 2} \times \text{Cost of Outcome 2})$$

$$= (0.99 \times \$0) + (0.01 \times \$20,000)$$

$$= \$0 + \$200 = \$200.$$

Now, assume that you, and everyone else, make $20,000 a year. With this salary, you can easily afford the $200 "expected" healthcare cost. The problem is, however, that no one's actual bill will be $200. If you stay healthy, your bill will be zero. But if you are unlucky and get sick, your bill will be $20,000, and this cost will force you, and most people who get sick, into personal bankruptcy, which is a ruinous event.

Now, suppose an insurance policy that pays all of your healthcare costs for the coming year is available for $250. Would you take the policy, even though it costs $50 more than your "expected" healthcare costs? Most people would. Because individuals are risk averse, they would be willing to pay a $50 premium over their expected benefit to eliminate the risk of financial ruin. In effect, policyholders are passing the costs associated with the risk of getting sick to the insurer.

Would an insurer be willing to offer the policy for $250? If the insurer could sell enough policies, it could take advantage of the *law of large numbers*. We know that it is impossible to predict the healthcare costs for the coming year for any one individual with any certainty because the cost will either be $0 or $20,000, and we will not know for sure until the year is over. For any individual, the expected cost of healthcare is $200, but the standard deviation is a whopping $1,990, so there is significant uncertainty about each individual's required expenditure.

However, if an insurance company sells a million policies, its expected total policy payout is one million times the expected payout for each policy, or $1,000,000 \times \$200 = \$200$ million. Furthermore, the law of large numbers tells us that the standard deviation of costs to an insurer with a large number of policyholders is $\sigma/\sqrt{n}$, where σ is the standard deviation for one individual and n is the number of individuals insured. Thus, payout uncertainty for the insurer, as measured by standard deviation, is only $1,990 / \sqrt{1,000,000} =$ $1.99 per subscriber, or $1.99 million in total. Given these data, we see that if there were no uncertainty in the $20,000 estimated medical cost per claim, the insurer could forecast its total claims quite precisely. It would collect 1,000,000 $\times \$250 = \$250$ million in health insurance premiums, pay out roughly $200 million in claims, and hence have about $50 million to cover administrative costs, provide a reserve in case realized claims are greater than predicted by its actuaries, and make a profit. Clearly, with a standard deviation of claims of about $2 million, the $50 million "cushion" should be sufficient to carry out a successful business. The problem for real-world insurers is their inability to forecast the cost of each claim.

Basic Characteristics of Insurance

The simple example of health insurance described above illustrates why individuals would seek health insurance, and why insurance companies would be formed to provide such insurance. Needless to say, the concept of insurance becomes much more complicated in the real world. Insurance is typically defined as having four distinct characteristics.

1. **Pooling of losses.** The *pooling*, or *sharing*, *of losses* is the heart of insurance. *Pooling* means that losses are spread over a large group of individuals so that each individual realizes the average loss of the pool rather than the actual loss incurred. In addition, pooling involves the grouping of a large number of homogeneous *exposure units* (people or things having the same risk characteristics) so that the law of large numbers can apply. Thus, pooling implies (1) the sharing of losses by the entire group, and (2) the prediction of future losses with some accuracy based on the law of large numbers.

2. **Payment only for random losses.** A *random loss* is one that is unforeseen and unexpected and occurs as a result of chance. Insurance is based on the premise that payments are made only for losses that are random. We will discuss the moral hazard problem, in which losses are not random, in a later section.

3. **Risk transfer.** An insurance plan almost always involves *risk transfer*. The sole exception to the element of risk transfer is *self-insurance*, which occurs when a business assumes a risk itself rather than insures the risk through an insurance company. (Self-insurance is discussed in a later section.) Risk transfer means that the risk is transferred from the insured to the insurer, which typically is in a better financial position to pay the loss than the insured because of the premiums collected

4. **Indemnification.** The final characteristic of insurance is *indemnification* for losses; that is, the reimbursement of the insured if a loss occurs. Within the context of health insurance, indemnification occurs when the insurer pays the insured, or the provider, in whole or in part, for the expenses related to an insured illness or injury.

Adverse Selection

One of the major problems facing insurers is *adverse selection*. Adverse selection occurs because those individuals and firms that are more likely to have claims are more inclined to purchase insurance than those that are less likely to have claims. For example, an otherwise healthy individual without insurance who needs a costly surgical procedure will likely seek health insurance if he or she can afford it, whereas an identical individual without the threat of surgery is much less likely to purchase insurance. Similarly, consider the likelihood of a 20-year old to seek health insurance versus the likelihood of a 60-year old. All else the same, the older individual, with much greater health risk due to age, is more likely to seek insurance.

If this tendency toward adverse selection goes unchecked, a disproportionate number of sick people, or those most likely to become sick, will seek health insurance, and the insurer will experience higher than expected claims. This increase in claims will trigger a premium increase, which only worsens the problem, because the healthier members of the plan will seek insurance from other firms at a lower cost or may totally forgo insurance. The adverse selection problem exists because of *asymmetric information*, which occurs when individual buyers of health insurance know more about their health status than do insurers.

Insurance companies attempt to control the adverse selection problem by underwriting provisions. *Underwriting* refers to the selection and classification of candidates for insurance. From a health insurance perspective, there are two extreme positions that can be taken by insurers regarding underwriting. First, assuming that insurers offer insurance in all 50 states, but not elsewhere, insurers can base premiums on national average statistics without regard to individual characteristics. Thus, each individual (or each individual's employer, if the firm provides the insurance) would pay the same health insurance premium regardless of age, gender, geographic location, line of work, smoking habits, genetic disposition, and so on. The premium charged for each individual would be sufficient in the aggregate to cover all expected outlays, plus administrative expenses, plus earn a profit for the insurer. In this situation, *cross-subsidies* clearly exist because young, healthy nonsmokers in relatively safe jobs would pay the same premiums as older, sickly smokers in relatively hazardous jobs. Thus, after taking administrative costs out of the insurance premium, healthy individuals would pay premiums that exceed their expected healthcare costs, while the sicker individuals would pay premiums that are less than their expected costs.

At the other extreme, if no information asymmetries existed and perfect information were available, insurers could charge a premium to each subscriber on the basis of that subscriber's expected healthcare costs, as was done in the illustration presented previously. Individuals who are expected to have higher costs would be charged higher premiums, and those with lower expected costs would be charged lower premiums. Of course, neither individuals nor insurers has perfect foresight, so the extreme of charging an insured individual on the basis of his or her expected healthcare costs is not actually attainable. However, insurers could take into account all factors that are proven to affect health status, and hence costs, when fixing insurance rates such as smoking habits, weight, cholesterol level, and hereditary factors.

What approach do health insurers take in practice? Initially, most health insurers used *community ratings*. Here, a single set of premiums, or rates, is offered to all members of a community without regard to age, gender, health status, and so on. Thus, rates reflected geographical differences, and potentially even ethnic and cultural differences if the community was dominated by a single ethnic or cultural group. However, within the community, rates represented an average of high- and low-risk individuals. Then, some insurers (particularly commercial insurers) started to offer *experience ratings*, whereby rates are set based on the claims experience of the specific group being insured.

For example, the Boeing Company might contract with a health insurer to insure all of Boeing's employees in the Seattle area. If Boeing's employees, who, as a group, tend to be younger and more educated, have lower healthcare costs than the community in general, then insurers competing for the contract that use experience ratings can offer Boeing lower rates than competitors that use community ratings. As more and more employers with low-risk employees seek health insurance based on experience ratings, the least costly groups are skimmed from the insurance pool, and those that remain have higher-than-average costs. Because the healthcare costs for those remaining are above the average for the community, insurers serving that population have no choice but to apply experience ratings, so higher premiums can be charged to the remaining groups. The trend, then, has been toward experience ratings and away from community ratings, although community ratings are still used.

Another way that health insurers protect themselves against adverse selection is by including *preexisting conditions* clauses in contracts. A preexisting condition is a physical or mental condition of the insured individual that existed prior to the issuance of the policy. A typical clause states that preexisting conditions are not covered until the policy has been in force for some period of time, say, one or two years. Preexisting conditions present a true problem for the health insurance industry. As we discussed previously, one of the key elements of insurance is randomness; that is, payouts on a policy should be in response to random events. If an individual has a preexisting condition, this key feature of insurance is violated. In regards to the preexisting condition, the insurer no longer bears random risk, but rather assumes the role of payer for the treatment of a known condition.

Because of the tendency of insurers to shy away from large predictable claims, Congress passed the *Health Insurance Portability and Accountability Act (HIPAA)* in 1996. Among other things, the HIPAA sets national standards, which can be modified within limits by the states, regarding what provisions can be included in health insurance policies. For example, under a group health policy, coverage to individuals cannot be denied or limited, nor can individuals be required to pay more, because of health status. Although preexisting condition clauses are not banned, there are limits as to what counts as a preexisting condition and how long it takes for coverage to begin. Also, time credit for preexisting conditions under one plan can be credited toward the exclusion period in a second plan, provided there is no break in coverage. Furthermore, health insurance cannot be canceled because the policyholder becomes sick, and individuals have the right to purchase inidividual insurance from the insurer that provided group insurance when they leave the firm. All in all, the provisions of the HIPAA give consumers of health insurance protection against arbitrary actions by insurers when health status changes for the worse.

Moral Hazard

The fact that insurance is based on the premise that payments are made only for random losses creates the problem of *moral hazard*. The most common illustration of moral hazard in a casualty insurance setting is the owner who deliberately sets a failing business on fire to collect the insurance. Moral hazard is also present in health insurance, but its form typically is not so dramatic—not too many people are willing to voluntarily sustain injury or illness for the purpose of collecting health insurance. However, undoubtedly there are people who purposely use healthcare services that are not medically required. For example, some people who live alone might visit a physician or a walk-in clinic for the social value of human companionship rather than to address a medical necessity. Also, some hospital discharges might be delayed for the convenience of the patient rather than for medical purposes. Finally, when the full cost, or most of the cost, is covered by insurance, individuals often are quick to agree to a $1,000 MRI scan or other high-cost procedure that may not be necessary. If the same test required total out-of-pocket payment, individuals would think twice before agreeing to such an expensive procedure unless the medical necessity was clearly understood. All in all, the fact that "somebody else" is paying the costs leads to a greater consumption of healthcare services than would occur if patients bore the costs.

Even more insidious is the impact of insurance on individual behavior. Individuals are less likely to take preventive actions when the costs of not taking those actions will be borne by insurers. Why worry about getting a flu shot if the monetary costs associated with the treatment are borne by the insurer, or why stop smoking if others will pay for the likely adverse health consequences? Clearly, the very fact that insurance exists causes individuals to forgo preventive actions and embrace unhealthy behaviors, both of which might be approached differently in the absence of insurance.

Insurers generally attempt to protect themselves from moral hazard claims by paying less than the full amount of healthcare costs borne by the insured. By making insured individuals bear some of the cost, there will be less of a tendency to consume unneeded services or engage in unhealthy behaviors. One way of doing this is to require a *deductible*. Medical policies usually contain some dollar amount that must be satisfied before benefits are paid. Although deductibles have some positive effect on the moral hazard problem, their primary purpose is to eliminate the payment of small claims, wherein the administrative cost of processing the claim may be larger than the claim itself. Although there are several types of deductibles, the most common form is the *calendar year deductible*. Here, the first $100 (or $250 or more) of medical expenses incurred each year is paid by the individual insured. Once the deductible is met, the insurer will pay all eligible medical expenses (less any copayments) for the remainder of the year.

The primary weapon that insurers have against the moral hazard problem is the *copayment*, which requires insured individuals to pay a certain percentage of eligible medical expenses—say, 20 percent—in excess of the deductible amount. For example, assume that George Maynard, who has employer-provided medical insurance that pays 80 percent of eligible expenses after the $100 deductible is satisfied, incurs $10,000 in medical expenses during the year. The insurer will pay $0.80 \times (\$10,000 - \$100) = 0.80 \times \$9,900 = \$7,920$, so George's responsibility is $\$10,000 - \$7,920 = \$2,080$.

The purposes of copayments are to reduce premiums and to prevent overutilization of healthcare services, and hence insurance benefits. Because insured individuals pay part of the cost, premiums can be reduced. Additionally, by being forced to pay some of the costs, insured individuals will presumably seek fewer and more cost-effective treatments and embrace a healthier lifestyle.

Some health insurance policies contain *stop-loss limits*, also called *out-of-pocket maximums*, whereby the insurer pays all covered costs, including the copayment, after the insured individual pays a certain amount of copayment costs, say, $2,000. Thus, if George had $50,000 of covered expenses above the deductible amount, his coinsurance share would be $10,000 if there were no stop-loss provision. If his policy contained a stop-loss amount of $2,000, George would only have to pay $2,000, and his insurer would pay the remaining $48,000 of costs. Of course, health insurance policies with stop-loss provisions are more costly than those without such features.

Finally, most insurance policies have policy limits; for example, $1,000,000 in total lifetime coverage, or $1,500 per year for mental health benefits, or $100 for eyeglasses. These limits are designed to control excessive use of certain services and to protect the insurer against catastrophic losses. Of course, a lifetime coverage limit means that subscribers must bear the risk of catastrophic losses.

Self-Test Questions

1. Briefly, explain the following characteristics of insurance:
   a. Pooling of losses
   b. Payment only for random losses
   c. Risk transfer
   d. Indemnification
2. What is adverse selection, and how do insurers deal with the problem?
3. What is the moral hazard problem?

Generic Reimbursement Methods

Regardless of the payer for a particular healthcare service, only a limited number of payment methods are used to reimburse providers. Payment methods fall into two broad classifications: (1) fee-for-service and (2) capitation. In *fee-for-service* payment methods, of which many variations exist, the greater the amount of services provided, the higher the amount of reimbursement. Under *capitation*, a fixed payment is made to providers for each covered life, regardless of the amount of services provided. In this section, the mechanics of alternative payment methods are first considered. The incentives created for providers under the alternative methods are then discussed. Finally, the risk implications of the alternative reimbursement methods are analyzed.

The Methods

The three primary fee-for-service methods of reimbursement are: (1) cost based, (2) charge based, and (3) prospective payment. In addition to the fee-for-service methods, some payers, especially managed care plans, pay by capitation. In this section, the methods are reviewed in more detail.

Cost-Based Reimbursement

Under *cost-based reimbursement*, the payer agrees to reimburse the provider for the costs incurred in providing services to the insured population. Reimbursement is limited to *allowable costs*, usually defined as those costs directly related to the provision of healthcare services. Nevertheless, for all practical purposes, cost-based reimbursement guarantees that a provider's total costs will be covered by payments from payers. Typically, the payer makes *periodic interim payments (PIPs)* to the provider, and a final reconciliation is made after the contract period expires and all costs have been processed through the provider's accounting system. During the early years (1966–1983), Medicare reimbursed providers on the basis of costs incurred.

Charge-Based Reimbursement

When payers pay *billed charges*, they pay according to the schedule of charge rates established by the provider. To a certain extent, this reimbursement system places payers at the mercy of providers in regards to the cost of healthcare services, especially in markets where competition is limited. In the very early days of health insurance, all payers reimbursed providers on the basis of billed charges. Some insurers still reimburse providers according to billed charges, but the trend for payers is toward other, less generous reimbursement methods. If this trend continues, the only payers that will be expected to pay billed charges are self-pay, or private-pay, patients.

Some payers that historically have reimbursed providers on the basis of billed charges now pay by *negotiated*, or *discounted*, *charges*. This payment method is frequently used by insurers that have established managed care plans such as HMOs and PPOs. Because HMOs and PPOs, as well as some conventional insurers, have bargaining power because of the large number of patients that they bring to a provider, they can negotiate discounts from billed charges. Such discounts generally range from 20 to 30 percent, or more, of billed charges.

Prospective Payment

In a *prospective payment system*, the rates paid by payers are determined before the services are provided. Furthermore, payments are not directly related to either reimbursable costs or billed charges. Four common units of payment are included in the category of prospective payment:

1. **Per procedure.** Under *per procedure* reimbursement, a separate payment is made for each procedure performed on a patient. Because of the high administrative costs associated with this method when applied to complex diagnoses, per procedure reimbursement is more commonly used in outpatient than in inpatient settings.

2. **Per diagnosis.** In the *per diagnosis* reimbursement method, the provider is paid a rate that depends on the patient's diagnosis. Diagnoses that require higher resource utilization, and, hence, are more costly to treat, have higher reimbursement rates. Medicare pioneered this basis of payment in its *diagnosis related group (DRG)* system, which it first used for hospital reimbursement in 1983. (Reimbursement on the basis of DRG is discussed in detail in the section on Medicare.)

3. **Per diem (per day).** If reimbursement is based on a *per diem* rate, the provider is paid a fixed amount for each day that service is provided, regardless of the nature of the services. This type of reimbursement is applicable only to inpatient settings. Note that per diem rates can be *stratified*. For example, a hospital may be paid one rate for a medical/surgical day, a higher rate for a critical care unit day, and yet a different rate for an obstetrical day. Stratified per diems recognize that providers incur widely different daily costs for providing different types of care.

4. **Global pricing.** Under *global pricing*, payers pay a single prospective payment that covers all services delivered in a single episode, whether the services are rendered by a single or by multiple providers. For example, a global fee may be set for all obstetric services associated with a pregnancy, including all prenatal and postnatal visits as well as the delivery, provided by a single physician. For another example, a global price may be paid for all physician and hospital services associated with a cardiac bypass operation.

Capitation   Up to this point, all the reimbursement methods presented have been fee-for-service methods; that is, providers are reimbursed on the basis of the amount of services provided. The service may be defined as a visit, a diagnosis, a hospital day, or in some other manner, but the key feature is that the more services that are performed, the greater the reimbursement amount. *Capitation*, although a form of prospective payment, is an entirely different approach to reimbursement, and hence deserves to be treated as a separate category. Under capitated reimbursement, the provider is paid a fixed amount per covered life per period (usually a month) regardless of the amount of services provided.

Because the payment is tied only indirectly to the amount of services provided, capitation dramatically changes the financial landscape of healthcare providers and, hence, has profound implications for financial management decision making. In fact, we devote a full chapter (Chapter 19) to capitation and its implications.

Nonpayment   Before we close this section, we think it worthwhile to address briefly the issue of nonpayment. If a user of healthcare services does not have insurance, then the responsibility for payment of total billed charges falls on the patient or the patient's family. Because people without health insurance tend to be poor, many of them find it difficult, if not impossible, to pay for healthcare services that can quickly amount to tens of thousands of dollars. Nonpaying patients fall into two categories. First, those who have the capacity, but are unwilling, to pay. The lost revenues attributable to the first class of nonpayer are called *bad debt losses*. The second group is made up of patients who are not able to pay. The lost revenues attributable to the second class of nonpayer are called *charity*, or *indigent, care losses*.

These classifications are important for two reasons. First, the two types of nonpayment are handled differently on the income statement. Second, it is important that not-for-profit providers be able to document their contributions to society, and one of the most important contributions is willingness to treat indigent patients.

Provider Incentives

Providers, like individuals and other businesses, react to the incentives created by the financial environment. For example, individuals can deduct mortgage interest from income for tax purposes, but they cannot deduct interest payments on personal loans. Loan companies have responded by offering home equity loans that are a type of second mortgage. The intent is not that such loans would be used to finance home ownership, as the tax laws intended, but rather the funds can be used for any purpose, including financing vacations, cars, and appliances. In this situation, tax laws created incentives for consumers to have mortgage debt rather than personal debt, and the mortgage loan industry responded accordingly.

In the same vein, it is interesting to briefly examine the incentives that alternative reimbursement methods have on provider behavior. Under cost-based reimbursement, providers are given a "blank check" to be used in acquiring assets and incurring operating costs. If payers reimburse providers for all costs, the incentive is to incur costs. Facilities will be lavish and conveniently located, and staff will be available to ensure that patients are given "deluxe" treatment. Furthermore, as in billed-charges reimbursement, services that may not truly be required will be provided because more services lead to higher costs, which mean higher revenues.

Under charge-based reimbursement, providers have the incentive to set high charge rates, which leads to high revenues. However, in competitive markets, there will be a constraint on how high providers can go. But, to the extent that insurers, rather than patients, are footing the bill, there is often considerable leeway in setting charges. Because billed charges is a fee-for-service type of reimbursement, in which more services result in higher revenue, a strong incentive exists to provide the highest possible amount of services. In essence, providers can increase utilization, and hence revenues, by *churning*—creating more visits, ordering more tests, extending inpatient stays, and so on. Although charge-based reimbursement does encourage providers to contain costs, the incentive is weak because charges can be more easily increased than costs can be reduced. Note, however, that discounted charge reimbursement places additional pressure on profitability, and hence creates increased incentive for providers to lower costs.

Under prospective payment reimbursement, provider incentives are altered. First, under per procedure reimbursement, the profitability of individual procedures will vary depending on the relationship between the actual costs incurred and the payment for that procedure. Providers, usually physicians, have the incentive to perform procedures that have the highest profit potential. Furthermore, the more procedures the better because each procedure typically generates additional profit. The incentives under per diagnosis reimbursement are similar. Providers, usually hospitals, will seek patients with diagnoses that have the greatest profit potential and discourage (even discontinue) services that have the least profit potential. Furthermore, to the extent that providers have some flexibility in assigning diagnoses to patients, an incentive exists to *upcode* diagnoses to another one that provides greater reimbursement.

In all prospective payment methods, providers have the incentive to reduce costs because the amount of reimbursement is fixed and independent of the costs actually incurred. When per diem reimbursement is used, particularly with hospitals, providers have an incentive to increase length of stay. Because the early days of a hospitalization are typically more costly to the provider than the later days, the later days are more profitable. However, as mentioned previously, hospitals have the incentive to reduce costs during each day of a patient's stay.

Under global pricing, providers do not have the opportunity to be reimbursed for a series of separate services, which is called *unbundling*. For example, a physician's treatment of a fracture could be bundled, and hence billed as one episode, or it could be unbundled with separate bills submitted for diagnosis, x-rays, setting the fracture, removing the cast, and so on. The rationale for unbundling is usually to provide more detailed records of treatments rendered, but often the result is higher total charges for the parts than would be charged for the entire package. Also, global pricing, when applied to multiple providers for a single episode of care, forces involved providers (e.g., physicians and a hospital) to jointly offer the most cost-effective treatment. Such a joint view of cost containment may be more effective than each provider separately attempting to minimize its treatment costs because lowering costs in one phase of treatment could increase costs in another.

Finally, capitation reimbursement totally changes the playing field by completely reversing the actions that providers must take to ensure financial success. Under all prospective payment methods, the key to provider success is to work harder, increase utilization, and hence increase profits; under capitation, the key to profitability is to work smarter and decrease utilization. As with prospective payment, capitated providers have the incentive to reduce costs, but now they also have the incentive to reduce utilization. Thus, only those procedures that are truly medically necessary should be performed, and treatment should take place in the lowest cost setting that can provide the appropriate quality of care. Furthermore, providers have the incentive to promote health, rather than just treat illness and injury, because a healthier population consumes fewer healthcare services.

Financial Risks to Providers

A key issue facing providers is the impact of various reimbursement methods on financial risk, which is a concept that is explained in detail in Chapters 5 and 13. For now, think of financial risk in terms of the effect that the reimbursement methods have on profit uncertainty—the greater the chances of losing money, the higher the risk. Cost- and charge-based reimbursements are the least risky for providers because payers more or less ensure that costs will be covered, and hence profits will be earned. In cost-based systems, costs are automatically covered. In charge-based systems, providers typically can set charges high enough to ensure that costs are covered, although discounts introduce uncertainty into the reimbursement process.

Regardless of the reimbursement method (except cost based), providers bear the cost-of-service risk in that costs can exceed revenues. However, a primary difference among the reimbursement types is the ability of the provider to influence the revenue/cost ratio. If providers set charge rates for each type of service provided, they can most easily ensure that revenues exceed costs. Furthermore, if providers have the power to set rates above those that would exist in a truly competitive market, charge-based reimbursement could result in higher profits than cost-based reimbursement.

Prospective payment adds a second dimension of risk to reimbursement contracts because the bundle of services needed to treat a particular patient may be more extensive than that assumed in the payment. However, when the prospective payment is made on a per procedure basis, risk is minimal because each procedure will produce its own revenue. When prospective payment is made on a per diagnosis basis, provider risk is increased. If, on average, patients require more intensive treatments, and for inpatients a longer length of stay (LOS) than assumed in the prospective payment amount, the provider must bear the added costs.

When prospective payment is made on a per diem basis, even when stratified, one daily rate usually covers a large number of diagnoses. Because the nature of the services provided could vary widely, both because of varying diagnoses as well as intensity differences within a single diagnosis, the provider bears the risk that costs associated with the services provided on any day exceed the per diem rate. However, patients with complex diagnoses and greater intensity tend to remain hospitalized longer, and per diem reimbursement does differentiate among different LOSs. However, the additional days of stay may be insufficient to make up for the increased resources consumed.

In addition, providers bear the risk that the payer, through utilization review process, will constrain LOS, and hence increase intensity during the days that a patient is hospitalized. Thus, under per diem, compression of services and shortened LOS can put significant pressure on providers' profitability.

Under global pricing, a more inclusive set of procedures, or providers, are included in one fixed payment. Clearly, the more services that must be rendered for a single payment, or the more providers that have to share a single payment, the more providers are at risk for intensity of services.

Finally, under capitation, providers assume all utilization and actuarial risks along with the risks assumed under the other reimbursement methods. The assumption of utilization risk has traditionally been an insurance, rather than a provider, function. In the traditional fee-for-service system, the financial risk of providing healthcare is shared between purchasers and insurers. Hospitals, physicians, and other providers bear negligible risk because they are paid on the basis of the amount of services provided. Insurers bear short-term risk in that payments to providers in any year can exceed the amount of premiums collected. However, poor profitability by insurers in one year usually can be offset by premium increases to purchasers the next year, so the long-term risk of financing the healthcare system is borne by purchasers. Capitation, however, places the burden of short-term utilization risk on providers.

When provider risk under different reimbursement methods is discussed in this descriptive fashion, an easy conclusion to make is that capitation is by far the riskiest to providers, while cost- and charge-based reimbursement are by far the least risky. Although this conclusion is not a bad starting point for analysis, financial risk is a complex subject, and its surface has just been scratched. One of the key issues throughout the remainder of this text is financial risk, so readers will see this topic over and over. For now, keep in mind that different payers use different reimbursement methods. Thus, providers can face conflicting incentives and differing risk, depending on the predominant method of reimbursement.

In closing, note that all prospective payment methods involve a transfer of risk from insurers to providers, which increases as the payment unit moves from per procedure to capitation. The added risk does not mean that providers should avoid such reimbursement methods; indeed, refusing to accept contracts with prospective payment provisions would be tantamount to organizational suicide for most providers. However, providers must understand the risks involved in prospective payment arrangements, especially the effect on profitability, and make every effort to negotiate a level of payment that is consistent with the risks incurred.

Self-Test Questions

1. Briefly, describe the following payment methods:
   a. Cost based
   b. Charge based and discounted charges
   c. Per procedure

    d. Per diagnosis

    e. Per diem

    f. Global

    g. Capitation

2. What is the major difference between fee-for-service reimbursement and capitation?

3. What provider incentives are created under each of the payment methods previously listed?

4. Which of these payment methods carry the least risk for providers? The most risk? Explain your answer.

Major Health Insurers (Third-Party Payers)

Up to this point, we have discussed the basic concept of insurance, some key elements of health insurance, and the general types of reimbursement methodologies. Now, we will provide a brief background of the major health insurers (third-party payers) and, more importantly, we will discuss some of the specific reimbursement methods that they use to pay healthcare providers.

Health insurance originated in Europe in the early 1800s, when mutual benefit societies were formed to reduce the financial burden associated with illness or injury. Today, health insurers fall into two broad categories: (1) private insurers and (2) public programs.

1. What are the two major classifications of health insurers?

Self-Test Question

Private Insurers

In the United States, the concept of public, or government, health insurance is relatively new, while private health insurance has been in existence since the turn of the century. In this section, we discuss the major private insurers—Blue Cross and Blue Shield, commercial insurers, and self-insurers.

Blue Cross and Blue Shield

Blue Cross and Blue Shield organizations trace their roots to the Great Depression, when both hospitals and physicians were concerned about their patients' abilities to pay healthcare bills.

Blue Cross originated as a group of separate insurance programs offered by individual hospitals. At the time, many patients were unable to pay their hospital bills, but most individuals, except the poorest, could afford to purchase some type of hospitalization insurance. Thus, the programs initially were designed to benefit hospitals as well as patients. The programs were all similar in structure: Hospitals agreed to provide a certain amount of services to program members who made periodic payments of fixed amounts to the hospitals whether services were used or not. In a short time, these programs were expanded from single hospital programs to community-wide multihospital plans called *hospital service plans*. The American Hospital Association (AHA) recognized the benefits of such plans to hospitals, so a close relationship was formed between the AHA and the organizations that offered hospital service plans.

In the early years, several states ruled that the sale of hospital services by prepayment did not constitute insurance, so the plans were exempt from regulations that govern the insurance industry. However, it was clear that the legal status of hospital service plans would be subject to future scrutiny unless their status was formalized. So the states, one by one, passed enabling legislation that provided for the founding of not-for-profit hospital service corporations that were exempt both from taxes and from the capital requirements mandated for other insurers. However, state insurance departments had, and continue to have, oversight over most aspects of the plans' operations. The Blue Cross name was officially adopted by most of these plans in 1939.

Blue Shield plans developed in a manner similar to that of the Blue Cross plans, except that the providers were physicians, instead of hospitals, and the professional organization was the American Medical Association (AMA), instead of the AHA. Today, there are about 50 Blue Cross and Blue Shield member organizations; some offer only one of the two plans, but most offer both plans. Member organizations are independent corporations that operate locally or statewide under license from a single national association that sets standards that must be met to use the Blue Cross and Blue Shield name. Collectively, the "Blues" provide healthcare coverage for about 75 million people in all 50 states, the District of Columbia, and Puerto Rico.

Historically, the individual state and local organizations have been not-for-profit corporations that enjoyed the full benefits accorded to that status, including freedom from taxes. But in 1986, Congress eliminated the Blues' tax exemption on the grounds that they operated "commercial-type" insurance activities. However, the plans were given some special deductions, which resulted in taxes that are generally less than those paid by commercial insurance companies. In spite of the change in tax status, the national association continued to require all Blues to operate entirely as not-for-profit corporations, although they could establish for-profit subsidiaries. In 1994, however, the national association lifted its traditional ban on member plans becoming investor-owned companies.

As of early 2000, three plans have converted to for-profit status: (1) Blue Cross of California, which is now a subsidiary of WellPoint Health Networks; (2) Blue Cross and Blue Shield of Georgia; and (3) Trigon Blue Cross and Blue Shield of Virginia. Because state laws require the assets of not-for-profit corporations to be used for charitable purposes in perpetuity, the conversion of ownership is a relatively complex endeavor. (We discuss the issues involved in conversion in Chapter 18.) To meet this requirement, plans that convert typically set up a charitable foundation to which they contribute a sum that is, in theory, equal to the value of the assets being converted. However, critics of conversions claim that the amounts contributed fall far short of the actual value of the tax exemptions that the not-for-profits received during their existence.

In spite of the conversion actions listed above, and the pending conversion by Empire Blue Cross and Blue Shield of New York, only a handful of state Blues likely will convert to for-profit status because of the legal problems inherent in conversion and because they already have the ability to create for-profit subsidiaries. The main rationale for converting or creating for-profit subsidiaries is having access to investor-supplied equity capital, which many believe is necessary for insurers to be competitive in today's healthcare market.

Because the Blue Cross and Blue Shield corporations operate independently, no one reimbursement method is universal to all of them. However, over the past few years the tendency has been to move away from cost-based and charge-based methods and toward prospective payment systems. For example, some of the Blues use hospital reimbursement methods that are similar to Medicare's prospective payment system based on diagnosis related groups, while other Blues use a two-tier system in which a per diem rate is paid for routine hospitalizations and negotiated charge-based rates are paid for nonroutine services.

Virtually all of the Blues now offer managed care plans along with more traditional indemnity insurance, and many plans are contracting exclusively with integrated delivery systems in certain service areas. In these situations, capitation often is the method of payment to providers.

Commercial Insurers

Commercial health insurance is issued by life insurance companies, by casualty insurance companies, and by businesses formed exclusively to write health insurance. Commercial insurance companies can be organized either as stock or mutual businesses. *Stock* businesses are shareholder owned, and can raise equity capital just like any other for-profit business. Furthermore, the stockholders assume the risks and responsibilities of ownership and management. A *mutual* business has no shareholders; its management is controlled by a board of directors elected by the firm's policyholders. Regardless of the form of ownership, commercial insurance businesses are taxable entities.

Commercial insurers moved strongly into health insurance following World War II. At that time, the United Auto Workers negotiated the first contract with employers where fringe benefits for employees were a major part of the contract. Like the Blues, the majority of individuals with commercial health insurance are covered under *group policies* with employee groups, professional and other associations, and labor unions. Group health coverage has the following advantages over individual coverage:

• Group coverage has low administrative costs because many individuals are insured under a single contract. This type of coverage lowers the costs associated with sales and administration of the contract. The group contract holder—say, the employer or labor union—usually pays a part of or the entire premium. Note, though, that employers that have costly employee health programs are usually forced by competitive pressures to offset higher healthcare costs with lower wages or reductions in other fringe benefits. Also, the competitive labor market forces employers to offer competitive aggregate benefits, although the benefit mix may differ.

- Generally, eligibility for a group plan does not depend on the insured individual's health status. The insurer bases its premiums on the overall health status of the group. Note, however, that the premiums paid by groups having a small number of members can be adversely affected by the poor health of one individual.
- In general, an individual's coverage cannot be canceled unless the individual leaves the group or the plan itself is terminated.

Commercial insurers have traditionally reimbursed healthcare providers on the basis of billed charges. However, with the dramatic increase in healthcare costs that has occurred over the past 20 years, the traditional providers of health insurance—employers and unions—have seen their healthcare premiums grow to almost unbelievable amounts. For example, the big three automakers estimate that about $700 of the cost of each car and truck produced results from employee healthcare costs. Clearly, this trend cannot continue, so the major purchasers of group health insurance have put pressure on the insurance companies to trim costs. This pressure, in turn, has forced commercial insurers to move toward other reimbursement methods and delivery systems, including managed care plans, that presumably have a better chance at controlling costs than does reimbursement on the basis of billed charges.

Self-Insurers   The third major form of private insurance is *self-insurance*. One could argue that all individuals who do not have any other form of health insurance are self-insurers, but this is not technically correct. Self-insurers make a conscious decision to bear the risks associated with healthcare costs, and then set aside funds to pay future costs as they occur. Individuals are not good candidates for self-insurance because they face too much uncertainty concerning future healthcare expenses. On the other hand, large groups, especially employers, are good candidates for self-insurance. Indeed, most large groups are self-insured today. For example, employees of the State of Florida are covered by health insurance that is administered by Blue Cross and Blue Shield of Florida, but the actual benefits to plan members are paid by the state. Blue Cross and Blue Shield is paid for administering the plan, but the state bears all risks associated with utilization and cost uncertainty.

Many firms today are even going one step further in their self-insurance programs by totally bypassing third-party payers. For example, Digital Equipment Corporation, a major computer maker, negotiates discounts directly with hospitals and physicians. Others, such as Deere & Company, a farm implements manufacturer, have set up health services subsidiaries to provide healthcare services to their employees. For the most part, these firms use the same techniques as managed care organizations, but they try to do things better and cheaper themselves by applying the kind of management attention to healthcare that they do to their core businesses.

1. Briefly, describe some different types of private insurers.
2. What reimbursement methods do private insurers commonly use?

Self-Test Questions

Public Insurers

The government is a major insurer and direct provider of healthcare services. For example, the government provides healthcare services directly to qualifying individuals through the Department of Veterans Affairs (VA), Department of Defense (DOD), and Public Health Service (PHS) medical facilities. In addition, the government either provides or mandates a variety of insurance programs, such as workers compensation and TRICARE, formerly called CHAMPUS (Civilian Health and Medical Program of the Uniformed Services). However, in this section, we focus on the two major government insurance programs: Medicare and Medicaid.

Medicare[2]

Medicare was established by the federal government in 1966 to provide medical benefits to individuals age 65 and older. Medicare consists of two separate coverages: (1) *Part A*, which provides hospital and some skilled nursing home coverage; and (2) *Part B*, which covers physician services, ambulatory surgical services, outpatient services, and certain other miscellaneous services. Part A coverage is free to all people eligible for social security benefits. Individuals who are not eligible for social security benefits can obtain Part A medical benefits by paying premiums of $301 per month (for 2000). Part B is optional to all individuals who have Part A coverage, and it requires a monthly premium of $45.50 (for 2000). About 97 percent of Part A participants purchase Part B coverage.

The Medicare program falls under the *Department of Health and Human Services (DHHS)*, which creates the specific rules of the program on the basis of enabling legislation. Medicare is administered by an agency under DHHS called the *Health Care Financing Administration* (*HCFA*, pronounced "hic-fah"). HCFA has eight regional offices that oversee the Medicare program and ensure that regulations are followed.

Administration of Medicare

    Medicare payments to healthcare providers are not made directly by HCFA, but rather by contractors at state or local level called *intermediaries* for Part A payments and *carriers* for Part B payments.[3] Intermediaries and carriers are typically either Blue Cross associations or commercial insurers. For example, Blue Cross Blue Shield of Florida is the HCFA intermediary for Florida, while Nationwide Mutual Insurance Company is the carrier for Ohio.

A Short History of Part A Reimbursement

From its inception in 1966 to 1983, hospital payments were based on a retrospective system that reimbursed hospitals for all reasonable costs. In general, reasonable costs were defined as (1) operating costs for labor and materials; (2) capital costs for depreciation, interest expense, lease payments, and return on equity for investor-owned hospitals; and (3) costs associated with medical educational programs. In effect, HCFA provided hospitals with blank checks that they could use to provide "gold-plated" services to Medicare beneficiaries.

For many providers, Medicare became the "goose that laid the golden egg." Per beneficiary Medicare spending rose from $648 in 1967 to about $5,000 (estimated) in 2000. Unfortunately, in its early years, Medicare provided no incentives whatever for providers to offer cost-effective services. If anything, Medicare encouraged overbuilding, "gold plating," excessive services, and overly long hospital stays. However, Medicare did lead to many positive results, although at a high price. First, Medicare fueled a hospital boom, which put a hospital nearby for most of the population. In addition, Medicare provided most elderly with access to healthcare services that only a small proportion had had before. Increased access is at least a partial reason why life expectancy has increased dramatically for the elderly—in 1966, a 65-year old could expect to live to about 70; today he or she can expect to live to about 83. Finally, Medicare was a major factor in the racial desegregation of hospitals because all providers had to desegregate to qualify for federal dollars.

Foundations of the Inpatient Prospective Payment System

On October 1, 1983, Congress established a new reimbursement system for Medicare Part A providers, called the *prospective payment system (PPS)*, in an attempt to curb spending. The intent of the PPS was (1) to reduce the growth in Medicare outlays, (2) to provide cost containment incentives to providers, and yet (3) to maintain the quality of care achieved under the old cost-based system. The basic concept of the PPS is to reimburse hospitals with a fixed sum for each admission based on the patient's diagnosis. If the hospital is able to provide the services for less than the fixed reimbursement amount, it can keep the difference. Conversely, if a Medicare patient costs the hospital more than the reimbursement amount, the hospital must bear the loss. Note that all hospitals are not paid under the PPS system; for example, specialty hospitals, such as psychiatric and children's hospitals, are still reimbursed on a retrospective cost basis. However, the vast majority of hospitals are paid under the system, so that will be the focus of our Medicare Part A reimbursement discussion.

The PPS was phased in over several years, and the initial fixed reimbursement rates were based on hospital costs at that time. Thus, upon implementation of PPS, hospitals were able to embark on cost-cutting measures that allowed them to deliver services to Medicare beneficiaries for less than the fixed payments, and many hospitals were able to generate large profits. For example, operating margins on Medicare patients during the first two years of PPS averaged over 13 percent.[4]

Unfortunately for hospitals, since the system's inception, PPS payments, on average, have not kept pace with hospital costs. In addition, once the most obvious cost cutting took place, it was difficult for hospitals to generate additional efficiency gains. Furthermore, the Balanced Budget Act of 1997 (BBA) placed significant restrictions on the growth in Medicare spending during the 1998–2002 period. Hospitals, through aggressive lobbying efforts, have been able to somewhat dilute the impact of the BBA. For example, the Balanced Budget Relief Act of 1999 (BBRA) restored some of the reductions in spending growth imposed by the BBA, but recent hospital payment growth rates still have been less than the growth in operating costs. The net result has been that the average hospital's operating margin on Medicare patients has fallen to the point that some hospitals are now losing money on Medicare inpatients.

The PPS has had a direct influence on hospital's lengths of stay. Prior to PPS, according to the AHA, the average hospital length of stay for Medicare patients was 10.3 days; now it is about 6.5 days. However, no evidence has been found to support the contention that Medicare patients are being discharged "quicker and sicker." Quicker yes, but probably not, at least on average, sicker. While the relationship between length of stay and quality is uncertain, shorter stays do often mean that Medicare patients or their families will have to worry sooner about finding posthospital services when they are needed.

The PPS also has had a profound impact on the provision of outpatient care. Because outpatient care is paid by Medicare Part B, it continued to be reimbursed on a cost basis after PPS was instituted for inpatient care. This reimbursement provided an incentive for hospitals to shift healthcare services from inpatient to outpatient. For example, while the inpatient activity at general acute care hospitals has fallen over the past decade, the number of outpatient visits has about doubled. Furthermore, Medicare spending for outpatient services has been growing three times as fast as spending for inpatient services. In effect, some of the cost savings expected from the PPS were lost because hospitals shifted inpatient services to outpatient services. As we describe in a later section, HCFA has implemented a prospective payment system for outpatient services to create a similar reimbursement system for both inpatient and outpatient care.

The Inpatient Prospective Payment System[5]

Under the PPS, a single payment for each patient covers the cost of routine inpatient care, special care, and ancillary services. The amount of the prospective payment is based on the patient's *diagnosis related group (DRG)* as assigned at discharge. (Originally, the attending physician had to attest, in writing, to the principal diagnosis, secondary diagnosis, and procedures performed. However, the requirement for physician certification was dropped in 1996.) The Medicare DRG payment generally covers all costs except medical education costs and bad debt costs, which we will discuss later along with capital costs.

The starting point in determining the amount of reimbursement is the DRG itself. HCFA has divided potential patient diagnoses into 24 *major diagnostic categories (MDCs)*, which roughly correspond to the major organ systems. Within the 24 MDCs, there are 511 DRGs.[6] To illustrate the nature of DRGs, consider Table 3.1, which contains relevant data for 2000 for ten of the most frequently used DRGs.

The individual DRG *relative weights* represent the average resources consumed in treating that particular diagnosis relative to resources consumed in treating the average diagnosis. Thus, the resources, and hence costs, associated with DRG 209—major joint and limb procedures—are over 2.1 times as much as the resources associated with the average diagnosis, while the resources associated with DRG 140—angina pectoris—are only 58 percent of the average diagnosis. To account for changes in resource consumption, treatment patterns, and technology, the DRG weights are *recalibrated,* or updated, annually.

The Medicare *case mix index* is a useful tool for judging the types of diagnoses that are being treated at a particular hospital. The index represents the average DRG weight for all Medicare patients treated in a specific period. Of course, the average DRG weight for an average hospital is 1.0. To illustrate the concept, consider that the recent case mix index for South Forest Medical

TABLE 3.1
2000 Data for Ten Frequently Used DRGs

DRG Name	DRG Number	MDC Number	Relative Weight	Average Length of Stay
Specific cerebrovascular disorders	14	1	1.1914	6.1 days
Simple pneumonia, age > 17	89	4	1.0855	6.1
Bronchitis and asthma with complications, age > 17	96	4	0.7943	4.8
Heart failure and shock	127	5	1.0144	5.4
Cardiac arrhythmia with complications	138	5	0.8154	4.0
Angina pectoris	140	5	0.5829	2.8
Esophagitis, age > 17	182	1	0.7821	4.3
Major joint and limb proc.	209	8	2.1175	5.2
Nutritional and metabolic disorders with complications, age > 17	296	10	0.8556	5.3
Psychoses	430	19	0.7881	8.4

Source: Federal Register, Volume 64, July 30, 1999.

Classification	Labor Related	Nonlabor Related
Large urban	$2,809	$1,142
Other areas	2,765	1,124

TABLE 3.2 National Average Standardized Amounts for 2000 (Rounded to the Nearest Dollar)

Source: *Federal Register*, Volume 64, July 30, 1999.

Center in Fort Lauderdale was 1.775, while that of Ponce De Leon Memorial Hospital in Arcadia, Florida, was 0.840. South Forest is treating much more complex cases that require greater services and longer lengths of stay than is Ponce De Leon.

HCFA classifies hospitals into one of two locational categories: (1) *large urban;* and (2) *other areas*, where other areas is itself a combination of two formerly separate categories: (1) other urban and (2) rural. Each year, HCFA publishes standardized national *labor-* and *nonlabor-related* costs per discharge for the two locational categories. For example, Table 3.2 contains the national average amounts for 2000. Most hospitals paid under PPS are reimbursed at the national rates; however, some hospitals, such as rural referral centers and hospitals with a disproportionate share of low-income patients, are subject to additional adjustments that effectively increase the reimbursement rates above those shown in Table 3.2.

The PPS rate computation is relatively simple given the standardized labor and nonlabor amounts, the local area wage index, and the DRG relative weight. To illustrate, consider Table 3.3, which displays the Medicare reimbursement computation for DRG 127—heart failure and shock—for a hospital located in Miami, Florida, which is designated a large urban area. The national large urban labor amount, $2,809, is first adjusted by the local *area wage index*, which is published periodically by HCFA and reflects relative labor costs across the United States. This product, $2,874, which is the labor amount adjusted for area wage rates, is then added to the national nonlabor amount. The result is the adjusted hospital rate, $4,016, which is the base rate applied to all diagnoses. Finally, the adjusted hospital rate is multiplied by the DRG relative weight to obtain the reimbursement amount. In our illustration, the DRG relative weight is 1.0144, which produces a DRG payment of $4,074 for a patient discharged from a Miami hospital with a diagnosis of heart failure and shock.

The PPS payment is based on the costs associated with an average patient for each diagnosis. Of course, for any given DRG in any given hospital, some patients will incur costs that are greater than average, while some will be less costly than average. If the patients select hospitals randomly—that is, if all of the sicker patients in a given DRG do not go a particular hospital—and if a large number of patients are treated by the hospital in each DRG, then the

TABLE 3.3
Sample
Medicare DRG
Payment

Hospital location	Large urban
Area wage index for Miami	1.0233
DRG description	127 (Heart failure and shock)
DRG relative weight	1.0144 (From Table 3.1)
Large urban labor amount	$2,809 (From Table 3.2)
Multiplied by area wage index	× 1.0233
Adjusted labor amount	$2,874
Plus nonlabor amount	+1,142 (From Table 3.2)
Adjusted hospital rate	$4,016
Multiplied by DRG relative weight	× 1.0144
Hospital reimbursement for DRG 127	$4,074

high-cost and low-cost patients will offset one another, and the hospital will experience average costs for each DRG.

Reimbursement on an arithmetic mean, or average cost basis, works well if the distribution of patient costs within each DRG is symmetrical, but the distribution is actually skewed to the right—patients with a "mild" case of heart failure and shock may incur a cost of half of the average amount, but patients with a "severe" case may incur a cost of five times the average amount.

To provide some cushion for the high costs associated with severely ill patients within each diagnosis, the PPS includes a provision for *outlier payments*. Outliers are classified into two categories: (1) *length of stay (LOS) outliers* and (2) *cost outliers*. Medicare will make additional payments when a patient's LOS or cost exceeds the established LOS or cost cutoff points.

In addition to the regular PPS payment and outlier payments, hospitals also receive a payment to account for capital costs, which include *depreciation expense*, *interest expense*, and *lease* and *rental expense*. The theory here is that the PPS payment accounts only for operating costs, and hospitals must bear the costs associated with raising the capital used to acquire the assets needed to provide the services. The capital payment rate is about $377 for 2000, and hence hospitals will receive an additional $377 for every Medicare discharge during the year. At one time, Medicare reimbursed for-profit hospitals for equity costs, so investor-owned hospitals received higher capital payments than not-for-profit hospitals, but such payments were discontinued some time ago.

Finally, there are additional payments for hospitals that have a medical education role, as well as payments for Medicare bad-debt losses that occur when patients do not make their copayments. There are several other types of Medicare payments such as payments for hospitals that have a disproportionate share of poor Medicare patients who are typically in ill health and, hence, cost more to treat than average Medicare patients. However, we will leave additional details on PPS reimbursement to other readings.

As we discussed earlier, the transition to a fixed payment system for inpatient care, while continuing to reimburse outpatient services on the basis of costs, created an incentive to increase the amount of outpatient services offered. Although this trend in general is not a bad one, outpatient services offered by hospitals often have higher costs than the same services offered in stand-alone settings. Thus, Medicare's long-run intent was to create a prospective payment system for hospital outpatient services similar to that for inpatient services. The intent was realized on August 1, 2000.

An Overview of the Hospital Outpatient Prospective Payment System (OPPS)

Instead of using DRGs as the basis for payment, hospital outpatient service reimbursement is based on ambulatory payment classifications (APCs). The system consists of about 350 APCs that specify surgical and nonsurgical procedures, visits to clinics and emergency departments, and ancillary services. The payment calculation is very similar to that for DRGs. In essence, each APC has a standard national payment rate (dollar amount) and national Medicare program percentage, which defines the amount paid by Medicare. The difference between the national payment rate and the amount paid by Medicare is the copayment amount. In the payment calculation, the payment is further divided into a labor-related component, which is 60 percent of the national payment rate; and a nonlabor component, which is the remaining 40 percent. The labor component is then adjusted by the specific hospital's PPS inpatient wage index. The end result is a total payment for the APC broken down into the amount paid by Medicare and the amount paid by the patient.

The actual calculation is not complex, but there are considerable complications within the OPPS that must account for many complexities such as multiple procedures conducted on a single patient, which is a common occurrence in outpatient settings. The system will undoubtedly be modified as problems are encountered during implementation. Still, the movement by Medicare to prospective payment for hospital outpatient services is here to stay.

The Balanced Budget Act of 1997 (BBA) mandated that both skilled nursing facility (SNF) care and home health care provided to Medicare patients be reimbursed on a prospective payment basis. While the prospective payment methods were being developed, Medicare payments to these providers were made under an interim system, which resulted in reimbursement amounts that were significantly less than under the old systems. Because, as we discuss later, state Medicaid plans often use the same methodologies as Medicare, the new systems have had a very detrimental effect on the profitability of both long-term care facilities and home health businesses. Many for-profit providers in these industries lost huge amounts of market capitalization when their stock prices plummeted. Even worse, many providers, both for-profit and not-for-profit, were forced into bankruptcy and closure. Of course, the industry trade

Medicare Re-imbursement for Nursing Homes and Home Health Care

organizations are lobbying hard for increased reimbursement rates, but there is no doubt that a lot of damage has been done.

Part B Reim-
bursement

Through 1991, Part B reimbursement to physicians and medical equipment suppliers was based on the concept of *reasonable charges*. In essence, Medicare defined a reasonable charge as the lowest of (1) the actual charge for the service performed, (2) the physician's customary charge, or (3) the prevailing charge for that service in the community. Medicare then paid providers 80 percent of the reasonable charge after the Medicare patient had satisfied his or her deductible amount. The patient was responsible for the 20 percent copayment.

However, Medicare changed its physician payment system beginning in 1992 to a *resource based relative value system (RBRVS)*. Under RBRVS, reimbursement is based on three resource components: (1) physician work, (2) practice expenses, and (3) malpractice insurance. Each of about 7,500 common procedure codes (HCPCs) have assigned relative value units for the three resource components, which are summed to get the total number of units per code. The total units for each code are multiplied by a conversion factor that equals the dollar value of one unit, then adjusted by cost indexes that reflect geographical differences in costs, to get the dollar reimbursement amount. The 2000 conversion factor—the dollar amount by which a service's "relative value" is multiplied to determine the fee—is $36.6137.

When the RBRVS payment system was first put into place, it appeared to have had two primary goals: (1) controlling Medicare costs for physician services and (2) closing the spread between specialist and primary care compensation by cutting Medicare payments for surgical and diagnostic procedures and increasing payments for office visits. The results, since 1992, indicate that the switch to the RBRVS has been more successful in controlling overall costs than in increasing the relative incomes of primary care physicians. Still, the gap has closed somewhat, and it appears that the increased financial incentive for primary care physicians is causing an increasing proportion of medical school graduates to choose primary care as a career.

Peer Review
Organizations

An integral part of the Medicare reimbursement system is the *Peer Review Organization (PRO)*. PROs are independent organizations contracted by HCFA at the state level to monitor the care, and the resulting reimbursement, provided by hospitals and other providers that treat Medicare patients. For example, the PRO for New York, IPRO, is a not-for-profit corporation that does Medicare review for HCFA as well as for New York and several other states.

Basically, PROs review hospital admissions patterns, lengths of stay, transfers, outlier cases, and quality of services. If a PRO determines that a hospital has misrepresented admission, discharge, or billing data, payment for the services related to that discharge may be denied. Patterns of behavior designed to circumvent PPS payment procedures could result in termination of the provider agreement. As with most oversight of this nature, a process is available by which hospitals and other Medicare providers can appeal PRO rulings.

The *Medicare Payment Advisory Commission (MedPAC)* is an independent organization that advises Congress on issues that affect Medicare. MedPAC was established by federal law in 1997 by the merger of two formerly separate commissions—(1) the Prospective Payment Assessment Commission (ProPAC) and the (2) Physician Payment Review Commission (PPRC). MedPAC has 17 members with a wide range of expertise in the financing and delivery of health services. The primary work of the Commission is to prepare two reports annually—(1) one that focuses on payment policies, including specific reimbursement amounts, and (2) one that addresses other issues. Because MedPAC is the principal "independent" advisor to Congress on Medicare payment issues, its influence over the program is significant.

*Medicare
Payment
Advisory
Commission
(MedPAC)*

Medicaid

Medicaid was begun in 1966 as a modest program to be jointly funded and run by the states and the federal government to provide a medical safety net for low income mothers and children, and for elderly, blind, and disabled individuals who receive benefits from the Supplemental Security Income program. Congress mandated that Medicaid cover hospital and physician care, but states were encouraged to expand on the basic package of benefits by either increasing the range of benefits or extending the program to the near poor through optional eligibility. A mandatory nursing home benefit was added in 1972.

States with large tax bases were quick to expand coverage to many of the optional groups, while states with limited abilities to raise funds for Medicaid were forced to construct limited programs. In 2000, total Medicaid expenditures were nearly $200 billion, with over $300 billion in expenditures forecasted as early as 2006. Of these total expenditures, the federal government picks up about 55 percent of the tab and the states pay for the remainder.

Because Medicaid is administered by the states, each state establishes its own reimbursement system for providers. Although historically Medicaid has reimbursed providers on a cost basis, more and more states are moving to per diem and fixed fee prospective rates similar to those instituted by Medicare. As Medicaid expenditures continue to rise at alarming rates, policymakers are struggling to find cost-effective ways to improve the program's access, quality, and reimbursement systems.

Hospitals recently have been very vocal in their claims that Medicaid reimbursement does not cover the costs of service, and some have even sued their state governments for increased payments on the grounds that Medicaid laws call for "fair market" rate reimbursement. Physicians historically have also fared badly under Medicaid because states have tried to cut Medicaid costs by freezing physicians' fees. Citing excess paperwork, high risks, and low fees, many physicians, particularly obstetricians and pediatricians, have either quit taking Medicaid patients or are limiting the numbers served.

Self-Test Questions

1. Briefly, describe the origins and purpose of Medicare.
2. What is the prospective payment system, and how does it work?
3. What is the outpatient prospective payment system, and how does it work?
4. How are physicians reimbursed for providing services to Medicare patients?
5. What are Peer Review Organizations?
6. What does MedPAC stand for, and what is its purpose?
7. What is Medicaid, and how is it administered?

Managed Care Plan Reimbursement Methods

Managed care plans use all of the reimbursement techniques used by third-party payers described in this chapter plus capitation. In addition, managed care plans often create financial incentives in their reimbursement systems that encourage minimizing the amount of services provided.[7] Because of the complexities of such reimbursement, and the fact that it completely changes provider incentives, we devote an entire chapter to the topic (see Chapter 19).

Self-Test Question

1. What reimbursement methodology is unique to managed care plans?

Other Issues

Two other issues that relate to reimbursement and the third-party-payer system merit discussion: (1) cost shifting and (2) case-mix management.

Cost Shifting

Providers of most services, from auto repair shops to fast-food restaurants to window repair businesses, charge all customers the same rate for similar services. Furthermore, the rates charged are set by supply and demand conditions in a competitive marketplace. However, in the provision of healthcare services, there is typically a wide range of reimbursement amounts for a single treatment protocol. For example, assume a hospital treats six different patients for heart failure and shock (DRG 127) in a single week. Table 3.4 contains a hypothetical reimbursement pattern for those six patients.

Reimbursement for this single DRG ranges from a high of $6,575 for private-pay, or self-pay, patients to a low of $0 for indigent patients. Assuming one patient from each payer (an even payer mix), the hospital is reimbursed $4,331, on average, which is only 3.1 percent above the $4,200 average cost of treatment. Thus, a hospital with this payer mix is barely breaking even on this DRG. Now, assume that this hospital's payer mix changes so that it now

Payer	Reimbursement Method	Reimbursement Amount
Private pay	Billed charges	$ 6,575
Commercial insurance	Billed charges less 10%	5,920
HMO/PPO	Billed charges less 20%	5,260
Medicare	Prospective payment	4,451[a]
Medicaid	Cost less 10%	3,780[b]
Indigent patient	No payment	0
Total reimbursement		$26,212
Average reimbursement		$ 4,331

TABLE 3.4
Typical Reimbursement Pattern

[a]Includes capital-related costs. See Table 3.3 and related discussion.
[b]Assumes $4,200 cost of treatment.

has one more Medicare patient and it loses its commercial insurance patient: its average reimbursement for this DRG now is only $3,977, which is $223 below costs.

Clearly, the hospital cannot allow this situation to persist, so it engages in *cost shifting*—that is, it increases its billed charges applicable to this DRG so that private-pay, commercially insured, and HMO/PPO patients pay even more than is indicated in Table 3.4. Thus, costs associated with patients whose reimbursement does not cover those costs are shifted to other payers who, at least temporarily, are willing to absorb, or pass on, the higher billings.

Cost shifting has been the remedy that many healthcare providers have used to maintain profitability in the face of higher indigent care loads and less-generous government reimbursement amounts. However, as the burden of cost shifting falls more and more heavily on just a few classes of payers, it has become more and more difficult to continue the practice. As private-pay rates increase and insurance rates increase for group health insurance, especially for medium and small businesses, these parties are finding it very difficult, if not impossible, to carry the burden of payers that are paying less than costs. Indeed, cost shifting has contributed to the movement to managed care plans, which in turn have adopted reimbursement methodologies, such as discounted fee-for-service and capitation, that make further cost shifting difficult, if not impossible.

Case-Mix Management

In addition to cost shifting, which is not sustainable in the long run, providers have been using *case-mix management* to try to control costs and enhance profitability. Case-mix management can be exercised at two levels. First, at the lowest level, it is used to lower the costs associated with a particular diagnosis by changing the mix of procedures applied to the diagnosis.[8] The provider— say, a hospital—examines the costs associated with treating a large number of patients with the same diagnosis. Typically, these costs will vary substantially on the basis of severity of illness and the particular treatments prescribed by attending physicians.

Although a complicated and challenging job, it is possible in many situations to identify lower-cost treatment protocols that result in outcomes that are just as good as those from higher-cost protocols. When these are identified, hospital managers and physicians can work together to adopt the lower-cost treatment patterns. Although this might lower revenues from third-party payers that continue to reimburse on a cost basis, more and more payers are moving to prospective payment or capitation, so lower costs translate directly into higher profits.

The second type of case-mix management involves changing the provider's overall patient mix by lowering the number of patients with diagnoses that typically result in losses and increasing the number with diagnoses that are highly profitable. For example, many services associated with heart disease have been, and continue to be, highly profitable. Thus, many hospitals have been very aggressive in their advertising campaigns to promote themselves as "your cardiac care center" or "leaders in the fight against heart disease." Conversely, hospitals are not promoting, and even attempt to discontinue, those services that are money losers. By doing so, hospitals are attempting to increase the percentage of high-profit treatments and decrease the percentage of treatments that result in losses.

Self-Test Questions

1. What is cost shifting?
2. Will providers be able to continue to cost shift in the future?
3. What is case-mix management?

Key Concepts

This chapter presented information on the insurance function, the third-party-payer system, and the reimbursement methodologies used by payers. Here are its key concepts:

- Health insurance is widely used in the United States because individuals are *risk averse* and insurance firms can take advantage of the *law of large numbers*.
- Insurance is based on four key characteristics: (1) *pooling of losses*, (2) *payment for random losses*, (3) *risk transfer*, and (4) *indemnification*.
- *Adverse selection* occurs when those individuals most likely to have claims purchase insurance, while those least likely to have claims do not.
- *Moral hazard* occurs when an insured individual purposely sustains a loss, as opposed to a random loss. In a health insurance setting, moral hazard is more subtle, producing such behaviors as seeking more services than needed and engaging in unhealthful behavior because the costs of the potential consequences are borne by the insurer.

- When payers pay *billed charges*, they pay according to the schedule of charge rates established by the provider.
- *Negotiated charges*, which are *discounted* from billed charges, are often used by insurers in conjunction with managed care plans such as HMOs and PPOs.
- Under a *retrospective cost* system, the payer agrees to pay the provider certain allowable costs that are incurred in providing services to the payer's enrollees.
- In a *prospective payment system*, the rates paid by payers are determined in advance and are not tied directly to either reimbursable costs or billed charges. Typically, prospective payments are made on the basis of the following service definitions: (1) *per procedure*, (2) *per diagnosis*, (3) *per diem* (per day), or (4) *global pricing.*
- The major private insurers are *Blue Cross and Blue Shield, commercial insurers,* and *self-insurers.*
- The government is a major insurer and direct provider of healthcare services. The two major forms of government health insurance are *Medicare* and *Medicaid.*
- In 1983, the federal government adopted the *prospective payment system (PPS)* for Medicare hospital inpatient reimbursement. Under PPS, the amount of the payment is fixed by the patient's *diagnosis-related group (DRG).*
- To provide some cushion for the high costs associated with severely ill patients within each diagnosis, the PPS includes a provision for *outlier payments.*
- In addition, hospitals receive a *fixed amount* for each Medicare discharge to cover *capital-related costs,* such as depreciation, interest charges, and lease payments, that are directly related to inpatient care.
- In 2000, Medicare reimbursement for hospital-based outpatient care was changed from a cost-based system to the *outpatient prospective payment system (OPPS).* The payment calculation is similar in nature to that for inpatients. Also, Medicare recently created prospective payment systems for both nursing home and home health care services that are much less generous than the previous cost-based systems.
- Physicians are reimbursed by Medicare using the *resource based relative value system (RBRVS).* Under RBRVS, reimbursement is based on three resource components: (1) *physician work,* (2) *practice expenses,* and (3) *malpractice insurance.* Each of these components is given a weighting for each of some 7,500 procedures. The weightings are summed and multiplied by a dollar conversion factor to determine the payment amount.
- *Peer Review Organizations (PROs)* are independent organizations contracted by HCFA at the state level to monitor the care, and the resulting reimbursement, provided by hospitals and other healthcare providers that treat Medicare patients.

- The *Medicare Payment Advisory Commission (MedPAC)* is an independent body that advises Congress on Medicare matters, including specific reimbursement amounts.
- *Cost shifting* results when a provider increases its billed charges to one set of payers to compensate for insufficient reimbursement from another set of payers.
- Providers employ *case-mix management* to try to control costs and enhance profitability. First, case-mix management is used to lower the costs associated with a particular diagnosis by changing the mix of procedures applied to the diagnosis. Second, case-mix management involves changing the diagnosis mix by lowering the number of patients with diagnoses that typically result in losses and increasing the number with diagnoses that are highly profitable.

The information in this chapter plays a vital role in financial decision making within heath services organizations. Thus, it will be used over and over in future chapters.

Selected References

Abbey, Duane C., and L. Lamar Blount. 1996. "Understanding the Financial Implications of APGs." *Healthcare Financial Management* (October): 51–55.

Coddington, Dean C., David J. Keene, Keith D. Moore, and Richard L. Clarke. 1991. "Factors Driving Costs Must Figure into Reform." *Healthcare Financial Management* (July): 44–62.

Duncan, Donn G., and Cheryl S. Servais. 1996. "Preparing for the New Outpatient Reimbursement System." *Healthcare Financial Management* (February): 42–49.

Duncan, Donn G. 1999. "Preparing for Medicare's APC System." *Healthcare Financial Management* (July): 40–45.

Forgione, Dana A., and Cynthia M. D'Annunzio. 1999. "The Use of DRGs in Health Care Payment Systems Around the World." *Journal of Health Care Finance* (Winter): 66–78.

Grimaldi, Paul L. 1998. "Medicare's New Capitation Method." *Journal of Health Care Finance* (Summer): 7–21.

———. 1993. "Capital Update Factor: A New Era Approaches." *Healthcare Financial Management* (February): 32–37.

———. 1992. "Changes in Medicare Capital PPS Rates and Rules." *Healthcare Financial Management* (December): 40–47.

Guterman, Stuart, Paul W. Eggers, Gerald Riley, Timothy F. Greene, and Sherry A. Terrell. 1988. "The First 3 Years of Medicare Prospective Payment: An Overview." *Health Care Financing Review* (Spring): 67–77.

Harris-Shapiro, Jon and Marcia S. Greenstein. 1999. "RBRVS—1999 Update." *Journal of Health Care Finance* (Winter): 48–52.

Herr, Wendy W. 1991. "Taking A Deep Breath Over Medicare Capital Payments." *Healthcare Financial Management* (April): 19–32.

Hottinger, Margaret, Cynthia L. Polich, and Marcie Parker. 1991. "At Risk: A Look at Managing Medicare Losses." *Healthcare Financial Management* (May): 23–32.

Hughes, Kathleen E. 1993. "Medicare Physician Payment Reform: A View from the Field." *Healthcare Financial Management* (November): 48–54.

Lamm, Richard D. 1990. "High-Tech Health Care and Society's Ability to Pay." *Healthcare Financial Management* (September): 20–30.

Leary, Renee and Dean E. Farley. 2000. "APCs: Reimbursement Implications." *Healthcare Financial Management* (January): 38–44.

Medicare Prospective Price Setting. 1988. Westchester, IL: Healthcare Financial Management Association.

Micheletti, Julie A., Thomas J. Shlala, and Charles E. Greenfield. 1993. "Optimizing Medicare Reimbursement in Skilled Nursing Facilities." *Healthcare Financial Management* (February): 38–42.

Ryan, J. Bruce and Scott B. Clay. 1995. "Understanding the Law of Large Numbers." *Healthcare Financial Management* (October): 22–24.

Smith, Dean G. 1992. "Provider Involvement in Managed Care Underwriting." *Topics in Health Care Financing* (Winter): 33–39

Selected Web Sites

There are a multitude of web sites that pertain to this chapter.

For an extensive source of information on the Medicare program, including information for both patients and providers, see the Health Care Financing Administration (HCFA) web site at *www.hcfa.gov*.

The Blue Cross and Blue Shield national organization web site contains a great deal of information on their organization and the licensed health plans; see *www.bluecares.com*.

For more information on the resource based relative value system (RBRVS), see *www.rbrvs.com*.

The Health Insurance Association of American (HIAA) provides generic information on health insurance; see *www.hiaa.org*.

For more information on Peer Review Organizations (PROs), see the web site for the New York PRO at *www.ipro.org*.

Finally, to learn more about the Medicare Payment Advisory Commission (MedPAC) as well as see some of the reports that they have prepared for Congress, see *www.medpac.gov*.

Notes

1. For more information on the basics of insurance, see one of the many excellent insurance textbooks. For example, George E. Rejda, *Principles of Risk Management and Insurance* (Glenview, IL: Addison-Wesley, 1997); or Emmett J. Vaughan and Therese M. Vaughan, *Fundamentals of Risk and Insurance* (New York: Wiley, 1999).

2. This section was coauthored by Michael J. McCue of Virginia Commonwealth University.

3. Over 95 percent of hospital claims are processed electronically. Many different electronic formats were being used, but the Health Insurance Portability and Accountability Act of 1996 (HIPAA) requires a single standard format. For example, the format for claims and enrollment data is the American National Standards Institute specification ANSI X12N. HCFA plans to consolidate the processing of Medicare claims at regional processing centers under a new system called the *Medicare Transaction System*. When completed, the system will allow hospitals to file electronic Medicare claims directly to HCFA. Other functions such as audits, customer service, and medical reviews will continue to be performed by the intermediaries.

4. An operating margin of 14 percent means that for each dollar of Medicare revenue, operating costs amounted to 86 cents, so the hospital made a 14-cent operating profit. In most industries, operating margins run less than 10 percent, so most managers would view a 14 percent margin as highly profitable.

5. Our purpose here is not to make you an expert in Medicare's PPS. Indeed, most hospitals, other than the smallest, have one or more specialist on the financial staff whose sole responsibility is to keep track of changes in Medicare reimbursement practices. However, some type of DRG-based prospective payment system is being used by many payers with many different types of providers; so some knowledge of the system is necessary for all healthcare managers.

6. The number of DRGs in Medicare's PPS changes frequently as diagnoses are refined. Originally, there were only 383 DRGs.

7. As this chapter was being written (June 2000), the U.S. Supreme Court ruled that patients cannot sue health maintenance organizations under federal law for improper medical treatment when doctors are given financial bonuses to reduce costs. The ruling was a major victory for the managed care industry which argued that the doctor–patient relationship is governed by state laws, which tend to be more favorable to the concept of managed care.

8. For a more detailed discussion of case-mix management at the treatment level, see Dalton A. Tong and Patricia L. Jones, "Physicians, Financial Managers Join Forces to Control Costs," *Healthcare Financial Management*, January 1990, 21–30.

Basic Financial Management Concepts

4

TIME VALUE ANALYSIS

Learning Objectives

After studying this chapter, readers should be able to:

- Explain why time value analysis is so important to healthcare financial management.
- Find the present and future values for lump sums, annuities, and uneven cash flow streams.
- Explain and apply the opportunity cost principle.
- Measure the return on an investment.
- Create an amortization table.
- Describe and apply stated, periodic, and effective annual interest rates.

Introduction

The financial value of any asset, whether a *financial asset*, such as a stock or a bond, or a *real asset*, such as a piece of diagnostic equipment or an ambulatory surgery center, is based on future cash flows. However, a dollar to be received in the future is worth less than a current dollar because a dollar in hand today can be invested, earn interest, and hence can be worth more than one dollar in the future. Even if no investment opportunities existed, a dollar in hand would still be worth more than a dollar to be received in the future because a dollar today can be used for immediate consumption, whereas a future dollar cannot. Because current dollars are worth more than future dollars, valuation analyses must account for cash flow timing differences.

The process of assigning appropriate values to cash flows that occur at different points in time is called *time value analysis*. However, the application of time value analysis to valuation situations is often called *discounted cash flow analysis* because, as you will see later in this chapter, finding present values is called *discounting*. Time value analysis is an important part of many healthcare financial management decisions because many financial analyses involve the valuation of future cash flows. In fact, of all the financial analysis techniques discussed in this text, none is more important than time value analysis. The concepts presented in this chapter are the cornerstones of financial analysis, so a thorough understanding of these concepts is essential to good financial decision making.

Time Lines

One important tool used in time value analysis is the *time line.* Time lines make it easier to visualize when the cash flows in a particular analysis occur. To illustrate the time line concept, consider the following five-period time line:

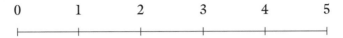

Time 0 is any starting point; Time 1 is one period from the starting point, or the end of Period 1; Time 2 is two periods from the starting point, or the end of Period 2; and so on. Thus, the numbers on top of the tick marks represent ends of periods. Often, the periods are years, but other time intervals such as quarters, months, or days are also used when needed to fit the timing of the cash flows being evaluated. If the time periods are years, the interval from 0 to 1 would be Year 1, and the tick mark labeled 1 would represent both the end of Year 1 and the beginning of Year 2. In many time value analyses, Time 0 (the starting point) is considered to be today, although the term "today" does not have to literally mean today's date.

Cash flows are shown on a time line directly below the tick marks, at the point in time that they are expected to occur. The interest rate that is relevant to the analysis is sometimes shown directly above the time line in the first period. (In rare cases, it may be appropriate to apply more than one interest rate in a time value analysis. In this situation, interest rates may be shown in multiple periods.) Additionally, unknown cash flows—the ones to be determined in the analysis—are sometimes indicated by question marks. To illustrate a completed time line, consider the following example:

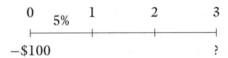

Here, the interest rate for each of the three periods is 5 percent, a *lump sum* (single amount) investment of $100 is made at Time 0, and the Time 3 value is to be determined. The $100 is an *outflow* because it is shown as a negative cash flow. (Outflows are often designated by parentheses rather than by minus signs.) In simple analyses, it is not really necessary to designate cash flows as inflows and outflows because the analyst is well aware of the economics of the situation. However, more complicated analyses require the correct cash flow designation, and many financial calculators require that signs be attached to cash flows in all analyses, even simple ones. Thus, to ensure that students are familiar with sign conventions, we will use them on most of our illustrations.

Time lines are essential when learning time value concepts, but even experienced analysts use time lines when dealing with complex problems. The time line may be an actual line, as used in this chapter, or it may be a series of columns, or rows, on a spreadsheet. Time lines will be used extensively in the remainder of this text, so get into the habit of creating time lines when conducting time value analyses.

Future Value of a Lump Sum (Compounding)

The process of going from today's values, or *present values*, to future values is called *compounding*. Although compounding is not used extensively in healthcare financial management, it is the best starting point for learning time value concepts. To illustrate *lump sum* compounding, which deals with a single-starting cash flow, suppose that the manager of Meridian Clinic deposits $100 of the clinic's excess cash in a bank account that pays 5 percent interest per year. How much would be in the account at the end of one year? At the end of five years? To begin, here are some terms used in the solutions:

- PV = $100 = present value, or beginning amount, of the account.
- I = 5% = interest rate the bank pays on the account per year. The interest amount, which is paid at the end of each year, is based on the balance at the beginning of the year. Expressed as a decimal, I = 0.05.
- INT = dollars of interest earned during each year, which equals the beginning amount multiplied by the interest rate. Thus, INT = PV × I.
- FV_N = future value, or ending amount, of the account at the end of N years. Whereas PV is the value now, or *present value*, FV_N is the value N years into the *future*, after the interest earned has been added to the account.
- N = number of years involved in the analysis.

To start, assume N = 1, so FV_N is calculated as follows:

$$FV_N = FV_1 = PV + INT$$
$$= PV + (PV \times I)$$
$$= PV \times (1 + I).$$

The future value at the end of one year, FV_1, equals the present value multiplied by (1.0 plus the interest rate). This future value relationship can be used to find how much $100 will be worth at the end of one year if it is invested in an account that pays 5 percent interest:

$$FV_1 = PV \times (1 + I) = \$100 \times (1 + 0.05) = \$100 \times 1.05 = \$105.$$

Now, what would be the value after five years? Here is a time line that shows the amount at the end of each year:

	0	1	2	3	4	5
		5%				
Beginning amount	−$100	?	?	?	?	?
Interest earned		$ 5	$ 5.25	$ 5.51	$ 5.79	$ 6.08
End of year amount		105	110.25	115.76	121.55	127.63

Note the following points:

- The account is opened with a deposit of $100. This is shown as an outflow at Year 0.
- Meridian earns $100 × 0.05 = $5 of interest during the first year, so the amount in the account at the end of Year 1 is $100 + $5 = $105.
- At the start of the second year, the account balance is $105. Interest of $105 × 0.05 = $5.25 is earned on the now larger amount, and the account balance at the end of the second year is $105 + $5.25 = $110.25. The Year 2 interest, $5.25, is higher than the first year's interest, $5, because $5 × 0.05 = $0.25 in interest was earned on the first year's interest.
- This process continues, and because the beginning balance is higher in each succeeding year, the interest earned increases in each year.
- The total interest earned, $27.63, is reflected in the final balance at the end of Year 5, $127.63.

To better understand the mathematics of compounding, note that the Year 2 value, $110.25, is equal to:

$$\begin{aligned} FV_2 &= FV_1 \times (1 + I) \\ &= PV \times (1 + I) \times (1 + I) \\ &= PV \times (1 + I)^2 \\ &= \$100 \times (1.05)^2 = \$110.25. \end{aligned}$$

Furthermore, the balance at the end of Year 3 is:

$$\begin{aligned} FV_3 &= FV_2 \times (1 + I) \\ &= PV \times (1 + I)^3 \\ &= \$100 \times (1.05)^3 = \$115.76. \end{aligned}$$

Continuing the calculation out to the end of Year 5 gives:

$$FV_5 = \$100 \times (1.05)^5 = \$127.63.$$

It is clear that a definite pattern exists in these future value calculations. In general, the future value of a lump sum at the end of N years can be found by applying this equation:

$$FV_N = PV \times (1 + I)^N.$$

Future values, as well as most other time value problems, can be solved three ways: (1) by using a regular calculator, (2) by using a financial calculator, and (3) by using a spreadsheet.

Regular calculator solution:
A regular (nonfinancial) calculator can be used, either by multiplying the PV by $(1 + I)$ for N times or by using the exponential function to raise $(1 + I)$ to the Nth power and then multiplying the result by the PV. The easiest way to find the future value of $100 after five years when compounded at 5 percent is to enter $100, then multiply this amount by 1.05 five times. If the calculator is set to display two decimal places, the answer would be $127.63:

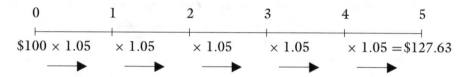

As denoted by the arrows, compounding involves moving to the **right** along the time line.

Financial calculator solution:
Financial calculators are preprogrammed to solve many types of time value problems. In effect, the future value equation is programmed directly into the calculator, so rather than actually perform the calculation, the user merely has to input the requisite starting values. Using a financial calculator, the future value is found using these time value input keys:[1]

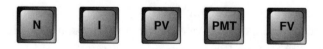

Note that these keys correspond to the five time value variables that are commonly used:

- N = number of periods.
- I = interest rate per period.
- PV = present value.
- PMT = payment (used only when the problem involves a series of equal cash flows).
- FV = future value.

Also, this chapter deals with time value analyses that involve only four of the variables at any one time. Three of the variables will be known, and the calculator will solve for the fourth, unknown variable. In Chapter 8, when bond valuation is discussed, all five variables will be included in the analysis.

To find the future value of $100 after five years when invested at 5 percent interest using a financial calculator, just enter $PV = -100$, $I = 5$, and $N = 5$, then press the FV key. The answer, 127.63 (rounded to two decimal places), will appear:

Inputs   5   5   −100

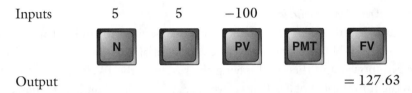

Output   = 127.63

Many financial calculators require that cash flows be designated as either inflows or outflows (entered as either positive or negative values). Let's apply this logic to the illustration: Meridian deposits the initial amount, which is an outflow to the business, and takes out, or receives, the ending amount, which is an inflow to the business. (If the PV was entered as 100, a positive value, the answer on a calculator using sign convention would be displayed as −127.63.)

Note that some calculators require the user to press a *Compute* key before pressing the FV key. Also, financial calculators permit specifying the number of decimal places that are displayed, even though 12, or more, significant digits are actually used in the calculations. Two places are generally used for answers in dollars or percentages, and four places for decimal answers. The final answer, however, should be rounded to reflect the accuracy of the input values; it makes no sense to say that the return on a particular investment is 14.63827 percent when the cash flows are highly uncertain. The nature of the analysis dictates how many decimal places should be displayed.

Spreadsheet solution:
Spreadsheet programs, such as Excel, Lotus 1-2-3, and Quattro Pro, are frequently used in time value analysis. Many common time value solutions are preprogrammed in the spreadsheet software, and users can create their own formulas to perform tasks that have not been preprogrammed. The preprogrammed time value formulas are called *functions,* or in some software, *@functions*—pronounced "at functions." Like any formula, a time value function consists of a number of arithmetic calculations combined into one statement. By using functions, spreadsheet users can save the time and tedium of building formulas from scratch.

Each function begins with a unique name that identifies the calculation to be performed, along with one or more *arguments* (the input values for the calculation) enclosed in parentheses. There is no spreadsheet function for finding the future value of a lump sum because it can be quickly calculated by formula. For example, the Excel formula for solving the Meridian Clinic example over five years is:

$$= 100^*(1.05)^{\wedge}5$$

Here, = tells the spreadsheet that a formula is being entered into the cell; * is the spreadsheet multiplication sign; and ^ is the spreadsheet exponential, or power, sign. When this formula is entered into a spreadsheet cell, the value 127.63 appears in the cell (when formatted to two decimal places).

In constructing spreadsheets, it typically is more useful to enter a formula that can accommodate changing input values than to embed these values into the formula, so it would be better to solve the above future value problem with this formula:

$$= A1^*(1 + B1)^{\wedge}C1$$

where the present value ($100) would be contained in Cell A1, the interest rate (0.05) in Cell B1, and the number of periods (5) in Cell C1. With this formula, future values easily can be calculated with different starting amounts, interest rates, or number of years. Finally, different spreadsheet programs use slightly different syntax in their time value functions. The examples presented in this text use Excel syntax.

The most efficient way to solve most problems involving time value is to use a financial calculator or a spreadsheet.[2] However, the basic mathematics behind the calculations must be understood to set up complex problems before solving them. In addition, the underlying logic must be understood to comprehend stock and bond valuation, lease analysis, capital budgeting analysis, and other important healthcare financial management topics.

To help you better understand time value solution techniques, we will use a more or less constant format in the illustrations presented in this chapter:

- We lay out the situation on a time line and show the equation that must be solved.
- We then present the regular calculator solution, if applicable.
- Next, we show how the equation can be solved with a financial calculator.
- Finally, we present the spreadsheet formula or function.

Graphic View of the Compounding (Growth) Process

Figure 4.1 shows how $1, or any other lump sum, grows over time at various rates of interest. The data used to plot the curves could be obtained by using any of the solution techniques described in the previous section. Note that the greater the rate of interest, the faster the growth rate. Thus, $100 on deposit for ten years at a 5 percent interest rate will grow to $162.89, but the same amount invested at 10 percent interest will grow to $259.37. The interest rate is, in fact, a growth rate: If a lump sum is deposited and earns 5 percent interest, the funds on deposit will grow at a rate of 5 percent per period. Note also that future value concepts are not restricted to bank deposits; they can be

FIGURE 4.1
Relationships
Among Future
Value, Interest
Rates, and
Time

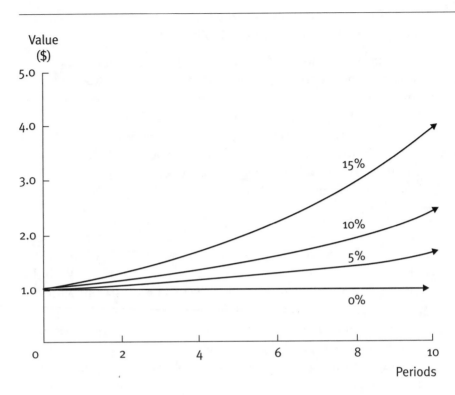

| | Interest Rate Plot Points | | |
Period	5%	10%	15%
1	1.0500	1.1000	1.1500
2	1.1025	1.2100	1.3225
3	1.1576	1.3310	1.5209
4	1.2155	1.4641	1.7490
5	1.2763	1.6105	2.0114
6	1.3401	1.7716	2.3131
7	1.4071	1.9487	2.6600
8	1.4775	2.1436	3.0590
9	1.5513	2.3579	3.5179
10	1.6289	2.5937	4.0456

applied to any growing, or declining, numerical value such as volume—say, clinic visits—population, or earnings per share.

The Power of Compounding

It is very important to understand what is commonly called "the power of compounding." In essence, this means that a relatively small starting value can grow to a large amount over a long period of time, even when the rate of growth (interest rate) is modest. For example, assume that a new parent places $1,000 in a mutual fund to help pay the child's college expenses, which are expected to begin in 18 years. The mutual fund—a balanced fund holding both stocks and bonds—is assumed to earn a return of 10 percent per year, which is a reasonable estimate by historical standards. After 18 years, the value of the mutual fund account would be $5,560, which is not an inconsequential sum.

Now, assume that the money was meant to help fund the child's retirement, which is assumed to occur 65 years into the future. The value of the mutual fund account at that time would be $490,371, or nearly a **half-million dollars**. Imagine that, $1,000 grows to nearly half a million all because of the power of compounding. The moral of this story is clear: When saving for retirement, or for any other purpose, start early.

1. What is compounding? What is interest on interest?
2. What is the basic equation for calculating the future value of a lump sum?
3. What are three solution techniques for solving lump sum compounding problems?
4. What is meant by the power of compounding?

Self-Test Questions

Present Value of a Lump Sum (Discounting)

Suppose that GroupWest Health Plans, which has premium income reserves to invest, has the opportunity to purchase a low-risk security that will pay $127.63 at the end of five years. A local bank is currently offering 5 percent interest on a five-year certificate of deposit (CD), and GroupWest's managers regard the security being offered as being as safe as the bank CD. The 5 percent interest rate available on the bank CD is GroupWest's *opportunity cost rate*. (Opportunity costs are discussed in detail in the next section.) How much would GroupWest be willing to pay for this security?

In the previous section, we learned that an initial amount of $100 invested at 5 percent per year would be worth $127.63 at the end of five years. Thus, GroupWest should be indifferent to the choice between $100 today and $127.63 to be received after five years. Today's $100 is defined as the *present value*, or *PV*, of $127.63 due in five years when the opportunity cost rate is 5 percent. If the price of the security being offered is anything less than $100, GroupWest should buy it. If the price is greater than $100, GroupWest should turn the offer down. If the price is exactly $100, GroupWest could buy it or turn it down because that is the security's "fair value." In general, the present value of a cash flow due N years in the future is the amount that, if it were on hand today, would grow to equal the future amount when compounded at the opportunity cost rate.

Finding present values is called *discounting*, and it is simply the reverse of compounding: If the PV is known, compound to find the FV; if the FV is known, discount to find the PV. Here are the solution techniques used to solve this discounting problem.

Time line:

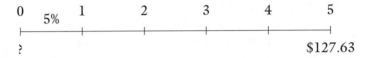

To develop the discounting equation, solve the compounding equation for PV:

$$\text{Compounding:} \quad FV_N = PV \times (1 + I)^N.$$

$$\text{Discounting:} \quad PV = \frac{FV_N}{(1 + I)^N}.$$

Regular calculator solution:
Enter $127.63 and divide it five times by 1.05:

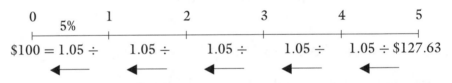

As shown by the arrows, discounting is moving to the **left** along a time line.

Financial calculator solution:

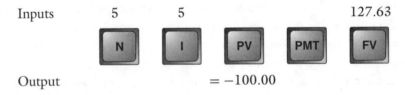

Spreadsheet solution:

Cell formula	$= 127.63/(1.05)\^5$
Cell display	100.00

Graphic View of the Discounting Process

Figure 4.2 shows how the present value of $1, or any other sum, to be received in the future diminishes as the years to receipt increase. Again, the data used to plot the curves can be developed by using any of the solution techniques. The graphs show (1) that the present value decreases and approaches zero as the payment date is extended further into the future, and (2) that the rate of decrease is greater the higher the interest (discount) rate.

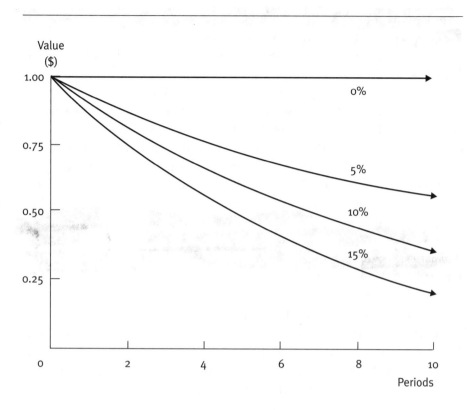

FIGURE 4.2
Relationships Among Present Value, Interest Rates, and Time

| Period | Interest Rate Plot Points | | |
	5%	10%	15%
1	.9524	.9091	.8696
2	.9070	.8254	.7561
3	.8638	.7513	.6575
4	.8227	.6830	.5718
5	.7835	.6209	.4972
6	.7462	.5634	.4323
7	.7107	.5132	.3759
8	.6768	.4665	.3269
9	.6446	.4241	.2843
10	.6139	.3855	.2472

Discounting at Work

At relatively high interest rates, funds due in the future are worth very little today, and even at moderate discount rates, the present value of a sum due in the distant future is quite small. To illustrate discounting at work, consider 100-year bonds. A bond is a type of debt security in which an investor loans some amount of principal, say, $1,000, to a borrower who promises to pay interest over the life of the bond and to return the principal amount at maturity. Typically, the longest maturities for bonds are 30–40 years, but in the early 1990s, several firms, including Columbia/HCA Healthcare (now HCA), issued 100-year bonds.

At first blush, it might appear that anyone who would buy a 100-year bond must be irrational because there is little assurance that the firm will even be around in 100 years to repay the amount borrowed. However, consider the present value of $1,000 to be received in 100 years. If the discount rate is 7.5 percent, which is roughly the interest rate that was set on the bond, the present value is a mere $0.72. Thus, the time value of money erodes the value of the principal repayment to the point that it is worth less than $1 when the bond is purchased. This tells us that the value of the bond stems mostly from the interest stream received in the early years of ownership, and that the payments expected during the later years of the bond contribute little to the bond's initial value.

Self-Test Questions

1. What is discounting? How is it related to compounding?
2. What are the three techniques for solving lump sum discounting problems?
3. What is the basic equation for calculating the present value of a lump sum?
4. How does the present value of an amount to be received in the future change as the time is extended and as the interest rate increases?

Opportunity Costs

In the last section, the *opportunity cost* concept was used to set the discount rate on GroupWest's investment. This concept plays a very important role in time value analysis. To illustrate the concept, suppose an individual found the winning ticket for the Florida lottery and now has $1 million to invest. Should the individual assign a cost to these funds? At first blush, it might appear that this money has zero cost because its acquisition was purely a matter of luck. However, as soon as the lucky individual thinks about what to do with the $1 million, he or she has to think in terms of the opportunity costs involved. By using the funds to invest in one alternative, for example, in the stock of HCA, the individual forgoes the opportunity to make some other investment, for example, buying U.S. Treasury bonds. Thus, there is an opportunity cost associated with any investment planned for the $1 million even though the lottery winnings were "free."

Because one investment decision automatically negates all other possible investments with the same funds, the cash flows expected to be earned from any investment must be discounted at a rate that reflects the return that could be earned on forgone investment opportunities. The problem is that the number of forgone investment opportunities is virtually infinite, so which one should be chosen to establish the opportunity cost rate? The opportunity cost rate to be applied in time value analysis is the rate that could be earned on alternative investments **of similar risk**. It would not be logical to assign a very low opportunity cost rate to a series of very risky cash flows, or vice versa. This concept is one of the cornerstones of financial management, so it is worth repeating. **The opportunity cost rate (i.e., the discount rate) applied to investment cash flows is the rate that could be earned on alternative investments of similar risk.**

Note that the opportunity cost rate does not depend on the source of the funds to be invested. Rather, the primary determinant of this rate is the riskiness of the cash flows being discounted. Thus, the same opportunity cost rate would be applied to a potential investment in HCA stock whether the funds were won in a lottery, taken out of petty cash, or obtained by selling off some land.

Generally, opportunity cost rates are obtained by looking at rates that could be earned, or more precisely, rates that are expected to be earned, on securities such as stocks or bonds. Securities are usually chosen to set opportunity cost rates because their expected returns are more easily estimated than rates of return on real assets such as HMOs, group practices, hospital beds, MRI machines, and the like. Furthermore, as discussed in Chapter 8, securities generally provide the minimum return appropriate for the amount of risk assumed, so securities returns provide a good benchmark for other investments.

To illustrate the opportunity cost concept, assume that Oakdale Community Hospital is considering building a nursing home. The first step in the financial analysis is to forecast the cash flows that the nursing home is expected to produce. These cash flows, then, must be discounted at some opportunity cost rate to determine their present value. Would the hospital's opportunity cost rate be (1) the expected rate of return on Treasury bonds; (2) the expected rate of return on the stock of Beverly Enterprises, which operates about 600 nursing homes and assisted living centers; or (3) the expected rate of return on pork belly futures? (Pork belly futures are investments that involve commodity contracts for delivery at some future time.) The answer is the expected rate of return on Beverly Enterprises' stock because that is the rate of return available to the hospital on alternative investments of similar risk. Treasury securities are low-risk investments, so they would understate the opportunity cost rate in owning a nursing home. Conversely, pork belly futures are very high-risk investments, so that rate of return is probably too high to apply to Oakdale's nursing home investment.[3]

The source of the funds used for the nursing home investment is **not relevant** to the analysis. Oakdale may obtain the needed funds by issuing tax-exempt debt, or by soliciting contributions, or it may have excess cash accumulated from profit retention. The discount rate applied to the nursing home cash flows depends only on the riskiness of those cash flows and the returns available on alternative investments of similar risk, not on the source of the investment funds.

At this point, you may question the ability of real-world analysts to assess the riskiness of a cash flow stream or to choose an opportunity cost rate with any confidence. Fortunately, the process is not as difficult as it may appear here because businesses have benchmarks that can be used as starting points. (Chapter 10 contains a discussion of how baseline opportunity cost rates are established for capital investments, while Chapter 13 presents a detailed discussion on how the riskiness of a cash flow stream can be assessed.)

Self-Test Questions

1. Why does an investment have an opportunity cost rate even when the funds employed have no explicit cost?
2. How are opportunity cost rates established?
3. Does the opportunity cost rate depend on the source of the investment funds?

Solving for Interest Rate and Time

In our examples thus far, four time value analysis variables have been used: PV, FV, I, and N. Specifically, the interest rate, I, and the number of years, N, plus either PV or FV have been initially given. However, if the values of any three of the variables are known, the value of the fourth can be found.

Solving for Interest Rate (I)

Suppose that Family Practice Associates (FPA), a primary care physicians' group practice, can buy a bank certificate of deposit (CD) for $78.35 that will return $100 after five years. In this case PV, FV, and N are known, but I, the interest rate that the bank is paying, is not known. Such problems are solved in this way:

Time line:

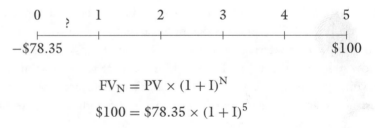

$$FV_N = PV \times (1 + I)^N$$
$$\$100 = \$78.35 \times (1 + I)^5$$

Financial calculator solution:

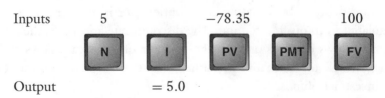

Spreadsheet solution:

Function	$= \text{RATE}(N, 0, PV, FV)$
Cell formula	$= \text{RATE}(5, 0, -78.35, 100)$
Cell display	5%

Here, a spreadsheet function named RATE is used to solve for I. Note that some spreadsheet programs display the answer in decimal form unless the cell is formatted to display in percent.

Solving for Time (N)

Suppose that the bank told FPA that a CD pays 5 percent interest each year, that it costs $78.35, and that at maturity the group would receive $100. How long must the funds be invested in the CD? In this case, PV, FV, and I are known, but N, the number of periods, is not known.

Time line:

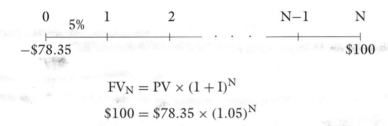

$$FV_N = PV \times (1 + I)^N$$
$$\$100 = \$78.35 \times (1.05)^N$$

Financial calculator solution:

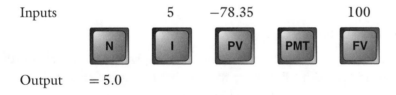

Output	$= 5.0$

Spreadsheet solution:

Function	$= \text{NPER}(I, 0, PV, FV)$
Cell formula	$= \text{NPER}(0.05, 0, -78.35, 100)$
Cell display	5.00

Note that interest rates usually are entered as decimals in function arguments.

The Rule of 72

The *Rule of 72* is a simple and quick method for judging the approximate effect of different interest rates on the growth of a lump sum deposit. It tells us that to find the number of years required to double the value of a lump sum, merely divide the number 72 by the interest rate paid. For example, if the interest rate is 10 percent, it would take $72/10 = 7.2$ years for the money in an account to double in value. The calculator solution is 7.27 years, so the Rule of 72 is relatively accurate, at least when reasonable interest rates are applied.

In a similar manner, the Rule of 72 can be used to determine the interest rate required to double the money in an account in a given number of years. To illustrate the concept, we find that an interest rate of $72/5 = 14.4\%$ is required to double the value of an account in five years. The calculator solution here is 14.9 percent, so the Rule of 72 again gives a reasonable approximation of the correct answer.

Self-Test Questions

1. What are some real-world situations that may require you to solve for interest rate or time?
2. What is the Rule of 72 and how is it used?

Annuities

Whereas lump sums are single cash flows, an *annuity* is a series of **equal** cash flows at **fixed intervals** for a specified number of periods. Annuity cash flows, which often are called *payments* and given the symbol *PMT*, can occur at the beginning or end of each period. If the payments occur at the end of each period as they typically do, the annuity is an *ordinary*, or *deferred*, or *regular annuity*. If payments are made at the beginning of each period, the annuity is an *annuity due*. Because ordinary annuities are by far the most common, the term *annuity* without further description usually means an ordinary annuity.

Ordinary Annuities

A series of equal payments at the end of each period constitute an ordinary annuity. If Meridian Clinic were to deposit $100 at the end of each year for three years in an account that paid 5 percent interest per year, how much would Meridian accumulate at the end of three years? The answer to this question is the future value of the annuity.

Time line:

0		1	2	3
	5%			
		−$100	−$100	−$100
				?

The future value of any annuity occurs at the end of the last period. Thus, for regular annuities, the future value coincides with the final payment.

Regular calculator solution:
One approach is to treat each individual cash flow as a lump sum, compound it to Year 3, then sum the future values:

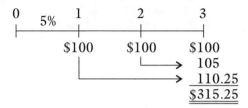

Financial calculator solution:

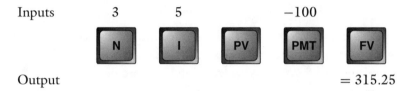

Inputs	3	5		−100	
	N	I	PV	PMT	FV

Output   = 315.25

In annuity problems, the PMT key is used in conjunction with either the PV or FV key.

Spreadsheet solution:

Function   = FV(I, N, PMT)

Cell formula   = FV(0.05, 3, −100)

Cell display $315.25

Suppose that Meridian Clinic was offered the following alternatives: (a) a three-year annuity with payments of $100 at the end of each year or (b) a lump sum payment today. Meridian has no need for the money during the next three years. If it accepts the annuity, it would deposit the payments in an account that pays 5 percent interest per year. Similarly, the lump sum payment would be deposited into the same account. How large must the lump sum payment be today to make it equivalent to the annuity? In other words, what is the present value of the annuity?

Regular calculator solution:

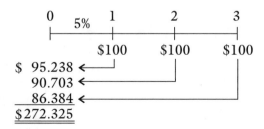

Financial calculator solution:

Inputs   3   5   −100

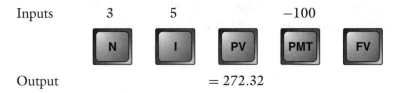

Output   = 272.32

Spreadsheet solution:

Function   = PV(I, N, PMT)

Cell formula   = PV(0.05, 3, −100)

Cell display $272.32

One especially important application of the annuity concept relates to loans with constant payments such as mortgages, auto loans, and many bank loans to businesses. Such loans are examined in more depth in a later section on amortization.

Annuities Due

If the three $100 payments in the previous example had been made at the beginning of each year, the annuity would have been an *annuity due*. When compared to an ordinary annuity, each payment is shifted to the left one year. Because the payments come in faster, an annuity due is more valuable than an ordinary annuity.

The future value of our example, assuming an annuity due, is found as follows:

Time line:

```
0        1        2        3
    5%
+--------+--------+--------+
-$100   -$100   -$100      ?
```

Note that the future value of an annuity due occurs one period after the final payment, while the future value of an ordinary annuity coincides with the final payment.

Regular calculator solution:

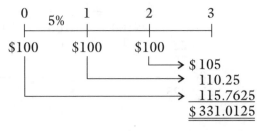

In the case of an annuity due, as compared with an ordinary annuity, all the cash flows are compounded for one additional period, and hence the future value of an annuity due is greater than the future value of a similar ordinary annuity by $(1 + I)$. Thus, the future value of an annuity due also can be found as follows:

$$FV \text{ (Annuity due)} = FV \text{ of a regular annuity} \times (1 + I)$$

$$= \$315.25 \times 1.05 = \$331.01.$$

Financial calculator solution:
Most financial calculators have a switch or key marked DUE or BEGIN that permits the switching of the mode from end-of-period payments (ordinary annuity) to beginning-of-period payments (annuity due). When the beginning-of-period mode is activated, the display will normally indicate the changed mode with the word BEGIN or another symbol. To deal with annuities due, change the mode to beginning of period and proceed as before. Because most problems will deal with end-of-period cash flows, do not forget to switch the calculator back to the END mode.

Spreadsheet solution:

Function	$= FV(I, N, PMT) * (1 + I)$
Cell formula	$= FV(0.05, 3, -100) * (1.05)$
Cell display	$331.01

The present value of an annuity due is found in a similar manner.

Time line:

```
    0       1        2        3
        5%
    |-------|--------|--------|
  -$100   -$100    -$100
    ?
```

Regular calculator solution:

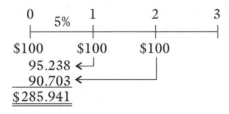

The present value of an annuity due can be thought of as the present value of an ordinary annuity that is compounded for one period, so it also can be found as follows:

$$PV(\text{Annuity due}) = PV \text{ of a regular annuity} \times (1 + I)$$
$$= \$272.32 \times 1.05 = \$285.94.$$

Financial calculator solution:
Activate the beginning of period mode (i.e., the BEGIN mode), then proceed as before. Again, because most problems will deal with end-of-period cash flows, do not forget to switch the calculator back to the END mode.

Spreadsheet solution:

Function	$= PV(I, N, PMT) * (1 + I)$
Cell formula	$= PV(0.05, 3, -100) * (1.05)$
Cell display	$285.94

Self-Test Questions

1. What is an annuity?
2. What is the difference between an ordinary annuity and an annuity due?
3. Which annuity has the greater future value: an ordinary annuity or an annuity due? Why?
4. Which annuity has the greater present value: an ordinary annuity or an annuity due? Why?

Perpetuities

Most annuities call for payments to be made over some finite period of time; for example, $100 per year for three years. However, some annuities go on indefinitely, or perpetually. Such annuities are called *perpetuities*. The present value of a perpetuity is found as follows:

$$PV \text{ (Perpetuity)} = \frac{\text{Payment}}{\text{Interest rate}} = \frac{PMT}{I}.$$

Perpetuities can be illustrated by some securities issued by General Healthcare, Inc. Each security promises to pay $100 annually in perpetuity (forever). What would each security be worth if the opportunity cost rate, or discount rate, was 10 percent? The answer is $1,000:

$$PV \text{ (Perpetuity)} = \frac{\$100}{0.10} = \$1,000.$$

Suppose interest rates, and hence the opportunity cost rate, rose to 15 percent. What would happen to the security's value? The interest rate increase would lower its value to $666.67:

$$PV \text{ (Perpetuity)} = \frac{\$100}{0.15} = \$666.67.$$

Assume that interest rates fell to 5 percent. The rate decrease would increase the perpetuity's value to $2,000:

$$PV \text{ (Perpetuity)} = \frac{\$100}{0.05} = \$2,000.$$

The value of a perpetuity changes dramatically when interest rates change. All securities' values are affected by interest rate changes, but some, like perpetuities, are more sensitive to interest rate changes than others, such as short-term government bonds. The risks associated with interest rate changes are discussed in more detail in Chapter 8.

1. What is a perpetuity?
2. What happens to the value of a perpetuity when interest rates increase or decrease?

Self-Test Questions

Uneven Cash Flow Streams

The definition of an annuity includes the words "constant amount," so annuities involve cash flows that are the same in every period. Although some financial decisions, such as bond valuation, do involve constant cash flows, most important healthcare financial analyses involve uneven, or nonconstant, cash flows. For example, the financial evaluation of a proposed outpatient clinic or MRI facility rarely involves constant cash flows.

In general, the term *payment (PMT)* is reserved for annuity situations, in which the dollar amounts are constant, and the term *cash flow (CF)* denotes either lump sums or uneven cash flows. Financial calculators are set up to follow this convention. When dealing with uneven cash flows, CF functions, rather than the PMT key, are used.

Present Value

The present value of an uneven cash flow stream is found as the sum of the present values of the individual cash flows of the stream. For example, suppose that Wilson Memorial Hospital is considering the purchase of a new x-ray machine. The hospital's managers forecast that the operation of the new machine would produce the following stream of cash inflows (in thousands of dollars):

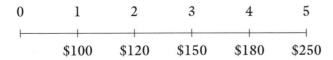

0	1	2	3	4	5
	$100	$120	$150	$180	$250

What is the present value of the new x-ray machine investment if the appropriate discount rate (i.e., the opportunity cost rate) is 10 percent?

Regular calculator solution:
The PV of each individual cash flow can be found using a regular calculator, then these values are summed to find the present value of the stream, $580,950:

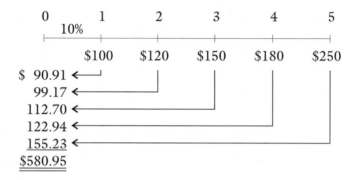

Financial calculator solution:
The present value of an uneven cash flow stream can be solved with most financial calculators by using the following steps:

- Input the individual cash flows, in chronological order, into the *cash flow registers*, usually designated as CF_0 and CF_j (CF_1, CF_2, CF_3, and so on) or just CF_j (CF_0, CF_1, CF_2, CF_3, and so on).
- Enter the discount rate.
- Push the *NPV* key.

For this problem, enter 0, 100, 120, 150, 180, and 250 in that order into the calculator's cash flow registers; enter $I = 10$; then push *NPV* to obtain the answer, 580.95. Note that an implied cash flow of zero is entered for CF_0.

Three points should be noted about the calculator solution. First, when dealing with the cash flow registers, the term *NPV*, rather than *PV*, is used to represent present value. The letter *N* in *NPV* stands for the word *net*, so *NPV* is the abbreviation for net present value. Net present value means the sum or net of the present values of a cash flow stream. In general, the stream will consist of both inflows and outflows, but the stream here contains all inflows.

Second, annuity cash flows within any uneven cash flow stream can be entered into the cash flow registers most efficiently on most calculators by using the N_j key. This key allows the user to specify the number of times a constant payment occurs within the stream. (Some calculators prompt the user to enter the number of times each cash flow occurs.)

Finally, amounts entered into the cash flow registers remain in those registers until they are cleared. Thus, if a problem had been previously worked with eight cash flows, and a new problem is worked with only four cash flows, the calculator assumes that the final four cash flows from the first calculation belonged to the second calculation. Be sure to clear the cash flow registers before starting a new problem.

Spreadsheet solution:
The NPV function calculates the present value of a stream, called a spreadsheet *range*, of cash flows. First, the cash flow values must be entered into consecutive cells in the spreadsheet. For example:

$$\text{Cell Address:} \quad \text{A10} \quad \text{B10} \quad \text{C10} \quad \text{D10} \quad \text{E10}$$
$$\text{Value:} \qquad\qquad 100 \quad\; 120 \quad\; 150 \quad\; 180 \quad\; 250$$

The NPV function then is placed in an empty cell, for example, A5:

Function	= NPV(I, range)
Cell formula	= NPV(0.10, A10:E10)
Cell display	$580.95

The NPV function assumes that cash flows occur at the **end** of each period, so NPV is calculated as of the **beginning** of the period of the first cash flow specified in the range, which is one period before the cash flow occurs. Because the cash flow specified as the first flow in the range is a Year 1 value, the calculated NPV occurs at the beginning of Year 1, or the end of Year 0, which is correct for this illustration. However, if a Year 0 cash flow is included in the range, the NPV would be calculated at the beginning of Year 0, or the end of Year −1, which typically is incorrect. This problem will be addressed in the next major section.

Future Value

The future value of an uneven cash flow stream is found by compounding each payment to the end of the stream and then summing the future values.

Regular calculator solution:
The future value of each individual cash flow can be found, using a regular calculator, by summing these values to find the future value of the stream, $935,630:

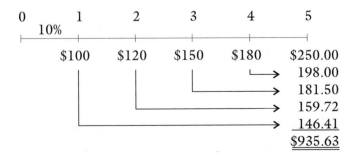

Financial calculator solution:
Some financial calculators have a net future value key (NFV) that, after the cash flows have been entered into the cash flow registers, can be used to obtain the future value of an uneven cash flow stream. However, there is generally more interest in the present value of a cash flow stream than in its future value because the present value represents the value of the investment today, which then can be compared to the cost of the investment, be it a stock, bond, x-ray machine, or new clinic.

Spreadsheet solution:
Most spreadsheet programs do not have a function that computes the future value of an uneven cash flow stream. However, future values can be found by building a formula in a cell that replicates the regular calculator solution.

Self-Test Questions

1. Give two examples of financial decisions that typically involve uneven cash flows.
2. Describe how present values of uneven cash flow streams are calculated using a regular calculator. Using a financial calculator. Using a spreadsheet.
3. What is meant by *net present value?*

Using Time Value Analysis to Measure Financial Returns

In most investments, an individual or business spends cash today with the expectation of receiving cash in the future. The financial attractiveness of such investments is measured by *financial return*, or just *return*. There are two basic ways of expressing financial return: (1) in dollar terms and (2) in percentage terms.

To illustrate the concept, let's reexamine the cash flows expected to be received if Wilson Memorial Hospital buys its new x-ray machine (shown on the time line in thousands of dollars). In the last section, we determined that the present value of these flows, when discounted at a 10 percent rate, is $580,950:

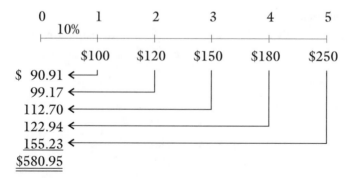

Dollar Return

The $580,950 calculated above represents the present value (in financial terms) of the cash flows that the x-ray machine is **expected** to provide to

Wilson Memorial Hospital. Note that these cash flows are not known with certainty, but rather represent the best estimates of the hospital's managers.

To measure the *dollar return* on the investment, the cost of the x-ray machine must be compared to the present value of the expected benefits (the cash inflows). If the machine is expected to cost $500,000, and the present value of the inflows is $580,950, then the expected dollar return on the machine is $580,950 − $500,000 = $80,950. Note that this measure of dollar return incorporates time value through the discounting process. Also, the opportunity cost inherent in the use of the $500,000 is accounted for because the 10 percent discount rate reflects the return that could be earned on alternative investments of similar risk. Thus, the x-ray machine is expected to produce a $80,950 return above that required for its riskiness as accounted for by the 10 percent opportunity cost rate.

The dollar return process can be combined into a single calculation by adding the cost of the x-ray machine to the time line:

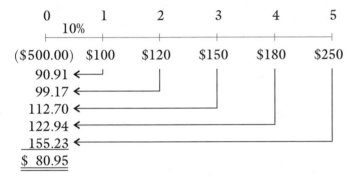

Financial calculator solution:
Now, with the investment outlay (cost) added to the time line, the following cash flows would be entered in the cash flow registers: −500, 100, 120, 150, 180, and 250 in that order. Then, enter I = 10 and push *NPV* to obtain the answer, 80.95.

Spreadsheet solution:
As in the financial calculator solution, the cost of the machine must be added to cash flow data. Here, it is added to the spreadsheet range:

Cell Address:	A10	B10	C10	D10	E10	F10
Value:	−500	100	120	150	180	250

The NPV function then is placed in an empty cell, for example, A5:

Function	= NPV (I, range)
Cell formula	= NPV (0.10, A10:F10)
Cell display	$73.59

Oops! We have a problem. As discussed earlier, the NPV function assumes that cash flows occur at the **end** of each period. Thus, NPV is calculated as of the **beginning** of the period of the first cash flow specified in the range, so the NPV incorrectly occurs at the beginning of Year 0, or the end of Year −1. One solution to the problem is to compound the calculated NPV one period at 10 percent. The effect is to move the NPV one year to the right along the time line. The spreadsheet cell would look like this:

Function	$= NPV(I, \text{range including } CF_0) * (1 + I)$
Cell formula	$= NPV(0.10, A10{:}F10) * 1.10$
Cell display	$80.95

A second solution is to change the range in the argument to force the first payment in the range to occur at Year 1, so the present value will be calculated at Year 0. However, because there is a Year 0 cash flow that must be included in the calculation, the Year 0 cash flow must be added to the spreadsheet-calculated NPV. This approach would look like this:

Function	$= NPV(I, \text{range without } CF_0) + \text{Year 0 Cell}$
Cell formula	$= NPV(0.10, B10{:}F10) + A10$
Cell display	$80.95

Rate of Return

The second way to measure the financial return on an investment is by *rate of return*, or *percentage return*. This measures the interest rate that must be earned on the investment outlay to generate the expected cash inflows. In other words, this measure provides the expected periodic rate of return on the investment. If the cash flows are annual, as in this example, the rate of return is an annual rate. In effect, we are solving for I—the interest rate that equates the present value of the cash inflows to the dollar amount of the cash outlay.

Mathematically, if the present value of the cash inflows equals the investment outlay, then the NPV of the investment is forced to $0. This relationship is shown here:

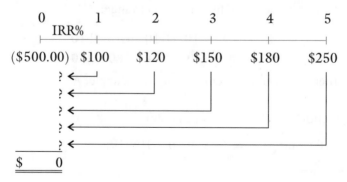

Note that the rate of return on an investment, particularly an investment in plant or equipment, typically is called the *internal rate of return* (*IRR*). Although a trial-and-error procedure could be used on a regular calculator to determine the rate of return, it is better to use a financial calculator or spreadsheet.

Financial calculator solution:
Use the same cash flows that were entered to solve for NPV: –500, 100, 120, 150, 180, and 250. However, now push the *IRR* button to obtain the answer, 15.3 percent.

Spreadsheet solution:
Use the same spreadsheet format as earlier:

Cell Address:	A10	B10	C10	D10	E10	F10
Value:	–500	100	120	150	180	250

But now, place the IRR function in an empty cell; for example, A6:

Function	= IRR (range, starting guess)
Cell formula	= IRR (A10:F10, 0.10)
Cell display	15.3

A starting guess is required to calculate the IRR because the methodology used by the spreadsheet IRR function is actually a trial-and-error process that requires a starting point.

We will have much more to say about investment returns in Chapters 8, 12, and 13. For now, an understanding of the basic concept is sufficient.

1. Differentiate between dollar return and rate of return.
2. Is the calculation of investment return an application of time value analysis? Explain your answer.

Self-Test Questions

Semiannual and Other Compounding Periods

In all the examples thus far, the assumption was that interest is compounded once a year, or annually. This is called *annual compounding*. Suppose, however, that Meridian Clinic puts $100 into a bank account that pays 6 percent annual interest, but it is compounded *semiannually*. How much would the clinic accumulate at the end of one year, two years, or some other period? Semiannual compounding means that interest is paid each six months, so interest is earned more often than under annual compounding.

To illustrate semiannual compounding, assume that the $100 is placed into the account for three years. The following situation occurs under **annual** compounding:

Time line:

$$
\begin{array}{ccccc}
0 & & 1 & 2 & 3 \\
& 6\% & & & \\
\vdash & & + & + & \dashv \\
-\$100 & & & & ?
\end{array}
$$

$$FV_N = PV \times (1 + I)^N = \$100 \times (1.06)^3$$

Regular calculator solution:

$$
\begin{array}{ccccc}
0 & & 1 & 2 & 3 \\
& 6\% & & & \\
\vdash & & + & + & \dashv \\
\$100 \times 1.06 & & \times 1.06 & \times 1.06 & = \$119.10 \\
& \longrightarrow & \longrightarrow & \longrightarrow &
\end{array}
$$

Financial calculator solution:

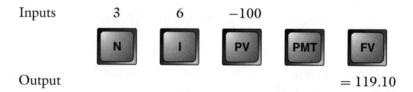

Inputs	3	6	−100		
	N	I	PV	PMT	FV
Output					= 119.10

Spreadsheet solution:

Cell formula	$= 100 * (1.06)\text{^}3$
Cell display	119.10

Now, consider what happens under **semiannual** compounding. Because interest rates usually are stated as annual rates, this situation would be described as 6 percent interest, compounded semiannually. With semiannual compounding, $N = 2 \times 3 = 6$ semiannual periods, and $I = 6/2 = 3\%$ per semiannual period. Here is the solution.

Time line:

$$
\begin{array}{cccccccc}
\text{Semiannual periods} & 0 & 1 & 2 & 3 & 4 & 5 & 6 \\
& 3\% & & & & & & \\
& \vdash & + & + & + & + & + & \dashv \\
& -\$100 & & & & & & ?
\end{array}
$$

$$FV_N = PV \times (1 + I)^N = \$100 \times (1.03)^6$$

Regular calculator solution:

Semiannual periods 0   1   2   3   4   5   6
                       3%

$100 × 1.03 × 1.03 × 1.03 × 1.03 × 1.03 × 1.03 = $119.41

Financial calculator solution:

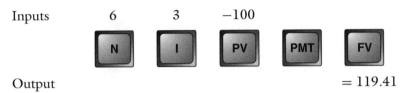

Inputs   6   3   −100

              N   I   PV   PMT   FV

Output   = 119.41

Spreadsheet solution:

Cell formula $= 100 * (1.03)^6$

Cell display   119.41

The $100 deposit grows to $119.41 under semiannual compounding, but only to $119.10 under annual compounding. This result occurs because interest on interest is being earned more frequently under semiannual compounding.

Throughout the economy, different compounding periods are used for different types of investments. For example, bank accounts often compound interest monthly or daily, most bonds pay interest semiannually, and stocks generally pay quarterly dividends.[4] Furthermore, the cash flows stemming from capital investments, such as new hospital wings or diagnostic equipment, can be analyzed in monthly, quarterly, or annual periods, or even some other interval. Time value analyses with different compounding periods must be put on a common basis for comparison, which is accomplished by the effective annual rate.

To begin the comparison, note that the *stated interest rate* in the Meridian Clinic semiannual compounding example is 6 percent, while the *effective annual rate* is the rate that produces the same ending value under annual compounding. In the example, the effective annual rate is the rate that would produce a future value of $119.41 at the end of Year 3 under **annual compounding**. The solution is 6.09 percent:

Inputs   3   −100   119.41

              N   I   PV   PMT   FV

Output   = 6.09

Thus, if one bank offered to pay 6 percent interest with semiannual compounding on a savings account, while another offered 6.09 percent with annual compounding, both banks would be paying the same effective annual rate because the ending value is the same under both sets of terms:

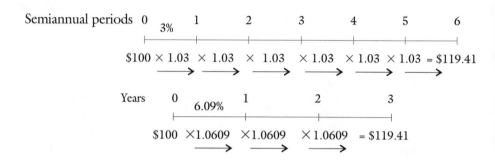

In general, the effective annual rate (EAR) can be determined, given the stated rate and number of compounding periods per year, by using this equation:

$$\text{Effective annual rate (EAR)} = (1 + I_{Stated}/M)^M - 1.0.$$

Here, I_{Stated} is the stated (i.e., the annual) interest rate and M is the number of compounding periods per year. The term I_{Stated}/M is the *periodic* interest rate, so the EAR equation can be restated as:

$$\text{Effective annual rate (EAR)} = (1 + \text{Periodic rate})^M - 1.0.$$

To illustrate use of the EAR equation, consider that the effective annual rate when the stated rate is 6 percent and semiannual compounding occurs is 6.09 percent:

$$EAR = (1 + 0.06/2)^2 - 1.0$$
$$= (1.03)^2 - 1.0$$
$$= 1.0609 - 1.0 = 0.0609 = 6.09\%.$$

Most financial calculators are programmed to calculate EAR, or given an EAR, to find the stated rate. This process is called *interest rate conversion*. In general, enter the stated rate first, then the number of compounding periods per year, and finally press the effective percent key.

As shown in the preceding calculations, semiannual compounding, or for that matter, any compounding that occurs more than once a year, can be handled two ways. First, the input variables can be expressed as periodic variables rather than annual variables. In the Meridian Clinic example, use N = 6 periods, rather than N = 3 years, and I = 3% per period, rather than I = 6% per year. Second, find the effective annual rate and then use this rate as an annual rate over the number of years. In the example, use I = 6.09% and N = 3 years.

For another illustration of the concept, consider the interest rate charged on credit cards. Many banks charge 1.5 percent per month and, in their advertising, state that their annual percentage rate (APR) is 18.0 percent.[5] However, the true cost rate to credit card users is the effective annual rate of 19.6 percent:

$$EAR = (1 + \text{ Periodic rate})^M - 1.0$$

$$= (1.015)^{12} - 1.0 = 0.196 = 19.6\%.$$

Compounding periods, other than annually, also can occur when dealing with annuities. To illustrate the concept, first consider the case of an ordinary annuity of $100 per year for three years discounted at 8 percent, compounded annually.

Time line:

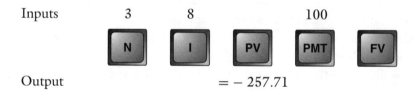

Financial calculator solution:

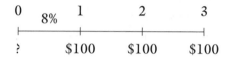

Inputs	3	8		100	
	N	I	PV	PMT	FV

Output   = − 257.71

Spreadsheet solution:

Function	= PV(I, N, PMT)
Cell formula	= PV(0.08, 3, 100)
Cell display	− $257.71

Suppose that the annuity calls for payments of $50 every six months for three years, and the interest rate is 8 percent, compounded semiannually:

Time line:

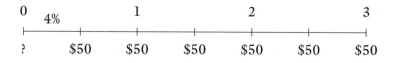

Financial calculator solution:

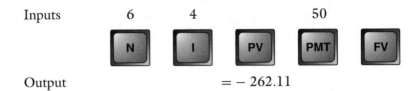

Inputs	6	4		50	
	N	I	PV	PMT	FV

Output   = − 262.11

Spreadsheet solution:

Function	= PV(I, N, PMT)
Cell formula	= PV(0.04, 6, 50)
Cell display	− $262.11

Semiannual payments come in earlier than annual payments, so the $50 semi-annual annuity is a little more valuable than the $100 annual annuity. However, an annuity with **annual payments**, but with **semiannual compounding**, cannot be treated in the same way because the discount rate period must match the annuity period. Thus, annual payments must be discounted using an annual rate, and when semiannual compounding occurs with annual payments, the correct rate to apply is the effective annual rate rather than the stated rate.

Self-Test Questions

1. What changes must be made in the calculations to determine the future value of an amount being compounded at 8 percent semiannually versus one being compounded at 8 percent annually?
2. Why is semiannual compounding better than annual compounding from an investor's standpoint?
3. How does the effective annual rate differ from the stated rate?

Amortized Loans

One important application of time value analysis involves loans that are to be paid off in equal installments over time, such as automobile loans, home mortgage loans, and most business debt other than very short-term loans and long-term bonds. If a loan is to be repaid in equal periodic amounts—monthly, quarterly, or annually—it is said to be an *amortized loan*. The word *amortize* comes from the Latin *mors*, meaning *death*, so an amortized loan is one that is killed off over time.

To illustrate the concept, suppose Santa Fe Healthcare System borrows $1 million from the Bank of New Mexico which will be repaid in three equal installments at the end of each of the next three years. The bank is to receive 6 percent interest on the loan balance that is outstanding at the beginning of each year. The first task in analyzing the loan is to determine the amount Santa Fe must repay each year, or the annual payment. To find this amount, recognize that the loan represents the present value of an annuity of PMT dollars per year for three years, discounted at 6 percent.

Time line:

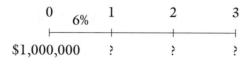

Financial calculator solution:

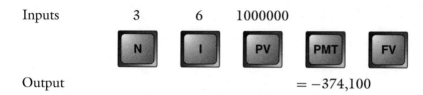

Spreadsheet solution:

Function	$= \text{PMT}(I, N, PV)$
Cell formula	$= \text{PMT}(0.06, 3, 1000000)$
Cell display	$- \$374,110$

Therefore, if Santa Fe pays the bank $374,110 at the end of each of the next three years, the percentage cost to Santa Fe, and the rate of return to the lender, will be 6 percent.

Each payment consists partly of interest and partly of repayment of principal. This breakdown is given in the *amortization schedule* shown in Table 4.1. The interest component is largest in the first year, and it declines as the outstanding balance of the loan is reduced over time. For tax purposes, a taxable business borrower reports the interest payments in Column 3 as a deductible expense each year, while the lender reports these same amounts as taxable income.

Financial calculators are often programmed to calculate amortization schedules; simply key in the inputs, then press one button to get each entry in Table 4.1.

Self-Test Questions

1. When constructing an amortization schedule, how is the periodic payment amount calculated?
2. Does the periodic payment remain constant over time?
3. Do the principal and interest components remain constant over time? Explain your answer.

A Review of Interest Rate Types

This chapter has covered many time value concepts, including three different types of interest rate. In this section, we review these rates.

TABLE 4.1
Loan
Amortization
Schedule

Year	Beginning Amount (1)	Payment (2)	Interest[a] (3)	Repayment of Principal[b] (4)	Remaining Balance (5)
1	$1,000,000	$ 374,110	$ 60,000	$ 314,110	$685,890
2	685,890	374,110	41,153	332,957	352,933
3	352,933	374,110	21,177	352,933	0
		$1,122,330	$122,330	$1,000,000	

[a]Interest is calculated by multiplying the loan balance at the beginning of each year by the interest rate. Therefore, interest in Year 1 is $1,000,000 × 0.06 = $60,000; in Year 2 is $685,890 × 0.06 = $41,153; and in Year 3 is $352,933 × 0.06 = $21,177.
[b]Repayment of principal is equal to the payment of $374,110 minus the interest charge for each year.

Stated Rate

The *stated rate* is the rate that is stated in financial contracts. Convention in the stock, bond, mortgage, commercial loan, consumer loan, and other markets calls for terms to be expressed in stated rates. A banker, broker, or mortgage lender will normally quote the stated rate. However, to be meaningful, the stated rate must indicate the number of compounding periods per year. For example, a bank savings account may offer 10 percent interest compounded quarterly, or a money market mutual fund may offer a 12 percent rate, with interest paid monthly. The stated rate is **not** used for calculations (i.e., never use I_{Stated} on a time line, in the calculator, or in a spreadsheet formula or function) **unless compounding occurs once a year** (M = 1). In this case, I_{Stated} = Periodic rate = Effective annual rate.

Periodic Rate

The periodic rate is the rate charged by a lender or paid by a borrower, or any other time value rate, expressed on a per period basis. It can be a rate per year, per six months, per quarter, per month, per day, or per any other time interval. For example, a bank may charge 1 percent per month on its credit card loans, or a finance firm may charge 3 percent per quarter on consumer loans. Periodic rate = I_{Stated}/M, which implies that I_{Stated} = Periodic rate × M, where M is the number of compounding periods per year. To illustrate the concept, consider the finance firm loan at 3 percent per quarter:

$$I_{Stated} = \text{Periodic rate} \times M = 3\% \times 4 = 12\%,$$

and

$$\text{Periodic rate} = I_{Stated}/M = 12\%/4 = 3\% \text{ per quarter.}$$

The periodic rate can be used when cash flows occur more frequently than once a year, and the number of cash flows per year corresponds to the number of compounding periods per year. Thus, if dealing with a retirement annuity that provides monthly payments; a semiannual payment bond; a consumer loan with quarterly payments; or with a credit card loan with monthly payments, the calculations would use Periodic rate = I_{Stated}/M. The implication in all these examples is that the interest compounding period is the same as the cash flow period. **The periodic rate can only be used directly in calculations when the cash flow period coincides with the interest rate compounding period (e.g., quarterly payments and quarterly compounding).**

Effective Annual Rate

This is the rate that, under annual compounding ($M = 1$), would produce the same results as a given stated rate with compounding more frequently than annual ($M > 1$). The effective annual rate (EAR) is found as follows:

$$\text{Effective annual rate (EAR)} = (1 + I_{Stated}/M)^M - 1.0$$
$$= (1 + \text{Periodic rate})^M - 1.0.$$

For example, suppose that either a 1 percent per month credit card loan or a 3 percent per quarter consumer loan could be used to make a purchase. Which one should be chosen? To answer this question, the cost rate of each alternative must be expressed as an EAR.

$$EAR_{\text{Credit card loan}} = (1 + 0.01)^{12} - 1.0 = (1.01)^{12} - 1.0$$
$$= 1.126825 - 1.0 = 0.126825 = 12.6825\%.$$

$$EAR_{\text{Consumer loan}} = (1 + 0.03)^4 - 1.0 = (1.03)^4 - 1.0$$
$$= 1.125509 - 1.0 = 0.125509 = 12.5509\%.$$

Thus, the consumer loan is slightly less costly than the credit card loan. This result should have been intuitive because although both loans have the same 12 percent stated rate, monthly payments would have to be made on the credit card, while under the consumer loan terms, only quarterly payments would have to be made.

The EAR is also used when the interest-rate compounding period occurs more often than the period between payments or cash flows. For example, if payments occur semiannually, but interest is compounded quarterly, then the EAR must be used. In this case, the EAR is really an "effective semiannual rate" calculated as $(1 + I_{Stated}/4)^2 - 1.0$, which is then applied to the semiannual payment stream.

1. Define the stated rate, the periodic rate, and the effective annual rate.
2. How are these three rates related?
3. Can you think of a situation where all three of these rates are the same?

Self-Test Questions

Fractional Time Periods

In all of the examples used in this chapter, we have assumed that payments occur at the beginning or the end of periods, but not *within* a period. However, many situations arise in which cash flows do occur within periods. For example, Meridian Clinic might deposit $100 in a bank that pays 10 percent interest compounded annually, and leave it in the bank for nine months, or 0.75 years. How much would be in the account at the end?

Time line:

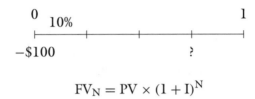

$$FV_N = PV \times (1 + I)^N$$

Regular calculator solution:

$$FV_N = \$100 \times (1.10)^{0.75} = \$100 \times (1.0741) = \$107.41.$$

Financial calculator solution:

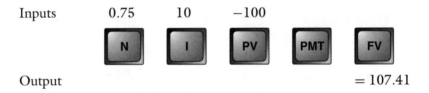

Spreadsheet solution:

Cell formula	$= 100 * (1.10)^{\wedge}0.75$
Cell display	107.41

Present values, annuities, and problems where you must find interest rates or numbers of periods with fractional time periods can all be handled with ease with a financial calculator or spreadsheet program. Indeed, financial calculators and spreadsheet programs have calendar functions specifically designed to deal with fractional time periods. However, any further discussion is beyond the scope of this text.

Self-Test Question

1. How are fractional time periods handled in discounted cash flow calculations?

Key Concepts

Financial decisions often involve situations in which future cash flows must be valued. The process of valuing future cash flows is called *time value analysis*. Here are the key concepts behind this type of analysis:

- *Times lines* are used to help analysts lay out the cash flows involved in a time value analysis.
- *Compounding* is the process of determining the *future value (FV)* of a lump sum or a series of payments.
- *Discounting* is the process of finding the *present value (PV)* of a future lump sum or series of payments.
- An *annuity* is a series of equal, periodic cash flows, which are often called *payments (PMT)*.
- An annuity that has payments occurring at the end of each period is called an *ordinary* annuity.
- If each annuity payment occurs at the beginning of the period rather than at the end, the annuity is an *annuity due*.
- A *perpetuity* is an annuity that lasts forever.
- If an analysis involving more than one cash value does not meet the definition of an annuity, it is called an *uneven cash flow stream*.
- The financial attractiveness of an investment is measured by its *return*.
- Returns can be measured either in *dollar* or *percentage* terms.
- The *stated rate* is the annual rate normally quoted in financial contracts.
- The *periodic rate* equals the stated rate divided by the number of compounding periods per year.
- If compounding occurs more frequently than once a year, it is often necessary to calculate the *effective annual rate*, which is the rate that produces the same results under annual compounding as compared with more frequent compounding.
- An *amortized* loan is one that is paid off in equal amounts over some specified number of periods. An *amortization schedule* shows how much of each payment represents interest, how much is used to reduce the principal, and the remaining balance on each payment date.

Time value analysis is one of the cornerstones of healthcare financial management, so readers should feel comfortable with this material before moving ahead.

Selected References

Owner's Manual for your calculator.
After-market reference manual for your spreadsheet software.
Help menu for your spreadsheet software.

Selected Web Sites

There are many web sites that contain online time value analysis calculators, see *www.centura.com/personal/calculator/index.cfm*. This page links to many different calculators that solve basic time value problems.

Selected Cases

The following case in *Cases in Healthcare Finance* can be assigned to help students learn more about time value analysis:

Case 9: Golden West Surgery Centers, which examines most of the time value analysis techniques discussed in this chapter.

Notes

1. On some financial calculators, the keys are buttons on the face of the calculator; on others, the time value variables are shown on the display after accessing the time value menu. Also, some calculators use different symbols to represent the number of periods and interest rate. For example, both lower and upper cases are used for N and I, while other calculators use N/YR and I/YR or I%/YR or some other variation. Finally, financial calculators today are quite powerful in that they can easily solve relatively complex time value of money problems, such as when intraperiod cash flows occur. To focus on concepts rather than mechanics, all the illustrations in this chapter and the remainder of the text assume that cash flows occur at the end or beginning of a period, and that there is only one cash flow per period. Thus, to follow the illustrations, financial calculators must be set to one period per year, and it is not necessary to use the calendar function.

2. Time value analyses also can be solved using mathematical multipliers obtained from tables. At one time, tables were the most efficient way to conduct time value analyses, but calculators and spreadsheets have made tabular solutions obsolete.

3. Actually, owning a single nursing home is riskier than owning the stock of a firm that has a large number of nursing homes with geographical diversification. Also, an owner of Beverly Enterprise's stock can easily sell the stock if things go sour, whereas it would be much more difficult for Oakdale to sell its nursing home. These differences in risk and liquidity suggest that the true opportunity cost rate is probably higher than the return that is expected from owning the stock of Beverly Enterprises. However, direct ownership of a nursing home implies control, while ownership of the stock of a large firm usually does not. Such control rights would tend to reduce the opportunity cost rate. The main point here is that in practice it may not be possible to obtain a "perfect" opportunity cost rate. Nevertheless, an imprecise one is better than none at all.

4. Some financial institutions even pay interest that is compounded *continuously*. However, continuous compounding is not relevant to healthcare financial management, so it will not be discussed here.

5. The *annual percentage rate (APR)* and *annual percentage yield (APY)* are terms defined in Truth in Lending and Truth in Savings Laws. APR is defined as Periodic rate × Number of compounding periods per year, so it ignores the consequences of compounding. Although the APR on a credit card with interest charges of 1.5 percent per month is $1.5\% \times 12 = 18.0\%$, the true effective annual rate as calculated in the text is 19.6 percent.

FINANCIAL RISK AND REQUIRED RETURN

Learning Objectives

After studying this chapter, readers should be able to:

- Explain in general terms the concept of financial risk.
- Define and differentiate between stand-alone risk and portfolio risk.
- Define and differentiate between corporate risk and market risk.
- Explain the CAPM relationship between risk and required return.

Introduction

Two of the most important concepts in healthcare financial management are financial risk and required return. What is financial risk, how is it measured, and what effect, if any, does it have on required return, and hence on managerial decisions? Because so much of financial decision making involves risk and return, it is impossible to gain a good understanding of healthcare financial management without having a solid appreciation of risk and return concepts.

If investors—both individuals and businesses—viewed risk as a benign fact of life, it would have little impact on decision making. However, decision makers are, for the most part, averse to risk, believing that risk is to be avoided. Furthermore, if risks must be taken, there must be a reward for doing so. Thus, investments of higher risk, whether an individual investor's security investment or a radiology group's investment in diagnostic equipment, must offer higher returns to make the investment financially attractive.

In this chapter, basic risk concepts are presented from the perspective of both individual investors and businesses. Healthcare managers must be familiar with both contexts because investors supply the capital that businesses need to function. In addition, the chapter discusses the relationship between risk and required rate of return. To be truly useful in financial decision making, it is necessary to know the impact of risk on investors' views of investment acceptability.

The Many Faces of Financial Risk

Unfortunately, a full discussion of financial risk would take many chapters, perhaps even an entire book, because financial risk is a very complicated subject. First of all, it depends on whether the investor is an individual or a business. Then, if the investor is an individual, it depends on the investment horizon, or the amount of time until the investment proceeds are needed. To make the situation even more complex, it may even be difficult to define, measure, or translate financial risk into something usable for decision making. For example, the risk that individual investors face when saving for retirement is the risk that the amount of funds accumulated will not be sufficient to fund the lifestyle expected during the full term of retirement. Needless to say, translating such a definition of risk into investment goals is not easy. The good news is that our primary interest concerns the financial risk inherent in making decisions within businesses. Thus, our discussion can focus on the fundamental factors that influence the riskiness of real asset investments.

Still, two factors come into play that complicate our discussion of financial risk. The first complicating factor is that financial risk is seen both by businesses and the investors in businesses. There is some risk inherent in the business itself that depends on the type of business. For example, pharmaceutical firms are generally acknowledged to face a great deal of risk, while healthcare providers typically have less risk. Then, investors (i.e., stockholders and creditors) bear the riskiness inherent in the business, but as modified by the nature of the securities they hold. For example, the stock of Beverly Enterprises is more risky than its debt, although the risk of both securities depends on the inherent risk of a business that operates in the long-term care industry. Not-for-profit firms have the same partitioning of risk with debtholders, but now the inherent riskiness of the business is split between creditors and the implied stockholders, who generally are considered to be the community at large.

The second complicating factor for our discussion results from the fact that the riskiness of an investment depends on the context in which it is held. For example, a stock held alone is riskier than the same stock held as part of a large portfolio of stocks. Similarly, a magnetic resonance imaging (MRI) system operated independently is riskier than the same system operated as part of a large, geographically diversified business that owns numerous types of diagnostic equipment.

Self-Test Question

1. What are the complications that arise when dealing with financial risk in a business setting?

Introduction To Financial Risk

Generically, *risk* is defined as "a hazard; a peril; exposure to loss or injury." Thus, risk refers to the chance that an unfavorable event will occur. If an individual engages in skydiving, he or she is taking a chance with injury or death; skydiving is risky. If an individual gambles at roulette, he or she is not risking injury or death, but is taking a *financial risk*. Even when an individual invests in stocks or bonds, he or she is taking a risk in the hope of earning a positive rate of return. Similarly, when a healthcare business invests in new assets, such as diagnostic equipment, new hospital beds, or a new managed care plan, it is taking a financial risk.

To illustrate basic financial risk, consider two potential personal investments. The first investment consists of a one-year, $1,000 face value U.S. Treasury bill that is bought for $950. Treasury bills are short-term federal debt securities that are sold at a *discount* (i.e., less than face value) and return *face*, or *par*, *value* at maturity. The investor expects to receive $1,000 at maturity in one year, so the anticipated rate of return on the T-bill investment is 5.3 percent. Using a financial calculator:

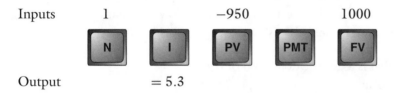

The $1,000 payment is fixed by contract (the T-bill promises to pay this amount), and the U.S. government is certain to make the payment except for a national disaster—a very unlikely event. Thus, there is virtually a 100 percent probability that the investment will actually earn the 5.3 percent rate of return expected. In this situation, the investment is defined as being *riskless*, or *risk free*.

Now, assume that the $950 is invested in a biotechnology partnership that will be terminated in one year. If the partnership develops a new commercially valuable product, its rights will be sold and $2,000 will be received from the partnership, for a rate of return of 110.53 percent:

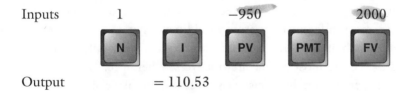

But if nothing worthwhile is developed, the partnership would be worthless, no money would be received, and the rate of return would be −100 percent:

Inputs	1		−950		0
	N	I	PV	PMT	FV
Output		= −100.00			

(Note that most financial calculators give no solution when the future value is entered as zero, but if a very small number, for example, 0.0001, is entered for the future value, the solution for interest rate is −100.00.)

Now, assume that there is a 50 percent chance that a valuable product will be developed. In this admittedly unrealistic situation, the expected rate of return—a statistical concept that will be discussed shortly—is the same 5.3 percent as on the T-bill investment: $(0.50 \times 110.53\%) + (0.50 \times [-100\%]) = 5.3\%$. However, the biotechnology partnership is a far cry from being riskless. If things go poorly, the entire $950 investment will be lost and the realized rate of return will be -100 percent. Because there is a significant chance of actually earning a return that is far less than expected, the partnership investment is described as being very risky.

Thus, financial risk is related to the probability of earning a return less than expected. The greater the chance of low or negative returns, the greater the amount of financial risk.

Self-Test Questions
1. What is a generic definition of risk?
2. Explain the general concept of financial risk.

Risk Aversion

Why is it so important to define and measure financial risk? The reason is that both individual and business investors, for the most part, dislike risk. Suppose you were given the choice between a sure $1 million and the flip of a coin for either $0 or $2 million. You, and just about everyone else, would likely "take the $1 million and run." An individual who takes the sure $1 million is *risk averse*; an individual who is indifferent between the two alternatives, or views them as the same, is *risk neutral*; and an individual who prefers the gamble to the sure thing is *risk seeker*.

Of course, people and businesses do gamble and take chances, so all of us typically exhibit some risk-seeking behavior at one time or another. However, most individual investors would never put a sizable proportion of their net worth at risk, and most business executives would never "bet the business," because most people are risk averse when it really matters.

What are the implications of risk aversion for financial decision making? First, given two investments with similar returns but differing risk, investors will favor the lower-risk alternative. Second, investors will require higher returns to invest in higher-risk investments. These typical outcomes of risk-averse behavior have a significant impact on many facets of financial decision making, and hence these results will appear time and time again in later chapters.

Self-Test Questions
1. What does "risk aversion" mean?
2. What are the implications of risk aversion for financial decision making?

Probability Distributions

The chance that an event will occur is called *probability of occurrence*, or just *probability*. For example, a weather forecast might predict a 40 percent chance of rain. Or, when rolling a single die, the probability of rolling a two is one out of six, or $1/6 = 0.1667 = 16.67\%$. If all possible outcomes related to a particular event are listed, and a probability is assigned to each outcome, the result is a *probability distribution*. In the example of the weather forecast, the probability distribution looks like this:

Outcome	Probability
Rain	0.40 = 40%
No rain	0.60 = 60%
	1.00 = 100%

In the example of the role of a die, the probability distribution looks like this:

Outcome	Probability
1	0.1667 = 16.67%
2	0.1667 = 16.67%
3	0.1667 = 16.67%
4	0.1667 = 16.67%
5	0.1667 = 16.67%
6	0.1667 = 16.67%
	1.0000 = 100.00%

All possible outcomes (i.e., the number of dots showing after the die roll) are listed in the left column, while the probability of each outcome is listed in the right column and is expressed as both decimals and percentages. If the probability distribution is complete, the probabilities must sum to 1.0, or 100 percent.

Probabilities can also be assigned to possible outcomes—in this case, returns—on both personal and business investments. If an individual buys stock, the return will usually come in the form of *dividends* and *capital gains* (selling the stock for more than the individual paid for it) or *losses* (selling the stock for less than the individual paid for it). Because all stock returns are uncertain, there is some chance that the dividends will not be as high as expected and that the stock price will not increase as much as expected or that it will even decrease. The higher the probabilities of dividends and stock price well below those expected, the higher the probability that the return will be significantly less than expected, and hence the greater the risk.

To illustrate the concept using a business investment, consider a hospital evaluating the purchase of a new MRI system. The cost of the system is an investment, and the net cash inflows that stem from patient utilization of the MRI provide the return. The net cash inflows, in turn, depend on the number of procedures, charge per procedure, payer discounts, operating costs, and so on. These values typically are not known with certainty, but rather are dependent on factors such as patient demographics, physician acceptance, local market conditions, labor costs, and so on. Thus, the hospital actually faces a probability distribution of returns, rather than a single return known with certainty. The greater the probability of returns well below the return anticipated, the greater the risk of the MRI investment.

Self-Test Questions

1. What is a probability distribution?
2. How are probability distributions used in financial decision making?

Expected and Realized Rates of Return

To be most useful, the concept of financial risk must be defined more precisely than just the chances of a return well below that anticipated. Table 5.1 contains the estimated return distributions developed by the financial staff of Norwalk Community Hospital for two proposed investments: (1) a MRI system and (2) a walk-in clinic. Here, each economic state reflects a combination of factors that dictate each project's profitability. For example, for the MRI project, the very poor economic state signifies very low physician acceptance and, hence, very low utilization, very high discounts on reimbursements, very high operating costs, and so on. The economic states are defined in a similar fashion for the walk-in clinic.

The *expected rate of return*, defined in the statistical sense, is the weighted average of the return distribution, where the weights are the probabilities of occurrence. For example, the expected rate of return on the MRI system, $E(R_{MRI})$, is 10 percent:

$$
\begin{aligned}
E(R_{MRI}) = {} & (\text{Probability of Return 1} \times \text{Return 1}) \\
& + (\text{Probability of Return 2} \times \text{Return 2}) \\
& + (\text{Probability of Return 3} \times \text{Return 3}) \text{ and so on} \\
= {} & (0.10 \times [-10\%]) + (0.20 \times 0\%) + (0.40 \times 10\%) \\
& + (0.20 \times 20\%) + (0.10 \times 30\%) \\
= {} & 10.0\%.
\end{aligned}
$$

TABLE 5.1
Norwalk Community Hospital: Estimated Returns for Two Proposed Investments

Economic State	Probability of Occurrence	Rate of Return if State Occurs MRI	Clinic
Very poor	0.10	−10%	−20%
Poor	0.20	0	0
Average	0.40	10	15
Good	0.20	20	30
Very good	0.10	30	50
	1.00		

Calculated in a similar manner, the expected rate of return on the walk-in clinic is 15 percent.

The expected rate of return is the average return that would result, given the return distribution, if the investment were randomly repeated many times. In this illustration, if 1,000 clinics were built in different areas, each of which faced the return distribution given in Table 5.1, the average return on the 1,000 investments would be 15 percent, assuming the returns in each area are independent of one another. However, only one clinic would actually be built, and the realized rate of return may be less than the expected 15 percent. Therefore, the clinic investment, as well as the MRI investment, is risky.

Expected rate of return expresses expectations for the future. When the managers at Norwalk Community Hospital analyzed the MRI investment, they expected it to earn 10 percent. However, assume that economic conditions took a turn for the worse and the very poor economic scenario actually occurred. In this case, the *realized rate of return,* which is the rate of return that the investment actually produced as measured at termination, would be a negative 10 percent. It is the potential of realizing a return of −10 percent on an investment that has an expected return of +10 percent that produces risk. Note that in many situations, especially those arising in text illustrations, the expected rate of return is not even achievable. For example, an investment that has a 50 percent chance of a 5 percent return and a 50 percent chance of a 15 percent return has an expected rate of return of 10 percent. Yet, there is zero probability of actually realizing the 10 percent expected rate of return.

Self-Test Questions

1. How is the expected rate of return calculated?
2. What is the economic interpretation of the expected rate of return?
3. What is the difference between the expected rate of return and the realized rate of return?

Stand-Alone Risk

We can look at the two distributions in Table 5.1 and intuitively conclude that the clinic is more risky than the MRI system because the clinic has a chance of a 20 percent loss, while the worst possible loss on the MRI system is 10 percent. This intuitive risk assessment is based on the *stand-alone risk* of the two investments; that is, we are focusing on the riskiness of each investment under the assumption that it would be the business's only asset (operated in isolation). In the next section, portfolio effects will be introduced, but for now, let us continue our discussion of stand-alone risk.

Stand-alone risk depends on the "tightness" of an investment's return distribution. If an investment has a tight return distribution, with returns falling close to the expected return, it has relatively low stand-alone risk. Conversely, an investment with a return distribution that is "loose," and hence has values well below the expected return, is relatively risky in the stand-alone sense.

It is important to recognize that risk and return are **separate** attributes of an investment. An investment may have a very tight distribution of returns, and hence very low stand-alone risk, but its expected rate of return might be only 2 percent. In this situation, the investment probably would not be financially attractive, in spite of its low risk. Similarly, a high-risk investment with a sufficiently high expected rate of return would be attractive.

To be truly useful, any definition of risk must have some measure, or numerical value, so we need some way to specify the "degree of tightness" of an investment's return distribution. One such measure is the *standard deviation*, which is often given the symbol "σ" (Greek lowercase sigma). Standard deviation is a common statistical measure of the dispersion of a distribution about its mean—the smaller the standard deviation, the tighter the distribution, and hence the lower the riskiness of the investment. To illustrate the calculation of standard deviation, consider the MRI investment's estimated returns listed in Table 5.1. Here are the steps:

1. The expected rate of return on the MRI, $E(R_{MRI})$, is 10 percent.
2. The *variance* of the return distribution is determined as follows:

$$\text{Variance} = (\text{Probability of Return 1} \times [\text{Rate of Return 1} - E(R_{MRI})]^2)$$
$$+ (\text{Probability of Return 2} \times [\text{Rate of Return 2} - E(R_{MRI})]^2) \text{ and so on}$$
$$= (0.10 \times [-10\% - 10\%]^2) + (0.20 \times [0\% - 10\%]^2) + (0.40 \times [10\% - 10\%]^2)$$
$$+ (0.20 \times [20\% - 10\%]^2) + (0.10 \times [30\% - 10\%]^2)$$
$$= 120.00.$$

Variance, like standard deviation, is a measure of the dispersion of a distribution about its expected value, but it is less useful than standard deviation because its measurement unit is percent or dollars **squared**, which has no economic meaning.

3. The standard deviation is defined as the square root of the variance:

$$\text{Standard deviation } (\sigma) = \sqrt{\text{Variance}}$$
$$= \sqrt{120.00} = 10.95\% \approx 11.0\%.$$

Using the same procedure, the clinic investment listed in Table 5.1 was found to have a standard deviation of returns of about 18 percent. Because the clinic investment's standard deviation of returns is larger than that of the MRI investment, the clinic investment has more stand-alone risk than the MRI investment.

As a general rule, investments with higher expected rates of return have larger standard deviations than investments with smaller expected returns. This situation occurs in our MRI and clinic example. In situations where expected rates of return on investments differ substantially, standard deviation may not give a good picture of one investment's stand-alone risk relative to another. The *coefficient of variation (CV)*, which is defined as the standard deviation of returns divided by the expected return, measures the risk per unit of return, and hence standardizes the measurement of stand-alone risk. To illustrate the concept, consider that the MRI investment has a CV of 1.10, while the clinic's CV is 1.20:

$$\text{Coefficient of variation } = \text{CV} = \frac{\sigma}{E(R)}.$$

$$\text{CV}_{\text{MRI}} = 11.0\%/10.0\% = 1.10.$$

$$\text{CV}_{\text{Clinic}} = 18.0\%/15.0\% = 1.20.$$

In this situation, the clinic investment has slightly more risk per unit of return, so it is riskier than the MRI as measured by both standard deviation and coefficient of variation. However, note that the clinic's stand-alone risk as measured by the coefficient of variation is not as great relative to the MRI as it is when measured by standard deviation. This difference in relative risk occurs because the clinic has a higher expected rate of return. Finally, note that coefficient of variation has no units; it is just a raw number.

Self-Test Questions

1. What is stand-alone risk?
2. What are some measures of stand-alone risk?
3. Is one measure better than another?

Portfolio Risk and Return

The preceding section developed a risk measure—standard deviation—that applies to investments held in isolation. However, most investments are not held in isolation. Instead, they are held as part of a collection, or *portfolio*, of investments. Individual investors typically hold portfolios of **securities** (i.e., stocks and bonds), while businesses generally hold portfolios of **projects** (i.e., product or service lines). When investments are held in portfolios, the primary concern of investors is not the realized rate of return on an individual investment, but rather the realized rate of return on the entire portfolio. Similarly, the riskiness of each individual asset in the portfolio is not important to the investor; what matters is the aggregate riskiness of the portfolio. Thus, the whole nature of risk, and how it is defined and measured, changes when one recognizes that investments are not held in isolation, but rather as parts of portfolios.

Portfolio Returns

Consider the returns estimated for the seven investment alternatives listed in Table 5.2. The individual investment alternatives (Investments A, B, C,

TABLE 5.2

Estimated Returns for Four Individual Investments and Three Portfolios

Economic State	Probability of Occurrence	Rate of Return if State Occurs						
		A	B	C	D	AB	AC	AD
Very poor	0.10	−10%	30%	−25%	15%	10%	−17.5%	2.5%
Poor	0.20	0	20	−5	10	10	−2.5	5.0
Average	0.40	10	10	15	0	10	12.5	5.0
Good	0.20	20	0	35	25	10	27.5	22.5
Very good	0.10	30	−10	55	35	10	42.5	32.5
	1.00							
Expected rate of return		10.0%	10.0%	15.0%	12.0%	10.0%	12.5%	11.0%
Standard deviation		11.0%	11.0%	21.9%	12.1%	0.0%	16.4%	10.1%

and D) could be projects under consideration by South West Clinics, Inc., or they could be stocks that are being evaluated as personal investments. The remaining three alternatives in Table 5.2 are portfolios. Portfolio AB consists of 50 percent invested in Investment A and 50 percent in Investment B (e.g., $10,000 invested in A and $10,000 invested in B), while Portfolio AC is an equal-weighted portfolio of Investments A and C, and Portfolio AD is an equal-weighted portfolio of Investments A and D. As shown in the bottom of the table, Investments A and B have 10 percent expected rates of return, while the expected rates of return for Investments C and D are 15 percent and 12 percent, respectively. Investments A and B have identical stand-alone risk (i.e., standard deviation), while Investments C and D have greater stand-alone risk than A and B.

The *expected rate of return on a portfolio, $E(R_{Portfolio})$,* is the weighted average of the expected returns on the assets that make up the portfolio, with the weights being the proportion of the total portfolio invested in each asset:

$$E(R_{Portfolio}) = (w_1 \times E[R_1]) + (w_2 \times E[R_2]) + (w_3 \times E[R_3]) \text{ and so on}$$

where w_1 is the proportion of Investment 1 in the overall portfolio and $E(R_1)$ is the expected rate of return Investment 1, and so on. Thus, the expected rate of return on Portfolio AB is 10 percent:

$$E(R_{AB}) = (0.5 \times 10\%) + (0.5 \times 10\%) = 5\% + 5\% = 10\%$$

while the expected rate of return on Portfolio AC is 12.5 percent and on AD is 11.0 percent.

Alternatively, the expected rate of return on a portfolio can be calculated by looking at the portfolio's return distribution. To illustrate the concept, consider the return distribution for Portfolio AC contained in Table 5.2. The portfolio return in each economic state is the weighted average of the returns on Investments A and C in that state. For example, the return on Portfolio AC in the very poor state is $(0.5 \times [-10\%]) + (0.5 \times [-25\%]) = -17.5\%$.

Portfolio AC's return in each other state is calculated similarly. Portfolio AC's return distribution now can be used to calculate its expected rate of return:

$$E(R_{AC}) = (0.10 \times [-17.5\%]) + (0.20 \times [-2.5\%]) + (0.40 \times 12.5\%)$$
$$+ (0.20 \times 27.5\%) + (0.10 \times 42.5\%)$$
$$= 12.5\%.$$

This is the same value as calculated from the expected rates of return of the two portfolio components:

$$(0.5 \times 10\%) + (0.5 \times 15\%) = 12.5\%.$$

After the fact, the actual, or realized, returns on Investments A and C will probably be different from their expected values, and hence the realized rate of return on Portfolio AC will likely be different from its 12.5 percent expected return.

Portfolio Risk: Two Assets

When an investor holds a portfolio of assets, the portfolio is in effect a stand-alone investment, so the riskiness of the **portfolio** is measured by the standard deviation of portfolio returns, which is the previously discussed measure of stand-alone risk. How does the riskiness of the individual investments in a portfolio combine to create the overall riskiness of the portfolio? Although the rate of return on a portfolio is the weighted average of the returns on the component investments, a portfolio's standard deviation (i.e., riskiness) is generally **not** the weighted average of the standard deviations of the individual components. The portfolio's riskiness may be smaller than the weighted average of each component's riskiness. Indeed, the riskiness of a portfolio may be less than the least risky portfolio component. Under certain conditions, a portfolio of risky assets may even be riskless.

A simple example can be used to illustrate this concept. Suppose that an individual is given the opportunity to flip a coin once; if it comes up heads, the individual wins $10,000, but if it comes up tails, he or she loses $8,000. This is a reasonable bet; the expected dollar return is $(0.5 \times \$10,000) + (0.5 \times [-\$8,000]) = \$1,000$. However, it is a highly risky proposition; the individual has a 50 percent chance of losing $8,000. Thus, because of risk aversion, most people would refuse to make the bet, especially if the $8,000 potential loss would result in financial hardship.

Alternatively, suppose that individual is given the opportunity to flip the coin 100 times, and he or she would win $100 for each head but lose $80 for each tail. It is possible, although extremely unlikely, that the individual would flip all heads and win $10,000. It is also possible, and also extremely unlikely, that he or she would flip all tails and lose $8,000. But the chances are very high that the individual would actually flip close to 50 heads and 50 tails and net about $1,000. Even if he or she flipped a few more tails than heads, the individual would still make money on the gamble.

Although each flip is a very risky bet in the stand-alone sense, collectively the individual has a low-risk proposition. In effect, the multiple flipping has created a portfolio of investments; each flip of the coin can be thought of as one investment, so the individual now has a 100-investment portfolio. Furthermore, the return on each investment is independent of the returns on the other investments; the individual has a 50 percent chance of winning on each flip of the coin regardless of the results of the previous flips. By combining the flips into a single gamble (i.e., into an investment portfolio), the gambler can reduce the risk associated with each bet. In fact, if the gamble consisted of a very large number of flips, almost all risk would be eliminated; the probability of a near-equal number of heads and tails would be extremely high, and the result would be a sure profit. The key to the risk reduction inherent in the portfolio is the fact that the negative consequences of tossing a tail can now be offset by the positive consequences of tossing a head.

To examine portfolio effects in more depth, consider Portfolio AB in Table 5.2. Each individual investment (A and B) is quite risky when held in isolation; each has a standard deviation of returns of 10 percent. However, a portfolio of the two investments has a rate of return of 10 percent in every possible state of the economy, and hence it offers a riskless 10 percent return. This result is verified by the value of zero for Portfolio AB's standard deviation of return. The reason Investments A and B can be combined to form a riskless portfolio is that their returns move exactly opposite one another. Thus, in economic states when A's returns are relatively low, those of B are relatively high, and vice versa, so the gains on one investment in the portfolio exactly offset losses in the other.

The movement relationship of two variables (i.e., their tendency to move either together or in opposition) is called *correlation*. The *correlation coefficient, r,* measures this relationship. Investments A and B can be combined to form a riskless portfolio because the returns on A and B are *perfectly negatively correlated,* which is designated by r = −1.0. In every state where Investment A has a return higher than its expected return, Investment B has a return lower than its expected return, and vice versa.

The opposite of perfect negative correlation is *perfect positive correlation,* which is designated by r = +1.0. Returns on two perfectly positively correlated investments move up and down together as the economic state changes. When the returns on two investments are perfectly positively correlated, combining the investments into a portfolio will not lower risk; the standard deviation of the portfolio is merely the weighted average of the standard deviations of the two components.

To illustrate the impact of perfect positive correlation, consider Portfolio AC in Table 5.2:

- Its expected rate of return, $E(R_{AC})$, is 12.5 percent
- The variance of the portfolio is 270:

$$\text{Variance} = (\text{Probability of Return 1} \times [\text{Rate of Return 1} - E(R_{AC})]^2)$$
$$+ (\text{Probability of Return 2} \times [\text{Rate of Return 2} - E(R_{AC})]^2) \text{ and so on}$$
$$= (0.10 \times [-17.5\% - 12.5\%]^2) + (0.20 \times [-2.5\% - 12.5\%]^2)$$
$$+ (0.40 \times [12.5\% - 12.5\%]^2) + (0.20 \times [27.5\% - 12.5\%]^2)$$
$$+ (0.10 \times [42.5\% - 12.5\%]^2)$$
$$= 270.00.$$

- Finally, Portfolio AC's standard deviation is 16.4 percent:

$$\sigma_{AC} = \sqrt{\text{Variance}}$$
$$= \sqrt{270.00} = 16.4\%.$$

Because of perfect positive correlation between the returns on A and C, Portfolio AC's standard deviation is the weighted average standard deviation of its components:

$$\sigma_{AC} = (0.5 \times 11.0\%) + (0.5 \times 21.9\%)$$
$$= 16.4\%.$$

There is no risk reduction in this situation. The risk of the portfolio is less than the risk of Investment C, but it is more than the risk of Investment A. Forming a portfolio does not reduce risk when the returns on the two components are perfectly positively correlated; the portfolio merely **averages** the risk of the two investments.

What happens when a portfolio is created with two investments that have positive, but not perfectly positive, correlation? Combining the two investments can eliminate some, but not all, risk. To illustrate the concept, consider Portfolio AD in Table 5.2. This portfolio has a standard deviation of returns of 10.1 percent, so it is risky. However, Portfolio AD's standard deviation is not only less than the weighted average of its components' standard deviations, $(0.5 \times 11\%) + (0.5 \times 12.1\%) = 11.6\%$, it is also less than the standard deviation of each component. The correlation coefficient between the return distributions for A and D is 0.53, which indicates that the two investments are positively correlated, but the correlation is less than +1.0. Thus, combining two investments that are positively, but not perfectly, correlated lowers risk but does not eliminate it.[1]

Because returns correlation is the factor that drives risk reduction, a logical question here is: What is the correlation among the returns on "real-world" investments? Generalizing about the correlations among real-world investment alternatives is difficult. However, it is safe to say that the return distributions of two randomly selected investments, whether they are real assets in a hospital's portfolio of projects or financial assets in an individual's investment portfolio, are virtually never perfectly correlated, and hence correlation coefficients are never −1.0 or +1.0. In fact, it is almost impossible to find actual investment opportunities with returns that are negatively correlated with one another or even to find investments with returns that are uncorrelated (r = 0). Because all investment returns are affected to a greater or lesser degree by general economic conditions, investment returns tend to be positively correlated with one another. However, because investment returns are not affected identically by general economic conditions, returns on most real-world investments are not perfectly positively correlated.

The correlation coefficient between the returns of two randomly chosen investments will usually fall in the range of +0.4 to +0.8. Returns on investments that are similar in nature, such as two inpatient projects in a hospital or two stocks in the same industry, will typically have return correlations at the upper end of this range. Conversely, returns on dissimilar projects or securities will tend to have correlations at the lower end of the range.

To illustrate real-world correlations, consider Table 5.3, which shows the correlation coefficients between several investment classes. The table uses securities—primarily stocks—to illustrate correlations because good data are just not available on other types of investments. Furthermore, the base for all correlations is the S&P 500 Index, which is a diversified portfolio of large-firm stocks. The data confirm the fact that even stocks that are considered to move counter to most other stocks—gold stocks—still have a significant positive correlation with the S&P 500 Index. Because all investments are affected to a greater or lesser degree by overall economic conditions, the correlations between returns on most investments are highly positive, but not perfectly so.

Portfolio Risk: Many Assets

Businesses are not restricted to two projects, and individual investors are not restricted to holding two-security portfolios. Most firms have tens, or even hundreds or thousands, of individual projects (i.e., product or service lines),

TABLE 5.3
Correlations Among Selected Pairs of Stock Investments

Investment 1	Investment 2	Correlation Coefficient
S&P 500	S&P 500	1.00
S&P 500	Domestic small stocks	0.79
S&P 500	Foreign stocks	0.53
S&P 500	Real estate	0.44
S&P 500	Treasury bonds	0.36
S&P 500	Gold stocks	0.30

Source: Walter Updegrave, "Why Diversification Pays," *Money Magazine*, December 1999.

and most individual investors hold many different securities, or mutual funds that may be composed of hundreds or even thousands of individual securities. Thus, what is most relevant to financial decision making is not what happens when two investments are combined into portfolios, but rather what happens when many investments are combined.

To illustrate the risk impact of creating large portfolios, consider Figure 5.1. The figure illustrates the riskiness inherent in holding randomly selected portfolios of one asset, two assets, three assets, four assets, and so on, considering the correlations that occur among real-world investments. The plot is based on **historical** annual returns on common stocks traded on the New York Stock Exchange (NYSE), but the conclusions reached are applicable to portfolios made up of any type of investment, including healthcare providers that offer many different types of services.

The riskiness inherent in holding an average one-asset portfolio is relatively high, as measured by the standard deviation of annual returns. The average two-asset portfolio has a lower standard deviation, so holding an average two-asset portfolio is less risky than holding a single asset of average risk. The average three-asset portfolio has an even lower standard deviation of returns, so an average three-asset portfolio is even less risky than an average two-asset portfolio. As more assets are randomly added to create larger portfolios, the average riskiness of the portfolio decreases. However, as more and more assets are added, the incremental risk reduction of adding even

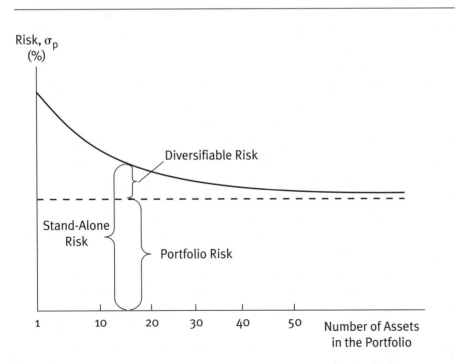

FIGURE 5.1
Portfolio Size and Risk

more assets decreases; and, regardless of how many assets are added, some risk always remains in the portfolio—even with a portfolio of thousands of assets, substantial risk remains.[2]

The reason all risk cannot be eliminated by creating a very large portfolio is that the returns on the component investments, although not perfectly so, are still positively correlated with one another. In other words, all investments, both real and financial, are affected to a lesser or greater degree by general economic conditions.

Diversifiable Risk Versus Portfolio Risk

Figure 5.1 shows what happens as investors create ever larger portfolios. As the size of a randomly created portfolio increases, the riskiness of the portfolio decreases. Thus, a large proportion of the stand-alone risk inherent in an individual investment can be eliminated if it is held as part of a large portfolio. For example, if a stock investor wanted to eliminate as much stand-alone risk inherent in owning NYSE stocks as possible, he or she would have to own over 2,000 stocks. Fortunately, it is not necessary for individuals to purchase all the stocks because mutual funds are available that mimic all of the major stock indexes. A portfolio that consists of a large number of stocks is called the *market portfolio* because it consists of the entire stock market, or at least one entire segment of the stock market. Recent studies have found that the market portfolio has only about one-half the standard deviation of an average stock. However, it is not necessary for individual investors to actually own the market portfolio to take advantage of the risk-reducing benefits of diversification. As illustrated in Figure 5.1, most of the benefit can be obtained by holding about 50 randomly selected stocks. Such a collection of investments is called a *well-diversified portfolio*.

The part of the stand-alone riskiness of a single investment that can be eliminated by diversification (i.e., by holding it as part of a well-diversified portfolio) is called *diversifiable risk*. The part of the riskiness of a single investment that cannot be eliminated by diversification is called *portfolio risk*. Thus, every investment, whether it be the stock of Beverly Enterprises held by an individual investor or an MRI system operated by a hospital, has some diversifiable risk that can be eliminated and some portfolio risk that cannot be diversified away.

Diversifiable risk, as seen by individuals who invest in stocks, is caused by events that are unique to a single business, such as new product or service introductions, strikes, and lawsuits. Because these events are essentially random and influence only one business, their effects can be eliminated by diversification. When one stock in a portfolio does worse than expected because of a negative event unique to that firm, another stock in the portfolio will do better than expected because of a firm-unique positive event. On average, bad events in some firms will be offset by good events in others, so lower than expected returns will be offset by higher than expected returns, leaving the investor with an overall portfolio return closer to that expected than would be the case if only a single stock were held.

The same logic can be applied to a business with a portfolio of projects. Perhaps hospital returns generated from inpatient surgery are less than expected because of the trend toward outpatient procedures, but this may be offset by returns that are greater than expected on state-of-the-art diagnostic services. (If the hospital offered both inpatient and outpatient surgery, it would be *hedging* itself against the trend toward more outpatient procedures because reduced demand for inpatient surgery would be offset by increased demand for outpatient surgery.)

The point to be made here is that the negative impact of random events that are unique to a particular firm, or to a particular product or service within a firm, can be offset by positive events in other firms or in other products or services. Thus, the risk caused by random, unique events can be eliminated by portfolio diversification. Individual investors can diversify by holding many securities, and businesses can diversify by operating many projects.

There are two important points to understand about diversifiable risk. First, not all investments benefit to the same degree from portfolio risk-reducing effects. Some have a large amount of diversifiable risk, and hence have a great deal of risk reduction when added to a well-diversified portfolio. Others do not benefit nearly as much from portfolio risk reduction.

Second, the degree of correlation to the portfolio affects the amount of risk reduction. For example, consider adding the stock of Tenet Healthcare, a hospital management firm, to two portfolios. The first portfolio consists of the stocks of 50 healthcare providers. The second portfolio consists of the stocks of 50 randomly selected firms from many different industries. Much less risk reduction will occur when the Tenet stock is added to the healthcare provider portfolio than when it is added to the randomly selected portfolio. The reason should be obvious. Tenet's returns are more highly correlated with healthcare providers than with firms in other industries.

When applied to real assets, this logic tells us that, potentially, there is more risk reduction inherent in adding a nursing home to a hospital business than there is adding it to a long-term care firm that already owns a large number of such investments. However, we should recognize that it is probably more difficult for managers of a hospital business to manage a nursing home than it is for managers of a firm that specializes in such investments.

Unfortunately, not all risk can be diversified away. Portfolio risk, the risk that remains even in well-diversified portfolios, stems from factors, such as wars, inflation, recessions, and high interest rates, that systematically affect all stocks in a portfolio or all products or services produced by a business. For example, the increasing power of managed care organizations could lower reimbursement levels for all services offered by a hospital. The portfolio risk inherent in single investments cannot be eliminated, so even well-diversified investors, whether they are individuals with large securities portfolios or diversified healthcare businesses with many different service lines, must deal with this type of risk.

Implications for Investors

The ability to eliminate a portion of the stand-alone riskiness inherent in individual investments has two significant implications for investors, which are listed below, whether the investor is an individual who holds securities or a business that offers products or services.

1. Holding a single investment is **not** rational. Holding a portfolio can eliminate much of the stand-alone riskiness inherent in individual investments. Investors who are risk averse should seek to eliminate all diversifiable risk. Individual investors can easily diversify their personal investment portfolios by buying either many individual securities or mutual funds that hold diversified portfolios. Businesses cannot diversify their investments as easily as individuals, but businesses that offer a diverse line of products or services are less risky than businesses that rely on a single product or service.

2. Because an asset held in a portfolio has less risk than when held in isolation, the traditional stand-alone risk measure of standard deviation is no longer appropriate for individual assets. Thus, it is necessary to rethink the definition and measurement of financial risk for such assets. (Note, though, that standard deviation remains the correct measure for the riskiness of an investor's portfolio because the portfolio is, in effect, a single asset held in isolation.)

Self-Test Questions

1. What is a portfolio of assets?
2. What is a well-diversified portfolio?
3. What happens to the risk of a single asset when it is held as part of a portfolio of assets?
4. Explain the differences between stand-alone risk, diversifiable risk, and portfolio risk.
5. Why should all investors hold portfolios rather than individual assets?
6. Is standard deviation the appropriate risk measure for an individual asset?
7. Is standard deviation the appropriate risk measure for an investor's portfolio of assets? Explain your answer.

Portfolio Risk of Business Assets

Businesses typically offer a myriad of different products or services, and thus can be thought of as having a large number (hundreds or even thousands) of individual activities. For example, most HMOs offer healthcare services to a large number of diverse groups of enrollees in numerous service areas, and many hospitals and hospital systems offer a large number of inpatient, outpatient, and even home health care services that cover a wide geographical area and treat a wide range of illnesses and injuries. Thus, healthcare managers operate a portfolio of individual products or services, or *projects*. Furthermore, when investors buy the stock of a healthcare business, they are really buying a portfolio of individual projects. So a well-diversified portfolio of 50 or more healthcare stocks is really a portfolio of tens of thousands of individual projects run by the firms whose stocks are held in the portfolio.

From this description, it is obvious that individual projects undertaken by investor-owned businesses actually reside in two different portfolios. First, a project is part of the business's overall portfolio of projects. For example, the Women's Center at North Florida Regional Medical Center is one of a thousand projects that make up HCA's portfolio of projects. Second, a project is one very small part of stockholders' well-diversified portfolios of security investments. Investors who own HCA stock own the Women's Center at North Florida Regional Medical Center along with thousands of other HCA projects, plus tens of thousands of projects owned by other firms in their stock portfolios.

Thus, the portfolio risk of a business project depends on one's perspective. A healthcare manager sees project riskiness from the standpoint of the business's portfolio of projects, while a stock investor sees the riskiness inherent in holding the project as part of a well-diversified stock portfolio. Because the context is different for each portfolio, the riskiness of a given project is also different. In the next two sections, these two types of portfolio risk are discussed in detail.

Corporate Risk: The Risk to Businesses

To begin, put your manager's hat on. What is the riskiness of a project to the business? Because the project is part of the business's portfolio of assets, and hence its diversifiable risk will be eliminated, stand-alone risk is **not** relevant. Rather, the relevant risk of a project to the business is its contribution to the business's overall risk, or the impact of the project on the variability of the business's overall rate of return. Some of the stand-alone riskiness of the project will be diversified away by combining the project with the business's other projects. The remaining portfolio risk, which uses the business's portfolio of projects as the benchmark, is called *corporate risk*.

To illustrate corporate risk, assume that Project P represents the expansion into a new service area by AtlantiCare, a for-profit HMO with many existing projects. Table 5.4 contains the estimated rate of return distributions both for Project P and for AtlantiCare as a whole. AtlantiCare's rate of return, like that of Project P, is uncertain and depends on future economic events. Overall, AtlantiCare's expected rate of return is 7.0 percent, with a standard deviation of 2.0 percent and a coefficient of variation of 0.3. Thus, looking at either the standard deviation or the coefficient of variation (stand-alone risk

TABLE 5.4
Estimated
Return
Distributions
for Project P
and AtlantiCare

State of the Economy	Probability of Occurrence	Rate of Return	
		Project P	AtlantiCare
Very poor	0.05	2.5%	1.0%
Poor	0.20	5.0	6.0
Average	0.50	10.0	7.0
Good	0.20	15.0	8.0
Very good	0.05	17.5	13.0
Expected return		10.0%	7.0%
Standard deviation		4.0%	2.0%
Coefficient of variation		0.4	0.3
Correlation coefficient		0.80	

measures), Project P is riskier than the HMO in the aggregate; that is, Project P is riskier than AtlantiCare's *average project*.

However, the relevant risk of Project P is not its stand-alone risk, but rather its contribution to AtlantiCare's overall riskiness. Project P's corporate risk depends not only on its standard deviation of returns, but also on the correlation between the returns on Project P and the returns on the HMO's average project (AtlantiCare's rate of return distribution). If Project P's returns were negatively correlated with the returns on AtlantiCare's other projects, which they are not, then accepting it would reduce the riskiness of the HMO's aggregate returns; and the larger Project P's standard deviation, the greater the risk reduction. (An economic state that results in a low return on AtlantiCare's average project would produce a high return on Project P, and vice versa, so the returns would offset one another and AtlantiCare's overall risk would be reduced.) In such a situation, Project P would actually have negative risk relative to the HMO's average project, in spite of its high stand-alone risk. In actuality, however, Project P's returns are positively correlated with AtlantiCare's aggregate returns, and the project has twice the standard deviation, so accepting it would increase the risk of AtlantiCare's aggregate returns.

The quantitative measure of a project's corporate risk is its *corporate beta*, or *corporate b*, which is the slope of the regression (scatter plot) line that results when the project's returns are plotted on the Y axis and the returns on the firm's average project are plotted on the X axis. Figure 5.2 contains this regression line, which is called the *corporate characteristic line*, for Project P. The slope (rise over run) of Project P's corporate characteristic line, which is Project P's corporate beta coefficient, is about 1.60, and it can be found algebraically as follows:

$$\text{Corporate } b_P = (\sigma_P/\sigma_F) \times r_{PF},$$

FIGURE 5.2
Corporate
Characteristic
Line for
Project P

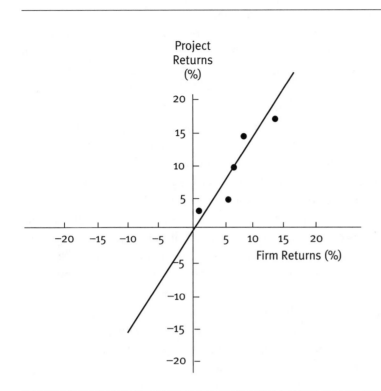

where

σ_P = standard deviation of Project P's returns,

σ_F = standard deviation of AtlantiCare's returns
(F stands for "firm"), and

r_{PF} = correlation coefficient between the returns on Project P
and AtlantiCare's returns.

Thus,

$$\text{Corporate } b_P = (4.0\%/2.0\%) \times 0.80 = 1.60.$$

A project's corporate beta measures the volatility of returns on the project **relative to the firm as a whole,** or relative to the firm's average project, which has a corporate beta of 1.0. (To estimate the corporate beta of the business's average project, the business's aggregate returns are plotted on both the X and Y axes, so the resulting slope of the corporate characteristic line is 1.0.)

If a project's corporate beta is 2.0, its returns are twice as volatile as the business's returns. Thus, if economic events lead to a 10 percent decrease in the business's profitability, the profitability of a project with a corporate beta of 2.0 would be expected to fall by 20 percent. Because of the higher relative volatility, adding such a project to the business will increase the overall volatility of the business's returns, and hence will increase the riskiness of the business. A corporate beta of 1.0 indicates that the project's returns have the same volatility as the business; and hence taking on the project would add identical risk to the business's existing projects. A corporate beta of 0.5 indicates that the project's returns are less volatile than the business's returns, so taking on the project would lower the overall risk of the business.

Finally, a negative corporate beta, which results when a project's returns are negatively correlated with the business's returns, indicates that the returns on the project move counter cyclical to the returns of the business. The addition of such a project to the business's portfolio of projects could reduce a firm's riskiness by a large amount (if the project is large enough). However, such projects are very hard to find because most projects are in a single line of business, or in related lines, so their returns are positively correlated.

With a corporate beta of 1.6, the returns on Project P are 1.6 times as volatile as the returns on AtlantiCare's average project. Thus, adding project P to AtlantiCare's portfolio of projects would increase the risk of the HMO, and hence Project P would be judged to have more corporate risk than AtlantiCare's average project. Note that Project P's stand-alone risk is twice as much as that of AtlantiCare (σ_P = 4% versus σ_F = 2%). However, Project P's corporate (portfolio) risk is only 1.6 times as much (b_P = 1.6 versus b_F = 1.0), so a large amount of Project P's stand-alone risk has been eliminated by portfolio effects.

Market Risk: The Risk to Owners (Stockholders)

The last section discussed the portfolio risk of projects as seen by the business. This section discusses the portfolio risk of projects as seen by the owners (for corporations, stockholders) of the business. Why should a healthcare manager be concerned about how a business's owners view risk? The answer is simple: Stock investors are the suppliers of equity capital to investor-owned businesses, so they set the rates of return that such businesses must pay to raise equity capital. These rates, in turn, set the minimum profitability that investor-owned businesses must earn on the equity portion of their real asset investments. Even managers of not-for-profit firms should have an understanding of how stock investors view risk because market-set required rates of return also establish the opportunity costs inherent in making not-for-profit investments. (We will have much more to say about this in Chapter 10.)

Because stock investors hold well-diversified portfolios of stocks, the relevant riskiness of an individual project undertaken by a business whose stock is held in the portfolio is its contribution to the overall riskiness of the portfolio. Thus, the riskiness of the Women's Center at North Florida Regional Medical Center to an individual investor who has a portfolio of 50 stocks, or to a trust officer who manages a 150-stock portfolio, or to a 500-stock mutual fund owner is the contribution that the project makes to the riskiness of the overall stock portfolio. Some of the stand-alone risk of the project will be diversified away by combining the project with all the other projects in the stock portfolio. The remaining portfolio risk is called *market risk*, which is defined as the contribution of a project to the riskiness of a well-diversified stock portfolio.

How should a project's market risk be measured? A project's *market beta*, or *market b*, measures the volatility of the project's returns relative to the returns on a well-diversified stock portfolio. Table 5.5 contains hypothetical estimates of the rate of return on a well-diversified portfolio of stocks, which is commonly called the *market portfolio*, or just *the market*, along with the returns on AtlantiCare's Project P. In practice, some stock index—say, the S&P 500 Index or the NYSE Index—is used as a proxy for the market portfolio. (The Standard & Poor's 500 is an index made up of 500 stocks across many industries, while the New York Stock Exchange Index is made up of the roughly 2,000 common stocks listed on the NYSE.)

The market beta of Project P is found by constructing the *market characteristic line* for the project, which is the regression (scatter plot) line that results from plotting the returns on Project P against the returns on the market. Project P's market characteristic line, which is shown in Figure 5.3, has a slope of 0.33, and hence Project P's market beta is 0.33.

Note that Project P's market beta can be calculated as follows:

$$\text{Market } b_P = (\sigma_P / \sigma_M) \times r_{PM},$$

where

σ_P = standard deviation of Project P's returns,

State of the Economy	Probability of Occurrence	Rate of Return		TABLE 5.5
		Project P	Market	Estimated Return Distributions
Very poor	0.05	2.5%	−15.0%	for Project P
Poor	0.20	5.0	5.0	and the Market
Average	0.50	10.0	15.0	
Good	0.20	15.0	25.0	
Very good	0.05	17.5	45.0	
Expected return		10.0%	15.0%	
Standard deviation		4.0%	11.4%	
Coefficient of variation		0.4	0.8	
Correlation coefficient			0.94	

FIGURE 5.3
Market
Characteristic
Line for Project
P

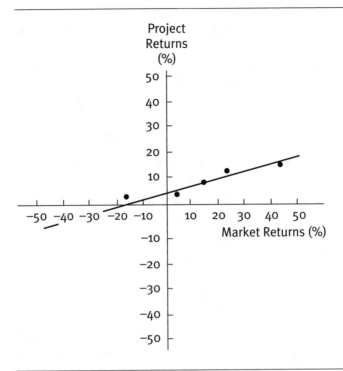

σ_M = standard deviation of the market's returns, and

r_{PM} = correlation coefficient of returns between Project P and the market.

Thus, using the data from Table 5.5,

$$\text{Market } b_P = (4.0\%/11.4\%) \times 0.94 = 0.33.$$

Project P's market beta measures its market risk, which is the risk relevant to AtlantiCare's well-diversified shareholders. Intuitively, a project's market beta measures the volatility of the project's returns relative to the returns on a well-diversified portfolio of stocks (the market portfolio), which has a beta of 1.0.

A project with a market beta of 2.0 has returns that are twice as volatile as the returns on the market, so adding it to a well-diversified portfolio will increase the portfolio's risk. A market beta of 1.0 indicates that the project's returns have the same volatility as the market, so adding such a project would have no impact on the riskiness of the market portfolio. A market beta of 0.5 indicates that the project's returns are half as volatile as the returns on the market, so adding such a project to a well-diversified portfolio would reduce its risk.

With a market beta of 0.33, Project P has only one-third the riskiness inherent in the market portfolio, and its acceptance by the HMO would reduce the riskiness of shareholder portfolios. (As you will see shortly, the beta of a portfolio is merely the weighted average of the betas of the individual components of the portfolio. Thus, adding a component with a lower beta than the portfolio average lowers the beta of the portfolio, and hence lowers the riskiness of the portfolio.)

As in our discussion of corporate risk, a negative market beta indicates that the returns on the project move countercyclically to the returns on the market—when the market's return goes up, the project's return goes down, and vice versa. Negative beta projects are valuable to stockholders because of their risk-reduction characteristics. However, negative market beta projects are rare because most projects' returns, as well as the market's returns, are positively correlated with the economy as a whole.

Note that Project P's stand-alone risk is about 35 percent of that of the market ($\sigma_P = 4\%$ versus $\sigma_M = 11.4\%$). However, Project P's portfolio (market) risk is only 33 percent as much as the market ($b_P = 0.33$ versus $b_M = 1.0$), so only a small amount of Project P's stand-alone risk has been eliminated by portfolio effects.[3]

Self-Test Questions

1. A project in a for-profit business is held as part of what two portfolios?
2. How is corporate risk defined?
3. What is a corporate beta and how is it determined?
4. How is market risk defined?
5. What is a market beta and how is it determined?

Portfolio Risk of Stocks (Entire Businesses)

Even though an individual investor's stock portfolio can be thought of as a portfolio of many separate projects, the portfolio actually consists of the stocks of firms, so individual investors are most concerned with the aggregate risk and return characteristics of the firms themselves. Thus, individual investors are concerned with the stock's market beta rather than the market betas of individual projects. A stock's market beta is the slope of the market characteristic line formed by regressing the business's aggregate returns against market returns. For example, using the data in Tables 5.4 and 5.5, we find AtlantiCare's market beta to be 0.17. Because the average stock has a market beta of 1.0, AtlantiCare's market beta is very low, and adding the stock of AtlantiCare to a well-diversified portfolio would tend to lower the overall riskiness of the portfolio.

When individual investors assess the riskiness of individual stocks, the relevant measure is the stock's market beta, and the reference value is the market portfolio's overall beta of 1.0. When investor-owned firms conduct project market risk analyses, the question that is relevant to managers is: How does the project's market risk compare to the market risk of the firm's average project? This question is answered by comparing the project's market beta to the business's market beta. Our illustrative Project P, with a market beta of 0.33, has significantly more market risk than AtlantiCare's average project, which has a market beta of only 0.17. Thus, although the market risk of Project P is quite low, the project's market risk relative to the market risk of the entire business is high.

1. What is the difference between a project's market beta and the business's, or stock's, market beta?

Portfolio Betas

Individual investors hold portfolios of stocks, each with its own market risk as measured by the stock's market beta coefficient, while businesses hold portfolios of projects, each with its own corporate and market betas. What impact does the beta of a portfolio component have on the overall portfolio's beta? The beta of any portfolio of investments is simply the weighted average of the individual investments' betas:

$$b_{Portfolio} = (w_1 \times b_1) + (w_2 \times b_2) + (w_3 \times b_3) + (w_i \times b_i) \text{ and so on.}$$

Here, $b_{Portfolio}$ is the beta of the portfolio, which measures the volatility of the entire portfolio; w_i is the fraction of the portfolio invested in each particular asset; and b_i is the beta coefficient of that asset.

To illustrate the concept, consider the following example. HCA might have a market beta of 1.2, which indicates that the returns on its stock are slightly more volatile than the returns on a well-diversified portfolio (with a beta of 1.0), and hence the stock is somewhat riskier than the average stock. But each project within HCA has its own market risk, as measured by each project's market beta. Some projects may have very high market betas, say, over 1.5, while other projects may have very low market betas, say, under 0.5. When all of the projects are combined, the overall market beta of the firm is 1.2. For ease of illustration, assume that HCA has only the following three projects:

Project	Market Beta	Dollar Investment	Proportion
A	0.5	$ 15,000	15.0%
B	1.0	30,000	30.0
C	1.5	55,000	55.0
		$100,000	100.0%

The weighted average of the project market betas, which is the firm's market beta, is 1.2:

$$b_{Portfolio} = (0.15 \times 0.5) + (0.30 \times 1.0) + (0.55 \times 1.5)$$
$$= 1.20.$$

Note that each project within HCA's fictitious portfolio of three projects also has a corporate beta that measures the volatility of the project's returns relative to that of the overall business. The weighted average of these project corporate betas must equal 1.00, which is the corporate beta of any business.

1. How is the beta of a portfolio related to the individual betas of the investments that make up the portfolio?

Self-Test Question

Relevance of the Risk Measures

Thus far, the chapter has discussed in some detail three measures of financial risk—stand-alone, corporate, and market—but it is still unclear which risk is the most relevant in financial decision making. It turns out that the risk that is relevant to any financial decision depends on the particular situation at hand. When the decision involves a single investment that will be held in isolation, stand-alone risk is the relevant risk. Here, the risk and return on the portfolio is the same as the risk and return on the single asset in the portfolio. In this situation, the riskiness faced by the investor, whether it be an individual considering a stock purchase or a business considering a MRI system investment, is defined in terms of returns less than expected, and the appropriate measure is the standard deviation or coefficient of variation of the return distribution.

In most decisions, however, the investment under consideration will not be held in isolation, but rather will be held as part of an investment portfolio. Individual investors normally hold portfolios of stocks, while businesses normally hold portfolios of real asset investments (projects). Thus, it is clear that portfolio risk is more relevant to real-world decisions than is stand-alone risk. However, there are three distinct ownership situations that affect the relevancy of portfolio risk.

Large Investor-Owned Businesses

For large investor-owned businesses, the primary financial goal is shareholder wealth maximization. This means that managerial decisions should focus on risk and return as seen by the business's stockholders. Because stockholders tend to hold large portfolios of securities, and hence a very large portfolio of individual projects, the most relevant risk of a project under consideration by a large for-profit firm is the project's contribution to a well-diversified stock portfolio (the market portfolio). Of course, this is the project's market risk. Many would argue, and we agree, that corporate and stand-alone risk cannot be disregarded in all situations. For example, corporate risk, which best measures the impact of the project on the financial condition of the business, clearly is relevant to the business's other stakeholders, such as managers, employees, creditors, and suppliers, who should not be totally ignored. Also, the failure of a project that is large, relative to the business, could bring down the entire firm. Under such circumstances, the project clearly has high risk to stockholders even if its market risk is low. The bottom line here is that market risk should be of primary importance in large investor-owned businesses, but corporate and stand-alone risk should not be ignored.

Small Investor-Owned Businesses

For small investor-owned businesses, the situation is more complicated. Take, for example, a three-physician group practice. Here, there is no separation between management and ownership and the equity investment position is complicated by the fact that the business is also the owners' employer. In this situation, the primary goal of the business is more likely to be maximization of the owners' overall well-being rather than strict shareholder wealth maximization. For example, owner/managers may value leisure time, as exemplified by three afternoons of golf, as being more important than additional wealth creation. To complicate the situation even more, shareholder wealth consists of both the value of the ownership position and the professional fees (salaries) derived from the business.

Thus, in small for-profit businesses, corporate risk is probably more relevant than market risk. The owner/managers would not want to place the viability of the business in jeopardy just to increase their expected ownership value by a small amount. Put another way, the owner/managers are not well diversified in regards to the business because a large proportion of their wealth comes from future employment earnings. Because of this, market risk loses relevance and corporate risk becomes most important. However, the potential relevancy of stand-alone risk as described in the previous section also applies.

Not-for-Profit Businesses

Not-for-profit businesses do not have stockholders, and their goals stem from a mission statement that generally involves service to society. In this situation, market risk clearly is not relevant; the concern to managers is the impact of the project on the riskiness of the business, which is measured by a project's corporate risk. Thus, the risk measure most relevant here is corporate risk. Again, however, the stand-alone risk of large projects that could sink the business is relevant.

Self-Test Question

1. Explain the situations in which each of the risk types—stand-alone, corporate, and market risk—are relevant.

Interpretation of the Risk Measures

It is important to recognize that none of the risk measures discussed can be interpreted without some standard of reference. For example, if we are focusing on stand-alone risk, does Project P's coefficient of variation of returns of 0.4 indicate high risk, low risk, or moderate risk? We don't know the answer without more information. However, knowing that AtlantiCare in the aggregate has a coefficient of variation of returns of 0.3 enables us to state that Project P has more stand-alone risk than the HMO's average project.

Similarly, Project P's corporate beta of 1.6, when compared to Atlanti-Care's overall corporate beta of 1.0 (by definition), indicates that the project has above-average corporate risk. Similarly, Project P's market beta of 0.33, when compared to AtlantiCare's market beta of 0.17, indicates that the project has above-average market risk. The point to remember is that in practice risk is always interpreted against some standard because without a standard it is impossible to make judgments.

Which risk is most relevant to AtlantiCare? As discussed in the previous section, market risk is most relevant because AtlantiCare is a large investor-owned business, and hence managers should be most concerned about the impact of new projects on stockholders' risk.

1. How are risk measures interpreted?

Self-Test Question

The Relationship Between Risk and Return

This chapter contains a great deal of discussion that focuses on defining and measuring financial risk. However, being able to define and measure financial risk is of no value in financial decision making unless risk can be related to return; that is, the answer to this question is needed: How much return is required to compensate investors for assuming a given level of risk? In this section, we focus on setting required rates of return on stock investments because the basic theory of risk and return was developed for stock investments. However, in later chapters the focus will be on setting required rates of return on individual projects within firms.

The relationship between the market risk of a stock, as measured by its market beta, and its required rate of return is given by the *Capital Asset Pricing Model (CAPM)*. To begin, some basic definitions are needed:

- $E(R_i)$ = Expected rate of return on Stock i, any stock.
- $R(R_i)$ = Required rate of return on Stock i. If $E(R_i)$ is less $R(R_i)$, the stock should not be purchased or it should be sold if it was owned. If $E(R_i)$ was greater than $R(R_i)$, the stock should be bought, and an individual should be indifferent about the purchase if $E(R_i) = R(R_i)$.
- RF = Risk-free rate of return. In a CAPM context, RF is generally measured by the return on long-term U.S. Treasury bonds.
- b_i = Market beta coefficient of Stock i. The market beta of an average-risk stock is $b_A = 1.0$.
- $R(R_M)$ = Required rate of return on a portfolio that consists of all stocks, which is the market portfolio. $R(R_M)$ is also the required rate of return on an average ($b_A = 1.0$) stock.

- RP_M = Market risk premium = $R(R_M) - RF$. This is the additional return over the risk-free rate required to compensate investors for assuming average ($b_A = 1.0$) risk.
- RP_i = Risk premium on Stock i = $[R(R_M) - RF] \times b_i = RP_M \times b_i$. Stock i's risk premium is less than, equal to, or greater than the premium on an average stock, depending on whether its beta is less than, equal to, or greater than 1.0. If $b_i = b_A = 1.0$, then $RP_i = RP_M$.

Using these definitions, the CAPM relationship between risk and required rate of return is given by the following equation, which is called the *Security Market Line (SML)*:

$$R(R_i) = RF + (R[R_M] - RF) \times b_i$$
$$= RF + (RP_M \times b_i).$$

To illustrate use of the SML, assume that the risk-free rate (RF) is 6 percent; the required rate of return on the market, $R[R_M]$, is 10 percent; and the market beta of Regis Healthcare is 1.1. According to the SML, the required rate of return on Regis stock is 10.4 percent:

$$R(R_{Regis}) = 6\% + (10\% - 6\%) \times 1.1$$
$$= 6\% + (4\% \times 1.1)$$
$$= 6\% + 4.4\% = 10.4\%.$$

If the expected rate of return, $E(R_{Regis})$, were 15 percent, investors should buy the stock because $E(R_{Regis})$ is greater than $R(R_{Regis})$. Conversely, if the expected rate of return were $E(R_{Regis}) = 8\%$, investors should sell the stock because $E(R_{Regis})$ is less than $R(R_{Regis})$.

A stock with a beta of 2.0, one that is riskier than Regis Healthcare, would have a required rate of return of 14 percent:

$$R(R_{b=2.0}) = 6\% + (4\% \times 2.0)$$
$$= 6\% + 8\% = 14\%$$

while an average stock, with $b_i = 1.0$, would have a required return of 10 percent, which is the same as the market return:

$$R(R_{b=1.0}) = 6\% + (4\% \times 1.0)$$
$$= 6\% + 4\% = 10\% = R(R_M).$$

A stock with below-average risk, for example, $b_i = 0.5$, would have a required return of 8 percent:

$$R(R_{b=0.5}) = 6\% + (4\% \times 0.5)$$
$$= 6\% + 2\% = 8\%.$$

The market risk premium, RP_M, depends on the degree of aversion that investors in the aggregate have to risk. In this example, T-bonds yielded RF = 6%, and an average share of stock had a required rate of return of $R(R_M)$ = 10%, so RP_M is 4 percentage points. If the degree of risk aversion increased, $R(R_M)$ might increase to 12 percent, which would cause RP_M to increase to 6 percentage points. Thus, the greater the overall degree of risk aversion, the higher the required rate on the market, and hence the higher the required rates of return on all stocks.

Also, values for the risk-free rate, RF, and the required rate of return on the market, $R(R_M)$, are influenced by inflation expectations. The higher the expectations of investors regarding inflation, the greater these values; hence, the greater the required rates of return on all stocks.

The SML is often expressed in graphical form, as in Figure 5.4, which shows the SML when RF = 6% and $R(R_M)$ = 10%. Here are the relevant points concerning the figure:

- Required rates of return are shown on the vertical axis, while risk as measured by market beta is shown on the horizontal axis.
- Riskless securities have b_i = 0; therefore, RF is the vertical axis intercept.
- The slope of the SML reflects the degree of risk aversion in the economy. The greater the average investor's aversion to risk (1) the steeper the slope of the SML, (2) the greater the risk premium for any stock, and (3) the higher the required rate of return on stocks.
- The Y axis intercept reflects the level of expected inflation. The higher

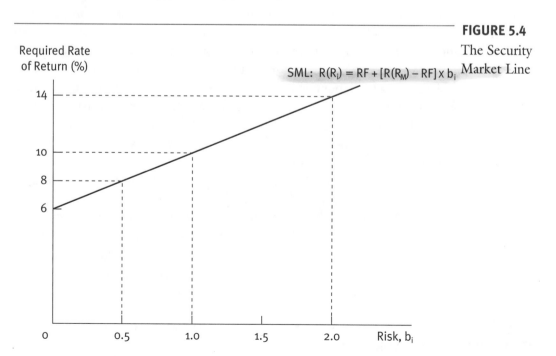

FIGURE 5.4

The Security Market Line

inflation expectations, the greater both RF and R(R$_M$). Thus, the higher the SML plots on the graph.

- The values previously calculated for the required rates of return on stocks with b$_i$ = 0.5, b$_i$ = 1.0, and b$_i$ = 2.0 agree with the values shown on the graph.

Both the SML and a firm's position on it change over time because of changes in interest rates, investors' risk aversion, and individual firm's betas. Thus, the SML, as well as a firm's risk, must be evaluated on the basis of current information. The SML, its use, and how its input values are estimated are covered in greater detail in Chapter 10.

Self-Test Questions

1. What is the Capital Asset Pricing Model (CAPM)?
2. What is the appropriate measure of risk in the CAPM?
3. Write out the equation for the Security Market Line (SML) and graph it.
4. Describe the SML.

Some Thoughts About Beta and the CAPM

The Capital Asset Pricing Model (CAPM) is more than just an abstract theory described in textbooks. It is widely used by analysts, investors, and corporate managers. However, despite its intuitive appeal, a number of serious concerns have surfaced concerning the CAPM. First, it is built on a very restrictive set of assumptions that does not conform well to real-world conditions. Second, it has been shown that it is impossible to prove; that is, studies that do demonstrate the linear relationship between market risk and required return prove nothing because the results stem from the mathematical properties of the model and not because it is theoretically correct. Third, some studies find no relationship between stocks' returns and market betas. Finally, the market betas that are actually used in the CAPM measure the historical relative volatility of a stock but conditions often change, so its future volatility, which is of real concern to investors, might be quite different from its past volatility.

In spite of these concerns, the CAPM is extremely appealing because it is simple and logical. It focuses on the impact that a single investment has on a portfolio, which in most situations is the correct way to think about risk. Furthermore, it tells us that the required rate of return on an investment is composed of the risk-free rate, which compensates investors for time value, plus a risk premium that is a function of investors' attitudes toward risk bearing in the aggregate and the specific portfolio risk of the investment being evaluated. Because of these points, the CAPM is an important conceptual tool. However, its actual use to set required rates of return must be viewed with some caution. We will have more to say about this in Chapter 10.

Self-Test Question

1. What are the pros and cons regarding the Capital Asset Pricing Model (CAPM)?

Earnings Volatility Versus Risk

Before closing this chapter, we should note the difference between earnings volatility and risk. Sun Coast Healthcare, an investor-owned hospital in Palm Beach, Florida, has a great deal of earnings volatility that stems from its highly seasonal business. Its volume, and hence revenues and earnings, is much higher in the winter months than in the summer months. However, this volatility does **not** constitute risk because it is predictable, so Sun Coast's stock price is not affected by the earnings volatility. Furthermore, if earnings during a peak winter season fell below expectations because of unusually warm weather in the Northeast, Sun Coast's stock price would not fall very much because the earnings drop would be correctly interpreted as a random event.

However, consider what would happen if a brand new competing hospital opened in the same service area. If peak earnings at Sun Coast were lower than expected because of the new competition, investors would perceive that normal volatility was not the cause, but rather long-term factors that had the potential to permanently lower Sun Coast's earnings stream were at work. In this situation, the stock price probably would fall significantly.

Note, however, that stock price volatility does imply risk because stock price volatility stems from uncertainty in future earnings. The bottom line here is that earnings volatility does not necessarily imply risk because predictable volatility is not risk. However, unpredictable volatility does imply risk because unpredictable earnings will lead to an unpredictable stock price.

1. What is the difference between earnings volatility and risk?

Self-Test Question

Key Concepts

This chapter has covered the very important concepts of financial risk and return. Here are its key concepts:

- Risk definition and measurement are very important in financial management because decision makers, in general, are *risk averse*, and hence require higher returns from investments that have higher risk.
- *Financial risk* is associated with the prospect of returns less than anticipated. The higher the probability of a return being far less than anticipated, the greater the risk.
- The riskiness of investments held in isolation, called *stand-alone risk*, can be measured by the dispersion of the rate of return distribution about its *expected value*. One commonly used measure of stand-alone risk is the *standard deviation* of the return distribution.
- Most investments are not held in isolation, but rather as part of *portfolios*. Individual investors hold portfolios of securities and businesses hold portfolios of projects (i.e., products and services).

- When investments with returns that are less than perfectly positively correlated are combined in a portfolio, risk is reduced. The risk reduction occurs because less-than-expected returns on some investments are offset by greater-than-expected returns on other investments. However, among real-world investments, it is impossible to eliminate all risk because the returns on all assets are influenced to a greater or lesser degree by overall economic conditions.
- The portion of the stand-alone risk of an investment that can be eliminated by holding the investment in a portfolio is called *diversifiable risk*, while the risk that remains is called *portfolio risk*.
- There are two different types of portfolio risk. *Corporate risk* is the riskiness of business projects when they are considered as part of a business's portfolio of projects. *Market risk* is the riskiness of business projects, or of the stocks of entire businesses, when they are considered as part of an individual investor's well-diversified portfolio of securities.
- Corporate risk is measured by a project's *corporate beta*, which reflects the volatility of the project's returns relative to the volatility of returns of the aggregate business.
- Market risk is measured by a project's, or stock's, *market beta*, which reflects the volatility of a project's, or stock's, returns relative to the volatility of returns on a well-diversified stock portfolio.
- *Stand-alone risk* is most relevant to investments held in isolation; *corporate risk* is most relevant to projects held by not-for-profit businesses and by small investor-owned businesses; and *market risk* is most relevant to projects held by large investor-owned firms.
- The *overall beta coefficient of a portfolio* is the weighted average of the betas of the components of the portfolio, where the weights are the proportion of the overall investment in each component. Therefore, the weighted average of corporate betas of all projects in a business must equal 1.0, while the weighted average of all projects' market betas must equal the market beta of the firm's stock.
- The *Capital Asset Pricing Model (CAPM)* is an equilibrium model that describes the relationship between market risk and required rates of return.
- The *Security Market Line (SML)* provides the actual risk/required rate of return relationship. The required rate of return on any Stock i is equal to the risk-free rate plus the market risk premium times the stock's market beta coefficient: $R(R_i) = RF + [R(R_M) - RF)] \times b_i = RF + (RP_M \times b_i)$.

This concludes our discussion of basic financial management concepts, which included time value analysis, financial risk, and required rate of return. The next chapter—Debt Financing—begins our coverage of capital acquisition.

Selected References

For a more complete discussion of financial risk, see Eugene F. Brigham, Louis C. Gapenski, and Michael C. Ehrhardt. 1999. *Financial Management: Theory and Practice*. Fort Worth, TX: Dryden Press, Chapters 5 and 6.

Selected Web Sites

There are a multitude of web sites that pertain to this chapter.

For stock market betas, see Market Guide at *www.marketguide.com*. Then, in the Search For box, enter the stock symbol for a firm (for example, HCA for HCA—The Healthcare Company) then click on Go. The firm's profile will appear. Beta is given under the Key Ratios and Statistics (Price and Volume) section.

Try *www.financialweb.com/rshindex.asp*. Then, under Search, type in the stock symbol and click on Go. Finally, under Fundamentals, click on Detailed Company Profile. Beta can be found in the Additional Information section.

Try Morningstar for information about the riskiness of mutual funds at *www. morningstar.com*. Then, click on Funds on the menu bar. Next, type in a fund symbol—for example, VFINX for the Vanguard 500 Index Fund—then click on Go. Finally, click on Ratings and Risk, which appears in the left column. The next screen will display several risk (volatility) measures including standard deviation.

Selected Cases

The following case in *Cases in Healthcare Finance* can be assigned to help students learn more about financial risk concepts:

Case 10: Academic Group Practice, Inc., which illustrates many of the concepts discussed in this chapter.

Notes

1. A portfolio of two investments will have lower risk than that of either one only when the correlation coefficient between the returns on the two investments is less than the ratio of the standard deviations constructed with the lower standard deviation in the numerator. For example, for Portfolio AD to have less risk than both A and D, the correlation coefficient between the returns on A and D must be less than $\sigma_A/\sigma_D = 11.0\%/12.1\% = 0.91$. The actual correlation coefficient is 0.53, so the condition is met in this example.
2. Although stocks actually can be combined with complex investments (derivatives) to form riskless portfolios, our emphasis here is on real-assets investments.
3. The amount of risk reduction that occurs when an asset is added to a portfolio is measured by the distance of the plot points from the characteristic line. The more the points plot away from the line, the greater the risk reduction when the

investment is added to the portfolio. In other words, the distance of the plot points from the line measures the amount of diversifiable risk. In this illustration, the points are farther from the line in Figure 5.2 than in Figure 5.3, so more risk reduction occurs when Project P is added to the corporate portfolio than when it is added to the market portfolio.

Capital Acquisition

DEBT FINANCING

Learning Objectives

After studying this chapter, readers should be able to:

- Describe how interest rates are set in the economy.
- Discuss the various types of debt, including both long-term and short-term, and their features.
- Discuss credit ratings and their importance.
- Explain the term structure of interest rates and its implications.
- Discuss the components that make up the interest rate on a debt security.

Introduction

If a business is to operate, it must have assets, and to acquire assets, it must raise *capital*. Capital comes in two basic forms: debt and equity. This chapter focuses on debt financing, while Chapter 7 focuses on equity financing. To illustrate the importance of debt financing to healthcare businesses, *Value Line* reports that, on average, providers finance their assets with roughly 5 percent short-term debt, 30 percent long-term debt, and 65 percent equity. Thus, over one-third of providers' financing comes from debt. In this chapter, many facets of debt financing are discussed, including important background information on how interest rates are set in the economy.

Unfortunately, the term "debt" can be interpreted in two ways. First, debt can refer to everything on the right side of a balance sheet that is not equity, including both interest-bearing debt and noninterest-bearing liabilities such as accruals and trade credit (accounts payable). For some purposes, this all-inclusive definition is appropriate. Second, debt can refer only to interest-bearing debt supplied by *creditors* such as banks and bondholders. For purposes of this chapter, we will use the second definition and confine our discussion to interest-bearing debt. Other types of liabilities, specifically accruals and trade credit, will be discussed in Chapter 16.

The Cost of Money

Capital in a free economy is allocated through the price system. The *interest rate* is the price paid to obtain debt capital, whereas in the case of equity capital in for-profit firms, investors' returns come in the form of *dividends* and *capital gains* or *losses*. The four most fundamental factors that affect the supply of and demand for investment capital, and hence the cost of money, are (1) investment opportunities, (2) time preferences for consumption, (3) risk, and (4) inflation.

To see how these factors operate, visualize the situation facing Lori Gibbs, an entrepreneur who is planning to start a new home health agency. Lori does not have sufficient personal funds to finance the business, so she must go to the debt markets for additional capital. If Lori estimates that the business will be highly profitable, she will be able to pay creditors a higher interest rate than if it is barely profitable. Thus, her ability to pay for borrowed capital depends on the business's *investment opportunities*. The higher the profitability of the business, the higher the interest rate that Lori can afford to pay lenders for use of their savings.

The interest rate that lenders will charge depends, in large part, on their *time preferences for consumption*. For example, one potential lender, Jane Wright, may be saving for retirement, so she may be willing to loan funds at a relatively low rate because her preference is for future consumption. Another person, John Davis, may have a wife and several young children to clothe and feed, so he may be willing to lend funds out of current income, and hence forgo consumption, only if the interest rate is very high. John is said to have a high time preference for consumption and Jane a low time preference. If the entire population of an economy were living right at the subsistence level, time preferences for current consumption would necessarily be high, aggregate savings would be low, interest rates would be high, and capital formation would be difficult.

The *risk* inherent in the prospective home health care business, and thus in Lori's ability to repay the loan, would also affect the return that lenders would require—the higher the perceived risk, the higher the interest rate. Investors would be unwilling to lend to high-risk businesses unless the interest rate was higher than on loans to low-risk businesses.

Finally, because the value of money in the future is affected by *inflation*, the higher the expected rate of inflation, the higher the interest rate demanded by savers. Note that to simplify matters, the illustration implied that savers would lend directly to businesses that need capital, but in most cases the funds would actually pass through a *financial intermediary* such as a bank or mutual fund.

Self-Test Questions

1. What is the "price" of debt capital?
2. What four factors affect the cost of money?

Interest Rate Levels

Like any free market, debt markets set prices on the basis of supply and demand. To illustrate the process, consider Figure 6.1, which shows how supply and demand interact in two debt markets—A and B. The going interest rate, designated I, is initially 10 percent for the low-risk securities in Market A. Borrowers whose credit is strong enough to qualify for this market can obtain funds at a cost of 10 percent. Riskier borrowers must obtain higher-cost funds in Market B. Investors who are more willing to take risks invest in Market B and expect to receive a 12 percent return, but also realize that they might receive much less if the borrower fails.

If the demand for funds in a market declines, as it typically does during a business recession, the demand curves will shift to the left, as shown in Curve D_2 in Market A. The market-clearing, or equilibrium, interest rate in

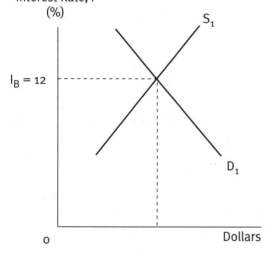

FIGURE 6.1

Interest Rates as a Funciton of Supply and Demand for Funds

this example declines to 8 percent. Similarly, you should be able to visualize what would happen if the Federal Reserve tightened credit: The supply curve, S_1, would shift to the left, which would raise interest rates and lower the level of borrowing in the economy.

Debt markets, indeed all capital markets, are interdependent. For example, if Markets A and B were in equilibrium before the demand shift to D_2 in Market A, then investors were willing to accept the higher risk in Market B in exchange for a *risk premium* of 12% − 10% = 2 percentage points. After the shift to D_2, the risk premium would initially increase to 12% − 8% = 4 percentage points. In all likelihood, this much larger premium would induce some of the lenders in Market A to move to Market B, which, in turn, would cause the supply curve in Market A to shift to the left, or up, and the supply curve in Market B to shift to the right. This transfer of capital between markets would raise the interest rate in Market A and lower it in Market B, thus bringing the risk premium back closer to its original level—2 percentage points.

There are many capital markets in the United States, including markets for short-term debt (*money markets*) and for long-term debt and equity (*capital markets*). These markets are further broken down into markets for home loans; farm loans; business loans for both taxable and tax-exempt firms; federal, state, and local government loans; and consumer loans. Within each category, there are regional markets as well as different types of submarkets. For example, within the business sector there are dozens of types of debt and also several sharply differentiated markets for common stocks. There is a price for each type of capital, and these prices change over time as shifts occur in supply and demand conditions.

Self-Test Questions

1. How do interest rates serve to allocate debt capital among borrowers?
2. How does risk affect interest rates?
3. What happens to the market-clearing, or equilibrium, interest rate when the loan demand changes?

Long-Term Debt

One of the most important ways of categorizing debt is by *maturity*, or the length of the loan. In general, debt is categorized as long-term or short-term. Although the definitions of "long" and "short" depend somewhat on the type of debt under discussion, in most situations *short-term debt* is defined as having a maturity of one year or less, while *long-term debt* has maturities greater than one year. Even when the focus is solely on long-term debt, there are still hundreds, if not more, different types. In this section, we briefly discuss the long-term debt instruments most commonly used by healthcare businesses.

Term Loans

A *term loan* is a contract under which a borrower agrees to make a series of payments, on specified dates, to the lender. These payments consist of *principal*, which pays back the amount borrowed, and *interest*, which provides the return to the lender for the use of the capital. In general, term loans are negotiated directly between the borrowing firm and a financial institution—generally, a bank, a mutual fund, an insurance company, or a pension fund. Thus, term loans are *private placements* as opposed to *public offerings*, which are typically used on bonds—the other major type of long-term debt. (The details of how securities are issued by businesses is discussed in Chapter 7.)

Most term loans have maturities in the range of two to seven years, with an average of about four years. Term loans usually are amortized in equal installments over the life of the loan, so part of the principal of the loan is retired with each payment. For example, Sacramento Cardiology Group has a $100,000 five-year term loan with Bank of America to fund the purchase of new diagnostic equipment. The interest rate on the fixed-rate loan is 10 percent, which obligates the Group to five end-of-year payments of $26,379.75. Thus, loan payments total $131,898.75, of which $31,898.75 is interest and $100,000 is repayment of principal.

Term loans have three major advantages over debt sold to the general public: (1) speed, (2) flexibility, and (3) low issuance costs. Because they are negotiated directly between the lender and the borrower, formal documentation is minimized. The key provisions of the loan can be worked out much more quickly, and with more flexibility, than can those for a public issue, and it is not necessary for a term loan to go through a complicated registration process. A further advantage of term loans over publicly held debt has to do with future flexibility. If many different investors hold a debt issue, it is virtually impossible to alter the terms of the agreement, even though new economic conditions may make such changes desirable. With a term loan, the borrower can generally negotiate with the lender to work out modifications in the contract.

The interest rate on a term loan can be either fixed for the life of the loan or variable. If fixed, the rate used will be close to the rate on bonds of equivalent maturity for firms of comparable risk. If variable, the rate is usually set at a certain number of percentage points over an index rate, such as the prime rate or the T-bill rate.[1] Then, when the index rate goes up or down, so does the rate on the outstanding balance of the term loan.

Although term loans have many advantages, there are two potential disadvantages. First, there is a limit to the size of a term loan. Although they can be quite large, such as when multiple banks combine to make a loan of $100 million or more, most term loans are relatively small, with an average of less than one million dollars. Also, lenders typically will not extend term loans to the maturity that businesses can attain in a bond financing, which makes term loans inappropriate for use in financing assets with long lives, such as clinic buildings or hospital wings.

Corporate Bonds

Like a term loan, a *bond* is a long-term contract under which a borrower agrees to make payments of interest and principal, on specific dates, to the holder of the bond. Although bonds are similar in some ways to term loans, a bond issue generally is registered with the Securities and Exchange Commission (SEC), advertised, offered to the public through investment bankers, and actually sold to many different investors. Indeed, thousands of individual and institutional investors may participate when a firm, such as HCA, sells a bond issue, while there is generally only one lender in the case of a term loan.

Bonds are categorized as either government (Treasury), corporate, or municipal. *Government*, or *Treasury, bonds* are issued by the U.S. Treasury and are used to raise money for the federal government.[2] *Corporate bonds* are issued by investor-owned firms, while *municipal bonds* are issued by governments and governmental agencies other than federal. In this section, the primary focus is on corporate bonds, but much of the discussion also is relevant to municipal bonds. The unique features of municipal bonds will be discussed in the next major section.

Although bonds generally have maturities in the range of 20 to 30 years, shorter maturities, as well as longer maturities, are occasionally used. In fact, in 1995, HCA issued $200 million of 100-year bonds, following the issuance of 100-year bonds by Disney and Coca-Cola in 1993. These ultra-long term bonds had not been used by any firm since the 1920s. Unlike term loans, bonds usually pay only interest over the life of the bond, with the entire amount of principal returned to lenders at maturity.

Most bonds have *fixed* interest rates, which locks in the current rate for the entire maturity of the bond, and hence minimizes interest payment uncertainty. However, some bonds have *floating, or variable, rates* that are tied to some interest rate index, so the interest payments move up and down with the general level of interest rates. Floating rate bonds are more prevalent when rates are high, or when the yield curve—which we discuss in a later section—has a steep upward slope, or both. In early 2000, A-rated investor-owned hospitals had to pay 7.9 percent on long-term, fixed rate bonds, but only had to pay 6.0 percent on floating rate bonds. Of course, floating rate bonds are riskier to the issuer because interest rates could rise in the future, but virtually all such debt has call provisions—which we discuss later—that permit issuers to replace the floating rate debt with fixed rate debt should conditions so dictate.

Mortgage Bonds   With a *mortgage bond*, the issuer pledges certain real assets as security for the bond. To illustrate the concept, consider the following example. Mid-Texas Healthcare System recently needed $50 million to purchase land and to build a new hospital. *First mortgage bonds* in the amount of $20 million, secured by a mortgage on the property, were issued. If the firm defaults on the bonds, the bondholders could foreclose on the hospital and sell it to satisfy their claims.

Mid-Texas could, if it so chose, also issue *second mortgage bonds* secured by the same $50 million hospital. In the event of bankruptcy and liquidation, the holders of these second mortgage bonds would have a claim against the property only after the first mortgage bondholders had been paid off in full. Thus, second mortgages are sometimes called *junior mortgages*, or *junior liens*, because they are junior in priority to claims of senior mortgages, or first mortgage bonds.

A *debenture* is an unsecured bond, and as such, it has no lien against specific **Debentures** property as security for the obligation. For example, Mid-Texas Healthcare System has $5 million of debentures outstanding. These bonds are not secured by real property, but are backed instead by the revenue-producing power of the corporation. Debenture holders are, therefore, general creditors whose claims, in the event of bankruptcy, are protected by property not otherwise pledged. In practice, the use of debentures depends on the nature of the firm's assets and general credit strength. If a firm's credit position is exceptionally strong, it can issue debentures—it simply does not need specific security. Debentures are also issued by firms with only a small amount of assets suitable as collateral. Finally, firms that have used up their capacity to borrow in the lower-cost mortgage market may be forced to use higher-cost debentures.

The term *subordinate* means "below" or "inferior." Thus, *subordinated debt* **Subordinated** has a claim on assets in the event of bankruptcy only after senior debt has **debentures** been paid off. Debentures may be subordinated either to designated notes payable—usually bank loans—or to all other debt. In the event of liquidation, holders of subordinated debentures cannot be paid until senior debt, as named in the debenture, has been paid. Subordinated debentures are normally quite risky, and hence carry interest rates that are much higher than the rate on top-quality debt.

1. Describe the primary features of the following long-term debt securities: **Self-Test**
   a. Term loan   **Question**
   b. Corporate bond
   c. First mortgage bond; junior mortgage
   d. Debenture; subordinated debenture

Municipal Bonds

Whereas corporate bonds are issued by investor-owned businesses, *municipal bonds,* or "munis," are issued by states and their political subdivisions, including counties and cities. Although most municipal bonds are backed by the taxing power of the issuing entity, *revenue bonds* are backed by the revenues derived from facilities, such as toll roads and airports, deemed to be beneficial to the community. In addition, not-for-profit healthcare providers are legally entitled to issue such securities through government-sponsored healthcare financing authorities.

Because the interest on municipal debt is exempt from federal income taxes, as well as state income taxes in the state of issue, investors are willing to accept lower interest rates on such debt than on comparable-risk taxable debt. To illustrate the concept, consider that in early 2000, the interest rate on an AAA-rated, long-term corporate bond was 7.4 percent, while the rate on a similar-risk healthcare muni was 6.2 percent. To an individual investor in the 40 percent federal-plus-state tax bracket, the muni bond's equivalent taxable yield is $6.2\%/(1 - 0.40) = 6.2\%/0.6 = 10.3\%$, or almost 3 percentage points above the corporate bond. It is easy to see why investors in high tax brackets are so enthusiastic about municipal bonds. On the surface, it might appear that the ability to obtain debt financing at relatively low rates (6.2 percent versus 7.4 percent in our example) creates a cost of financing advantage for not-for-profit providers. However, as we will discuss in Chapter 11, this advantage is offset by the ability of taxable providers to deduct interest expense from taxable income.

The issuance of municipal bonds by healthcare providers is big business. In 1999, 430 healthcare issues came to market, raising $21.4 billion of debt capital. In 1998, the highest year on record, 668 issues worth $32.8 billion were issued. The largest single issue in 1999, $2.4 billion, was by Ascension Health, a St. Louis-based system created by the merger of Daughters of Charity (St. Louis, Missouri) and Sisters of St. Joseph (Ann Arbor, Michigan). Although municipal bonds typically are used to finance capital assets, such as hospital renovations and outpatient facilities, Ascension used its bonds primarily to restructure its outstanding debt. In this case, older, higher interest-rate debt, some of it short term, was replaced on the balance sheet by the new issue.

Most municipal bonds are sold in *serial* form; that is, a portion of the issue comes due periodically, anywhere from six months after issue to 30 years or more. Municipal bonds usually are issued in denominations of $5,000, or integral multiples of $5,000, and although most municipal bonds are tax exempt, some are taxable to investors. Whereas the vast majority of federal government (Treasury) and corporate bonds are held by institutions, about half of all healthcare municipal bonds outstanding are held by individual investors.

In contrast to corporate bonds, municipal bonds are not required to be registered with the SEC. However, prior to bringing municipal debt to market, issuers are required to prepare an *official statement* that contains relevant financial information about the issuer and the nature of the bond issue. In addition, issuers are required to (1) provide annual financial statements that update the information contained in the official statement, and (2) release information on material events that could affect bond values as such events occur. This information is not sent directly to investors, but rather goes to data banks that can be easily accessed by investment bankers, mutual fund managers, and institutional investors. In effect, by making the information available to investment bankers who handle public trades, any individual who wants to buy or sell a municipal bond will also have access to current information that affects the bond's value.

To illustrate the use of municipal bonds by a healthcare provider, consider the $56 million in municipal bonds issued in March 2000 by the Bay Area Health Facilities Authority. The Authority is a public body created under Florida's Health Facilities Authorities Law for the sole purpose of issuing health facilities municipal revenue bonds for qualifying healthcare providers. For this particular bond issue, the provider is Palm Coast Medical Center, a not-for-profit hospital, and the primary purpose of the issue was to raise funds to build and equip a new children's hospital. The bonds are secured solely by the revenues of Palm Coast Medical Center, so the municipal conduit agency—the Bay Area Health Facilities Authority—has no responsibility whatever regarding the interest or principal payments on the issue.

The bonds are rated AAA, not on the basis of the financial strength of Palm Coast Medical Center, but rather because the bonds are insured by the Municipal Bond Investors Assurance Corporation (MBIA). (Municipal bond insurance, which is called *credit enhancement*, will be discussed in more detail later in the chapter.) Table 6.1 shows the maturities and interest rates associated with the issue.

Note the following points:

- The issue is a serial issue; that is, the $56 million in bonds is composed of 13 series, or individual issues, with maturities ranging from one year to 30 years.

Maturity[a]	Amount	Approximate Interest Rate
2001	$ 705,000	4.0%
2002	740,000	4.6
2003	785,000	4.7
2004	825,000	4.8
2005	880,000	5.0
2006	925,000	5.1
2007	985,000	5.2
2008	1,050,000	5.3
2009	1,115,000	5.4
2010	1,190,000	5.5
2015	5,590,000	5.8
2020	9,435,000	6.1
2030	31,775,000	6.2
	$56,000,000	

TABLE 6.1
Palm Coast Medical Center Municipal Bond Issue: Maturities, Amounts, and Interest Rates

[a]All serial issues mature on March 1 of the listed year.

- Because the yield curve on municipal bonds was normal, or upward sloping, at time of issue, the interest rates increase across series as the maturities increase.
- The bonds that mature in 2015, 2020, and 2030 have sinking fund provisions, which we discuss in a later section, whereby the hospital must place a specified dollar amount with a trustee each year to ensure that funds are available to retire the issues as they become due.
- Although it is not shown in the table, the hospital's *debt service requirements*—that is, the total amount of principal and interest that it has to pay on the issue—are relatively constant over time. The purpose of structuring the series so that the debt service requirements are spread evenly over time is to match the maturity of the issue to the maturity of the asset being financed. Think about it this way: The children's hospital has a life of about 30 years, and during this time, it will be generating revenues more or less evenly, and its value will decline more or less evenly. Thus, the hospital has structured the debt series so that the debt service requirements can be met by the revenues associated with the children's hospital. At the end of 30 years, the debt will be paid off, and Palm Coast Medical Center will probably be planning for a replacement facility that would be funded, at least in part, by a new debt issue.

Current law limits the amount of tax-exempt bonds that can be issued by nonacute care providers to $150 million. Thus, while not-for-profit hospitals and hospital systems can issue an unlimited amount of municipal bonds, not-for-profit "nonhospital" facilities, such as nursing homes, HMOs, and clinics, are capped at $150 million. In addition, the cap applies to nonhospital facilities that are developed by acute care hospitals. The cap places an artificial limit on the ability of not-for-profit nonhospital corporations to obtain favorable financing, and hence to consolidate and form integrated delivery systems, so lobbyists for managed care, nursing home, and other nonhospital providers have been arguing for a change in the law to eliminate the restriction.

Self-Test Questions

1. What is the primary motivation for investors to purchase municipal bonds?
2. Describe the major differences between corporate and municipal bonds?
3. What is a serial issue and why is it used?

Short-Term Debt

Thus far, we have focused on long-term debt. However, as pointed out in the introduction to this chapter, healthcare providers use 5 percent short-term debt in their total financing mix. This section provides some of the details associated with short-term financing.

Short-term credit has three primary advantages over long-term debt. First, a short-term loan can be obtained much faster than long-term credit.

Lenders will insist on a more thorough financial examination before extending long-term credit, and the loan agreement will have to be spelled out in considerable detail because a lot can happen during the life of a ten-year term loan or a 30-year bond. Thus, businesses that require funds in a hurry look to the short-term markets.

Second, if the need for funds is seasonal or cyclical (i.e., temporary), a firm may not want to commit to long-term debt for the following three reasons:

1. Issuance costs are generally high when raising long-term debt, but are trivial for short-term credit. Although long-term debt can be repaid early, provided the loan agreement includes a prepayment provision, prepayment penalties can be expensive. Accordingly, if a firm thinks its need for funds may diminish in the near future, it should choose short-term debt for the flexibility it provides.
2. Long-term loan agreements always contain restrictive covenants that constrain the firm's future actions. Short-term credit agreements are generally much less onerous in this regard.
3. The interest rate on short-term debt generally is lower than the rate on long-term debt because, as we discuss in a later section, the yield curve normally is upward sloping. Thus, when coupled with lower issuance costs, short-term debt can have a significant total cost advantage over long-term debt.

In spite of these advantages, short-term credit has one serious disadvantage: It subjects the firm to more risk than does long-term financing. First, if a firm borrows on a long-term basis, its interest costs will be relatively stable over time, but if it uses short-term credit, its interest expense can fluctuate widely, at times possibly going quite high. For example, the short-term rate (the prime rate) that banks charge large corporations more than tripled over a two-year period in the early 1980s, rising from 6.25 to 21 percent. Many businesses that had borrowed heavily on a short-term basis simply could not meet their rising interest costs; as a result, bankruptcies hit record levels during that period. The exposure to increasing interest rates is called *roll-over risk*.

Second, the principal amount on short-term debt comes due on a regular basis. If the financial condition of a business temporarily deteriorates, the business may find itself unable to repay this debt when it matures. Furthermore, the business may be in such a weak financial position that the lender will not extend the loan. Such a scenario can result in severe problems for the borrower, which, like unexpectedly high-interest rates, could force the business into bankruptcy. The risk that a business will not be able to roll over, or renew, its short-term debt is called *renewal risk*.

Types of Short-Term Debt

The two most common types of short-term debt are commercial paper and bank loans.

Commercial Paper

Commercial paper is a type of unsecured debt issued by large, strong firms, and sold primarily to other businesses, to insurance companies, to pension funds, to money market mutual funds, and to banks. Although the amount of commercial paper outstanding is smaller than bank loans outstanding, this form of financing has grown rapidly in recent years.

Maturities of commercial paper generally vary from one to nine months, with an average of about five months.[3] The rate on commercial paper fluctuates with supply and demand conditions—it is determined in the market place, varying daily as conditions change. Recently, commercial paper rates have generally ranged from 1½ to 2½ percentage points below the stated prime rate, and about ½ of a percentage point above the rate on short-term Treasury debt (the T-bill rate).

The use of commercial paper is restricted to businesses that are exceptionally good credit risks. Dealers prefer to handle the paper of firms whose net worth is $100 million or more and whose annual borrowing exceeds $10 million. One potential problem with commercial paper is that a debtor who is in temporary financial difficulty may receive little help because commercial paper dealings are generally less personal than are bank relationships. Thus, banks are generally more able and willing to help a good customer weather a temporary storm than is a commercial paper dealer. On the other hand, using commercial paper permits a business to tap a wide range of credit sources, including financial institutions outside its own area and industrial corporations across the country, which can reduce interest costs.

Bank Loans

Commercial banks, whose short-term loans generally appear on firms' balance sheets as notes payable, are the primary source of short-term financing. Although banks make longer-term loans, the bulk of their lending is on a short-term basis; about two-thirds of all bank loans mature in a year or less. Bank loans to businesses are frequently written as 90-day notes, so the loan must be repaid or renewed at the end of 90 days. When a bank loan is approved, a loan agreement is executed that specifies:

- the amount borrowed;
- the interest rate;
- the repayment schedule, which can involve either a lump sum or a series of installments;
- any collateral that might have to be put up as security for the loan; and
- any other terms and conditions to which the bank and the borrower may have agreed.

When the agreement is signed, the bank credits the borrower's checking account with the amount of the loan, while both cash and notes payable increase on the borrower's balance sheet.

Banks sometimes require borrowers to maintain a checking account balance equal to 10 to 20 percent of the face amount of the loan. This requirement is called a *compensating balance,* and such balances raise the effective interest rate on the loan. For example, suppose that Pine Garden nursing home needs an $80,000 short-term bank loan to meet temporary cash needs. If the loan requires a 20 percent compensating balance, then the nursing home must borrow $100,000 to obtain a usable $80,000, assuming that the business does not have an "extra" $20,000 around to use as a compensating balance. If the stated interest rate is 8 percent, the effective cost rate is actually 10 percent: $0.08 \times \$100,000 = \$8,000$ in interest expense divided by $80,000 of usable funds.

A *line of credit*, sometimes called a *revolving credit agreement* or just *revolver*, is a formal understanding between the bank and the borrower, which indicates the maximum credit the bank will extend to the borrower over some specified period of time. For example, in December, a bank loan officer might indicate to Pine Garden's manager that the bank regards the nursing home as being good for up to $80,000 during the coming year. If on January 10, Pine Garden's manager decides to borrow $15,000 from the line, this borrowing would be called *taking down* $15,000 of the credit line. This take down would be credited to the nursing home's checking account at the bank, and before repayment of the $15,000, Pine Garden could borrow additional amounts up to a total of $80,000 outstanding at any one time. Lines of credit are generally for one year, and borrowers typically have to pay an up-front commitment fee of about 0.5 to 1 percent of the total amount of the line. Many businesses have a continuing relationship with a bank, which allows them to automatically renew the credit line year after year. However, if the business's financial condition deteriorates, the bank has the right to deny renewal.

Revolvers typically involve large sums over longer periods. To illustrate the concept, consider the following example. In 1999, Colorado Healthcare negotiated a revolving credit agreement for $100 million with a group of banks. The banks were formally committed for four years to lend the firm up to $100 million if the funds were needed. Colorado Healthcare, in turn, paid an annual commitment fee of one-quarter of 1 percent on the unused credit to compensate the banks for making the commitment. Thus, if Colorado Healthcare did not take down any of the $100 million commitment during a year, it would still be required to pay a $250,000 annual fee in monthly installments of $20,833.33. If it borrowed $50 million on the first day of the agreement, the unused portion of the credit line would fall to $50 million, and the annual fee would fall to $125,000. But, interest would have to be paid on the money Colorado Healthcare actually borrowed. As a general rule, the rate of interest on credit lines is pegged to the prime rate, so the cost of the loan varies over time as interest rates change. Colorado Healthcare's rate was set at prime plus 0.5 percentage points.

Secured Short-Term Debt

Given a choice, it is ordinarily better to borrow on an unsecured basis because the administrative costs associated with secured loans are often high. However, weak businesses may find that they can borrow only if they put up some form of security to protect the lender, or that by using security they can borrow at a much lower rate.

Several kinds of *collateral*, or security, can be employed including marketable securities, land or buildings, equipment, inventory, and accounts receivable. Marketable securities make excellent collateral, but businesses that need short-term credit generally do not hold large marketable securities portfolios. Both real property (i.e., land and buildings) and equipment are good forms of collateral. However, because of maturity matching, such assets are generally used as security for long-term debt rather than for short-term credit. Therefore, most secured short-term business borrowing involves the use of accounts receivable or inventories as collateral.

Accounts receivable financing involves either the pledging of receivables or the selling of receivables. Such financing is provided by commercial banks or by one of the large industrial finance firms such as GE Capital. The *pledging* of accounts receivable is characterized by the fact that the lender not only has a claim against the dollar amount of the receivables, but also has recourse against the pledging firm. This means that if the individual, or third-party payer, who owes the receivable does not pay, the business that borrows against the receivable must take the loss. Therefore, the risk of default on the accounts receivable pledged remains with the borrowing firm. When receivables are pledged, the payer is not ordinarily notified about the pledging, and payments are made on the receivables in the same way as when receivables are not used as loan security.

The second form of receivables financing is *factoring*, or *selling accounts receivable*. In this type of secured financing, the receivables account is actually "purchased" by the lender, generally without recourse to the borrowing business. In a typical factoring transaction, the buyer of the receivables pays the seller about 90 to 95 percent of the face value of the receivables. When receivables are factored, the individual, or third-party payer, who owes the receivable is often notified of the transfer and is asked to make payment directly to the firm that bought the receivables. Because the factoring firm assumes the risk of default on bad accounts, it must perform a credit check on the receivables prior to the purchase. Accordingly, *factors*, which are the firms that buy receivables, can provide not only money but also a credit department for the borrower. Incidentally, the same financial institutions that make loans against pledged receivables also serve as factors. Thus, depending on the circumstances and the wishes of the borrower, a financial institution will provide either form of receivables financing.

Because healthcare providers tend to carry relatively large amounts of receivables, such firms are prime candidates for receivables financing. For example, hospitals alone have accounts receivable that total nearly $15 billion. The selling of these receivables, especially by hospitals that are experiencing liquidity problems, represents one way to reduce carrying costs and stimulate cash flow.

To illustrate receivables financing for hospitals, consider the program recently instituted between Chase Manhattan Bank and Presbyterian Hospital, New York City's largest hospital. This program provides $15 million in advance funding of receivables over a three-year period. Presbyterian sells its accounts receivable to Chase for cash. In turn, Chase obtains the cash it needs by selling commercial paper. The payers of the receivables technically make payments directly to Chase, although Chase actually pays Presbyterian a fee to service the receivables accounts. Chase charges an up-front fee for the program, and then charges an interest rate of about 1 to 1.5 percent above the prime rate on the amount advanced.

Interestingly, the expanding volume of healthcare receivables financing has created a new class of receivables-backed securities. For example, Prudential Securities recently placed $40 million in medium-term, taxable, AAA-rated notes issued by a firm that was created solely to buy receivables from cash-strapped providers. The notes are backed by the Medicare, Medicaid, and commercial insurance receivables of 21 hospitals nationwide. Under the plan, the hospitals sell their receivables to the firm each week, and hence get cash in less than ten days versus the 60–70 days commonly required to collect from third-party payers.

Although receivables financing is a way to reduce current assets, and, hence, financing costs, critics contend that such programs are too expensive. Because of costs involved, most receivables financing programs are used by providers that have serious liquidity problems, although programs are being developed that can provide benefits even to well-run providers that are not facing a liquidity crunch. Although the illustrations here have focused on the use of receivables financing by hospitals, such financing is also used by medical group practices and other healthcare providers.

Receivables financing dominates healthcare providers' use of secured financing, but other healthcare businesses, such as equipment manufacturers and pharmaceutical firms, are more likely to obtain credit secured by business inventories. If a firm is a relatively good credit risk, the mere existence of the inventory may be sufficient to obtain an unsecured loan. However, if the firm is a relatively poor risk, the lending institution may insist upon security, which can take the form of a blanket lien against all inventory or either trust receipts or warehouse receipts against specific inventory items. The *inventory blanket lien* gives the lending institution a lien against all the borrower's inventories.

However, the borrower is free to sell inventories, so the value of the collateral can be reduced below the level that existed when the loan was granted.

Because of the inherent weakness of the blanket lien, another procedure for inventory financing was developed. The *security instrument*, also called a *trust receipt*, is an instrument that acknowledges that the goods are held in trust for the lender. When trust receipts are used, the borrowing firm signs and delivers a trust receipt upon receiving funds from the lender. The goods pledged as collateral can be stored in a public warehouse or held on the premises of the borrower. The trust receipt acknowledges that the goods are held in trust for the lender and that any proceeds from the sale of trust goods must be transmitted to the lender at the end of each day.

Self-Test Questions

1. What are the advantages and disadvantages of short-term versus long-term debt?
2. Explain the difference between roll-over risk and renewal risk.
3. How might a hospital that expects to have a temporary cash shortage during the coming year make sure that needed funds will be available?
4. What are some types of current assets that might be pledged as security for short-term loans?

Debt Contracts

Debt contracts, which spell out the rights of the borrower and lender(s), have different names depending on the type of debt. The contract between the issuer and bondholders is called an *indenture*. Indentures tend to be long—some run several hundred pages in length. For other types of debt, a similar, but much shorter, document called a *loan agreement* or *promissory note* is used. Healthcare managers are most concerned about the overall cost of debt, including issuance costs, as well as any provisions that may restrict the business's future actions. In this section, some debt contract features are discussed that could affect either the business's future flexibility or the interest rate on the issue.

Restrictive Covenants

Many debt contracts include provisions, called *restrictive covenants*, that are designed to protect creditors from managerial actions that would be detrimental to the creditors' best interests. For example, the Palm Coast Medical Center bond issue described earlier contains several restrictive covenants, including the covenant that the issuer must maintain a minimum current ratio of 2.0. The current ratio is defined as current assets divided by current liabilities, so a current ratio of 2.0 indicates that current assets are twice as large as current liabilities. Because the current ratio measures a business's liquidity— the ability to meet current cash obligations as they become due—a minimum current ratio provides some assurance to bondholders that the interest and principal payments coming due can be covered. If Palm Coast violates any of its restrictive covenants, say, by allowing its current ratio to drop below 2.0, it is said to be in *technical default*. ("Regular" default occurs when an interest or principal payment is *missed*, or not paid on time.)

Trustees

When debt is supplied by a single creditor, there is a one-to-one relationship between the lender and borrower. However, bond issues can have thousands of lenders, so a single voice is needed to represent bondholders. This function is performed by a *trustee*, usually an institution such as a bank, which represents the bondholders and ensures that the terms of the indenture are being carried out. The trustee is responsible for trying to keep the covenants from being violated and for taking appropriate action if a violation does occur. What constitutes appropriate action varies with the circumstances. A trustee has the power to *foreclose* on an issue in default, which makes the full amount of principal and unpaid interest due and payable immediately. However, insisting on immediate payment may result in bankruptcy and possibly large losses on the bonds. In such a case, the trustee may decide that the bondholders would be better served by giving the issuer a chance to work out its problems, which would avoid forcing the business into bankruptcy.

Call Provisions

A *call provision* gives the issuer the right to call a bond for *redemption* prior to maturity; that is, the issuer can pay off the bondholders in entirety and *redeem*, or *retire*, the issue. If it is used, the call provision generally states that the firm must pay an amount greater than the initial amount borrowed. The additional sum required is defined as the *call premium*.

Many callable bonds offer a period of call protection, which protects investors from a call just a short time after the bonds are issued. For example, the 20-year callable bonds issued by Vanguard Healthcare in 1999 are not callable until 2009, which is ten years after the original issue date. This type of call provision is known as a *deferred call*.

The call privilege is valuable to the issuer but potentially detrimental to bondholders, especially if the bond is issued in a period when interest rates are cyclically high. In general, bonds are called when interest rates have fallen because the issuer usually replaces the old, high-interest issue with a new, lower-interest issue, and hence reduces annual interest expense. When this occurs, investors are forced to reinvest the principal returned in new securities at the then current (lower) rate. As readers will see later, the added risk to investors of a call provision causes the interest rate on a new issue of callable bonds to exceed that on a similar new issue of noncallable bonds.

If a bond, or other debt security, has a call provision and interest rates drop, the issuer has to make a decision, called a *refunding decision*, as to whether or not to call the issue. In essence, the decision involves a cost/benefit analysis wherein the costs are the administrative and issuance costs associated with calling one bond and issuing another, and the benefits are lower future interest payments. We will discuss refunding decisions in some detail in Chapter 8.

Sinking Funds

A *sinking fund* is a provision that provides for the systematic retirement of a bond issue. Typically, sinking fund provisions require the issuer to retire (i.e., redeem) a portion of the issue in each year. (A serial issue of municipal bonds can be thought of as a type of sinking fund.)

On some occasions, the issuer of bonds with a sinking fund may be required to deposit money with a trustee, who invests the funds and then uses the accumulated sum to retire the entire bond issue when it matures. Sometimes, the stipulated sinking fund payment is tied to the level of revenues or earnings in each year, but usually it is a mandatory fixed amount. If it is mandatory, a failure to meet the sinking fund requirement places the issue in technical default.

Although a sinking fund is designed to protect the bondholders by assuring that the issue is retired in an orderly fashion, it must be recognized that, like a call provision, a sinking fund may at times work to the detriment of bondholders. However, securities that provide for a sinking fund are regarded as being safer than those without sinking funds, and that fact tends to balance the risk of a sinking fund call. Thus, sinking fund provisions generally have little effect on an issue's interest rate.

Self-Test Questions

1. Describe the following debt contract features:
   a. Bond indenture
   b. Restrictive covenant
   c. Trustee
   d. Call provision
   e. Sinking fund
2. What is the difference between technical default and "regular" default?
3. What impact does a call provision have on an issue's interest rate?
4. How do sinking fund provisions differ from call provisions?

Credit Ratings

Since the early 1900s, corporate and municipal bonds, as well as other types of debt, have been assigned credit ratings that reflect their probability of going into default. In addition to individual debt issues, a business's overall financial capacity, or *creditworthiness*, can also be rated. The three major credit rating agencies are Fitch IBCA (Fitch), Moody's Investors Service (Moody's), and Standard & Poor's Corporation (S&P).[4] On large issues, more than one agency will rate the debt, while on smaller deals, one agency is sufficient.

In general, the ratings of these agencies are consistent with one another, although occasionally the agencies will give different ratings to the same firm or issue. Although there are minor variations in the rating grades among the three agencies, the S&P issue ratings, given in Table 6.2, are representative. Furthermore, in the discussion to follow, reference to the S&P code implies similar ratings by the other agencies as well.

Note that debt with a BBB and higher rating is called *investment grade*, which is the lowest rated debt that many institutional investors are permitted by law to hold. Double B and lower debt, called *junk debt*, is more speculative in nature because it has a much higher probability of going into default than does higher-rated debt.

TABLE 6.2
S&P Issue
Credit Ratings

Rating	Description
AAA	The highest rating assigned. Issuer's capacity to meet the debt obligation is extremely strong.
AA	This rating differs from AAA by only a small degree. Issuer's capacity to meet the debt obligation is very strong.
A	The obligation is somewhat more susceptible to adverse changes in circumstances and economic conditions than those with higher ratings. However, the issuer's capacity to meet its financial commitment is still strong.
BBB	The obligation has adequate protection. However, adverse economic conditions or changing circumstances are more likely to lead to a weakened capacity of the issuer to meet its obligation. Note that debt rated lower than BBB is regarded as having significant speculative characteristics.
BB	This rating is less vulnerable to nonpayment than other speculative issues. However, ongoing uncertainties or exposure to adverse conditions could lead to inadequate capacity to meet the financial commitment.
B	The issuer currently has the capacity to meet the obligation, but adverse conditions will likely lead to inadequate capacity.
CCC	This issue is currently vulnerable to nonpayment. The ability of the issuer to meet its obligation is dependent upon favorable conditions. Unfavorable conditions are likely to lead to nonpayment.
CC	This obligation is highly vulnerable to nonpayment.
C	Typically used on an obligation when a bankruptcy petition has been filed, but payments are still being made.
D	The obligation is in default.

Note: The credit rating agencies use "modifiers" for ratings below triple A. For example, S&P uses a plus and minus system. Thus, within the A rating category, A+ designates the strongest, and A- the weakest.

Rating Criteria

Although the rating assignments are subjective, they are based on both qualitative characteristics and quantitative factors. Clearly, financial analyses are an important consideration in the rating process. In addition, the quality and effectiveness of management, organizational structure, competitiveness of the service area, risks associated with medical staff and third-party-payer relationships, and local demographic and economic considerations all influence credit ratings.

Analysts at the rating agencies have consistently stated that no precise formula is used to set a credit rating—many factors are taken into account, but not in a mathematically precise manner. Statistical studies have supported this contention. Researchers who have tried to predict debt ratings on the basis of quantitative data alone have had only limited success, which indicates that the agencies do indeed use a good deal of subjective judgment in the rating process.

Importance of Credit Ratings

Credit ratings are important both to businesses and to investors. First, a credit rating is an indicator of the default risk of the debt, or of the business as a whole, so the rating has a direct, measurable influence on the interest rate required by investors, and hence on the firm's cost of debt capital. Second, most corporate bonds are purchased by institutional investors rather than by individuals. Many of these institutions are restricted by law or charter to investment-grade securities. Also, most individual investors who buy municipal bonds are unwilling to take high risks in their bond purchases. Thus, if an issue has a rating below BBB, the issuer will have a harder time trying to sell the debt because the number of potential purchasers is reduced. As a result of their higher risk and more restricted market, low-grade debt typically carries much higher interest rates than does high-grade debt. (We will illustrate the impact of credit rating on interest rate in the next major section.)

Changes in Ratings

A change in a credit rating will have a significant effect on the business's ability to obtain debt capital, and on the cost of that capital. Rating agencies continually review current information about issuers and debt that has been rated. If a major change occurs in an issuer's near-term or long-term credit outlook, the issuer's ratings are placed under review for possible change. For example, S&P will announce that a firm, or issue, has been placed on *CreditWatch* with either a positive or negative implication. Such an announcement provides warning to investors that a firm, or one or more of its issues, is under review and a ratings change could occur. If circumstances dictate such a change, the rating agency will later announce an upgrade or downgrade.

To illustrate the CreditWatch system, consider Innovative Clinical Solutions, Inc. The firm was originally founded as PhyMatrix Corporation, a physician practice management firm. However, the firm reorganized in early 1999. It changed its name, shed its physician practice assets, and created three new business lines: (1) clinical studies, (2) healthcare research, and (3) network management. The firm was initially placed on CreditWatch on May 27, 1998, with negative implications, following the firm's announcement that it was exploring strategic alternatives. Then, on February 11, 2000, S&P announced that it had lowered Innovative Clinical Solutions's corporate credit and bank loan ratings from B+ to B-, and its subordinated debt rating from B- to CCC. The announcement also indicated that the ratings remained on CreditWatch with negative implications. According to S&P, the rating actions reflected concerns surrounding the firm's weakening financial profile and continued losses, as well as the challenges encountered during restructuring. Downgrades such as these are not viewed with joy by debtholders, who can see the value of their holdings plummet because of increased credit (default) risk.

Recent years have not been kind to the financial conditions of many healthcare businesses, especially not-for-profit hospitals and healthcare systems. Moody's reported that in 1999 not-for-profit hospitals experienced their second straight year of record-setting downgrades—$13.4 billion of debt in 1999 versus $11 billion in 1998. Looking at another measure of changes in credit quality, downgrades outpaced upgrades by roughly five to one over the same period, based on value of debt regraded. According to Moody's, the outlook for the next few years remains gloomy; however, there is some reason to believe that the worst is over. Specifically, a more favorable pricing environment and partial relief from the cutbacks contained in the Balanced Budget Act of 1997 may help hospitals in the long run.

In addition to the routine review of credit ratings, an announcement that a firm plans to sell a new debt issue, or to merge with another firm and pay for the acquisition by issuing new debt, will trigger agency reviews and possibly lead to a rating change. Thus, if a business's situation has deteriorated somewhat, but its debt has not been reviewed and downgraded, it may choose to use a term loan or short-term debt rather than to finance through a public bond issue that would require regrading. Such a strategy is intended to postpone a rating agency review until the situation has had time to improve.

1. Who are the major rating agencies?
2. What are some criteria that the rating agencies use when assigning ratings?
3. What impact do debt ratings have on the cost of debt to the issuing firm?

Self-Test Questions

Credit Enhancement

Credit enhancement, or *bond insurance*, which is primarily available for municipal bonds, is a means of upgrading the rating of a lower-rated bond to AAA. Credit enhancement is offered by several credit insurers including the three largest: Municipal Bond Investors Assurance (MBIA) Corporation; AMBAC

Indemnity Corporation; and Financial Guaranty Insurance Corporation, a subsidiary of GE Capital. Currently, almost 70 percent, which is up from about 60 percent a few years ago, of all new healthcare municipal issues carry bond insurance.

Here is how credit enhancement works. Regardless of the inherent credit rating of the issuer, the bond insurer guarantees that bondholders will receive the promised interest and principal payments. Thus, bond insurance protects investors against default by the issuer. Because the insurer gives its guarantee that payments will be made, the bond carries the credit rating of the insurance firm rather than that of the issuer. For example, Palm Coast Medical Center has an A rating, so new bonds issued by the hospital without credit enhancement would likely also be rated A. However, its 2000 serial municipal bond issue summarized in Table 6.1 carries an AAA rating because it is insured by MBIA.

Credit enhancement gives the issuer access to the lowest possible interest rate, but not without a cost. Bond insurers typically charge an up-front fee of about 35 to 125 basis points of the total debt service over the life of the bond. The lower the hospital's inherent credit rating and the worse the outlook for the industry, the higher the cost of bond insurance. Most of the newly issued insured municipal bonds have an underlying credit rating of AA or A. The remainder are still of investment grade, rated BBB. Interestingly, increasing competition in the market for credit enhancement as well as the reduced risk that results from larger insurer portfolios has lowered fees over time. Still, credit enhancement fees can vary significantly as industry conditions change. For example, the fees charged to AA-rated hospitals surged from only 35 basis points in early 1998 to 80 basis points in early 2000, which represents a 129 percent increase. Increasing uncertainty about the future operating environment of hospitals has increased the price of insuring default risk.

Upon careful analysis, it appears that the insurance costs on many issues fully negate the value inherent in lower-interest payments. Still, such "economically neutral" deals often appeal to issuers because insurance protects investors, and the reputation of the issuer, against future uncertainty. A provider with a solid rating today—say, A+—could easily fall on hard times 20 or so years down the road. Credit enhancement allows the issuer's creditworthiness to decline without having to explain the reasons to the investment community.

However, bond insurers are quick to take action when the underlying credit quality of an insured issue starts to fall. In the mildest cases, bond insurers demand quarterly or even monthly audited financial statements. If the situation worsens, it is common practice among credit insurers to pressure hospitals to merge, cut costs, or implement other actions that will improve their ability to make the debt payments, and hence reduce the probability that the insurer will have to come to the rescue.

Thus far, municipal bond issuers have defaulted on very few insured issues. However, there has been an upturn in both corporate and municipal healthcare bond defaults in 1998 and 1999, and some insurance analysts question the ability of bond insurers to cover default payments should a severe recession occur. Furthermore, the market as a whole has some reservations about bond insurance because interest rates on AAA insured issues tend to be slightly higher than rates on otherwise similar bonds that carry an uninsured AAA rating.

Self-Test Questions

1. What does "credit enhancement" mean?
2. How is bond insurance priced?
3. Why would not-for-profit healthcare issuers seek bond insurance?

Interest Rate Components

Although interest rates are actually set by the interaction of supply and demand, the suppliers of debt capital (creditors) base their supply decisions for each debt security on the basis of a minimum required rate of return (interest rate), which depends on several components. By understanding these components, it is possible to gain insights on why interest rates change over time, differ among borrowers, and even differ on separate issues by the same borrower.

Real Risk-Free Rate (RRF)

The base upon which all interest rates are built is the *real risk-free rate* (*RRF*). This is the rate that investors would demand on a debt security that is totally **riskless** when there is **no inflation**. Although difficult to measure, the RRF is thought to fall somewhere in the range of 2 to 4 percent. In the real world, inflation is rarely zero, and most debt securities have some risk; thus, the actual interest rate on a given debt security will typically be higher than the real risk-free rate.

Inflation Premium (IP)

Inflation has a major impact on interest rates because it erodes the purchasing power of the dollar and lowers the value of investment returns. Creditors, who are the suppliers of debt capital, are well aware of the impact of inflation. Thus, they build an *inflation premium* (*IP*) into the interest rate that is equal to the expected inflation rate over the life of the security.

For example, suppose that the real risk-free rate was RRF = 3%, and that inflation was expected to be 4 percent, and hence IP = 4%, during the next year. The rate of interest on a one-year riskless debt security would be 3% + 4% = 7%. The combination of the RRF and IP is called the *risk-free rate* (*RF*). Thus, the risk-free rate incorporates inflation expectations, but it does not incorporate any risk factors. In this example, RF = 7%.

The rate of inflation built into interest rates is the rate of inflation **expected in the future**, not the rate experienced in the past. Thus, the latest reported figures may show an annual inflation rate of 3 percent, but that is for a past period. If investors expect a 6 percent inflation rate in the future, then 6 percent would be built into the current rate of interest. Also, the inflation rate built into the inflation premium is the average rate of inflation expected **over the life of the security**. Thus, the inflation rate built into a one-year bond is the expected inflation rate for the next year, but the inflation rate built into a 30-year bond is the average rate of inflation expected over the next 30 years.

Default Risk Premium (DRP)

The risk that a borrower will default—not make the payments promised—has a significant impact on the interest rate set on a debt security. This risk, along with the possible consequences of default, is captured by a *default risk premium* (*DRP*). Treasury securities have no default risk; thus, they carry the lowest interest rates on taxable securities in the United States. For corporate and municipal bonds, the higher the bond's rating, the lower its default risk. All else the same, the lower the default risk, the lower the DRP and, hence, the interest rate.

Table 6.3 lists the interest rates on some representative long-term bonds with different ratings in early 2000. The difference between the interest rate on a T-bond and that on a corporate bond with similar maturity, liquidity, and other features is the *default risk premium (DRP)*. Therefore, if the bonds listed were otherwise similar, the default risk premium would be DRP = 7.4% − 6.3% = 1.1 percentage points for AAA corporate bonds, 7.7% − 6.3% = 1.4 percentage points for AA corporate bonds, 7.9% − 6.3% = 1.6 percentage points for A corporate bonds, and so on. As discussed previously, bonds that are rated below BBB are called *junk bonds*, and such bonds tend to have large default risk premiums. The default risk premiums for tax-exempt healthcare bonds use AAA-rated bonds as the base, so they are not "pure" default risk premiums as in the case of corporate bonds, which can be compared to default-free Treasury securities.

In addition to the probability of default, the DRP incorporates a second risk factor, called *recovery risk*. To illustrate recovery risk, consider an issuer that has both mortgage bonds and subordinated debentures outstanding, each carrying the same default rating. Yet, if default occurred, the mortgage bondholders would have a much better chance of recovering the full amount due to them than would the debenture holders. Thus, the DRP would be higher on the debenture than on the mortgage bond, even though both bonds had the same credit rating.

Default risk premiums change over time as the degree of investors' risk aversion changes. For example, if investors believe that businesses will face a tougher operating environment in the future than in the immediate past, DRPs will increase. Thus, the spread between AAA-rated and BBB-rated municipal hospital issues was only 30 basis points in early 1998, but it increased to 120 basis points by early 2000 as the impact of the BBA of 1997 took hold.

Rating	Interest Rate	
	Taxable[a]	Tax-Exempt[b]
U.S. Treasury	6.3%	—
AAA	7.4	6.2%
AA	7.7	6.4
A	7.9	6.7
BBB	8.4	7.4
BB	10.1	8.8
B	12.5	10.2
CCC	14.8	11.8

TABLE 6.3
Representative Long-Term Interest Rates in Early 2000

[a]The non-Treasury taxable bonds are corporate issues by industrial firms.
[b]The tax-exempt bonds are municipal issues by not-for-profit hospitals.
Sources: Bridge Information Systems and FMS, Inc.

Liquidity Premium (LP)

A *liquid* asset is one that can be sold quickly at a predictable fair market price, and thus can be converted to a known amount of cash on short notice. Active markets, which provide liquidity, exist for Treasury securities and for the stocks and bonds of larger corporations. Securities issued by small businesses, including healthcare providers that issue municipal bonds, are somewhat *illiquid:* They can be sold to raise cash, but not very quickly and not at a predictable price. Furthermore, illiquid assets require more effort to sell, and hence have relatively high *transactions costs.* (Transactions costs include commissions, fees, spreads between asking and selling prices, and other expenses associated with selling an investment.) Securities issued by very small businesses, which typically only have a local presence, are very illiquid.

If a security is illiquid, investors will add a *liquidity premium* (*LP*) when they set their required interest rate. It is very difficult to measure liquidity premiums with precision, but a differential of at least 2 percentage points is thought to exist between the least liquid and the most liquid financial assets of similar default risk and maturity.

Price Risk Premium (PRP)

As we will demonstrate in Chapter 8, the market value (price) of a long-term bond declines sharply when interest rates rise. Because interest rates can and do rise, all long-term bonds, including Treasury bonds, have an element of risk called *price risk*. For example, if an individual bought a 30-year Treasury bond in January 1999 for $1,000 when the long-term interest rate on Treasury securities was 5.1 percent, and held it for only one year, until January 2000, when T-bond rates were 6.7 percent, the value of the bond would have declined to about $800. This decline would represent a loss of about 20 percent, which demonstrates that long-term bonds—even U.S. Treasury bonds—are not riskless.

As a general rule, the bonds of any organization, from the U.S. government to HCA to Palm Coast Medical Center, have more price risk the longer the maturity of the bond. Therefore, a *price risk premium* (*PRP*), which is higher the longer the term to maturity, must be included in the interest rate. The effect of price risk premiums is to raise interest rates on long-term bonds relative to those on short-term bonds. This premium, like the others, is extremely difficult to measure, but it seems to vary over time; it rises when interest rates are more volatile and uncertain and falls when they are more stable. In recent years, the price risk premium on 30-year T-bonds has been in the range of 1/2 to 2 percentage points.

Call Risk Premium (CRP)

Bonds that are callable are riskier for investors than those that are noncallable because callable bonds have uncertain maturities. To compensate for bearing call risk, investors charge a *call risk premium* (*CRP*) on callable bonds. The amount of the premium depends on such factors as the interest rate on the bond, current interest rate levels, and time to first call. Historically, call risk premiums have been in the range of 30 to 50 basis points.

Combining the Components

When all the interest rate components listed above are taken into account, the interest rate on any debt security is expressed as follows:

$$\text{Interest rate} = \text{RRF} + \text{IP} + \text{DRP} + \text{LP} + \text{PRP} + \text{CRP}.$$

To illustrate, assume that RRF is 2 percent and inflation is expected to average 3 percent in the coming year. Because T-bills have no default, liquidity, or call risk, and almost no price risk, the interest rate on a one-year T-bill would be 5 percent:

$$\text{Interest rate}_{\text{T-bill}} = \text{RRF} + \text{IP} + \text{DRP} + \text{LP} + \text{PRP} + \text{CRP}$$
$$= 2\% + 3\% + 0 + 0 + 0 + 0 = 5\%.$$

As discussed previously, the combination of RRF and IP is the risk-free rate, so RF = 5%. In general, the rate of interest on short-term Treasury securities (T-bills) is used as a proxy for the **short-term** risk-free rate.

Consider another illustration, the callable 30-year bonds issued by HCA. Assume that these bonds have an inflation premium of 4 percent; default risk, liquidity, and price risk premiums of 1 percent each; and a call risk premium of 40 basis points. Under these assumptions, the HCA bonds would have an interest rate of 9.4 percent:

$$\text{Interest rate}_{30-\text{year bonds}} = \text{RRF} + \text{IP} + \text{DRP} + \text{LP} + \text{PRP} + \text{CRP}$$

$$= 2\% + 4\% + 1\% + 1\% + 1\% + 0.4\% = 9.4\%.$$

When interest rates are viewed as the sum of a base rate plus premiums for inflation and risk, it is easy to visualize the underlying economic forces that cause interest rates to vary among different issues and over time.

1. Write out the equation for the required interest rate on a debt security.
2. What is the difference between the real risk-free rate, RRF, and the risk-free rate, RF?
3. Do the interest rates on Treasury securities include a default risk premium? A liquidity premium? A price risk premium? Explain your answer.
4. Does the default risk premium incorporate only the probability of default? Explain your answer.
5. What is price risk? What type of debt securities would have the largest price risk premium?

Self-Test Questions

The Term Structure of Interest Rates

At most times, short-term interest rates are lower than long-term rates. However, at some times, short-term rates are higher than long-term rates. The relationship between long- and short-term rates, which is called the *term structure of interest rates*, is important to healthcare managers, who must decide whether to borrow by issuing long- or short-term debt, and to investors, who must decide whether to buy long- or short-term debt. Thus, it is important to understand how interest rates on long- and short-term debt are related to one another, and what causes shifts in their relative positions.

To examine the current term structure, look up the interest rates on debt of various maturities by a single issuer (usually the U.S. Treasury) in a source such as the *Wall Street Journal* or the *Federal Reserve Bulletin*. For example, the tabular section of Figure 6.2 presents interest rates for Treasury securities of different maturities on three dates. The set of data for a given date, when plotted on a graph, is called a *yield curve*. As shown in the figure, the yield curve changes both in position and in shape over time.

Figure 6.2 shows yield curves for U.S. Treasury securities, but the curves could have been constructed for similarly rated corporate or municipal (i.e., tax-exempt) bonds, if the data were available. In each case, the yield curve would be approximately the same shape, but would differ in vertical position. For example, had the yield curve been constructed for Beverly Enterprises, a for-profit nursing home operator, it would fall above the Treasury curve because interest rates on corporate debt include default risk premiums, while Treasury rates do not. Conversely, the curve for Palm Coast Medical Center, a not-for-profit hospital, would probably fall below the Treasury curve because the tax-exemption benefit, which lowers the interest rate on tax-exempt securities, generally outweighs the default risk premium. In every case, however, the riskier the issuer (i.e., the lower the bonds are rated), the higher the yield curve plots on the graph.

Historically, long-term rates have generally been above short-term rates, so usually the yield curve has been upward sloping. An *upward sloping curve* would be expected if the inflation premium is relatively constant across all maturities because the price risk premium applied to long-term issues will push long-term rates above short-term rates. Because an upward-sloping yield curve is most prevalent, this shape is also called a *normal yield curve*, as illustrated by the curve for March 1995. Conversely, a yield curve that

FIGURE 6.2

U.S. Treasury Bond Interest Rates on Three Dates

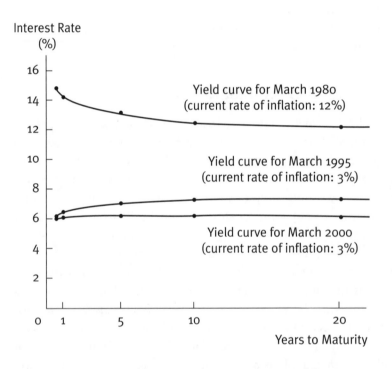

Term to Maturity	Interest Rate		
	March 1980	*March 1995*	*March 2000*
6 months	15.0%	6.2%	6.0%
1 year	14.0	6.5	6.2
5 years	13.5	7.0	6.5
10 years	12.8	7.2	6.4
20 years	12.5	7.3	6.4
30 years	12.4	7.4	6.2

slopes downward is called an *inverted,* or *abnormal, yield curve.* Thus, in Figure 6.2, the yield curve for March 1980 illustrates an inverted curve. Additionally, yield curves can be "kinked" or exhibit other shapes, such as the curve shown for March 2000.[5] However, at most of the time by far, the yield curve is normal.

Healthcare managers use yield curve information to help make decisions regarding debt maturities. To illustrate the concept, assume for the moment that it is March 1995, and that the yield curve for that month in Figure 6.2 applies to Palm Coast Medical Center. Now, assume that the hospital plans to issue $10 million of debt to finance a new outpatient clinic with a 20-year life. If it borrowed in 1995 on a short-term basis—say, for one year—Palm Coast's interest cost for that year would be 6.5 percent, or $650,000. If it used long-term (30-year) financing, its cost would be 7.4 percent, or $740,000. Therefore, at first glance, it would seem that Palm Coast should use short-term debt.

However, if the hospital uses short-term debt, it will have to renew the loan every year at the then current short-term rate. Although unlikely, it is possible that interest rates could return to their March 1980 levels. If this happened, at some time in the future the hospital could be paying 14 percent, or $1,400,000, per year. Conversely, if Palm Coast used long-term financing in 1995, its interest costs would remain constant at $650,000 per year, so an increase in interest rates in the economy would not hurt the hospital.

Does this suggest that businesses should always avoid short-term debt? Not necessarily. If Palm Coast had borrowed on a long-term basis for 7.4 percent in March 1995, it would be at a major disadvantage if interest rates remained low. Its interest expense would be locked in at $740,000 a year, while any competitors that used short-term debt that cost 6.2 percent would be able to continually renew the debt at the lower rate, or even less. Conversely, inflation expectations could push interest rates up to record levels. If that situation occurred, all borrowers would wish that they had borrowed on a long-term basis in 1995.

Financing decisions would be easy if managers could develop accurate forecasts of future interest rates. Unfortunately, predicting future interest rates with consistent accuracy is somewhere between difficult and impossible—people who make a living by selling interest rate forecasts say it is difficult, but many others say it is impossible. Sound financial policy, therefore, calls for using a mix of long- and short-term debt, as well as equity, in such a manner that the business can survive in all but the most severe, and hence unlikely, interest rate environments. Furthermore, the optimal financing policy depends in an important way on the maturities of the firm's assets: In general, to reduce risk, managers try to match the maturities of the financing with the maturities of the assets being financed. The issue of optimal debt maturities will be addressed in more detail in Chapter 11.

Self-Test Questions

1. What is a yield curve and what information is needed to create this curve?
2. What is the difference between a normal yield curve and an abnormal one?
3. If short-term rates are lower than long-term rates, why may a business still choose to finance with long-term debt?
4. Explain the following statement: "A firm's financing policy depends in large part on the nature of its assets."

Advantages and Disadvantages of Debt Financing

From the viewpoint of the issuer, there are several advantages to using debt financing as opposed to equity financing:

- The cost of debt is independent of a business's earnings, so creditors do not participate if profits soar. This statement means that all of the "excess" value created by good business decisions accrues to the owner(s) of for-profit businesses.
- Because of the tax-deductibility of interest for investor-owned businesses, and the ability of not-for-profit firms to issue tax-advantaged (municipal) debt, the risk-adjusted component cost of debt is lower than that of common stock.
- The owners of a for-profit business do not have to share control with creditors.
- Debt financing allows not-for-profit businesses to offer more services than they could using only equity financing.

The major disadvantages are as follows:

- Because debt service (interest plus principal repayment) is a fixed charge, a decline in operating income could result in default and possibly even bankruptcy.
- As we discuss in Chapter 11, the use of debt financing increases the riskiness of the business, and hence increases both debt and equity costs.
- Debt has a fixed maturity date, and hence has to be repaid when due. If the business's financial capacity at the time of a large principal repayment is limited, financial problems can result.
- Debt contracts, especially those for long-term debt, often contain covenants that restrict managerial actions.
- The amount of debt that can be raised at "reasonable" interest rates is limited.

Self-Test Question

1. What are the primary advantages and disadvantages of debt financing as compared to equity financing?

Key Concepts

This chapter provides an overview of debt financing, including how interest rates are determined and the characteristics of the major types of debt securities. Here are its key concepts:

- Any business must have assets if it is to operate, and to acquire assets, the business must raise *capital*. Capital comes in two basic forms: (1) *debt* and (2) *equity (or fund)* capital.
- Capital is allocated through the price system; a price is charged to "rent" money. Lenders charge *interest* on funds they lend, while equity investors receive *dividends* and *capital gains* in return for letting the firm use their money.
- Four fundamental factors affect the cost of money: (1) *investment opportunities*, (2) *time preferences for consumption*, (3) *risk*, and (4) *inflation*.
- *Term loans* and *bonds* are long-term debt contracts under which a borrower agrees to make a series of interest and principal payments on specific dates to the lender. A term loan is generally sold to one, or a few, lenders, while a bond is typically offered to the public and sold to many different investors.
- Many different types of bonds exist including *mortgage bonds, debentures, subordinated debentures,* and *municipal bonds.* Prevailing interest rates, the bond's riskiness, and tax consequences determine the return required on each type of bond.
- *Revenue bonds* are municipal bonds in which the revenues derived from projects, such as roads or bridges, airports, water and sewage systems, and not-for-profit healthcare facilities are pledged as security for the bonds.
- The advantages of short-term credit are the *speed* of arranging such loans, increased *flexibility,* and the fact that short-term *interest rates* are generally *lower* than long-term rates. The principal disadvantage of short-term credit is the *extra risk* that borrowers must bear because lenders can demand payment on short notice, and the cost of the loan will increase if interest rates rise.
- *Bank loans* are an important source of short-term credit. When a bank loan is approved, a *promissory note* is signed.
- Banks sometimes require borrowers to maintain *compensating balances,* which are deposit requirements set at between 10 and 20 percent of the loan amount. Compensating balances raise the effective rate of interest on bank loans.
- *Lines of credit*, or *revolving credit agreements*, are formal understandings between the bank and the borrower in which the bank agrees to extend some maximum amount of credit to the borrower over some specified period.
- Sometimes a borrower will find that it is necessary to borrow on a *secured basis,* in which case the borrower uses assets, such as real estate, securities, equipment, inventories, or accounts receivable, as collateral for the loan.
- *Restrictive covenants* are placed in loan agreements to protect creditors from detrimental actions by borrowers.
- A *call provision* gives the issuer the right to redeem the bonds prior to maturity under specified terms, usually at a price greater than the maturity

value (the difference is a *call premium*). A firm will call a bond issue and refund it if interest rates fall sufficiently after the bond has been issued.

- A *sinking fund* is a provision that requires the issuer to retire a portion of the bond issue each year. The purpose of the sinking fund is to provide for the orderly retirement of the issue. No call premium is paid to the holders of bonds called for sinking fund purposes.
- Bonds are assigned *ratings* that reflect the probability of their going into default. The higher a bond's rating, and the greater the probability of recovering bondholder capital should default occur, the lower its interest rate.
- *Credit enhancement*, or *bond insurance*, upgrades a municipal bond rating to AAA. Regardless of the inherent credit rating of the issuer, the bond insurer guarantees that bondholders will receive the promised interest and principal payments.
- The *interest rate* on a debt security is composed of the real risk-free rate (RRF) plus premiums that reflect inflation (IP), default risk (DRP), liquidity (LP), price risk (PRP), and call risk (CRP):

$$\text{Interest rate} = RRF + IP + DRP + LP + PRP + CRP.$$

- The relationship between the yields on securities and the securities' maturities is known as the *term structure of interest rates*. The *yield curve* is a graph of this relationship.
- Debt has several advantages and disadvantages when compared to equity financing. The primary advantages are fixed payments, lower costs, and no control rights, whereas the primary disadvantage is the additional risk that debt financing brings to the business.

Debt provides a major source of capital for health services organizations. Thus, it is necessary for healthcare managers to be familiar with debt concepts. In the next chapter, we discuss equity financing, the second major type of capital.

Selected References

Aderholdt, John M., and Charles R. Pardue. 1989 "A Guide to Taxable Debt Financing Alternatives." *Healthcare Financial Management* (July): 58–66.

Carlile, Larry L., and Bruce M. Serchuk. 1995. "The Coming Changes in Tax-Exempt Health Care Finance." *Journal of Health Care Finance* (Fall): 1–42.

Cleverley, William O., and Paul C. Nutt. 1984. "The Decision Process Used for Bond Rating—and Its Implications." *Health Services Research* (December): 615–637.

Culler, Steven D. 1993a. "Assessing Hospital Credit Risk: A Banker's View." *Topics in Health Care Financing* (Summer): 35–43.

———. 1993b. "A Creditor's Perspective on the Hospital Industry." *Topics in Health Care Financing* (Summer): 12–20.

Demby, Hillary J. 1995. "Overcoming Financial Challenges with Bond Insurance." *Healthcare Financial Management* (March): 48–49.

Harris, John P., and Jeannette B. Price. 1988. "Finding Money Under Your Nose Using New Capital Techniques." *Healthcare Financial Management* (July): 24–30.

McCue, Michael J., and Jan P. Clement. 1996. "Assessing the Characteristics of Hospital Bond Defaults." *Medical Care* (November): 1121–1132.

Mullner, Ross, Dale Matthews, Joseph D. Kubal, and Stephen Andes. 1983. "Debt Financing: An Alternative for Hospital Construction Funding." *Healthcare Financial Management* (April): 18–24.

Nemes, Judith. 1991. "Dealing with the Authorities." *Modern Healthcare* (October 14):22–29.

Prince, Thomas R., and Ramachandran Ramanan. 1994. "Bond Ratings, Debt Insurance, and Hospital Operating Performance." *Topics in Health Care Financing* (Fall): 36–50.

Sims, William B. 1984. "Financing Strategies for Long-Term Care Facilities." *Healthcare Financial Management* (March): 42–54.

Sterns, Jay B.1994. "Emerging Trends in Health Care Finance." *Journal of Health Care Finance* (Winter): 1–10.

Tobin, William C., and Larry A. Kryzaniak. 1998. "Using Real-Estate-Based Financing to Access Capital." *Healthcare Financial Management* (July): 58–60.

West, David A. 1983. "Debt Financing in the 1980s: Is the Risk for Non-Profit Hospitals Too Great?" *Healthcare Financial Management* (April): 56–62.

Selected Web Sites

There are a multitude of web sites that pertain to this chapter.

For both tabular term structure data and a graph of the yield curve, see *www.bloomberg.com/markets/C13.html.*

For current (updated daily) interest rate information, see the Federal Reserve site at *www.bog.frb.fed.us/releases/H15/update.* Note that this site includes data on commercial paper, corporate bonds, and other rates in addition to the rates on Treasury securities.

For yields (interest rates) on AAA-rated insured municipal bonds of varying maturities, see *www.bloomberg.com/markets/psamuni.html.*

The Standard and Poor's web site provides a great deal of information on bond ratings. To see the ratings section, go directly to *www.standardpoor.com/ratings/index/htm.*

To learn more about bond insurance (credit enhancement), see the MBIA site at *www.mbia.com.*

Selected Cases

There are no cases that focus on the institutional details of debt financing. However, the following case in *Cases in Healthcare Finance* can be assigned to help students understand bond valuation, which is covered in Chapter 8:

Case 11: Potomac Healthcare (A), which focuses on the valuation of corporate bonds, as opposed to the managerial decisions inherent in floating a bond issue.

In addition, here is another case that focuses on related (Chapter 8) material:

Case 16: Boston Enterprises, which focuses on the bond refunding decision.

Notes

1. The *prime rate* is the base rate that banks charge on loans to businesses. Theoretically, the prime rate is set separately by each bank, but in practice all banks follow the lead of the major New York City banks, so there usually is a single prime rate in the United States. The prime rate changes—sometimes quite rapidly—to changing economic conditions, primarily inflation expectations. In early 2000, the prime rate was 8.75 percent. T-bills are discussed in the next footnote.
2. Treasury bonds, or T-bonds, have original maturities at issue of 10–30 years. The Treasury also issues *notes*, called T-notes, which have maturities of 1–10 years, and *bills*, called T-bills, which have maturities of less than one year. Note that the names of Treasury securities are fixed at issue even though their maturities shorten over time. Thus, a 30-year T-bond that was issued 25 years ago now has only five years remaining to maturity, but it is still classified as a bond, not a note.
3. The maximum maturity without SEC registration is 270 days. Also, commercial paper can only be sold to "sophisticated" investors; otherwise, SEC registration would be required even for maturities of 270 days or less.
4. A fourth rating agency, Duff & Phelps, was acquired by Fitch IBCA in 2000. Also, note that Moody's and S&P dominate the credit-rating industry, handling about 85 percent of all bond deals.
5. For a discussion of the forces that influence the shape of the yield curve, see Eugene F. Brigham, Louis C. Gapenski, and Michael C. Ehrhardt, *Financial Management: Theory and Practice* (Fort Worth, TX: Dryden Press, 1999), Chapter 4.

EQUITY FINANCING AND INVESTMENT BANKING

Learning Objectives

After studying this chapter, readers should be able to:

- Describe the key features associated with preferred stock financing.
- Explain the rights and privileges associated with common stock ownership.
- Discuss the procedures for selling new common stock.
- Describe the market for common stock.
- Explain how not-for-profit businesses obtain equity financing.

Introduction

Debt financing concepts were discussed in Chapter 6, including how interest rates are set in the economy, types of debt, and how various debt features affect the interest rate on any particular issue. The second source of capital to healthcare businesses is *equity financing*. Within investor-owned, or for-profit, firms, equity financing is obtained from shareholders through the sale of *stock* and by retaining earnings within the business. The equivalent financing in not-for-profit firms, sometimes called *fund capital*, is raised through contributions, grants, and by retaining earnings. From a financial perspective, common stock and fund financing serve the same basic purpose, so the generic term *equity* will be used to refer to all nondebt capital, regardless of a business's ownership.

In this chapter, we discuss the same general issues as in Chapter 6, but the focus is on equity financing. In addition, we will provide some supplemental information on how securities are sold, or the investment banking process.

Preferred Stock

Preferred stock, which can be issued only by investor-owned firms, is a hybrid—it is similar to bonds in some respects and to common stock in other ways. Accountants classify preferred stock as equity, so it is shown on the balance sheet as an equity account. However, from a financial management perspective, preferred stock is probably closer in nature to debt than to equity. Preferred stock imposes a fixed charge on the firm, and hence it has the same impact on the riskiness of the business as does debt financing. However, unlike interest on debt, if a payment is missed on preferred stock, the holders do not have the legal right to force the business into bankruptcy.

Basic Features

Preferred stock usually has a stated *par*, or *face*, *value*—often $100. The *dividend* on preferred stock, which is the equivalent to interest on a debt security, typically is paid quarterly. When a preferred issue is sold, the dividend is stated either as some percentage of par value or as so many dollars per share. For example, in 2000, Regent Healthcare, a large for-profit integrated system, sold 50,000 shares of $100 par value preferred stock, raising a total $5 million of new capital. This issue had a stated dividend of 10 percent, so the annual dollar dividend was $10, or $2.50 each quarter. Preferred dividends are generally fixed at issue, so Regent's preferred dividend will remain at $10 per year regardless of interest rate changes over time. Thus, if the required rate of return on Regent's preferred increases to 12 percent, the value of the stock will fall, just as it will with debt securities.

Although preferred stock contains a promise to pay the stated dividend, issuers do not have the contractual obligation to make the payment. Thus, like common stock, preferred stock dividends are declared each quarter by the business's board of directors; and if the issuer's financial condition deteriorates, the board can elect to *omit*, or *pass*, the dividend. However, most preferred issues are *cumulative*, which means that the cumulative total of all unpaid preferred dividends must be paid before dividends can be paid on the firm's common stock. Unpaid preferred dividends are called *arrearages*, and all arrearages must be paid before common dividends can be paid.

Preferred stock typically carries no voting privileges, so preferred stock-holders have no ownership rights. However, most preferred issues stipulate that preferred stockholders can elect a minority of directors—say, 3 out of 12—if the preferred dividends are passed. Even though nonpayment of preferred dividends will not bankrupt a firm, businesses issue preferred stock with every intention of paying the promised dividends. Passing a dividend usually pre-cludes the payment of common dividends and places preferred stockholders on the board. Furthermore, firms with preferred dividends in arrears have a difficult time selling new debt, and find it almost impossible to sell new common or preferred stock.

Investors regard preferred stock as being riskier than debt for two reasons: (1) Preferred dividends will be omitted before interest payments because default on interest payments has more serious consequences; and (2) in the event of bankruptcy and liquidation, preferred stockholders' claims are junior (subordinate) to debtholders' claims. Accordingly, investors require a higher rate of return on a firm's preferred stock than on its bonds. However, preferred stock has tax advantages to corporate buyers because 70 percent of the preferred dividends received by a corporation are exempt from corporate taxes. Thus, a corporate buyer of Regent's preferred stock in the 40 percent tax bracket would pay 40 percent taxes on 30 percent of the preferred dividend for an effective tax rate of only $0.40 \times 0.30 = 0.12 = 12$ percent. If the corporate buyer purchased Regent's debt, it would have to pay taxes on the interest earned at the full 40 percent rate. Because of this tax advantage to corporate buyers, dividend rates on preferred stock are pushed down to the point where before-tax returns are actually lower on preferred stocks than on lower-risk bonds. For this reason, almost all ordinary preferred stock is sold to corporate, rather than individual, investors.

Almost half of all preferred stock sold in recent years is *convertible*, which means that the preferred stock can be converted, or exchanged, into a set number of shares of common stock. The number of common shares obtained by conversion is fixed when the preferred is issued so that immediate conversion makes no financial sense. Over time, however, if the price on the firm's common stock rises, a point is reached when the holders of the preferred stock will be better off if they convert the preferred into common.

Some older preferred stocks are similar to perpetual bonds in that they have no maturity date. However, all preferred stock issued today has either a sinking fund or call provisions that limit the life of the issue. For example, many preferred shares have a sinking fund that calls for the retirement of 2 percent of the issue each year, which means that the average maturity of the issue is 25 years, and that the issue will be totally refunded in 50 years.

Advantages and Disadvantages of Preferred Stock Financing

There is a lot more that could be said about preferred stock, particularly about the type that is convertible into common stock. However, this type of equity is not a major source of funding for healthcare businesses, so we will conclude our discussion with the advantages and disadvantages of "regular" preferred stock.[1] From the viewpoint of the issuer, there are three primary advantages:

1. Unlike debt financing, the obligation to pay preferred dividends is not contractual, so passing (omitting) a preferred dividend cannot force a business into bankruptcy.
2. By issuing preferred stock, rather than common stock, the firm avoids the dilution of adding more shares of common stock as well as the additional sharing of control.
3. Because preferred stock often has a longer maturity than debt, preferred stock pushes principal repayments further into the future than typically occurs with debt issues.

There are two major disadvantages, however:

1. Preferred stock dividends are not deductible from taxable income by the issuer, so the after-tax cost on a preferred issue is higher than the cost of a similar debt issue. However, the fact that preferred stock has tax advantages to corporate buyers means that the difference in cost is not as great as it first appears.

2. Although preferred dividends can be passed, investors expect them to be paid. If they are not, there are negative consequences for the issuer, so preferred dividends impose a more stringent fixed cost on a business than do common dividends. Thus, like the use of debt, the use of preferred stock increases the financial risk of a business and, hence, its cost of common stock.

Self-Test Questions

1. What are the general features of preferred stock?
2. Should preferred stock be considered as equity or debt financing? Explain your answer.
3. Who are the major purchasers of nonconvertible preferred stock? Why?
4. What are the advantages and disadvantages of preferred stock financing?

Rights and Privileges of Common Stockholders

Common stockholders are the owners of for-profit corporations, and, as such, have certain rights and privileges. The most important of these rights and privileges are discussed in this section.

Claim on Residual Earnings

The reason that most people buy common stocks is to gain the right to a proportionate share of the residual earnings of the firm. A firm's net income, which is the residual earnings after all expenses have been paid, belongs to the firm's common stockholders. For many firms, particularly mature ones, some portion of net income will be paid out to common stockholders as *dividends*. Although the predominant timing of dividend payments is quarterly, some firms are now changing to annual dividends to reduce the administrative costs associated with such payments. The portion of net income that is retained within the firm will be invested in new assets, which presumably will increase the firm's earnings over time, and hence contribute to even greater dividends in the future. (We will have much more to say about dividends and other distributions to owners in Chapter 17.)

An increasing dividend stream means that the firm's stock will be more valuable in the future than it is today because dividends will be higher, say, in five years, than they are today. Thus, common stockholders typically expect to be able to sell the stock they purchased at some time in the future at a higher price than they paid for it, and hence realize a *capital gain*. To illustrate the payment of dividends, consider Table 7.1, which lists the annual per share dividend payment and earnings, as well as the average annual stock price, for Big Sky Healthcare from 1990 through 2000. Over the ten growth periods, Big Sky's dividend grew by 275 percent, or at an average annual growth rate of 14.1 percent. At the same time, the firm's stock price grew by 247 percent, which is an average annual growth rate of 13.2 percent.

TABLE 7.1
Big Sky
Healthcare:
Dividends,
Earnings, and
Stock Price,
1990–2000

Year	Annual per Share Dividend	Annual per Share Earnings	Average Annual Stock Price
1990	$0.20	$0.48	$ 7.70
1991	0.23	0.55	10.95
1992	0.23	0.52	11.00
1993	0.23	0.58	10.40
1994	0.48	0.85	15.30
1995	0.52	1.10	18.70
1996	0.58	1.25	20.60
1997	0.58	0.45	19.50
1998	0.65	1.35	23.20
1999	0.70	1.50	24.40
2000	0.75	1.55	26.70

Note that Big Sky's dividend growth was not a constant 14.1 percent each year. Many firms hold the dividend constant for several years to allow earnings to climb to a point where they can support a higher dividend payment. For example, Big Sky kept its dividend at $0.23 a share from 1991 through 1993, while earnings per share were flat at about $0.55.

In general, managers are very reluctant to reduce dividends because investors interpret lower dividends as a signal that management forecasts poor times ahead.[2] Thus, when Big Sky saw its earnings per share tumble from $1.25 in 1996 to $0.45 in 1997, it maintained its $0.58 per share dividend. Big Sky was able to pay a cash dividend that exceeded earnings in 1997 because the firm's cash flow, which is roughly equal to Net income + Depreciation, easily supported the dividend. When earnings picked up again in 1998, Big Sky increased its dividend to $0.65.

Over the entire period, Big Sky has proved to be a good investment for stockholders. For example, assume that you bought the stock for $7.70 in 1990, received a $0.20 dividend payment, and then sold the stock one year later for $10.95. For simplicity, assume that the dividend payment was paid at the end of the one-year holding period rather than quarterly. Thus, you paid $7.70, and one year later you received $10.95 + $0.20 = $11.15. The total return earned was Total profit/Amount of investment = ($11.15 − $7.70)/$7.70 = 0.448 = 44.8%. (Or, using a financial calculator, enter PV = 7.70[or − 7.70], FV = 11.15, N = 1, and press I to get 44.8 percent.) Note, however, that investors who bought Big Sky's stock in 1992 or 1996 and then sold it one year later would have had a capital loss, rather than a capital gain, on the sale. Of course, they would have received quarterly dividends over the one-year holding period. We will have much more to say about stock valuation in Chapter 8.

Control of the Firm

Common stockholders have the right to elect the firm's directors, who in turn elect the officers who will manage the business. In small, privately owned corporations, the major stockholders typically assume all of the management leadership positions. However, in large, publicly owned firms, managers typically have some stock, but their personal holdings are insufficient to allow them to exercise voting control. Thus, the management of most publicly owned firms can be removed by the stockholders if they decide a management team is not effective.

Various state and federal laws stipulate how stockholder control is to be exercised. First, corporations must hold an election of directors periodically, usually once a year, and take votes at the annual meeting. Frequently, one third of the directors are elected each year for a three-year term. Each share of stock has one vote; thus, the owner of 1,000 shares has 1,000 votes.[3] Stockholders can appear at the annual meeting and vote in person, but typically they transfer their right to vote to a second party by means of a *proxy*. Management always solicits stockholders' proxies and usually gets them. However, if the common stockholders are dissatisfied with current management, an outside group may solicit the proxies in an effort to overthrow management and take control of the business. This is known as a *proxy fight*.

The question of corporate control in large firms has become a central issue in recent years. The frequency of proxy fights has increased, as have attempts by one corporation to take over another by purchasing a majority of the outstanding stock. A *hostile takeover* occurs when such a control change takes place without approval by the managers of the firm being bought.

Obviously, managers who do not have majority control are very concerned about proxy fights and hostile takeovers. One of the most common tactics to thwart hostile takeovers is to place a *poison pill* provision in the corporate charter. A poison pill typically permits stockholders of the firm that is taken over to buy shares of the firm that instituted the takeover at a greatly reduced price. Obviously, shareholders at the acquiring firm do not want an outside group to get bargain-priced stock, so such provisions effectively stop hostile takeovers. Although poison pill provisions of this type might appear to be illegal, they have withheld many court challenges. The ultimate effect of poison pills is to force acquiring firms to get the approval of the managers of the other firm prior to the takeover. Although the stated reason for poison pills is to protect shareholders against a hostile takeover at a price that is too low, many people believe that they protect managers more than stockholders.

The Preemptive Right

Common stockholders often have the right, called the *preemptive right*, to purchase any new shares sold by the corporation. In some states, the preemptive right is mandatory; in others, it can be specified in the corporate charter.

The purpose of the preemptive right is twofold. First, it protects current stockholders' power of control. If it were not for this safeguard, the management of a corporation under criticism from stockholders could secure its position by issuing a large number of additional shares and purchasing these shares itself. Management would thereby gain a controlling position in the corporation and frustrate the outside stockholders.

The second, and more important, reason for the preemptive right is that it protects stockholders against a dilution of value. For example, suppose HealthOne HMO has 1,000 shares outstanding at a price of $100 per share, so the total market value of the firm is $100,000. If an additional 1,000 shares were sold at $50 a share, or for $50,000, it would raise the total market value of HealthOne's stock to $150,000. When the new total market value is divided by the new number of shares outstanding, a value of $75 per share is obtained. HealthOne's old stockholders lose $25 per share, and the new stockholders have an instant profit of $25 per share. Thus, selling common stock at a price below the current market price dilutes its market value and, hence, transfers wealth from the present stockholders to those who purchase the new shares. The preemptive right prevents such occurrences.

1. In what forms do common stock investors receive returns?
2. How do common stockholders exercise their right of control?
3. What is the preemptive right, and what is its purpose?

**Self-Test
Questions**

Types of Common Stock

Although most firms issue only one type of common stock, multiple types may be used in some instances.

Classified Stock

Classified stock is sometimes used to meet the special needs of corporations, especially start-up businesses. Generally, when special classifications of stock are used, one type is designated *Class A*, another *Class B*, and so on. Small, new firms seeking to obtain funds from outside sources frequently use different types of common stock. For example, when Genetic Research, Inc., went public in 1998, its Class A stock was sold to the public and paid a token dividend, but carried no voting rights for five years. Its Class B stock was retained by the organizers of the firm and carried full voting rights for five years; but dividends could not be paid on the Class B stock until the firm had established its earning power by building up retained earnings to a designated level. The firm's use of classified stock allowed the public to take a position in a conservatively financed growth firm and to earn a small amount of dividend income, while the founders retained absolute control during the crucial early stages of the firm's development. At the same time, outside investors were protected against excessive withdrawals of funds by the original owners. As is often the case in such situations, the Class B stock was also called *founders' shares.*

Note that "Class A," "Class B," and so on, have no standard meanings. Most corporations have no classified shares, but a firm that does could designate its Class B shares as founders' shares and its Class A shares as those sold to the public, while another could reverse these designations. Other firms could use the A and B designations for entirely different purposes.

In general, voting rights is one of the distinguishing features of classified stock. For example, suppose that Big East Healthcare had two classes of stock that differed only with respect to voting rights: Class V had such rights, while Class N did not. As you would expect, the Class V stock would be more valuable than the Class N stock, typically by about 2 to 5 percent. Thus, if the Class N stock were selling at $100 per share, the Class V stock might sell for $104.

Tracking Stock

In a *spin-off*, some portion of an existing firm is set up as a separate firm, and stock of the newly formed firm is distributed to existing shareholders of the original parent firm. The end result is that the original shareholders now own the stock of two independent firms. As an alternative to a spin off, a firm may opt to issue tracking stock. *Tracking stock* is used when a parent firm wants to separate the performance of a particular segment from the rest of the business, yet continue to retain control of that segment. As one observer stated, "The parent [firm] can have its cake and sell it too." For the most part, tracking stock has been used by firms that have a high-growth Internet subsidiary along with slower-growth business lines. However, it is possible that someday it might be used by investor-owned healthcare businesses.

Typically, a firm will create some number of shares whose value is tied solely to the performance of the subsidiary; issue a portion—say, 30 percent—to the parent firm's stockholders; and retain the remainder within the firm. Thus, the tracking stock becomes publicly held and trades separately from the stock of the parent firm although the parent retains control. At some later time, the firm may sell additional shares of the tracking stock to raise money for the subsidiary. Another way of creating a tracking stock is to initially sell the tracking shares to the public through an initial public offering (IPO) rather than distribute the shares to the current shareholders of the parent. In this method, new capital is raised immediately upon creation of the tracking shares.

Trackers possess many of the same features as "regular" stock. For example, firms can declare dividends on tracking stock. Also, firms must file separate financial data for the tracking stock. One of the biggest advantages of tracking stock is that it allows a firm to align the compensation of the subsidiary's managers directly to the stock performance of that business line. Additionally, it is sometimes the case that tracking stock "unlocks" the value of a fast-growing subsidiary, which otherwise is hidden within a much larger firm. Furthermore, tracking stock allows investors to buy shares only in the portion of the overall business that they might be interested in.

However, for control purposes, tracking stock shareholders are considered to be shareholders of the parent firm and not of the division being tracked. Thus, another firm cannot acquire the subsidiary by buying up the tracking stock. This means that tracking stockholders have no chance of earning a takeover premium on the business. Finally, investors in tracking stocks must recognize that the board of directors of the parent firm controls both the parent and the business being tracked; and if a conflict of interest arises between the parent firm and the subsidiary, it might be resolved in favor of the parent and to the detriment of the subsidiary. For example, a parent could raise, say, $200 million, from a tracking stock IPO, and use the bulk of the proceeds outside of the tracking subsidiary. This, and similar, action transfers wealth from the tracking stockholders to the parent firm stockholders.

1. Name several types of classified stock and explain their uses.
2. How would the values of voting and non-voting stock differ?
3. What is tracking stock and how is it used?

Self-Test Questions

Procedures for Selling New Common Stock

New stock usually is sold to raise equity capital. In addition, new stock sometimes is distributed to current shareholders without raising additional funds, for example, in a spin off. When stock is issued to raise new equity capital, the new shares may be sold in one of six ways:

1. On a pro rata basis to existing stockholders through a rights offering;
2. Through investment bankers to the general public in a public offering;
3. To a single buyer, or a very small number of buyers, in a private placement;
4. To employees through employee stock purchase plans;
5. Through a dividend reinvestment plan; and
6. Through direct purchase plans.

The following sections provide more information on these methods.

Rights Offerings

As discussed in the preceding section, common stockholders often have the *preemptive right* to purchase any additional shares sold by the firm. If the preemptive right is contained in a particular firm's charter, the firm must offer any newly issued commons stock to existing stockholders. If the charter does not prescribe a preemptive right, the firm can choose to sell to its existing stockholders or to the public at large. If it sells to the existing stockholders, the stock sale is called a *rights offering*. Each stockholder is issued an option to buy a certain number of new shares at a price below the existing market price, and the terms of the option are listed on a certificate called a *stock purchase right*, or simply a *right*. If a stockholder does not wish to purchase any additional shares in the firm, then he or she can sell the rights to some other person who does want to buy the stock.[4]

Public Offerings

If the preemptive right exists in a firm's charter, it must sell new stock through a rights offering. If the preemptive right does not exist, the firm may choose to offer the new shares to the general public through a *public offering*. We discuss procedures for public offerings in detail in a later section.

Private Placements

In a *private placement,* securities are sold to one or a few investors—generally institutional investors. Private placements are most common with bonds, but they also occur with stocks. The primary advantages of private placements are lower issuance costs and greater speed because the shares do not have to go through the SEC registration process.

The primary disadvantage of a private placement is that because the securities generally will not have gone through the SEC registration process, they must be sold initially to a large, "sophisticated" investor—usually an insurance firm, mutual fund, or pension fund. Furthermore, in the event that the original purchaser wants to sell the securities, they must be sold to other large, "sophisticated" investors. However, the SEC currently allows any institution with a portfolio of $100 million or more to buy and sell private placement securities. Because there are thousands of institutions with assets that exceed this limit, private placements are becoming more and more popular with issuers.

To illustrate a private equity placement, consider the situation facing Healtheon/WebMD in early 2000. Healtheon needed cash quickly to help pay for an acquisition. At the same time, the managers at Janus funds were flush with cash that they wanted to invest in the stocks of fast-growing firms. Within 24 hours, a win-win deal was struck in which Healtheon sold $930 million of newly issued stock directly to the Janus funds. The deal was good for Healtheon because it got its equity infusion without bearing the costs of going through an investment banker, which for this issue would have been about $30 million. In addition, Healtheon did not have to spend the time and money to do a "roadshow" to convince prospective investors to buy the issue. Janus was able to acquire a sizable chunk of a fast-growing Internet firm without having to battle other institutional investors for a share of the new issue. Additionally, Janus was able to buy the stock at a discount to what it would have cost if a public placement were used.

Employee Purchase Plans and ESOPs

Many firms have plans that allow employees to purchase stock on favorable terms. First, under executive incentive *stock option plans*, key managers are given options to purchase stock. These managers generally have a direct, material influence on the firm's fortunes, so if they perform well, the stock price will go up and the options will become valuable. Second, there are plans for lower-level employees. For example, Texas HealthPlans, Inc., a regional investor-owned HMO, permits employees who are not participants in its stock option plan to allocate up to 10 percent of their salaries to its *stock purchase plan*, and the funds are then used to buy newly issued shares at 85 percent of the market price on the purchase date. Often the firm's contribution— in this case, the 15 percent discount—is not vested in an employee until five years after the purchase date. Thus, the employee cannot realize the benefit of the firm's contribution without working an additional five years. This type of plan is designed both to improve employee performance and to reduce turnover.

A third type of plan is related to the second one, but here the stock bought for employees is purchased out of a share of the firm's profits. Under an *Employee Stock Ownership Plan (ESOP)*, firms can claim a tax credit equal to a percentage of wages, provided that the funds are used to buy newly issued stock for the benefit of employees. The amount of the credit varies from year to year, depending on the whims of Congress: Currently it is 1/2 of 1 percent of total wages. Because of their favorable tax treatment, and because they are thought to create a more loyal and productive workforce, many firms have created ESOPs in recent years. Now, over 10,000 firms have such plans that cover over 12 million employees.

Dividend Reinvestment Plans

During the 1970s, many large firms instituted *dividend reinvestment plans (DRIPs)*, whereby stockholders can automatically reinvest their dividends in the stock of the paying corporation. There are two types of DRIPs: (1) Plans that involve only "old" stock that is already outstanding, and (2) plans that involve newly issued stock. In either case, the stockholder must pay income taxes on the amount of the dividends, even though stock, rather than cash, is received.

Under both types of DRIP, stockholders must choose between continuing to receive cash dividends or using the cash dividends to buy more stock in the corporation. Under the "old" stock type of plan, a bank, which acts as a trustee, takes the total funds available for reinvestment from each quarterly dividend, purchases the corporation's stock on the open market, and allocates the shares purchased to the participating stockholders on a pro rata basis. The brokerage costs of buying the shares are low because of volume purchases, so these plans benefit small stockholders who do not need cash for current consumption.

The "new" stock type of DRIP provides for dividends to be invested in newly issued stock; hence, these plans raise new capital for the firm. No fees are charged to participating stockholders, and some firms offer the new stock at a discount of 3 to 5 percent below the prevailing market price. The firms absorb these costs as a trade-off against the issuance costs that would be incurred if the stock were sold through investment bankers rather than through the DRIP.

Direct Purchase Plans

In recent years, many firms have established *direct purchase plans*, which allow individual investors to purchase stock directly from the firm. Many of these plans grew out of DRIPs, which were expanded to allow participants to purchase shares in excess of the dividend amount. In direct purchase plans, investors usually pay little or no brokerage fees, and many plans offer convenient features such as fractional share purchases, automatic purchases by bank debit, and quarterly statements.

Although employee purchase plans, DRIPs, and direct purchase plans are an excellent way for employees and individual investors to purchase stock, they typically do not raise large sums of new capital for the business, so other methods must be used when equity needs are great.

Self-Test Questions

1. What is a rights offering?
2. What is a private placement and what are its primary advantages over a public offering?
3. Briefly, what are employee stock purchase plans?
4. What is a dividend reinvestment plan?
5. What is a direct purchase plan?

The Market for Common Stock

Some corporations are so small that their common stock is not actively traded; rather, it is owned by only a few people who usually are the managers. Such firms are said to be *privately held*, or *closely held*, and the stock is said to be a *closely held stock*.

The stocks of most small, publicly owned firms, as well as some large firms, are not listed on any exchange, and hence are said to be *unlisted*. Such stocks trade in the *over-the-counter (OTC)* market. However, most large, publicly owned firms apply for listing on an exchange. These stocks are said to be *listed*. As a general rule, firms are first listed on a regional exchange, such as the Pacific or Midwest; then they move up to the American (AMEX); and finally, if they grow large enough, to the "Big Board"—New York Stock Exchange (NYSE).

For example, American Healthcare Management, a King of Prussia, Pennsylvania-based firm that owns or manages 16 hospitals in nine states, recently listed on the NYSE. The firm, which had previously traded on the AMEX, believed that listing on the NYSE increases the trading of its shares and makes it more visible to the investment community, which presumably will have a positive impact on the price of its stock. Over five thousand stocks are traded in the OTC market versus about three thousand on the NYSE. But, because of the larger size of its listed firms, the NYSE has, until recently, dominated the OTC market in terms of market value and the number of shares traded. However, the recent surge in trading among the stocks of Internet and other "new economy" firms has caused trading in the OTC market to surge to the point where it now has higher volume, both in number of share and dollar terms, than does the NYSE.

Institutional investors, such as pension funds, insurance firms, and mutual funds, own about 60 percent of all common stocks. However, the institutions buy and sell relatively actively, so they account for about 75 percent of all transactions. Thus, the institutions have the greatest influence on the prices of individual stocks.

Stock market transactions can be classified into three distinct categories:

1. **The new issue market.** A small firm typically is owned by its management and a handful of private investors. At some point, if the firm is to grow further, its stock must be sold to the general public, which is defined as *going public*. The market for stock that is in the process of going public is often called the *new issue market*, and the issue is called an *initial public offering (IPO)*. To illustrate the concept, consider that in 1999 Healtheon, an online healthcare network, raised $40 million in an IPO by selling 5 million shares at $8 per share. The business had about 54 million shares held by insiders, so the IPO left the firm with about 59 million shares outstanding. On the first day of trading, the stock price closed at $31, giving the new public investors, as well as the original insiders, many reasons to celebrate.

2. **The primary market.** In 2000, Pacific Eldercare, which operates 79 nursing homes in ten states, sold 3.1 million shares of new common stock, thereby raising $31.2 million of new equity financing. Because the shares sold were newly created, the issue was defined as a *primary market* offering, but because the firm was already publicly held, the offering was not an IPO. Corporations prefer to obtain equity by retaining earnings because of the issuance costs and market pressure associated with the sale of new common stock. Still, if a firm requires more equity funds than can be generated from retained earnings, a stock sale may be required.

3. **The secondary market.** If the owner of 100 shares of HCA sells his or her stock, the trade is said to have occurred in the *secondary market*. Thus, the market for *outstanding*, or used, shares is defined as the secondary market. Almost 15 million shares of HCA were bought and sold on the NYSE in 1999, but the firm did not receive a dime from these transactions.

Self-Test
Questions

1. What is an initial public offering (IPO)?
2. What is the difference between selling HCA shares in the primary market and selling the firm's shares in the secondary market?

The Decision to Go Public

Most businesses start as proprietorships or partnerships, and then, if they are successful and grow, they find it useful to convert to a corporation. Initially, the stock of most corporations is owned by the business's founders, key employees, and often a few investors—usually *venture capitalists*—who may or may not be actively involved in management.[5] However, if growth continues, at some point most firms go public. The advantages and disadvantages of public stock ownership are discussed next.

Advantages of Going Public

- **Permits founder diversification.** As a firm grows and becomes more valuable, its founders often have most of their wealth tied up in their ownership position. By selling some of their stock during the initial public offering, or sometime thereafter, the founders can better diversify their holdings, thereby reducing the riskiness of their personal portfolios.
- **Increases liquidity.** The stock of a closely held firm is very illiquid: It has no ready market. If one of the owners wants to sell some shares to raise cash, he or she finds that it is difficult to find a buyer, and even if one can be found, there is no established price on which to base the sale. Going public creates the liquidity that solves these problems.
- **Facilitates raising new corporate cash.** If a privately held firm needs to raise new equity, it must either get it from the current owners, who may not want to put additional capital into the business, or shop around for other investors. However, often the firm finds it difficult to get outsiders to contribute equity capital to a closely held business because they are at the mercy of the founders who have a controlling interest. To illustrate the concept, consider that the founders, who typically are the managers, can vote themselves excessive compensation packages, have private self-serving dealings with the business, and even withhold the business's financial information from outside investors. There are few positions as vulnerable as being an outside stockholder in a closely held firm. Going public, which requires both public disclosure and regulation by the SEC, greatly reduces these problems, and hence makes it much easier for the business to raise equity capital.
- **Establishes a value for the business.** There are several reasons why it is useful for the marketplace to establish the equity value of a business. For one thing, when the owner of a closely held business dies, tax appraisers must set a value on the ownership position. If the value is too high, the estate is treated unfairly, but if the value is too low, the taxpayers lose. A

firm that is publicly held has an established value. Similarly, if a firm gives incentive stock options to key employees, they cannot estimate a value for those options unless the stock is publicly traded.

Disadvantages of Going Public

- **Cost of reporting.** A publicly owned firm must file quarterly and annual reports with the SEC and various state agencies. Such reports are costly to produce, especially for smaller firms that do not have the internal resources to prepare them.
- **Disclosure.** In most situations, management of large firms would prefer to keep operating and financial data private rather than have them available to the firm's competitors. Similarly, the owners of smaller firms may not want to disclose their net worth, and because a publicly owned firm must disclose the number of shares owned by its officers, directors, and major stockholders, it is easy for anyone to estimate the net worth of the insiders or at least that portion due to ownership of the business.
- **Self-dealings.** The owners/managers of closely held firms have many opportunities for various types of questionable, but legal, self-dealings including the payment of above-market salaries; nepotism; personal transactions with the business, such as lease arrangements; overgranting of stock options and warrants; and other fringe benefits that go far beyond what the marketplace sets as reasonable. Such self-dealings become harder and harder to sustain when a firm becomes public and ultimately creates a board of directors that exercises true oversight.
- **Inactive market/low price.** If the corporation is very small, its shares will not be frequently traded; its stock will not really be liquid; and its market price often is a poor measure of the stock's true value. In addition, security analysts will not follow the stock. If this situation persists, much of the benefit associated with going public is not actually realized.
- **Control.** In many businesses, the most dramatic increase in shareholder wealth occurs when a proxy fight or hostile takeover takes place. In addition, these acts motivate managers to pursue stockholder wealth maximization with some zeal. Conversely, such acts often result in removal of the managers at the acquired firm. If the managers maintain a controlling interest, their jobs are secure. In most cases, going public ultimately leads to loss of control by the founding owners/managers.

Conclusions on Going Public

There are no hard and fast rules regarding when, or even if, a closely held firm should go public. This decision is different for each business and should be made on the basis of the unique circumstances surrounding the business and its stockholders. If a firm does decide to go public, either by selling new common stock to raise capital or by the sale of stock held by insiders, the key issue is setting the price at which the shares will be offered. The current owners want the price to be as high as possible because the higher the price, the smaller the proportion of the firm that they will have to relinquish to obtain a specified dollar amount of equity financing. On the other hand, potential buyers want the price set as low as possible. We will discuss the process of setting the price on an IPO in a later section.

1. What are the primary advantages of going public?
2. What are the disadvantages?

The Decision to List

The decision to go public is truly a milestone in a firm's life—it marks a major change in the relationship between the business and its owners. The decision to *list* the stock on an exchange rather than have it traded in the over-the-counter market, on the other hand, is not a significant event in the life of a business. The firm will have to file a few new reports and abide by the rules of the exchange; the brokers who handle sales of the stock will have to use a different process; and the stock's price will be quoted under an exchange listing rather than in the over-the-counter section.

To have its stock listed, a firm must meet the exchange's minimum requirements regarding size, number of shareholders, and number of shares held by outsiders—called *float*. These requirements become more stringent as a firm moves from the regional exchanges to the AMEX to the NYSE. Float is important to an exchange because shares held by insiders trade much less frequently than do shares held by outsiders. If the float is small, there will be limited trading and the exchange will gain little from the listing. Also, the firm must agree to disclose certain information to help the exchange track trading patterns in an effort to minimize the likelihood that the stock is being manipulated.[6] If the minimum requirements are met, the firm merely applies to the exchange, pays a relatively small fee, and is then listed on that exchange.

Many people believe that listing is beneficial both to the firm and its stockholders. Listed firms receive a certain amount of free advertising and publicity, and their listed status may enhance their prestige and reputation. These factors, as well the additional safeguards against manipulation, may have a positive impact on sales and stock price. However, in recent years, improvements in telecommunications and digital processing of trades have lowered transactions costs to the point where differences between trading on the exchanges and on the over-the-counter market are now inconsequential. In fact, the over-the-counter market now has more stocks listed and a larger dollar volume of trades than does the NYSE. As a result, some very large firms, including MCI, Intel, and Apple, which almost certainly would have been listed on the NYSE in times past, have elected to remain in the over-the-counter market.

1. What are some of the considerations involved in the decision to list a stock?

Self-Test Question

Advantages and Disadvantages of Common Stock Financing

In this section, we briefly discuss the advantages and disadvantages of financing with common stock.

Advantages of Common Stock

- **No fixed charges.** Common stock does not obligate the business to fixed charges. If the business does not generate sufficient earnings, it does not have to pay dividends on its common stock. Conversely, if the firm used debt financing, it must make the promised interest and principal payments regardless of the earnings level.
- **No maturity date.** Common stock has no maturity date; it is permanent capital that does not have to be "paid back."
- **Creates additional debt capacity.** Because equity financing strengthens the position of creditors, common stock financing increases access to the debt markets and lowers the cost of debt.
- **May be easier to sell.** Common stock can, at times, be sold more easily than debt, especially when the firm is small and growing rapidly, which almost by definition makes it risky. It appeals to some investors because (1) it offers a higher expected rate of return than does preferred stock or debt; (2) it provides a better hedge against inflation than does fixed return securities; and (3) it has tax advantages over preferred stock and debt investments.[7]

Disadvantages of Common Stock

- **Dilutes control.** The sale of common stock normally gives voting rights to new investors, which dilutes the control of current owners. For this reason, equity financing often is avoided by small firms whose owner/managers may be unwilling to share control with outsiders. However, as we discussed in a previous section, a special class of common stock can be used that does not confer voting rights.
- **Dilutes value.** Debt financing has a fixed cost, and hence creditors do not share in the success of a business beyond what is promised in the debt agreement. New common stock, however, "dilutes the equity" in the sense that there are more claims on the residual earnings of the business.
- **Issuance costs.** As discussed in the next section, the costs associated with a new stock issue are higher than the costs associated with a similar-sized preferred stock or debt issue.
- **Negative signaling.** The sale of new common stock may be perceived by investors as a negative signal, which would put downward pressure on the

stock price. The reason for such an interpretation is the assumption that managers know more about future prospects for the firm than do outside shareholders. Furthermore, it is in the firm's best interest to issue new common stock when it is overvalued in the marketplace. Thus, a new stock issue, especially one by mature firms, can be interpreted as a signal that managers believe the stock to be overvalued.

Self-Test Question

1. What are the advantages and disadvantages associated with common stock financing?

Securities Regulation and the Investment Banking Process

In this section, we describe the regulation of securities markets, the way securities are issued, and the role that investment bankers play in the issuance process.

Regulation of Securities Markets

Sales of new securities, and also sales in the secondary markets, are regulated by the *Securities and Exchange Commission (SEC)* and, to a lesser extent, by each of the 50 states. Here are the primary elements of SEC regulation:

- The SEC has jurisdiction over all **interstate** offerings of new securities to the public in amounts of $1.5 million or more.
- Newly issued securities must be registered with the SEC at least 20 days before they are publicly offered. The *registration statement* provides financial, legal, and technical information about the firm to the SEC, and the *prospectus* summarizes this information for investors. SEC lawyers and accountants analyze both the registration statement and the prospectus; if the information is inadequate or misleading, the SEC will delay or stop the public offering.
- After the registration has become effective, new securities may be offered, but any sales solicitation must be accompanied by the prospectus. Preliminary, or *"red herring," prospectuses* may be distributed to potential buyers during the 20-day waiting period, but no sales may be finalized during this time. The "red herring" prospectus contains all the key information that will appear in the final prospectus except the price, which is generally set after the market closes the day before the new securities are actually sold to the public.
- If the registration statement or prospectus contains misrepresentations or omissions of material facts, any purchaser who suffers a loss may sue for damages. Severe penalties may be imposed on the issuer or its officers, directors, accountants, engineers, appraisers, underwriters, and all others who participated in the preparation of the registration statement or prospectus.

- The SEC also regulates all national stock exchanges. Firms whose securities are listed on an exchange must file annual reports similar to the registration statement with both the SEC and the exchange.
- The SEC has control over corporate *insiders*. Officers, directors, and major stockholders must file monthly reports of changes in their holdings of the stock of the corporation.
- The SEC has the power to prohibit manipulation by such devices as *pools* (large amounts of money used to buy or sell stocks to artificially affect prices) or *wash sales* (sales between members of the same group to record artificial transaction prices).
- The SEC has control over the form of the proxy statement and the way the firm uses it to solicit votes.

Control over the use of credit to buy securities (primarily common stock) is exercised by the Federal Reserve Board through *margin requirements*, which specify the maximum percentage of the purchase price that can be financed by brokerage borrowings. The current margin requirement is 50 percent, so stock investors can borrow up to half of the cost of a stock purchase from his or her broker. (Of course, the entire amount on account with the broker could be borrowed from another source, so margin requirements only control broker-supplied debt capital.) If the stock price of a stock bought on margin falls, then the margin money (50 percent of the original value) becomes more than half the current value, and the investor is forced to put up additional personal funds. Such a demand for more personal money is known as a *margin call*. The amount of additional funds required depends on the *maintenance margin*, which is set by the broker supplying the loan. When a large proportion of trades are on margin and the stock market begins a retreat, the volume of margin calls can be substantial. Because most investors who buy on margin do not have a large reserve of personal funds, they are forced to sell some stock to meet margin calls, which, in turn, can accelerate the market decline.

States also have some control over the issuance of new securities within their boundaries. This control is usually exercised by a "corporation commissioner" or someone with a similar title. State laws relating to security sales are called *blue sky laws* because they were put into effect to keep unscrupulous promoters from selling securities that offered the "blue sky," but which actually had little or no assets or cash flows behind them.

The securities industry itself realizes the importance of stable markets, sound brokerage firms, and the absence of price manipulation. Therefore, the various exchanges work closely with the SEC to police transactions and to maintain the integrity and credibility of the system. Similarly, the *National Association of Securities Dealers (NASD)* cooperates to police trading in the over-the-counter market. These industry groups also cooperate with regulatory authorities to set net worth and other standards for securities firms, to develop insurance programs to protect the customers of brokerage houses, and the like.

In general, government regulation of securities trading, as well as industry self-regulation, is designed to ensure (1) that investors receive information that is as accurate as possible, (2) that no one artificially manipulates the market price of a given security, and (3) that corporate insiders do not take advantage of their position to profit in their firms' securities at the expense of others. Neither the SEC, the state regulators, nor the industry itself can prevent investors from making foolish decisions or from having bad luck, but they can, and do, help investors obtain the best data possible for making sound investment decisions.

The Investment Banking Process

The investment banking process takes place in two stages.

Stage I Decisions

At Stage I, the firm itself makes some initial, preliminary decisions, including the following:

- **Dollars to be raised.** How much new capital is needed?
- **Type of securities used.** Should common stock, bonds, some other security, or a combination of securities be used? Furthermore, if common stock is to be issued, should it be done as a rights offering, by a direct sale to the general public, or by a private placement? If the sale will be by a public offering, the next two decisions must be made.
- **Competitive bid versus negotiated deal**. Should the firm simply offer a block of its securities for sale to the highest bidding investment banker, or should it negotiate a deal with an investment banker? These two procedures are called *competitive bids* and *negotiated deals,* respectively. Only about 100 of the largest firms, whose securities are already well known to the investment banking community, are in a position to use the competitive bidding process. The investment banks must do a large amount of investigative work to bid on an issue unless they are already quite familiar with the firm, and such costs would be too high to make it worthwhile unless the banker were sure of getting the deal. Therefore, except for the largest firms, offerings of stocks or bonds are generally on a negotiated basis.
- **Selection of an investment banker**. Most deals are negotiated, so the firm must select an investment banker. This choice can be an important decision for a firm that is going public. On the other hand, an older firm that has already "been to market" will have an established relationship with an investment banker. However, it is easy to change bankers if the firm is dissatisfied. Different investment banking houses are better suited for different firms. The older, larger "establishment houses," such as Morgan Stanley Dean Witter, deal mainly with large, established firms. Other investment banking houses specialize in smaller firms, or new issues,

technology firms, or some other niche of the equity markets. To get some idea of the major players in the investment banking business, see Table 7.2, which lists the top ten underwriters of U.S. debt and equity for 1999.

Stage II decisions, which are made jointly by the firm and its selected investment banker, include the following:

Stage II Decisions

- **Reevaluating the initial decisions.** The firm and its banker will reevaluate the initial decisions regarding the size of the issue and the type of securities to use. For example, the firm may have decided initially to raise $50 million by selling common stock, but the investment banker may convince management that under current market conditions the firm would be better off to limit the stock issue to $25 million and to raise the other $25 as debt.
- **Contractual basis of sale.** The firm and its investment banker must decide whether the banker will work on a *best efforts* basis or will *underwrite* the issue. In a best efforts sale, the banker does not guarantee that the securities will be sold or that the firm will get the cash it needs; it only guarantees that it will put forth its best efforts to sell the issue. On an underwritten issue, the firm does get a guarantee because the banker agrees to buy the entire issue and then resell the stock to its customers. Bankers bear significant risk in underwritten offerings because if the price of the security falls between the time the security is purchased from the issuer and the time of resale to the public, the investment banker must bear the loss. For example, on one IBM bond deal, interest rates rose sharply after the deal had been set, but before the bonds had been sold. The bankers lost about

TABLE 7.2
Top Ten Underwriters of U.S. Debt and Equity for 1999

Underwriter	Dollar Amount of Securities Managed (In Billions of Dollars)
Merrill Lynch	$ 332
Salomon Smith Barney	268
Morgan Stanley Dean Witter	211
Goldman Sachs	192
Credit Suisse First Boston	181
Lehman Brothers	170
Chase Manhattan	109
J.P. Morgan	91
Bear Stearns	86
Bank of America Securities	76
Top ten total	$1,716
Industry total	$2,149

Source: The *Wall Street Journal*, January 3, 2000, page R24.

$15 million on the underwriting. Had the offering been on a best-efforts basis, IBM, rather than the investment banker, would have been the loser.

- **Banker's compensation and other expenses.** The investment banker's compensation must be negotiated. Also, the firm must estimate the other issuance expenses it will incur in connection with the issue, such as lawyers' fees, accountants' costs, and printing and engraving expenses. In an underwritten issue, the banker will buy the issue from the firm at a discount below the price at which the securities are to be offered to the public; this "spread" is set to cover the banker's costs and to provide a profit. In a best-efforts sale, fees to the investment banker are normally set as some percentage of the dollar volume sold.

   Table 7.3 gives an indication of the issuance costs associated with public issues of bonds and common stock. As the table shows, costs as a percentage of the proceeds are higher for stocks than for bonds, and costs are higher for small than for large issues. The relationship between size of issue and issuance cost is primarily a result of the existence of fixed costs, which are certain costs that must be incurred regardless of the size of the issue, so the percentage cost is quite high for small issues.

- **Setting the offering price.** If the firm is already publicly owned, the offering price will be based on the existing market price of its stock or the yield on its bonds. Typically, the investment banker buys the securities at a prescribed number of points below the closing price on the last day of registration. Usually, such agreements have *escape clauses* that provide for

TABLE 7.3
Issuance Costs as a Percentage of Gross Proceeds

Size of Issue (Millions of Dollars)	Common Stock	Bonds
2–9.99	13.28%	4.39%
10–19.9	8.72	2.76
20–39.99	6.93	2.42
40–59.99	5.87	2.38
60–79.99	5.18	2.34
80–99.99	4.73	2.16
100–199.99	4.22	2.31
200–499.99	3.47	2.19
500 and up	3.15	1.64

Notes:
a. Issuance costs tend to rise somewhat when interest rates are cyclically high, which indicates that money is in relatively tight supply; when this happens, investment bankers will have a relatively hard time placing issues with investors. Thus, the figures shown in this table represent averages, as the costs actually vary somewhat over time.
b. The issuance costs listed for common stocks are for new stock offerings by publicly owned firms. Issuance costs on initial public offerings are significantly higher, ranging from about 32 percent for small issues to about 15 percent on large issues.
Source: Inmoo Lee, Scott Lochhead, Jay Ritter, and Quanshui Zhao, "The Costs of Raising Capital," *The Journal of Financial Research,* Spring 1996.

the contract to be voided if the price of the security drops below some preset amount. The purpose of such clauses is to allow the issuing firm to withdraw the issue if the price sinks to a point that the needed amount of money would not be raised.

The investment banker will have an easier job if the issue is priced relatively low; but the issuer of the securities naturally wants as high a price as possible. Some conflict of interest on price, therefore, arises between the investment banker and the issuer. If the issuer is financially sophisticated and makes comparisons with similar security issues, the investment banker will be forced to price close to the market.

If the firm is going public, there is no established price for the stock, and hence the investment banker will have to estimate the equilibrium price at which the stock will sell after it is issued. If the offering price is set below the true equilibrium price, as with most IPOs, the stock price will rise sharply on the first day of trading. For example, Healtheon's IPO was priced at $8, but the stock closed at $31 on the first day of trading. When this rise happens, the firm and the existing stockholders give away too many shares to raise the new capital, and there is a wealth transfer from existing stockholders to the IPO buyers. Conversely, if the stock price falls on the first day of trading, there is a wealth transfer from the new buyers to the old shareholders. Thus, it is important that the equilibrium price estimate be as good as possible.[8]

Selling Procedures

Once the firm and its investment banker have decided how much money to raise, the types of securities to issue, and the basis for pricing the issue, they will prepare and file a registration statement and a prospectus. It generally takes about 20 days for the issue to be approved by the SEC. The final price of the stock, or the interest rate on a bond issue, is set at the close of business on the day the issue clears the SEC, and the securities are offered to the public the following day.

Investors are required to pay for securities within ten days, and the investment banker must pay the issuing firm within four days of the official commencement of the offering. Typically, the banker sells the securities within a day or two after the offering begins; but on occasion, the banker miscalculates, sets the offering price too high, and thus is unable to move the issue. At other times, the market declines during the offering period, forcing the banker to reduce the price of the stock or bonds. In either instance, on an underwritten offering, the firm receives the dollar amount that was agreed on, so the banker must absorb any losses incurred.

Because they are exposed to large potential losses, investment bankers typically do not handle the purchase and distribution of issues single handedly unless the issue is a very small one. If the sum of money involved is large, investment bankers form *underwriting syndicates* in an effort to minimize the risk each banker carries. The banking house that sets up the deal is called the *lead*, or *managing, underwriter*. In addition to the underwriting syndicate, on larger offerings, still more investment bankers are included in a *selling group*, which handles the distribution of securities to individual investors. The selling group includes all members of the underwriting syndicate, plus additional dealers who take relatively small percentages of the total issue from the members of the underwriting syndicate. Thus, the underwriters act as wholesalers, while members of the selling group act as retailers. The number of houses in a selling group depends partly on the size of the issue, but also on the number and types of buyers. For example, the selling group that handled a recent $92 million municipal bond issue for Adventist Health System/Sunbelt consisted of three members, while the one that sold $1 billion in junk (B-rated) bonds for National Medical Enterprises consisted of eight members.[9]

A new selling procedure has recently emerged that does not require an underwriting syndicate. In an *unsyndicated stock offering*, the managing underwriting, acting alone, sells the issue entirely to one or more institutional investors. This type of offering can be thought of as a private placement through an investment banker. (As discussed previously, it is possible to do a private placement without using an investment banker at all.) The motivating force behind this type of offering is, of course, money. The fees that issuers pay on a syndicated offering can run about 1 percentage point higher than on an unsyndicated offering. Furthermore, although total fees are lower on an unsyndicated offering, the lead, and only, underwriter usually ends up with more because they do not have to share the fees with an underwriting syndicate.

Once an issue is sold, the job of the investment banker may not be over. In the case of an IPO, the investment banker is obligated to maintain a market in the stock to establish its liquidity. This means that the banker must hold an inventory of shares and stand ready to buy and sell the stock if no matching orders materialize for the trades initiated in the secondary market. This action by investment bankers keeps its corporate customers happy, and hence leads to future IPO business.

Shelf Registrations

The selling procedures described to this point apply to most security sales. However, under SEC Rule 415, larger firms that issue securities frequently may file a master registration statement with the SEC and then file only a short-form update prior to each offering. Under this rule, it is possible to make the decision today and sell the securities tomorrow. The "quick" procedure is called a *shelf registration* because the firm puts its new securities "on the shelf" when it does the master registration and can take them "off the shelf" and sell them to investors when it believes that conditions are "right." Businesses with less than $150 million market value in float—stock held by outside investors—cannot use shelf registrations. The reason for this limitation is to protect investors who may not be able to get adequate financial data about a smaller firm in the short time between the announcement of the offering and the actual sale. Shelf registrations are advantageous to the issuer because overall costs are lower, and the firm has more control over the timing of the issue.

1. What are the key features of securities markets regulation?
2. What types of decisions must be made by the issuer and its investment banker?
3. What is the difference between an underwritten and a best-efforts issue?
4. Are there any conflicts that might arise between the issuer and the investment banker when setting the offering price on a stock issue?
5. What is a shelf registration?

Self-Test Questions

Equity in Not-for-Profit Firms

Investor-owned businesses have two sources of equity financing: (1) retained earnings and (2) new stock sales. Not-for-profit businesses can, and do, retain earnings, but they do not have access to the equity markets; that is, they cannot sell stock to raise equity capital. Not-for-profit businesses can, however, raise equity capital through *government grants* and *charitable contributions*. Federal, state, and local governments are concerned about the provision of healthcare services to the general population. Therefore, these entities often make grants to not-for-profit providers to help offset the costs of services rendered to patients who cannot pay for those services. Sometimes these grants are nonspecific, but often providers are required to offer specific services such as neonatal intensive care to needy infants.

As for charitable contributions, individuals, as well as firms, are motivated to contribute to health services organizations for a variety of reasons including concern for the well-being of others, the recognition that often accompanies large contributions, and tax deductibility. Because only contributions to not-for-profit firms are tax deductible, this source of funding is, for all practical purposes, not available to investor-owned health services organizations. Although charitable contributions are not a substitute for profit retentions, charitable contributions can be a significant source of fund capital. For example, the Association for Health Care Philanthropy reported that total gifts to not-for-profit hospitals in recent years have averaged over $5 billion per year, of which about half represented immediate cash contributions.

Most not-for-profit hospitals received their initial, start-up equity capital from religious, educational, or governmental entities, and today some hospitals continue to receive funding from these sources. However, since the 1970s, these sources have provided a much smaller proportion of hospital funding, forcing not-for-profit hospitals to rely more on retained earnings and charitable contributions. Furthermore, federal programs such as the Hill-Burton Act, which provided large amounts of funds for hospital expansion following World War II, have been discontinued, and state and local governments, which are also facing significant financial pressures, are finding it more and more difficult to fund grants to healthcare providers.

Finally, as we discussed in Chapter 2, there is a growing trend among legislative bodies and tax authorities to force not-for-profit hospitals to "earn" their favorable tax treatment by providing a certain amount of charity care to indigent patients. Even more severe, some cities have pressured not-for-profit hospitals to make "voluntary" payments to the city to make up for the lost property tax revenue. All of these trends tend to reduce the ability of not-for-profit health services organizations to raise equity capital by grants and contributions; hence, the result is increased reliance on making money "the old fashioned way"—by earning it.

On the surface, it appears that investor-owned firms have a significant advantage in raising equity capital. In theory, new common stock can be issued at any time and in any amount. Conversely, charitable contributions are much less certain. The planning, solicitation, and collection periods can take years, and pledges are not always collected, so funds that were counted on may not materialize. Also, the proceeds of new stock sales may be used for any purpose, but charitable contributions may be *restricted*, in which case they can be used only for a designated purpose.

However, managers of investor-owned firms do not have complete freedom to raise capital in the equity markets. If market conditions are poor and the stock is selling at a low price, then a new stock issue can be harmful to the firm's current stockholders. Additionally, a new stock issue can be viewed by investors as a signal by management that the firm's stock is overvalued, so new stock issues tend to have a negative impact on the firm's stock price. The bottom line here is that investor-owned businesses, especially those in fast growing industries and markets, do have a financing advantage over not-for-profit businesses. However, the advantage is not so great as to create market dominance. If the advantage were significant, it is likely that we would find many less not-for-profit businesses in the healthcare sector than currently exist.

Self-Test Questions
1. What are the sources of equity (fund capital) to not-for-profit businesses?
2. Do investor-owned businesses have a significant financing advantage over not-for-profit businesses?

Key Concepts

This chapter contains a wealth of material on equity financing and how securities are brought to market. Here are its key concepts:

- The most important *common stockholder* rights are a claim on the firm's residual earnings, control, and the preemptive right.
- New common stock may be sold by for-profit corporations in six ways: (1) on a pro rata basis to existing stockholders through a *rights offering;* (2)

through investment bankers to the general public in a *public offering*; (3) to a single buyer, or small number of buyers, in a *private placement;* (4) to employees through an *employee stock purchase plan;* (5) to shareholders through a *dividend reinvestment plan;* and (6) to individual investors by *direct purchase.*

- A *closely held corporation* is one that is owned by a few individuals who typically are the firm's managers.
- A *publicly owned corporation* is one that is owned by a relatively large number of individuals who are not actively involved in its management.
- Securities markets are regulated at the national level by the *Securities and Exchange Commission (SEC)* and at the state level by state agencies, which are often called *corporation commissions.*
- An *investment banker* assists in the issuing of securities by helping the business determine the size of the issue and the type of securities to be used; by establishing the selling price; by selling the issue; and in some cases, by maintaining an after-market for the securities.
- Not-for-profit firms do not have access to the equity markets. However, *charitable contributions*, which are tax deductible to the donor, and *governmental grants* constitute unique equity sources for not-for-profit firms.

This concludes our discussion of the institutional features associated with debt and equity financing. However, two chapters remain in the capital acquisition section. In the next chapter, we illustrate how securities are valued and how businesses make debt redemption decisions.

Selected References

Becker, Scott, Robert J. Pristave, and Emily H. Liebers. 1996. "Taking the Provider-Driven Company Public: A Primer on Business and Legal Issues." *Journal of Health Care Finance* (Summer): 71–80.

Dunn, Kenneth C., Geoffrey B. Shields, and Joanne B. Stern.1991. "The Dynamics of Leveraged Buy-Outs, Conversions, and Corporate Reorganizations of Not-For-Profit Health Care Institutions." *Topics in Health Care Financing* (Spring): 5–20.

Flaherty, Mary Pat. 1991. "Planned Giving Programs as a Source of Financing: Creating a 'Win-Win' Situation for a Health Care Organization and Its Donors." *Topics in Health Care Financing* (Spring): 70–81.

Shields, Geoffrey B., and George C. McKann. 1991. "Raising Health Care Capital Through the Public Equity Markets." *Topics in Health Care Financing* (Fall): 21–36.

Smith, Dean G., John R. C. Wheeler, and Jan P. Clement. 1995. "Fundraising, Government Grants and Donations to Non-Profit Hospital Charities." *Health Services Management Research* (August): 198–208.

Sykes, C. Scott, Jr. 1991. "The Role of Equity Financing in Today's Health Care Environment." *Topics in Health Care Financing* (Fall): 1–4.

Wallace, Cindy. 1985. "Not-For-Profits Competing for Capital by Selling Stock in Alternative Ventures." *Modern Healthcare* (August 16): 32–38.

Selected Web Sites

There are a multitude of web sites that pertain to this chapter.

To learn more about stock exchanges, see the NYSE site at *www.nyse.com*. Here, you can research listing requirements as well learn how the NYSE works.

To learn more about the over-the-counter market, see the NASDAQ site at *www.nasdaq.com*.

To learn about regulation, see the SEC site at *www.sec.gov*. In addition to providing a great deal of information about the SEC, the site also features recent firm filings. Click on the EDGAR Database icon in the left column of the page.

To learn more about dividend reinvestment plans, see the DRIP investor site at *www.dripinvestor.com*.

To learn more about investment banking, see any of the investment banker's—listed in Table 7.2—web sites. For example, see the Morgan Stanley Dean Witter site at *www.msdw.com*.

Selected Cases

There are no cases available that focus on equity financing or investment banking. However, the following case in *Cases in Healthcare Finance* can be assigned to help students learn equity valuation (covered in Chapter 8):

Case 12: Potomac Healthcare (B), which focuses on the mechanics of equity valuation.

Notes

1. For more information on other types of preferred stock, particularly convertible preferred, see Eugene F. Brigham, Louis C. Gapenski, and Michael C. Ehrhardt, *Financial Management: Theory and Practice* (Forth Worth, TX: Dryden Press, 1999), Chapter 20.

2. The folk wisdom among corporate managers is that "like diamonds, dividends are forever." The reason is that a dividend cut, or worse yet an omission, will trigger a sell-off that will substantially lower the firm's stock price and place management in a precarious position. Thus, dividends typically are cut only under extreme circumstances and after all other options have been exhausted.

3. In the typical voting procedure, a stockholder who owns 1,000 shares could cast 1,000 votes for each director whose seat was contested. An alternative voting procedure, called *cumulative voting*, is used at some firms. Here, the 1,000-share stockholder would get 3,000 votes if three seats were being contested, and he or she could cast all of them for one director. Cumulative voting helps small groups of shareholders to get a voice on the board.

4. For more details on the mechanics of a rights offer, see Eugene F. Brigham, Louis C. Gapenski, and Phillip R. Daves, *Intermediate Financial Management* (Forth Worth, TX: Dryden Press, 2000), Chapter 13.

5. *Venture capitalists* are individuals and firms that supply capital to small, start-up businesses that do not have the track record necessary to obtain capital from banks or public markets. This type of financing is referred to as *first round* financing. The capital may be in the form of debt or equity, but debt investments usually are accompanied by stock options or some other "equity kicker" that gives the venture capitalist an ownership position in the business. Although many venture capital investments never pan out, those that do typically create huge returns when the venture capitalists "cash out" after the succesful firm has gone public.

6. It is illegal for anyone to manipulate the price of a stock. During the 1920s, and earlier, syndicates would be formed for the sole purpose of buying and selling stocks among one another at pre-arranged prices so that the public would believe that the stock was worth more or less than its true value. The exchanges, with the enouragement and support of the SEC, utilize sophisticated computer programs to help spot any trading irregularities that suggest manipulation. Additionally, various disclosures, including transactions by insiders, are required.

7. If a stock is held for more than one year, any profit is classified as a long-term capital gain and, hence, taxed at a lower rate than is ordinary income. Furthermore, taxes are not paid until the stock is sold.

8. IPOs are almost always underpriced, and, in some cases, the underpricing is huge. Various theories have been put forth to explain this phenomenon. The best explanation seems to be that (1) both the current stockholders and the investment bankers want to create excitement about the firm, and a big price run-up does that; (2) a small percentage of the stock generally is offered to the public, so current stockholders give away less than it first appears; and (3) IPO firms generally plan to have follow-on stock issues in the near future, and the best way to ensure the success of future issues is to have a successful IPO.

9. Large security issues are announced in the *Wall Street Journal,* and other publications, by advertisements placed by the underwriters called *tombstones.* Check several recent issues of the *Journal* to see if there are any healthcare issues advertised.

8

SECURITIES VALUATION, MARKET EFFICIENCY, AND DEBT REFUNDING

Learning Objectives

After studying this chapter, readers should be able to:

- Describe how securities in general are valued.
- Value debt securities as well as calculate their yields to maturity.
- Value stocks as well as calculate their expected rates of return.
- Explain the concept of market efficiency and its implications for investors and managers.
- Conduct a debt refunding analysis.

Introduction

Now that you understand the basic features both of debt and equity securities, the next step is to learn how investors value these securities. Your reaction at this point might be: "Why should I have to worry about security valuation when what I really want to learn is managerial decision making?" Security valuation concepts are important to healthcare managers for many reasons. Here are just a few:

- The lifeblood of any business is capital. In fact, the most common reason for small business failures is insufficient capital. Therefore, it is vital that healthcare managers understand how investors make investment allocation decisions.
- For investor-owned businesses, stock price maximization is an important, if not primary goal, so healthcare managers of for-profit businesses must know how investors value the firm's securities to understand how managerial actions affect stock price.
- For healthcare managers to make financially sound investment decisions regarding real assets (plant and equipment), it is necessary to estimate the business's cost of capital, and security valuation is a necessary skill in this process. We will discuss the cost of capital in Chapter 10.
- All healthcare managers must grapple with the decision of how much debt, as opposed to equity, financing should the business use. An understanding of stock and bond valuation is critical to this decision, so the concepts presented in this chapter will be used again in Chapter 11.

- Real assets, such as hospital beds and diagnostic equipment, are valued in the same general way as securities. Thus, security valuation provides healthcare managers with an excellent foundation to learn real asset valuation, which is the heart of capital investment decision making within businesses. Thus, the general concepts present in this chapter are crucial to a good understanding of Chapters 12 and 13.

The General Valuation Model

In most situations, individuals and institutions buy assets (make investments) for one reason: to receive the cash flows that the asset is expected to produce. Because the values of investment opportunities stem from streams of expected cash flows, most investments are valued by the same four-step process:

1. **Estimate the expected cash flow stream.** Estimating the cash flow stream involves estimating both the expected cash flows and the periods in which they are expected to occur. For some types of investments, such as bonds, the estimation process is quite easy—the interest and principal repayment stream is fixed by contract. For other types of investments, such as a new service line, the estimation process can be very difficult.
2. **Assess the riskiness of the cash flow stream.** As with estimating the cash flows, in some situations, such as an investment in Treasury securities, it will be fairly easy to assess the riskiness of the estimated cash flow stream. In other situations it may be quite difficult.
3. **Set the required rate of return.** Once the riskiness is assessed, the opportunity cost principle is applied to set the required rate of return. By investing in one asset, the funds are no longer available to invest in alternative assets of similar risk. Thus, the required rate of return on the cash flow stream is established on the basis of the risk assessment and the returns available on alternative investments of similar risk.
4. **Discount the expected cash flows and sum the present values.** Each cash flow is now discounted at the asset's required rate of return and the present values are summed to find the value of the asset.

The following time line formalizes the general valuation process:

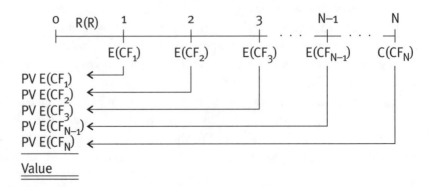

Here, $E(CF_t)$ is the expected cash flow in each Period t; $R(R)$ is the required rate of return (i.e., the opportunity cost rate) on the asset; and N is the number of periods for which cash flows are expected. The periods can be months, quarters, semiannual periods, or years, depending on the frequency of the cash flows expected from the investment.

The general valuation model can be applied to both financial assets (securities), such as stocks and bonds, and real (physical) assets, such as buildings, equipment, and even whole businesses. The key to its use is that it must be possible to estimate the cash flows expected from the investment with some confidence. Each asset type requires a somewhat different application of the general valuation model, but the basic approach remains the same. In this chapter, the general valuation model is applied to three types of securities: (1) bonds, (2) preferred stock, and (3) common stock. In the chapters that follow, the model will be applied to real assets and to entire businesses.

1. What is the general valuation model?
2. Under what conditions can it be used?

**Self-Test
Questions**

Debt Valuation

Unless there are some unusual features, debt securities are valued by applying the general valuation model without much modification. We will use bonds to illustrate debt valuation, but the techniques discussed in the following sections are applicable to most types of debt.

Definitions

To begin our discussion of bond (debt) valuation, it is useful to review some basic bond concepts:

- **Par value**. The *par*, or *face*, *value* is the stated value of the bond. It is often set at $1,000 or $5,000. The par value generally represents the amount of money the business borrows (per bond) and promises to repay at some future date.
- **Maturity date.** Bonds generally have a specified *maturity date* on which the par value will be repaid. For example, Big Sky Healthcare, a for-profit hospital system, issued $50 million worth of $1,000 par value bonds on January 1, 2001. The bonds will mature on December 31, 2015, so they had a 15-year *maturity* at the time they were issued. The effective maturity of a bond declines each year after it was issued. Thus, at the beginning of 2002, Big Sky's bonds will have a 14-year maturity, and so on.
- **Coupon rate.** A bond requires the issuer to pay a specific amount of interest each year or, more typically, each six months. The rate of interest is called the *coupon interest rate*, or just *coupon rate*. The rate may be variable, in which case it is tied to some index such as 2 percentage points above the prime rate. More commonly, the rate will be fixed over the life

(maturity) of the bond. For example, Big Sky's bonds have a 10 percent coupon rate, so each $1,000 par value bond pays $0.10 \times \$1,000 = \$100$ in interest each year. The dollar amount of annual interest, in this case $100, is called the *coupon payment*. The term *coupon* goes back to the time when all bonds were *bearer bonds*. Such bonds had small coupons attached, one for each interest payment. To collect an interest payment, bondholders would remove (i.e., "clip") a coupon and send it to the issuer, or take it to a bank, where it would be exchanged for the dollar payment. Today, all bonds are *registered bonds*, and the issuer (through an *agent*) automatically sends interest payments to the registered owner.

- **New issues versus outstanding bonds.** A bond's value is determined by its coupon payment—the higher the coupon payment, other things held constant, the higher its value. At the time a bond is issued, its coupon rate is generally set at a level that will cause the bond to sell at its par value. In other words, the coupon rate is set to match investors' required rate of return on the bond (i.e., the *going rate*). A bond that has just been issued is called a *new issue*. After the bond has been on the market for a while, about a month, it is classified as an *outstanding bond*, or a *seasoned issue*. New issues sell close to par, but because a bond's coupon payment is generally fixed, changing economic conditions, and hence interest rates, will cause a seasoned bond to sell for more or less than its par value.

- **Debt service requirements.** Firms that issue bonds are concerned with their total debt service requirements, which include both interest expense and repayment of principal. For Big Sky, the debt service requirement is $0.10 \times \$50$ million $= \$5$ million per year until maturity. In 2015, the firm's debt service requirement will be $5 million in interest plus $50 million in principal repayment, for a total of $55 million. In Big Sky's case, only interest is paid until maturity, so the entire principal amount must be repaid at that time. As we discussed in Chapter 6, many municipal bonds are serial issues structured so that the debt service requirements are relatively constant over time. In this situation, the issuer pays back a portion of the principal during each year.

The Basic Bond Valuation Model

Bonds call for the payment of a specific amount of interest for a specific number of years, and for the repayment of par on the bond's maturity date. Thus, a bond represents an annuity plus a lump sum, and its value is found as the present value of this cash flow stream:

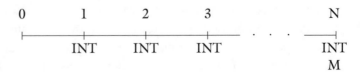

$$Value = \frac{INT}{[1+R(R)]^1} + \frac{INT}{[1+R(R)]^2} + \cdots + \frac{INT+M}{[1+R(R)]^N}.$$

Here,

INT = dollars of interest paid each year = Coupon rate × Par value.

M = par, or maturity, value.

R(R) = required rate of return on the bond, which, in general, depends on

the returns available on alternative investments of similar risk.

For bonds, these returns depend on the real risk-free rate,

inflation expectations, and the riskiness of the security.

N = number of years until maturity. N declines each year after the

bond is issued.

Here are the cash flows from Big Sky's bonds on a time line:

0	1	2		13	14	15
	$100	$100	· · ·	$100	$100	$ 100
						1,000

If the bonds had just been issued, and the coupon rate was set at the going interest rate for bonds of this risk, then R(R) = 10%. Because the value of the bond is merely the present value of its cash flows, discounted to Time 0 at a 10 percent discount rate, the value of the bond at issue was $1,000:

Present value of a 15-year, $100 payment annuity at 10 percent	= $ 760.61
Present value of a $1,000 lump sum discounted 15 years	= 239.39
Value of bond	= $1,000.00

The value of the bond can be found using most financial calculators as follows:

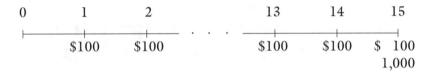

Inputs   15   10   −100   −1000

[N]   [I]   [PV]   [PMT]   [FV]

Output   = 1,000

Input N = 15, I = 10, PMT = −100, and FV = −1000, and then press the PV key to get the answer, 1,000. (The cash flows were treated as outflows so that the value would be displayed as a positive number.) Note that in bond valuation, all five time-value-of-money keys on a financial calculator are used because bonds involve both an annuity and a lump sum.

If R(R) remained constant at 10 percent over time, what would be the value of the bond one year after it was issued? Now, the term to maturity is only 14 years—that is, N = 14. As seen below, the bond's value remains at $1,000:

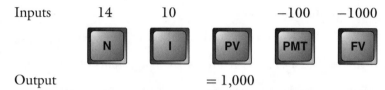

Inputs   14   10   −100   −1000

Output   = 1,000

Suppose that interest rates in the economy fell after the Big Sky bonds were issued, and, as a result, R(R) decreased from 10 percent to 5 percent. The coupon rate and par value are fixed by contract, so they remain unaffected by changes in interest rates, but, now, the discount rate is 5 percent rather than 10 percent. At the end of the first year, with 14 years remaining, the value of the bond would be $1,494.93:

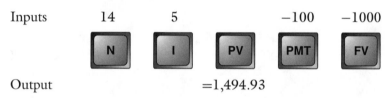

Inputs   14   5   −100   −1000

Output   =1,494.93

The arithmetic of the bond value increase should be clear: Lower discount rates lead to higher present values, but what is the logic behind it? The fact that R(R) has fallen to 5 percent means that if an individual had $1,000 to invest, he or she could buy new bonds like Big Sky's—every day some 10 to 20 firms sell new bonds—except that these new bonds would only pay $50 in interest each year. Naturally, he or she would favor $100 to $50, and would be willing to pay more than $1,000 for Big Sky's bonds. All investors would recognize this rationale; as a result, the Big Sky bonds would be bid up in price to $1,494.93, at which point they would provide the same rate of return as new bonds of similar risk, 5 percent.

Assuming that interest rates stay constant at 5 percent over the next 14 years, what would happen to the value of a Big Sky bond? It would fall gradually from $1,494.93 at present to $1,000 at maturity, when the firm will redeem each bond for $1,000. This point can be illustrated by calculating the value of the bond one year later, when it has only 13 years remaining to maturity:

Inputs   13   5   −100   −1000

N	I	PV	PMT	FV

Output   = 1,469.68

The value of the bond with 13 years to maturity is $1,469.68.

If an individual purchased the bond at a price of $1,494.93, and then sold it one year later with interest rates still at 5 percent, he or she would have a capital loss of $25.25. The rate of return on the bond over the year consists of an *interest*, or *current*, *yield* plus a *capital gains yield*:

Current yield   = $100/$1,494.93   =   0.0669 =   6.69%
Capital gains yield = −$25.25/$1,494.93 = −0.0169 = −1.69%
Rate of return, or
    total yield   = $74.75/$1,494.93 =   0.0500 =   5.00%

Had interest rates risen from 10 to 15 percent during the first year after issue rather than fallen, the value of Big Sky's bonds would have declined to $713.78 at the end of the first year. If interest rates held constant at 15 percent, the bond would have a value of $720.84 at the end of the second year, so the total yield to investors would be:

Current yield   = $100/$713.78   =   0.1401 = 14.01%
Capital gains yield = $7.06/$713.78   =   0.0099 = 0.99%
Rate of return, or
    total yield   = $107.06/$713.78   =   0.1500 = 15.00%

Figure 8.1 graphs the values of the Big Sky bond over time, assuming that interest rates will remain constant at 10 percent, fall to 5 percent and then remain at that level, and rise to 15 percent and remain constant at that level. The figure illustrates the following important points:

- Whenever the required rate of return on a bond equals its coupon rate, the bond will sell at its par value.
- When interest rates, and hence required rates of return, fall after a bond is issued, the bond's value rises above its par value, and the bond sells at a *premium*.
- When interest rates, and hence required rates of return, rise after a bond is issued, the bond's value falls below its par value, and the bond sells at a *discount*.
- Bond prices on outstanding issues and interest rates are inversely related. Increasing rates lead to falling prices, and decreasing rates lead to increasing prices.
- The price of a bond will always approach its par value as its maturity date approaches, provided the issuer does not default on the bond.

Note, however, that interest rates do **not** remain constant over time, so, in reality, a bond's price fluctuates both as interest rates in the economy fluctuate and the bond's term to maturity decreases. Still, regardless of interest rate movements, a bond's value will approach its par value as the maturity date gets closer and closer.

FIGURE 8.1

Time Path of the Value of a 15-Year, 10% Coupon, $1,000 Par Value Bond When Interest Rates are 5%, 10%, and 15%

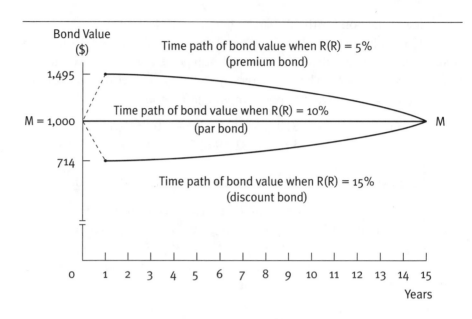

	Bond Value at		
Year	R(R) = 5%	R(R) = 10%	R(R) = 15%
0	—	$1,000.00	—
1	$1,494.93	1,000.00	$ 713.78
2	1,469.68	1,000.00	720.84
3	1,443.16	1,000.00	728.97
.	.	.	.
.	.	.	.
.	.	.	.
13	1,092.97	1,000.00	918.71
14	1,047.62	1,000.00	956.52
15	1,000.00	1,000.00	1,000.00

Zero Coupon Bonds

Some bonds, called *zero coupon bonds,* pay no interest at all during the life of the bond, so an investor's cash flows consist solely of the return of par value at maturity. Because there are no interest payments, when the bond is issued its value is much less than par value, so the bond originally sells at a discount. Thus, zero coupon bonds also are called *original issue discount bonds.*

Zero coupon bonds are valued in the same way as regular (coupon) bonds, recognizing that there are no coupon payments to contribute to the bond's value. To illustrate this concept, assume that Big Sky's 15-year bond issue discussed in the previous section was a zero coupon bond. Assuming a 10 percent required rate of return, the bond's value would be $239.39:

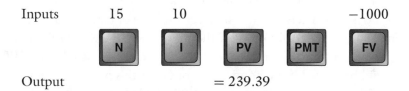

Inputs   15   10   −1000

N   I   PV   PMT   FV

Output   = 239.39

Note that this amount is merely the present value of the maturity payment that was calculated in the previous section.

Zero coupon bonds have some advantages as well as disadvantages when compared to coupon bonds. The primary advantage to issuers is that no payments have to be made to bondholders until the maturity date. As we will discuss in a later section, the primary advantage to buyers is that there are no coupon payments to reinvest.

Yield to Maturity

Up to this point, a bond's required rate of return and cash flows have been used to determine its value. In reality, investors' required rates of return on securities are not observable, but security prices can be easily determined— at least on those securities that are actively traded—by looking in the local newspaper or the *Wall Street Journal*. Suppose that the Big Sky bond had 14 years remaining to maturity, and the bond was selling at a price of $1,494.93. What percentage rate of return, or *yield to maturity (YTM)*, would be earned if the bond was bought at this price, held to maturity, and no default occurred? To find the answer, 5 percent, use a financial calculator as follows:

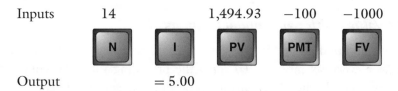

Inputs   14   1,494.93   −100   −1000

N   I   PV   PMT   FV

Output   = 5.00

The YTM can be thought of as the expected rate of return on the bond.[1] It is similar to the total rate of return discussed in the previous section. For a bond that sells at par, the YTM consists entirely of an interest yield, but if the bond sells at a discount or premium, the YTM consists of the current yield plus a positive or negative capital gains yield.

Yield to Call

Bonds that are callable have both a YTM and a *yield to call (YTC)*. The YTC is similar to the YTM, except that it assumes that the bond will be called. Thus, the YTC is calculated like the YTM, except that N reflects the number of years until the bond will be called, as opposed to years to maturity, and M reflects the call price, rather than the maturity value.

For example, suppose the Big Sky bond had ten years of call protection when it was issued. There are now nine years to date of first call, and the bond is selling at a price of $1,494.93. Furthermore, there is a $100 call premium that must be paid if the issue were called at the earliest possible date. What YTC would be earned if the bond were bought at this price and held to first call, at which time it was redeemed for $1,000 + $100 = $1,100? The answer is 4.2 percent:

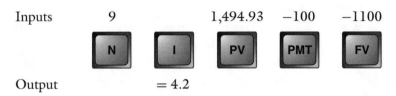

Inputs   9   1,494.93   −100   −1100

            [N]   [I]   [PV]   [PMT]   [FV]

Output   = 4.2

The question now facing potential investors of this bond is should they expect to earn its 5.0 percent YTM or its 4.2 percent YTC. Of course, the answer depends on whether or not the bond will be called. There is no way of knowing with certainty today when, or even if, the bond will be called. But we know that the bond is selling at a large premium now, and if interest rates do not change much over the next nine years, the bond is likely to be selling for more than $1,100 when first callable. If indeed that is the situation, it is likely that the bond will be called, and hence the YTC is probably a better estimate of the expected rate of return than is the YTM. On the other hand, if the bond were currently selling at a discount, and interest rates were expected to be relatively constant over the next nine years, it is likely that the bond would not be called and the YTM would be the appropriate measure of the return on the bond.

Bond Values with Semiannual Coupons

Virtually all bonds issued in the United States actually pay interest semiannually, or every six months. To apply the preceding valuation concepts to semiannual bonds, the bond valuation procedures must be modified as follows:

- Divide the annual interest payment, INT, by two to determine the dollar amount paid **each six months**.
- Multiply the number of years to maturity, N, by two to determine the number of **semiannual interest periods**.
- Divide the annual required rate of return, R(R), by two to determine the **semiannual required rate of return**.

To illustrate the use of the semiannual bond valuation model, assume that the Big Sky bonds pay $50 every six months rather than $100 annually. Thus, each interest payment is only half as large, but there are twice as many of them. When the going rate of interest is 5 percent annually, the value of Big Sky's bonds with 14 years left to maturity is $1,499.12:

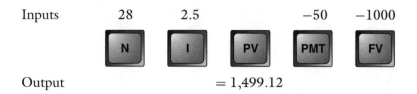

Output   = 1,499.12

Similarly, if the bond were actually selling for $1,400 with 14 years to maturity, its YTM would be 5.80 percent:

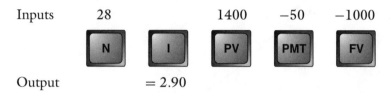

Output   = 2.90

The value for I, 2.90 percent, is the **periodic (semiannual) YTM**, so it is necessary to multiply it by two to get the annual YTM. The effective annual YTM on the bond is somewhat greater than the 5.80 percent that was calculated.[2] However, it is convention in the bond markets to quote all rates on a stated (annual) basis, so the procedures outlined in this section are correct when bonds—all of which have semiannual coupons—are being compared. However, when the returns on securities that have different periodic payments are being compared, all rates of return should be expressed as effective annual rates.

Interest Rate Risk

Interest rates change over time, which causes two types of investment risk that fall under the general classification of *interest rate risk*. First, an increase in interest rates leads to a decline in the values of outstanding bonds. Because interest rates can rise, bondholders face the risk of losses on their holdings. This risk is called *price risk*. Second, many bondholders buy bonds to build funds for future use. These bondholders reinvest the interest and principal cash flows as they are received. If interest rates fall, bondholders will earn a lower rate on the reinvested cash flows, which will have a negative impact on the future value of their holdings. This risk is called *reinvestment rate risk*.

To illustrate price risk, suppose you bought some of Big Sky's 10 percent bonds when they were issued at a price of $1,000. As illustrated earlier, if interest rates rise, the value of the bonds will fall. An investor's exposure to price risk depends on the maturity of the bonds. Figure 8.2, which shows the values of one-year and 14-year bonds at several different market interest rates, illustrates price risk. Notice how much more sensitive the value of the 14-year bond is to changes in interest rates. For bonds with similar coupons, the longer the maturity of the bond, the greater its price change in response to a given change in interest rates. Thus, bonds with longer maturities are exposed to more price risk.[3]

FIGURE 8.2

Value of Long-
and Short-Term
10% Annual
Coupon Rate
Bonds at
Different
Market Interest
Rates

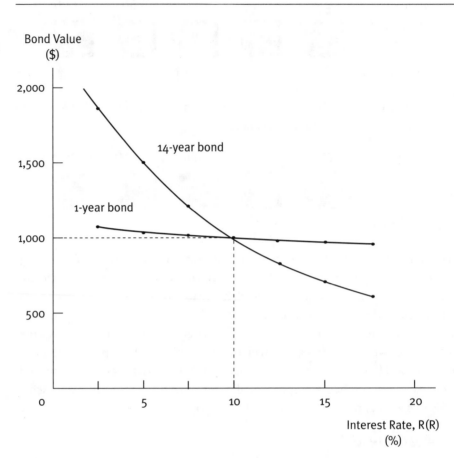

| Current Market | Bond Value | |
Interest Rate, R(R)	1-Year Bond	14-Year Bond
2.5%	$1,073.17	$1,876.82
5.0	1,047.62	1,494.93
7.5	1,023.26	1,212.23
10.0	1,000.00	1,000.00
12.5	977.78	838.45
15.0	956.52	713.78
17.5	936.17	616.25

Although a one-year bond exposes the buyer to less price risk than a
14-year bond, the one-year bond carries with it more reinvestment rate risk;
that is, if the holding period is more than one year, investing in a one-year
bond means that the principal and interest will have to be reinvested at the
end of the first year. If interest rates fall, the return earned during the second

year will be less than the return earned during the first year. Reinvestment rate risk is the second dimension of interest rate risk.

Clearly, bond investors face both price risk and reinvestment rate risk as a result of interest rate fluctuations over time. Which risk is most meaningful to a particular investor depends on the circumstances; but in general, interest rate risk, including both price and reinvestment rate risk, is reduced by matching the maturity of the bond with the anticipated *investment horizon*. For example, suppose Hilldale Community Hospital received a $5 million contribution that it will use in five years to build a new neonatal care center. By investing the contribution in five-year bonds, the hospital would minimize its interest rate risk because it would be matching its investment horizon. Price risk would be minimized because the bond will mature in five years, and hence Hilldale will receive par value regardless of the level of interest rates at that time. Reinvestment rate risk is also minimized because only the interest on the bond would have to be reinvested, which is a less risky situation than if both principal and interest had to be reinvested. If Hilldale invested in a zero coupon bond, reinvestment rate risk would be eliminated.

Interest rate risk is but one of many financial risks facing healthcare businesses. Fortunately, there are various techniques that can be used to mitigate such risks. We will discuss financial risk management in some detail in Chapter 20.

Self-Test
Questions

1. How are bonds valued?
2. What is a zero coupon bond?
3. What is meant by a bond's yield to maturity (YTM)? By its yield to call (YTC)?
4. Differentiate between price risk and reinvestment rate risk.

Preferred Stock Valuation

Most preferred stocks entitle their owners to regular, fixed dividend payments. If the stock is **perpetual preferred**—payments are expected to last forever—then the stock can be valued using the simple formula for valuing a perpetuity:

$$E(P_p) = \frac{D_p}{R(R_p)}.$$

Here, $E(P_p)$ is the value (expected price) of the preferred stock, D_p is the preferred dividend, and $R(R_p)$ is the required rate of return on the preferred stock. For example, Regent Healthcare's perpetual preferred dividend is $10 per year. If interest rates rose since the stock was issued, and the required rate of return is now 12 percent, the value of the stock would be $83.33:

$$E(P_p) = \frac{\$10}{0.12} = \$83.33.$$

The required rate of return on the issue would be determined in the same manner as for debt, as we discussed in Chapter 6.

In reality, preferred dividends typically are paid quarterly, so the holder of Regent's preferred stock actually receives a quarterly dividend of $10/4 = $2.50. The value of the preferred stock could be calculated on the basis of this quarterly dividend if we recognize that the quarterly required rate of return would be 12%/4 = 3%:

$$E(P_p) = \frac{\$2.50}{0.03} = \$83.33.$$

In theory, investors would now look at the current stock price. If it is greater than $83.33, the preferred stock should not be purchased, while if it is less than $83.33, the stock is attractive.

Although calculating the value of a preferred stock is a reasonable approach to making the investment decision, most investors make preferred stock investment decisions on the basis of expected rate of return. This approach is similar to that used by debt investors, who make decisions on the basis of yield to maturity. The expected rate of return on preferred stock, $E(R_p)$ can be determined easily by rearranging the valuation equation:

$$E(R_p) = \frac{D_p}{P_p}.$$

For example, the rate of return on Regent's preferred stock, if it is currently selling for $85, is 11.8 percent:

$$E(R_p) = \frac{\$10}{\$85} = 11.8\%.$$

Using the quarterly dividend of $2.50 and a price of $85 gives a quarterly expected rate of return of 2.94 percent. This expected rate of return is then multiplied by four to give a stated (annual) rate of 11.8 percent.[4] If an investor has a required rate of return on the stock of less than 11.8, it should be purchased. Conversely, if the required rate of return is greater than 11.8 percent, the stock should not be bought.

Although there are some perpetual preferred issues that remain outstanding forever, virtually all preferred stock issued today has either a sinking fund or a call provision that limits the stock's maturity. When the maturity is limited, preferred stock is valued using the debt valuation techniques described previously.

Self-Test Questions

1. What is a perpetual preferred stock and how is it valued?
2. How are nonperpetual preferred stocks valued?

Common Stock Valuation

For many reasons, the valuation of common stocks is a difficult and perplexing process. To begin, the type of model used depends on the characteristics of the firm being valued. In general, there are three distinct types of firms:

1. Start-up firms generally pay no dividends because all earnings must be reinvested in the business to fund growth. To make matters worse, start-up firms often take years to make a profit, so there is no track record of positive earnings to use as a basis for a cash flow forecast. Under such conditions, the general valuation model cannot be applied because the value of such firms stems from potential opportunities rather than from existing product or service lines. Even if most of the opportunities do not materialize, one or two could turn into blockbusters and, hence, create a highly successful firm. With such firms, option pricing techniques, which we briefly introduce in Chapter 20, at least in theory, can be used to value the stock. In reality, valuations on these firms are not much better than a shot in the dark, and hence stock prices are based more on qualitative factors, including emotions, than on anything else. The end result is that typically stock prices of such firms are highly volatile.
2. As a firm passes through its initial start-up phase, it often reaches a point where it has more or less predictable positive earnings, but still requires reinvestment of these earnings, so no dividends are paid. In such cases, it is possible to value the entire firm, as well as the stock of the firm, on the basis of the expected earnings stream. In such a valuation, the expected earnings stream is discounted, or *capitalized*, to find the current value of the firm. Then, the value of the debt is stripped off to estimate the value of the common stock. We will illustrate this method of valuing common stock in Chapter 18 when we discuss business valuation.
3. More mature firms generally pay a relatively predictable dividend, and hence the future dividend stream can be forecasted with reasonable confidence. In such cases, the common stock can be valued on the basis of the present value of the expected dividend stream. We illustrate this approach in the following sections.

Definitions

Common stocks with a predictable dividend stream can be valued using the general valuation model, with a focus on expected dividends. Before we present the model, here are some definitions that will be needed:

- $E(D_t)$ = Dividend the stockholder **expects** to receive at the end of Year t. D_0 is the most recent dividend, which has already been paid and is known with certainty; $E(D_1)$ is the first dividend expected and for valuation purposes is assumed to be paid **at the end** of one year; $E(D_2)$ is the dividend expected at the end of two years; and so forth. $E(D_1)$ represents the **first** cash flow a new purchaser of the stock will receive. D_0, the dividend that has just been paid, is known with certainty, but all future dividends are expected values, so the estimate of any $E(D_t)$ may differ among investors.[5]

- P_0 = Actual *market price* of the stock today.
- $E(P_t)$ = Expected price of the stock at the end of each Year t. $E(P_0)$ is the *value* of the stock today, as seen by a particular investor based on his or her estimate of the stock's expected dividend stream and riskiness; $E(P_1)$ is the price expected at the end of one year; and so on. Thus, whereas P_0 is fixed and is identical for all investors, $E(P_0)$ will differ among investors depending on each investor's assessment of the stock's riskiness and dividend stream. $E(P_0)$, each investor's estimate of the value today, could be above or below P_0, the current stock price, but an investor would buy the stock only if his or her estimate of $E(P_0)$ were equal to or greater than P_0.
- $E(g_t)$ = Expected growth rate in dividends in each future Year t. Different investors may use different $E(g_t)$s to evaluate a firm's stock. In reality, $E(g_t)$ is normally different for each Year t. However, the valuation process will be simplified by assuming that $E(g_t)$ is constant across time.
- $R(R_s)$ = Required rate of return on the stock, considering both its riskiness and the returns available on other investments.
- $E(R_s)$ = Expected rate of return on the stock. $E(R_s)$ could be above or below $R(R_s)$; but an investor would buy the stock only if his or her $E(R_s)$ were equal to or greater than $R(R_s)$. Note that $E(R_s)$ is an **expectation**. A return of $E(R_s) = 15\%$ may be expected if HCA stock were purchased today. If either conditions in the market or prospects at HCA take a turn for the worse, however, the realized return may be much lower than that expected—perhaps even negative.
- $E(D_1)/P_0$ = Expected *dividend yield* on a stock during the first year. If a stock is expected to pay a dividend of \$1 during the next 12 months, and if its current price is \$10, then its expected dividend yield is $\$1/\$10 = 0.10 = 10\%$.
- $[E(P_1) - P_0]/P_0$ = Expected *capital gains yield* on the stock during the first year. If the stock sells for \$10 today, and if it is expected to rise to \$10.50 at the end of the year, then the expected capital gain is $E(P_1) - P_0 = \$10.50 - \$10.00 = \$0.50$; and the expected capital gains yield is $[E(P_1) - P_0]/P_0 = \$0.50/\$10 = 0.050 = 5\%$.

Expected Dividends as the Basis for Stock Values

In the preceding discussion of debt valuation, the value of a bond was found by adding the present value of the interest payments over the life of the bond to the present value of the bond's maturity, or par, value. In essence, a bond's value is the present value of the cash flows expected from the bond. Stock prices using the dividend valuation model are likewise determined as the present value of a stream of cash flows, and the basic stock valuation equation is similar to the bond valuation equation. What are the cash flows that stocks provide to their holders? First, consider an investor who buys a stock with the intention of holding it in his or her family forever. In this situation, all the investor and his or her heirs will receive is a stream of dividends, and the value of the stock today is calculated as the present value of an infinite stream of dividends.

Consider the more typical case in which an investor expects to hold the stock for a finite period and then sell it. What would be the value of the stock in this case? The value of the stock is again the present value of the expected dividend stream. To see this, recognize that for any individual investor, expected cash flows consist of expected dividends plus the expected price of the stock when it is sold. However, the sale price received by the current investor will depend on the dividends some future investor expects to receive. Therefore, for all present and future investors in total, expected cash flows must be based on expected future dividends. To put it another way, unless a business is liquidated or sold to another concern, the cash flows it provides to its stockholders consist only of a stream of dividends; therefore, the value of a share of its stock must be the present value of that expected dividend stream.

The validity of this concept can also be confirmed by asking the following question: Suppose that an investor buys a stock and expects to hold it for one year. He or she will receive dividends during the year plus the value $E(P_1)$ when selling out at the end of the year, but what will determine the value of $E(P_1)$? It will be determined as the present value of the dividends during Year 2 plus the stock price at the end of that year, which in turn will be determined as the present value of another set of future dividends and an even more distant stock price. This process can be continued ad infinitum, and the ultimate result is that the value of a stock is the present value of its expected dividend stream, regardless of the holding period of the investor who performs the analysis. Occasionally, stock shares could have additional value, such as the value of a controlling interest when an investor buys 51 percent of a firm's outstanding stock, or the added value brought about by a takeover bid. However, in this model, the sole value inherent in stock ownership stems from the dividends expected to be paid by the firm to its shareholders.

Investors periodically lose sight of the long-run nature of stocks as investments, and forget that to sell a stock at a profit, he or she must find a buyer who will pay the higher price. Suppose that a stock's value is analyzed on the basis of expected future dividends and the conclusion is that the stock's market price exceeded a reasonable value. If an investor buys the stock anyway, he or she would be following the "bigger fool" theory of investment: The investor may be a fool to buy the stock at its excessive price, but he or she believes that when ready to sell an even bigger fool can be found.

The concept of the value of a stock being the present value of the expected dividend stream holds, regardless of the pattern of growth. It is not even necessary to project the stream for more than 40 or 50 years. Because of the time value of money, dividends beyond that point contribute an insignificant amount to a stock's value today. Needless to say, it is generally not possible to have much confidence in dividend values projected over a 40- or 50-year period, so stock valuation using the dividend valuation model must be viewed as something of an approximation.

Constant Growth Stock Valuation

Often, the projected stream of dividends follows a systematic pattern; hence, it is possible to develop a simplified (i.e., easier to evaluate) version of the dividend valuation model. This section discusses the most common simplifying assumption: *constant growth.*

Although the dividends of only a few firms actually grow at a constant rate, the assumption of constant growth is often made because it makes the forecasting of individual dividends over a long time period unnecessary. Furthermore, many mature businesses come close to meeting constant growth assumptions. For a constant growth firm, the expected dividend growth rate is constant for all years, so $E(g_1) = E(g_2) = E(g_3)$ and so on, which implies that $E(g_t)$ becomes merely $E(g)$. Under this assumption, the dividend in any future Year t may be forecasted as $E(D_t) = D_0 \times [1 + E(g)]^t$, where D_0 is the last dividend paid, and hence is known with certainty, and $E(g)$ is the constant expected rate of dividend growth. Alternatively, each year's dividend is $E(g)$ percent greater than the previous dividend, so $E(D_t) = E(D_{t-1}) \times [1 + E(g)]$.

To illustrate the concept, consider the following example. If Minnesota Health Systems (MHS), Inc., just paid a dividend of $1.82 (i.e., $D_0 = \$1.82$), and if investors expect a 10 percent constant dividend growth rate, the dividend expected in one year will be $E(D_1) = \$1.82 \times 1.10 = \$2.00$; $E(D_2)$ will be $\$1.82 \times (1.10)^2 = \$2.20$; and the dividend expected in five years will be $E(D_5) = D_0 \times [1 + E(g)]^5 = \$1.82 \times (1.10)^5 = \$2.93$. This method of estimating future dividends could be used to estimate MHS's expected future cash flow stream (i.e., the dividends) for some time into the future, say, 50 years. Then, the present values of this stream can be summed to find the value of MHS's stock.

The Value of a Constant Growth Stock 💾

However, when $E(g)$ is assumed to be constant, a stock can be valued using a simplified model called the *constant growth model*:

$$E(P_0) = \frac{D_0 \times [1 + E(g)]}{R(R_s) - E(g)} = \frac{E(D_1)}{R(R_s) - E(g)}$$

where $R(R_s)$ is the required rate of return on the stock. If $D_0 = \$1.82$, $E(g) = 10\%$, and $R(R_s) = 16\%$ for MHS, the value of its stock would be $33.33:

$$E(P_{MHS}) = \frac{\$1.82 \times 1.10}{0.16 - 0.10} = \frac{\$2.00}{0.06} = \$33.33.$$

A necessary condition for the derivation of the constant growth model is that the required rate of return on the stock is greater than the constant dividend growth rate—that is, $R(R_s)$ is greater than $E(g)$. If the constant growth model is used when $R(R_s)$ is not greater than $E(g)$, the results will be meaningless. However, to qualify as a constant growth stock, dividends must be expected to grow at the constant growth rate forever, or at least for a very long time. Although stocks can have $E(g)$ greater than $R(R_s)$ for short periods, $E(g)$ cannot exceed $R(R_s)$ over the long run because $E(g)$ measures long-term growth. Although the constant growth model is applied here to stock valuation, it can be used in any situation in which cash flows are growing at a constant rate.

How does an investor determine his or her required rate of return on a particular stock, $R(R_s)$? One way is to use the Security Market Line (SML) of the Capital Asset Pricing Model, which we discussed in Chapter 5. Assume that MHS's market beta, as reported by a financial advisory service, is 1.5. Assume also that the risk-free interest rate (the rate on long-term Treasury bonds) is 7 percent, and the required rate of return on the market is 13 percent. According to the SML, the required rate of return on MHS's stock is 16.0 percent:

$$R(R_{MHS}) = RF + [R(R_M) - RF] \times b_{MHS}$$
$$= 7\% + (13\% - 7) \times 1.5$$
$$= 7\% + (6\% \times 1.5)$$
$$= 7\% + 9\% = 16\%.$$

Remember, in the SML, RF is the risk-free rate; $R(R_M)$ is the required rate of return on the market, or the required rate of return on a $b = 1.0$ stock; and b_{MHS} is MHS's market beta.

Growth in dividends occurs primarily as a result of growth in earnings per share (EPS). Earnings growth, in turn, results from a number of factors including the inflation rate in the economy and the amount of earnings the firm retains and reinvests. Regarding inflation, if output in units is stable, and if both sales prices and input costs increase at the inflation rate, EPS also will grow at the inflation rate. EPS will also grow as a result of the reinvestment, or plowback, of earnings. If the firm's earnings are not all paid out as dividends (i.e., if a fraction of earnings is retained), the dollars of investment behind each share will rise over time, which should lead to growth in productive assets, and hence growth in earnings and dividends.

When using the constant growth model, the most critical input is $E(g)$—the expected constant growth rate in dividends. Investors can make their own E(g) estimates on the basis of historical dividend growth, but E(g) estimates are also available from brokerage and investment advisory firms.

Expected Rate of Return on a Constant Growth Stock

The constant growth model can be rearranged to solve for $E(R_s)$, the *expected rate of return*. In the model's normal form, $R(R_s)$ is the required rate of return; but when the model is transformed, the expected rate of return, $E(R_s)$, is found. This transformation requires that the required rate of return equal the expected rate of return, or $R(R_s) = E(R_s)$. This equality holds if the stock is in equilibrium, which is a condition that will be discussed later in the chapter. After solving the constant growth model for $E(R_s)$, this expression is obtained:

$$E(R_s) = \frac{D_0 \times [1 + E(g)]}{P_0} + E(g) = \frac{E(D_1)}{P_0} + E(g).$$

If an investor buys MHS's stock today for $P_0 = \$33.33$ and expects the stock to pay a dividend $E(D_1) = \$2.00$ one year from now, and for dividends to grow at a constant rate $E(g) = 10\%$ in the future, the expected rate of return on that stock is 16 percent:

$$E(R_{MHS}) = \frac{\$2.00}{\$33.33} + 10\% = 6\% + 10\% = 16\%.$$

In this form, $E(R_s)$, the expected total return on the stock, consists of an expected dividend yield, $E(D_1)/P_0 = 6.0\%$, plus an expected growth rate or capital gains yield, $E(g) = 10\%$.

Suppose this analysis had been conducted on January 1, 2001, so $P_0 = \$33.33$ is MHS's January 1, 2001 stock price, and $E(D_1) = \$2.00$ is the dividend expected at the end of 2001. What is the value of $E(P_1)$, the firm's expected stock price at the end of 2001 (the beginning of 2002)? The constant growth model would again be applied, but this time the 2002 dividend, $E(D_2) = E(D_1) \times [1 + E(g)] = \$2.00 \times 1.10 = \$2.20$, would be used:

$$E(P_1) = \frac{E(D_2)}{R(R_{MHS}) - E(g)} = \frac{\$2.20}{0.06} = \$36.67.$$

Notice that $E(P_1) = \$36.67$ is 10 percent greater than $P_0 = \$33.33$: $\$33.33 \times 1.10 = \$36.67$. Thus, a capital gain of $\$36.67 - \$33.33 = \$3.34$ would be expected during 2001, which produces a capital gains yield of 10 percent:

$$\text{Capital gains yield} = \frac{\text{Capital gain}}{\text{Beginning price}} = \frac{\$3.34}{\$33.33} = 0.100 = 10\%.$$

If the analysis were extended, in each future year the expected capital gains yield would always equal $E(g)$ because the stock price would grow at the 10 percent constant dividend growth rate. The expected dividend yield in 2002 (Year 2) could be found as follows:

$$\text{Dividend yield} = \frac{E(D_2)}{E(P_1)} = \frac{\$2.20}{\$36.67} = 0.060 = 6\%.$$

The dividend yield for 2003 (Year 3) could also be calculated, and again it would be 6 percent. Thus, for a constant growth stock, the following conditions must hold:

- The dividend is expected to grow forever, or at least for a long time, at a constant rate, $E(g)$.
- The stock price is expected to grow at this same rate.
- The expected dividend yield is a constant.
- The expected capital gains yield is also a constant and it is equal to $E(g)$.
- The expected rate of return in any Year t, which is equal to the expected dividend yield plus the expected capital gains yield (growth rate), is expressed by this equation: $E(R_t) = [E(D_{t+1})/E(P_t)] + E(g)$.

The term *expected* should be clarified—it means expected in a statistical sense. Thus, if MHS's dividend growth rate is expected to remain constant at 10 percent, this means that the growth rate in each year can be represented by a probability distribution with an expected value of 10 percent, and not that the growth rate is expected to be exactly 10 percent in each future year. In this sense, the constant growth assumption is reasonable for many large, mature businesses.

Nonconstant Growth Stock Valuation

Some firms exhibit constant dividend growth, or at least growth close enough to apply the constant growth model. However, many businesses do not. For example, some businesses that have not yet fully matured, but which have a solid dividend record, may be growing much faster today than they will over the long term. However, at some point in time, as the business matures, the growth will fall to some steady-state rate. Also, some dividend-paying firms may temporarily suspend the dividends because of a temporary downturn, but may have every intention of picking up the dividends when conditions improve. If a business is not expected to exhibit more or less constant growth in dividends in the future, the constant growth model cannot be used.

To find the value of a nonconstant growth stock, assuming that the growth rate will eventually stabilize to some steady-state rate, we proceed as follows:

- Estimate the stock's dividend stream on a year-by-year basis, stopping with the first dividend in the constant growth phase.
- Find the present value of the dividends during the period of nonconstant growth.
- Find the expected price of the stock at the end of the nonconstant growth period, at which point it has become a constant growth stock, and discount this price back to the present.

• Add the dividend and price components to find the value of the stock.

To illustrate the process for valuing nonconstant growth stocks, suppose the following facts exist:

$R(R_s)$ = stockholders' required rate of return = 16%.

N = years of nonconstant growth = 3.

$E(g_n)$ = rate of growth in dividends during the nonconstant growth period = 30%. (Note that the growth rate during the nonconstant growth period could vary from year to year.)

$E(g_c)$ = steady-state (constant) growth rate after the nonconstant period = 10%.

D_0 = last dividend paid = $1.82.

The valuation process, which is tedious but not difficult, is explained in the steps below:

1. Find the expected dividends during the nonconstant growth phase (Years 1, 2, and 3 in this case) plus the first dividend of the steady-state constant growth phase (Year 4) by multiplying each dividend by one plus the growth rate expected in the coming year:

$$D_0 = \$1.82.$$
$$D_1 = D_0 \times 1.30 = \$1.82 \ \times 1.30 = \$2.366.$$
$$D_2 = D_1 \times 1.30 = \$2.366 \times 1.30 = \$3.076.$$
$$D_3 = D_2 \times 1.30 = \$3.076 \times 1.30 = \$3.999.$$
$$D_4 = D_3 \times 1.10 = \$3.999 \times 1.10 = \$4.399.$$

2. Find the present values of the dividends that occur during the nonconstant growth phase, remembering that D_0 just occurred, so it does not contribute to the stock's value:

$$\text{PV } D_1 = \$2.366/(1.16)^1 = \$2.040.$$
$$\text{PV } D_2 = \$3.076/(1.16)^2 = \$2.286.$$
$$\text{PV } D_3 = \$3.999/(1.16)^3 = \$2.562.$$

3. The stock price expected at the end of Year 3 (the beginning of Year 4) can be found using the constant growth model because dividends are expected to grow at a constant rate of 10 percent in Year 4 and beyond. Note that this price captures the value of all the dividends beyond Year 3.

Calculate the stock price at the end of Year 3, and then discount this value to Year 0:

$$E(P_3) = \frac{D_4}{R(R_s) - E(g)} = \frac{\$4.399}{0.16 - 0.10} = \$73.317.$$

$$PV\ E(P_3) = \$73.32/(1.16)^3 = \$46.971.$$

4. Add the present values to find the value of the stock today:

$$E(P_0) = \$2.040 + \$2.286 + \$2.562 + \$46.971$$

$$= \$53.859 \approx \$53.86.$$

Although this illustration illustrates *supernormal growth*, in which the dividends are currently growing at a higher rate than the steady-state rate, the procedures illustrated here can be used with any pattern of nonconstant growth. The key to the use of this model is that the dividend stream must, at some not-to-distant point in time, return to constant growth.

Self-Test Questions

1. What are three potential methods for valuing common stocks and when does each apply?
2. Write out and explain the dividend valuation model for a constant growth stock in both the valuation and expected rate of return forms.
3. What are the assumptions of the constant growth model?
4. What are the key features of constant growth regarding dividend yield and capital gains yield?
5. Explain the key features of the nonconstant growth model.

Security Market Equilibrium

Investors will want to buy a security if its expected rate of return exceeds its required rate of return or, put another way, when its value exceeds its current price. Conversely, investors will want to sell a security when its required rate of return exceeds its expected rate of return (i.e., when its current price exceeds its value). When more investors want to buy a security than to sell it, its price is bid up. When more investors want to sell a security than to buy it, its price falls. In *equilibrium*, these two conditions must hold:

1. The expected rate of return on a security must equal its required rate of return to the marginal investor. This means that no investor who owns the stock believes that its expected rate of return is less than its required rate of return, and no investor who does not own the stock believes that its expected rate of return is greater than its required rate of return.
2. The market price of a security must equal its value to the marginal investor.

If these conditions do not hold, trading will occur until they do. Of course, security prices are not constant. A security's price can swing wildly as new information becomes available to the market that changes investors' expectations concerning the security's cash flow stream, or risk, or when the general level of returns (i.e., interest rates) change. However, evidence suggests that securities prices, especially of securities that are actively traded, such as those issued by the U. S. Treasury or by large firms, adjust rapidly to disequilibrium situations. Thus, most people believe that the bonds of the U. S. Treasury and the bonds and stocks of major corporations are generally in equilibrium. The key to the rapid movement of security prices toward equilibrium is informational efficiency, which is discussed in the next section.

Self-Test Questions

1. What is meant by security market equilibrium?
2. What securities are most likely to be in equilibrium?

Informational Efficiency

A securities market—say, the market for long-term U. S. Treasury bonds—is *informationally efficient* if (1) all information relevant to the values of the securities traded can be obtained easily and at low cost, and (2) the market contains many buyers and sellers who act rationally on this information. If these conditions hold, current market prices will have embedded in them all information of possible relevance; hence, future price movements will be based solely on **new** information as it becomes known.

The *Efficient Markets Hypothesis (EMH),* which has three forms, formalizes the theory of informational efficiency:

1. The *weak form* of the EMH holds that all information contained in **past price movements** is fully reflected in current market prices. Therefore, information about recent trends in a security's price, or a bond's yield, is of no value in choosing which securities will "outperform" other securities.
2. The *semistrong form* of the EMH holds that current market prices reflect all **publicly available information**. Therefore, it makes no sense to spend hours and hours analyzing economic data and financial reports because whatever information you might find, good or bad, has already been absorbed by the market and imbedded in current prices.
3. The *strong form* of the EMH holds that current market prices reflect **all relevant information**, whether publicly available or privately held. If this form holds, then even investors with "inside information," such as corporate officers, would find it impossible to earn abnormal returns—that is, returns in excess of that justified by the riskiness of the investment.

The EMH, in any of its three forms, is a hypothesis rather than a proven law, so it is not necessarily true. However, hundreds of empirical tests have been conducted to try to prove, or disprove, the EMH, and the results are relatively consistent. Most tests support the weak and semistrong forms of the EMH for well-developed markets such as the U.S. markets for large firms' stocks and bond issues and for Treasury securities. Supporters of these forms of the EMH note that there are some 100,000 or so full-time, highly trained, professional analysts and traders operating in these markets. Furthermore, many of these analysts and traders work for businesses such as Citibank, Fidelity Investments, Merrill Lynch, Prudential, and the like, which have billions of dollars available to take advantage of undervalued securities. Finally, as a result of disclosure requirements and electronic information networks, new information about these heavily followed securities is almost instantaneously available. Therefore, security prices in these markets adjust almost immediately as new developments occur, and hence prices reflect all publicly available information.

Virtually no one, however, believes that the strong form of the EMH holds. Studies of legal purchases and sales by people with inside information indicate that insiders can make abnormal profits by trading on that information. It is even more apparent that insiders can make abnormal profits if they trade illegally on specific information that has not been disclosed to the public, such as a takeover bid, a research and development breakthrough, and the like.

The EMH has important implications both for securities investment decisions and for business financing decisions. Because security prices appear to generally reflect all public information, most actively followed and traded securities are in equilibrium and fairly valued. Being in equilibrium, however, does not mean that new information could not cause a security's price to soar or to plummet, but it does mean that most securities are neither undervalued nor overvalued. Therefore, over the long run, an investor with no inside information can only expect to earn a return on a security that compensates him or her for the amount of risk assumed. In the short run, for example, a year, an investor can only expect to earn a return that is the same as the average for securities of equal risk. In other words, investors should not expect to "beat the market" after adjusting for risk. Also, because the EMH applies to most bond markets, bond prices, and hence interest rates, reflect all current public information. Consistently forecasting future interest rates is impossible because interest rates change in response to new information, and this information could either lower or raise rates.

For managers, the EMH indicates that managerial decisions generally should not be based on perceptions about the market's ability to properly price the firm's securities or on perceptions about which way interest rates will go. In other words, managers should not try to time security issues to try to catch stock prices while they are high or interest rates while they are low. However, in some situations, managers may have information about their own firms that is unknown to the public. This condition is called *asymmetric information*, which can affect managerial decisions. For example, suppose a drug manufacturer has made a breakthrough in AIDS research, but wants to maintain as much secrecy as possible about the new drug. During final development and testing, the firm might want to delay any new securities offerings because securities could probably be sold under more favorable terms once the announcement is made. Managers can, and should, act on inside information for the benefit of their firms, but inside information cannot legally be used for personal profit.

Are markets really efficient? If markets were not efficient, the better managers of stock and bond mutual funds and pension plans would be able to consistently outperform the broad averages over long periods of time. In fact, very few managers can consistently better the broad averages, and during most years, mutual fund managers, on average, underperform the market. In any year, some mutual fund managers will outperform the market and others will underperform the market—this is known with certainty. But, for an investor to beat the market by investing in mutual funds, he or she must identify the successful managers beforehand, which seems very difficult, if not impossible, to do.

In spite of the evidence, many theorists, and even more Wall Street experts, believe that pockets of inefficiency do exist. In some cases, entire markets may be inefficient. For example, the markets for the securities issued by small firms may be inefficient because there are neither enough analysts ferreting out information on these companies nor sufficient numbers of investors trading these securities. Many people even believe that individual securities traded in efficient markets are occasionally priced inefficiently, or that investor emotions can drive prices too high during raging bull markets or too low during whimpering bear markets. Indeed, if investors are driven more by greed and emotion than by rational assessments of security values, it may be that markets are not really as efficient as claimed by supporters of the EMH.

We really don't know whether it is possible to beat the market by skill or whether it is just a matter of luck. Nevertheless, it is wise for both investors and managers to consider the implications of market efficiency when making investment and financing decisions. If investors want to believe that they can beat the market, fine, but they should least recognize that there is a lot of evidence that tells us that most people that try ultimately fail.

Self-Test Questions

1. What two conditions must hold for markets to be efficient?
2. Briefly, what is the Efficient Markets Hypothesis (EMH)?
3. What are the implications of the EMH for investors and managers?

The Risk/Return Trade-Off

Most financial decisions involve alternative courses of action. For example, should a hospital invest its excess funds in Treasury bonds that yield 6 percent or in HCA bonds that yield 9 percent? Should a group practice buy a replacement piece of equipment now or wait until next year? Should a joint venture outpatient diagnostic center purchase a small, limited-use MRI system or a large, and more expensive, multipurpose system?

Generally, the alternative courses of action will have different expected rates of return, and one may be tempted to automatically accept the alternative with the higher expected return. However, this approach to financial decision making would be incorrect. In efficient markets, those alternatives that offer higher returns will also entail higher risk. The correct question to ask when making financial decisions is not which alternative has the higher expected rate of return, but which alternative has the higher return **after adjusting for risk**. In other words, which alternative has the higher return over and above the return commensurate with that alternative's riskiness?

To illustrate the *risk/return trade-off*, suppose HCA stock has an expected rate of return of 14 percent, while its bonds yield 9 percent. Does this mean that investors should flock to buy the firm's stock and ignore the bonds? Of course not. The higher expected rate of return on the stock merely reflects the fact that the stock is riskier than the bonds. Those investors who are not willing to assume much risk will buy HCA's bonds, while those that are less risk averse will buy the stock. From the perspective of HCA's managers, financing with stock is less risky than using debt, so the firm is willing to pay the higher cost of equity to limit the firm's risk exposure.

In spite of the efficiency of major securities markets, the markets for products and services (i.e., the markets for real assets such as MRI systems) are usually not efficient; hence, returns are not necessarily related to risk. Thus, hospitals, group practices, and other healthcare businesses can make real-asset investments and achieve returns in excess of those required by the riskiness of the investment. Furthermore, the market for *innovation* (i.e., the market for ideas) is not efficient. Thus, it is possible for people like Bill Gates, the founder of Microsoft, to become multibillionaires at a relatively young age. However, when excess returns are found in the product, service, or idea markets, new entrants quickly join the innovators, and competition over time will usually force rates of return down to efficient market levels. The result is that later entrants can only expect returns that are commensurate with the risks involved.

1. Explain the meaning of the term *risk/return trade-off.*   **Self-Test**
2. In what markets does this trade-off hold?   **Questions**

Debt Refunding

If a debt issue is callable, and if interest rates drop, the issuer may elect to lower its interest expense by issuing new debt and using the proceeds to call (retire) the existing issue. Such an action is called a *refunding*. There are costs involved in refunding, but there is also one major benefit: The issuer reduces the dollar amount of interest payments that it must make in the future. Thus, a refunding analysis is a classical application of discounted cash flow cost/benefit analysis—the issuer should refund the bond if the present value of the refunding savings exceeds the present value of the costs of refunding.

The easiest way to examine the refunding decision is through an example. Suppose Minnesota Health Systems (MHS), Inc., an investor-owned corporation, has a $60 million bond issue outstanding that has a 15 percent annual coupon and 20 years remaining to maturity.[6] This 30-year issue, which was sold ten years ago, had flotation costs of $3 million that MHS has been amortizing on a straight-line basis over the 30-year original life of the issue. (Flotation costs, which were discussed in Chapter 7, are the printing, accounting, legal, and investment banker expenses associated with new securities issues.) The bond has a call provision with a ten-year call deferral, so the bond can now be called, but a 10 percent call premium is required. MHS's investment bankers have assured the firm that it can sell a new $60–$70 million issue of 20-year annual coupon bonds at an interest rate of 12 percent. Flotation costs on a new issue would amount to $4 million. MHS's marginal federal-plus-state tax rate is 40 percent. Should MHS refund the $60 million of 15 percent bonds?

The following steps outline the decision process; the steps are summarized in worksheet form in Table 8.1.

- **Calculate the investment outlay required to refund the issue.**
  a. *Call premium on the old issue.*
     Before tax: $0.10 \times \$60,000,000 = \$6,000,000$.
     After tax: $\$6,000,000 \times (1 - T) = \$6,000,000 \times 0.60 = \$3,600,000$.
     Although MHS must spend $6 million on the call premium,
     this is a tax-deductible expense in the year the call is made.
     Because the firm is in the 40 percent marginal tax bracket, it saves
     $0.40 \times \$6,000,000 = \$2,400,000$ in taxes, for an after-tax cost of only
     $3,600,000. This amount is shown as a cost, or outflow, on Line 1 of
     Table 8.1.
  b. *Flotation costs on the new issue.*
     Flotation costs on the new issue are $4,000,000, as shown on Line 2
     of the worksheet. For tax purposes, flotation costs must be amortized,
     or spread, over the 20-year life of the new bond, and then used to
     reduce taxable income in each year. The amortization cash flows will
     be discussed later.
  c. *Flotation costs on the old issue.*
     The flotation costs on the old issue were amortized and deducted
     from taxable income, just as we will do on the new issue flotation
     costs. However, if the refunding takes place, tax laws permit MHS to
     immediately expense that portion of the old issue flotation costs that
     have not yet been expensed. Because ten years have passed since the old
     30-year bond was originally issued, only one-third of the $3 million
     flotation costs have been expensed for tax purposes, leaving two-thirds,

TABLE 8.1 Bond Refunding Worksheet

	Amount Before Tax	Amount After Tax	Present Value at 7.2%
Investment Outlay at $t = 0$			
1. Call premium on the old issue	($6,000,000)	($3,600,000)	($3,600,000)
2. Flotation costs on new issue	(4,000,000)	(4,000,000)	(4,000,000)
3. Tax savings on old issue flotation costs	2,000,000	800,000	800,000
4. Net investment outlay			($6,800,000)
Annual Flotation Cost Tax Effects			
5. Benefit from new issue flotation costs	$200,000	$80,000	$834,505
6. Lost benefit on old issue flotation costs	(100,000)	(40,000)	(417,252)
7. Present value of amortization tax effects			$417,253
Savings Due to Refunding			
8. Interest payment on old issue	$9,000,000	$5,400,000	
9. Interest payment on new issue	7,200,000	4,320,000	
10. Net interest savings		$1,080,000	$11,265,817
NPV of Refunding Decision			
11. NPV of refunding decision			$4,883,070

or $2 million, unexpensed. This immediate deduction from taxable income would create a $0.40 \times \$2,000,000 = \$800,000$ tax savings, or inflow, which is shown on Line 3.

  d. *Total after-tax investment outlay.*
    The total investment outlay required at Time 0 to refund the bond issue is $6,800,000, which is shown on Line 4.

- **Determine the net effect of flotation cost amortization.**
  a. *New issue flotation cost amortization.*
    With total flotation costs of $4 million on the new issue, the annual taxable income deduction is $\$4,000,000/20 = \$200,000$. Because MHS is in the 40 percent tax bracket, it has a tax savings of $0.40 \times \$200,000 = \$80,000$ a year for 20 years. In a refunding analysis, all cash flows must be discounted at the after-tax cost of new debt, which is $12\% \times (1 - T) = 12\% \times 0.6 = 7.2\%$. The present value of the

new issue flotation cost tax savings, when discounted at 7.2 percent, is $834,505, which is shown as a savings, or inflow, on Line 5. As in all cases, the primary consideration in choosing a discount rate is the riskiness of the cash flow stream. In a bond refunding, the cash flows are relatively safe because they are fixed by contract, so a relatively low discount rate should be chosen. What market rate reflects relatively low risk? The answer is the rate of return required on MHS's bonds, so it is chosen as the basis for the discount rate used in the refunding analysis.

b. *Old issue flotation cost amortization*

If the refunding takes place, MHS loses the opportunity to continue to expense the old flotation costs over time, so the $2,000,000/20 = $100,000 reduction in annual taxable income is lost. Thus, MHS loses the annual tax savings of $0.40 \times \$100,000 = \$40,000$ for the next 20 years. The present value of these lost savings, which is an opportunity cost of refunding, is $417,252, which is shown on Line 6. Note that because of the refunding, the remaining old flotation costs provide an immediate tax savings, shown on Line 3, rather than annual savings, shown on Line 6. Thus, the $800,000 - $417,252 = $382,748 net savings simply reflect the difference between the present value of tax benefits to be received in the future without the refunding versus the immediate benefit if the refunding takes place.

c. *Total amortization effect.*

The net effect of the amortization of flotation costs on the old and new debt issues is $417,253 on a present value basis. This amount is shown on Line 7.

- **Calculate the annual interest savings.**

  a. *Interest expense on old issue.*

  The annual after-tax interest on the old issue is $5,400,000, which is shown on Line 8: $0.15 \times \$60,000,000 \times 0.60 = \$5,400,000$.

  b. *Interest expense on new issue.*

  The annual after-tax interest on the new issue is $4,320,000, which is shown on Line 9: $0.12 \times \$60,000,000 \times 0.60 = \$4,320,000$.

  c. *Annual interest savings.*

  The annual interest savings is $1,080,000, which is shown on Line 10: $5,400,000 - \$4,320,000 = \$1,080,000$.

  d. *PV of annual savings.*

  The present value of $1,080,00 per year for 20 years, when discounted at 7.2 percent, is $11,265,817. This amount is also shown on Line 10.

- **Calculate the net present value (NPV) of the refunding.**

Net investment outlay	($ 6,800,000)
Amortization tax effects	417,253
Interest savings	11,265,817
NPV of refunding	$ 4,883,070

Because the net present value of the refunding is positive, the present value of the inflows exceeds the present value of the outflows. Thus, it would be profitable for MHS to refund the old bond issue.

Several other points should be noted. First, because the refunding is advantageous to MHS, it must be disadvantageous to bondholders; they must give up their 15 percent bonds and reinvest the proceeds in securities that have a lower interest rate. This points out the danger of a call provision to bondholders, and it also explains why bonds without a call provision have lower interest rates than callable bonds. Second, although it is not emphasized in the example, we assumed that the firm raises the investment required to undertake the refunding operation (the $6,800,000 shown on Line 4) as debt. Typically, businesses raise the investment outlay by increasing the amount of the new issue, which is easily done because the new issue has a lower interest rate, and hence additional principal can be taken on. In this example, MHS might sell $67,000,000 of new bonds. Third, we set up the example so that the new issue had the same maturity as the remaining life of the old issue. Often, the old bonds have only a relatively short term to maturity—say, five to ten years—while the new bonds have a longer maturity—say, 25 to 30 years. In this situation, a replacement chain analysis is required. Fourth, not-for-profit firms conduct refunding analyses in exactly the same way as that presented in Table 8.1. The only difference is that the tax rate is zero, and hence there are no direct tax effects to consider in the analysis.

Finally, although the analysis shows that the refunding would be profitable now, it might be even more profitable if MHS waits and refunds later. If interest rates fall further, then it might pay to delay the refunding. The mechanics of calculating the NPV of refunding is relatively simple, but the decision on when to refund is not simple at all because it requires a forecast of future interest rates. Thus, the refund now versus refund later decision is more a matter of judgment than of quantitative analysis.

To illustrate the timing decision, assume that MHS's managers forecast that long-term interest rates have a 50 percent probability of remaining at their present level of 12 percent over the next year. However, there is a 25 percent probability that rates could fall to 10 percent, and a 25 percent probability that rates could rise to 14 percent. The refunding analysis could then be repeated, as previously, but assuming it would take place one year from now when the old bonds have only 19 years to maturity. (We assume also that the new issue would have a 19-year maturity.) We performed the analysis and found the NPV distribution one year from now given in Table 8.2:

Note that if rates rose to 14 percent next year, the NPV of refunding would be negative, so MHS would not refund the issue and the realized NPV at a 14 percent interest rate would be $0. Thus, the expected NPV of refunding

TABLE 8.2

Interest Rate
and Bond
Refunding
Forecast

Probability	Interest Rate	NPV of Refunding One Year from Now
25%	10%	$13,737,916
50	12	4,607,124
25	14	(3,067,344)

next year is $5,738,041, versus $4,883,070 if refunding takes place now:

$$(0.25 \times \$13,737,916) + (0.50 \times \$4,607,124) + (0.25 \times \$0) = \$5,738,041.$$

Even though the expected NPV of refunding in one year is higher, MHS's managers would probably decide to refund today. First, when $5,738,041 is discounted back one year to today at some rate—say, a 10 percent rate—the NPV of refunding in one year drops to $5,216,401. More important, the NPV of refunding in one year is only an expected NPV because it depends on future interest rates, while the NPV of refunding today is known with some certainty. MHS's managers would opt to delay the refunding only if the expected NPV today from refunding later is sufficiently above the refund-now NPV to compensate for the risks involved.

Clearly, the decision to refund now versus refund later is complicated by the fact that there would be numerous opportunities to refund in the future, rather than just a single opportunity one year from now. Furthermore, the decision must be based on a large set of interest rate forecasts, which is a daunting task in itself. Fortunately, managers who make bond refunding decisions are advised by sophisticated investment bankers, who can now use the values of derivative securities to estimate the value of a bond's embedded call option. If the call option is worth more than the NPV of refunding today, the issue should not be immediately refunded. Rather, the issuer should either delay the refunding to take advantage of the information obtained from the derivative market or actually create a derivative transaction to lock in the value of the call option.

Key Concepts

This chapter provides an overview of security valuation, including debt re-funding. Here are its key concepts:

- Bonds call for the payment of a specific amount of *interest* for a specific number of years, and for the *repayment of par* on the bond's maturity date. Like many assets, a bond's value is simply the present value of the expected cash flow stream.

- The annual rate of return on a bond consists of an *interest*, or *current*, *yield* plus a *capital gains yield*. Assuming constant interest rates, if the bond is selling at a *discount*, the capital gains yield is positive; if the bond is selling at a *premium*, the capital gains yield is negative.

- A bond's *yield to maturity (YTM)* is the rate of return earned on a bond if it is held to maturity and no default occurs. The YTM for a bond that sells at par consists entirely of an interest yield, but if the bond sells at a discount or premium, the YTM consists of the current yield plus a positive or negative capital gains yield.

- Bondholders face *price risk* because bond values change when interest rates change. In general, the longer the maturity of the bonds, the greater the price risk.

- Bondholders face *reinvestment rate risk* when the investment horizon exceeds the maturity of the bond issue.

- The *value* of a share of stock using the dividend valuation model is found by *discounting* the stream of *expected dividends* by the stock's required rate of return.

- The value of a stock whose dividends are expected to grow at a constant rate for many years is found by applying the *constant growth model*:

$$E(P_0) = \frac{D_0 \times [1 + E(g)]}{R(R_s) - E(g)} = \frac{E(D_1)}{R(R_s) - E(g)}.$$

- The *expected rate of return* on a stock consists of an *expected dividend yield* plus an *expected capital gains yield*. For a constant growth stock, both the expected dividend yield and the expected capital gains yield are constant over time, and the expected rate of return can be found by this equation:

$$E(R_s) = \frac{D_0 \times [1 + E(g)]}{P_0} + E(g) = \frac{E(D_1)}{P_0} + E(g).$$

- The *Efficient Markets Hypothesis (EMH)* holds that (1) stocks are always in equilibrium and fairly valued; (2) it is impossible for an investor to consistently beat the market; and (3) managers should not try to forecast future interest rates or time security issues.

- In efficient markets, alternatives that offer higher returns must also have higher risk; this is called the *risk/return trade-off*. The implication is that investments must be evaluated on the basis of both risk and return.

- If a debt issue is callable, and if interest rates drop, the issuer may elect to lower its interest expense by issuing new debt and using the proceeds to call (retire) the existing issue. Such an action is called a *refunding*.

- A refunding analysis is a classical application of discounted cash flow cost/benefit analysis—the issuer should refund the bond if the present value of the refunding savings exceeds the present value of the costs of refunding.

This concludes our discussion of the traditional forms of financing—debt and equity—and how these securities are valued. In the next chapter, we discuss an alternative to traditional financing: lease financing.

Selected References

Many investment textbooks cover the valuation of securities in detail. For example, see

Radcliffe, Robert C. 1997. *Investment: Concepts, Analysis, and Strategy.* Reading, MA: Addison-Wesley.

The seminal modern work on stock valuation is Williams, John Burr. 1938. *The Theory of Investment Value.* Cambridge, MA: Harvard University Press.

Selected Web Sites

The web sites that pertain to this chapter generally involve data that are used in security valuation.

To obtain analyst growth forecasts for use in the constant growth stock valuation model, see the Zacks site at *www.zacks.com.* Here, you can use the Estimates capability on the upper left of the page, along with a stock symbol, to see analysts' forecasts.

To obtain stock betas, refer to the selected web sites section of Chapter 5.

Selected Cases

There are three cases in *Cases in Healthcare Finance* that are applicable to this chapter:

Case 11: Potomac Healthcare (A), which focuses on bond valuation.

Case 12: Potomac Healthcare (B), which covers stock valuation.

Case 16: Boston Enterprises, which focuses on debt refunding.

Notes

1. If the probability of default on the bond is much above zero, the expected rate of return on the bond is less than the YTM. Also, the calculation of YTM assumes that the coupon payments are reinvested at the YTM rate. Thus, if over the life of the bond, interest rates are above the YTM, the realized rate of return will be higher than the YTM. Similarly, if interest rates over time are less than the YTM, the realized return will be less than the YTM.

2. The effective annual YTM is $(1.029)^2 - 1.0 = 1.0588 - 1.0 = 0.0588 = 5.88\%$, as compared to the stated rate of 5.80%.

3. In reality, price risk is more related to a debt security's *duration* than to its maturity. Duration, which can be thought of as the average maturity of a debt issue including both interest and principal payments, is discussed in Chapter 20.

4. The effective annual rate, which includes the effect of quarterly compounding, is 12.3 percent.

5. Stocks generally pay dividends quarterly, so, theoretically, we should evaluate them on a quarterly basis. However, in stock valuation, most analysts work on an annual basis because the data generally are not precise enough to warrant the refinement of a quarterly model.

6. We are using annual coupon bonds to simplify the mathematics of the illustration. The same techiques, with minor modification, would be applied to semiannual coupon bonds.

LEASE FINANCING

Learning Objectives

After studying this chapter, readers should be able to:

- Describe the different types of leases.
- Explain how lease financing affects both financial statements and taxes.
- Conduct a basic lease analysis from the perspectives of both the lessee and lessor.
- Discuss the factors that create value in lease transactions.

Introduction

Businesses generally own fixed assets, but it is the use of the buildings and equipment that is important to the business, not their ownership. One way to obtain the use of assets is to raise debt or equity capital, and then use this capital to buy the assets. An alternative way to obtain the use of assets is to lease them. Prior to the 1950s, leasing was generally associated with real estate—land and buildings. Today, however, it is possible to lease almost any kind of asset, and leasing is used extensively in the health services industry. In fact, in 1999 alone, healthcare providers leased almost $6 billion worth of medical equipment, which amounted to about 40 percent of all medical equipment used in the industry. In addition to medical equipment, there has been increasing use of leasing to fund information technology, which is consuming a larger and larger proportion of capital expenditures within healthcare businesses.[1]

Before we begin our discussion of lease financing, note that there are two parties to any lease transaction. The user of a leased asset is called the *lessee*, while the owner of the property, usually the manufacturer or a leasing company, is called the *lessor*. (The term "lessee" is pronounced "less-ee," not "lease-ee," and "lessor" is pronounced "less-or.")

Types of Leases

Historically, leases have been informally classified into one of three categories: (1) operating leases, (2) financial leases, and (3) combination leases. In this section, we will discuss these informal classifications. In later sections, we will discuss more formal classifications used by accountants and by the Internal Revenue Service (IRS).

Operating Leases

Operating leases, sometimes called *service leases,* generally provide for both financing and maintenance in addition to use of the asset. IBM was one of the pioneers of operating lease contracts, and computers and office copying machines, together with automobiles, trucks, and medical diagnostic equipment, are the primary types of assets involved in operating leases. Ordinarily, operating leases require the lessor to maintain and service the leased equipment, and the cost of the maintenance is built into the lease payments.

Another important characteristic of operating leases is the fact that they are not fully amortized. In other words, the payments required under the lease contract are not sufficient for the lessor to recover the full cost of the equipment. However, the lease contract is written for a period considerably less than the expected economic life of the leased asset, and the lessor expects to recover all costs eventually by lease renewal payments, by releasing the equipment to other lessees, or by sale of the equipment.

A final feature of operating leases is that they frequently contain a *cancellation clause* that gives the lessee the right to cancel the lease and to return the equipment before the expiration of the basic lease agreement. This is an important consideration to the lessee because it means that the equipment can be returned if it is rendered obsolete by technological developments or if it is no longer needed because of a decline in the lessee's business.

Financial Leases

Financial leases, which are also called *capital leases,* are differentiated from operating leases in that (1) they typically do not provide for maintenance service; (2) they typically are not cancelable; (3) they are generally for a period that approximates the economic life of the asset; and, hence, (4) they are fully amortized—that is, the lessor receives rental payments equal to the full cost of the leased asset plus a return on the funds employed.

In a typical financial lease, the lessee selects the specific item it requires, and then it negotiates the price and delivery terms with the manufacturer. The lessee then arranges to have a leasing firm (lessor) buy the equipment from the manufacturer, and the lessee simultaneously executes a lease agreement with the lessor. The lessee is generally given an option to renew the lease at a reduced rate upon expiration of the initial lease agreement. However, under a "pure" financial lease, the initial lease cannot be cancelled. Also, the lessee generally pays the insurance premiums and any property taxes due on the leased property.

The terms of the lease call for full amortization of the lessor's investment, plus a rate of return on the unamortized balance, which is close to the percentage rate the lessee would have paid on a secured term loan. For example, if a radiology group practice would have to pay 10 percent for a term loan to buy a x-ray machine, then a rate of about 10 percent would be built into the lease contract by the lessor. The parallel to borrowing is obvious in a financial lease. Under a secured loan arrangement, the lender would normally receive a series of equal payments just sufficient to amortize the loan and to provide a specified rate of return on the outstanding loan balance. Under a financial lease, the lease payments are set up exactly the same way—the payments are just sufficient to return the full purchase price to the lessor, plus a stated return on the lessor's investment.

A *sale and leaseback* is a special type of financial lease, often used with real estate, that can be arranged by a user that currently owns some asset. Here, the user sells the asset to another party and simultaneously executes an agreement to lease the property back for a stated period under specific terms. In a sale and leaseback, the lessee receives an immediate cash payment in exchange for a future series of lease payments that must be made to rent the use of the asset sold.

Combination Leases

Although the distinction between operating and financial leases has historical significance, today many lessors offer leases under a wide variety of terms. Therefore, in practice, leases often do not fit exactly into the operating lease or financial lease category, but rather combine some features of each. To illustrate the concept, note that many of today's financial leases contain cancellation clauses, which historically have been associated only with operating leases. However, when used in financial leases these clauses generally include prepayment provisions whereby the lessee must make penalty payments sufficient to enable the lessor to recover some or all of the remaining lease payments.

1. What is the difference between an operating lease and a financial lease?
2. What is a sale and leaseback?
3. What is a combination lease?

Self-Test Questions

Tax Effects

For both investor-owned and not-for-profit healthcare businesses, tax effects can play an important role in the lease-versus-buy decision.

Investor-Owned Businesses

For investor-owned businesses, the full amount of lease payments is a tax-deductible expense for the lessee **provided that the IRS agrees that a particular contract is a genuine lease and not simply a loan that is called a lease.** This makes it important that a lease contract be written in a form acceptable to the IRS. A lease that complies with all of the IRS requirements for taxable businesses is called a *guideline,* or *tax-oriented, lease.* In a guideline lease, ownership tax benefits accrue to the lessor, but the lessee's lease payments are fully tax deductible. A lease that does not meet the tax guidelines is called a *non-tax-oriented lease.* For this type of lease, the lessee can only deduct the implied interest portion of each lease payment. However, the lessee is effectively the owner of the leased equipment; thus, the lessee can take the tax depreciation.

The main provisions of the tax guidelines are as follows:

• The lease term, including any extensions or renewals at a fixed rental rate, must not exceed 80 percent of the estimated useful life of the equipment at the commencement of the lease transaction. Thus, at the projected end of the lease, the property must have an estimated remaining life equal to at least 20 percent of its original life. Furthermore, the remaining useful life must not be less than one year. This requirement limits the maximum term of a lease to 80 percent of the asset's useful life. Note that an asset's useful life is normally much longer than its tax depreciation class life.

• The equipment's estimated value (in constant dollars without adjustment for inflation) at the projected expiration of the lease must equal at least 20 percent of its value at the start of the lease. Note that the estimated value of the asset at the end of the lease is called the *residual value*. This requirement also has the effect of limiting the maximum lease term.

• Neither the lessee nor any related party can have the right to purchase the property from the lessor at a fixed price predetermined at the lease's inception. However, the lessee can be given a fair market value purchase option.

• Neither the lessee nor any related party can pay or guarantee payment of any part of the price of the leased equipment. Simply put, the lessee cannot make any investment in the equipment, other than through the lease payments.

• The leased equipment must not be "limited use" property, which is equipment that can only be used by the lessee or a related party at the end of the lease.

The reason for the IRS's concern about lease terms is that, without restrictions, a business could set up a "lease" transaction that calls for very rapid lease payments, which would be deductible from taxable income. The effect would be to depreciate the equipment over a much shorter period than the IRS allows in its depreciation guidelines. For example, suppose that New England Laboratories, Inc., an investor-owned corporation that owns clinical laboratories in New Hampshire, Maine, Massachusetts, and Vermont, planned to acquire a $2 million computer that has a three-year life for tax purposes. According to current tax laws (Modified Accelerated Cost Recovery System, or MACRS), the annual depreciation allowances would be $660,000 in Year 1; $900,000 in Year 2; $300,000 in Year 3; and $140,000 in Year 4. If New England Laboratories were in the 40 percent federal-plus-state tax bracket, the depreciation would provide a tax savings of $0.40 \times \$660,000 = \$264,000$ in Year 1; $360,000 in Year 2; $120,000 in Year 3; and $56,000 in Year 4, for a total savings of $800,000. At a 6 percent discount rate, the present value of these tax savings would be $757,441.

Now, suppose the firm could acquire the computer through a one-year lease arrangement with Bank of Boston for a payment of $2 million, with a one-dollar purchase option. If the $2 million payment were treated as a lease payment, it would be fully deductible, so it would provide a tax saving of $0.40 \times \$2,000,000 = \$800,000$ versus a present value of only $757,441 for the depreciation shelters associated with ownership. Thus, the lease payment and the depreciation would both provide the same total amount of tax savings—40 percent of $2 million, or $800,000; but the savings would come in faster, and hence have a higher present value, with the one-year lease. Therefore, if just any type of contract could be called a lease and given tax treatment as a lease, then the timing of the tax shelters could be speeded up, compared with ownership depreciation tax shelters. This speed up would benefit businesses; but it would be costly to the government, and hence to individual taxpayers. For this reason, the IRS has established the rules described above for defining a lease for tax purposes.

Even though leasing can be used only within limits to speed up the effective depreciation schedule, there still are times when very substantial tax benefits can be derived from a leasing arrangement. For example, if an investor-owned hospital has a very large construction program that has generated so much accelerated depreciation that it has no current tax liabilities, then depreciation shelters are not very useful. In this case, a leasing company set up by a very profitable business, like General Electric, can buy the equipment, receive the depreciation shelters, and then share these benefits with the hospital by charging lower lease payments.[2] This issue will be discussed in detail later in the chapter, but the point to be made now is that if businesses are to obtain tax benefits from leasing, the lease contract must be written in a manner that will qualify it as a true lease under IRS guidelines. Any questions about the tax status of a lease contract must be resolved by the potential lessee prior to signing the contract.

Not-for-Profit Businesses

Not-for-profit businesses also benefit from tax laws, but in a different way. Because not-for-profit firms do not obtain tax benefits from depreciation, the ownership of assets has no tax value. However, lessors, which are all taxable businesses, do benefit from ownership. In effect, when assets are owned by not-for-profit firms the depreciation tax benefit is lost; while when assets are leased, the tax benefit is realized, but by the lessor rather than the lessee. This realized benefit, in turn, can be shared with the lessee in the form of lower rental payments. Note, however, that the cost of tax-exempt debt to not-for-profit firms can be lower than the after-tax cost of debt to taxable firms; so leasing is not automatically less costly to not-for-profit firms than borrowing in the tax-exempt markets and buying.

A special type of financial transaction has been created for not-for-profit businesses called a *tax-exempt lease*. Legally, such a "lease" is not really a lease, but these transactions have all of the general characteristics of leases. The major difference between a tax-exempt lease and a conventional lease is that the implied interest portion of the lease payment is not classified as taxable income to the lessor. Thus, a portion of the lease payment received by the lessor is exempt from federal income taxes. The rationale for this tax treatment is that the interest paid on most debt financing used by not-for-profit organizations is tax-exempt to the lender, and a lessor is, in actuality, a lender. Tax-exempt leases provide a greater after-tax return to lessors than do conventional leases, so some of this "extra" return could be passed back to the lessee in the form of lower lease payments. Thus, the lessee's payments on tax-exempt leases could be lower than when the asset is acquired by a not-for-profit business through a conventional lease.

Self-Test Questions

1. What is the difference between a tax-oriented lease and a non-tax-oriented lease?
2. What are some provisions that would make a lease non-tax-oriented?
3. Why should the IRS care about lease provisions?
4. What is a tax-exempt lease?

Financial Statement Effects

Under certain conditions, neither the leased asset nor the liabilities under the lease contract appear on the lessee's balance sheet. For this reason, leasing is often called *off-balance sheet financing*. This point is illustrated in Table 9.1 by the balance sheets of two hypothetical firms—B and L. Initially, the balance sheets of both firms are identical, and they both have debt ratios of 50 percent. Next, each firm decides to acquire a fixed asset that costs $100. Firm B borrows $100 and buys the asset, so both an asset and a liability go on its balance sheet, and its debt ratio rises from 50 to 75 percent. Firm L leases the equipment. The lease may call for fixed charges as high or even higher than the loan, and the obligations assumed under the lease may have equal or even more potential to force the business into bankruptcy; but the firm's debt ratio remains at only 50 percent.

To correct this problem, accounting rules require firms that enter into financial leases to restate their balance sheets to report the leased asset as a fixed asset and the present value of the future lease payments as a liability. This process is called *capitalizing* the lease, and hence such a lease is called a *capital lease*. The net effect of capitalizing the lease is to cause Firms B and L to have similar balance sheets, both of which will, in essence, resemble the one shown for Firm B.[3]

The logic here is as follows. If a firm signs a capital lease contract, its obligation to make lease payments is just as binding as if it had signed a loan agreement; the failure to make lease payments has the potential to bankrupt a firm just as the failure to make principal and interest payments on a loan

TABLE 9.1
Effects of
Leasing on
Balance Sheets

Before Asset Increase:

Firms B and L			
Current assets	$ 50	Debt	$ 50
Fixed assets	50	Equity	50
Total assets	$100		$100
Debt/assets ratio			50%

After Asset Increase:

Firm B, Which Borrows and Buys					Firm L, Which Leases			
Current assets	$ 50	Debt	$150		Current assets	$ 50	Debt	$ 50
Fixed assets	150	Equity	50		Fixed assets	50	Equity	50
Total assets	$200		$200		Total assets	$100		$100
Debt/assets ratio			75%		Debt/assets ratio			50%

can result in bankruptcy. Therefore, under most circumstances, a capital lease has the same impact on a firm's financial condition as does a loan. This being the case, if a firm signs a capital lease agreement, it has the effect of raising the firm's effective debt ratio. Therefore, if the firm had previously established a target capital structure, and if there is no reason to think that the optimal capital structure has changed, then using lease financing requires additional equity support exactly like debt financing. Another way of saying the same thing is that leasing uses up *debt capacity*.

Note, however, that there are some legal differences between loans and leases, mostly involving the rights of lessors versus lenders when a business in financial distress reorganizes or liquidates. In most financial distress situations, lessors fare better than lenders, so lessors may be more willing to deal with firms in poor financial condition than are lenders. At a minimum, lessors may be willing to accept lower rates of return than lenders when dealing with financially distressed firms because risks are lower.

If disclosure of the lease in our Table 9.1 example were not made, then Firm L's investors could be deceived into thinking that its financial position is stronger than it really is. Thus, even before firms were required to place financial leases on the balance sheet, they were required to disclose the existence of long-term leases in footnotes to their financial statements. At that time, it was debated whether or not investors fully recognized the impact of leases and, in effect, see that Firms B and L were in essentially the same financial position. Some people argued that leases were not fully recognized, even by sophisticated investors. The question of whether investors were truly deceived was debated but never resolved. Those who believe strongly in efficient markets thought that investors were not deceived and that footnotes were sufficient, while those who questioned market efficiency thought that all leases should be capitalized. Current accounting requirements represent a compromise between these two positions, although one that is tilted heavily toward those who favor capitalization.

A lease is classified as a capital lease, and thus is capitalized and shown directly on the balance sheet, if one or more of the following conditions exist:

- Under the terms of the lease, ownership of the property is effectively transferred from the lessor to the lessee.
- The lessee can purchase the property at less than its true market value when the lease expires.
- The lease runs for a period equal to or greater than 75 percent of the asset's life. Thus, if an asset has a ten-year life and the lease is written for eight years, the lease must be capitalized.
- The present value of the lease payments is equal to or greater than 90 percent of the initial value of the asset. The discount rate used to calculate the present value of the lease payments must be the lower of (1) the rate used by the lessor to establish the lease payments, which is discussed later in the chapter; or (2) the rate of interest which the lessee would have to pay for new debt with a maturity equal to that of the lease. Note that any maintenance payments embedded in the lease payment must be stripped out prior to checking this condition.

These rules, together with strong footnote disclosure rules for operating leases, are sufficient to insure that no one will be fooled by lease financing. In effect, a financial lease for a particular asset has the same economic consequences for the business as a loan in which the asset is pledged as collateral. Thus, leases are regarded as debt for capital structure purposes, and they have roughly the same effects as debt on the financial condition of the firm.

In closing, note that the rules that accountants follow in making the decision as to whether or not to capitalize a lease are not identical to the rules that the IRS follows to decide whether or not the lease is a guideline lease. In most cases, however, leases that meet IRS guidelines are operating leases that will not be capitalized, while leases that do not meet IRS guidelines are financial leases that will be capitalized. Remember, however, that even operating (noncapitalized) leases must be disclosed in the footnotes to the firm's financial statements.

Self-Test Questions
1. Why is lease financing sometimes called off-balance sheet financing?
2. How are leases accounted for in a business's financial statements?

Evaluation by the Lessee

Leases are evaluated by both the lessee and the lessor. The lessee must determine whether leasing an asset is less costly than obtaining equivalent alternative financing and buying the asset; and the lessor must decide what the lease payments must be to produce a rate of return consistent with the riskiness of the investment. This section focuses on the analysis by the lessee.

We should note that a degree of uncertainty exists regarding the theoretically correct way to evaluate lease-versus-purchase decisions, and some very complex decision models have been developed to aid in the analysis. However, the simple analysis given here, coupled with judgment, is sufficient to avoid situations where a lessee enters into a lease agreement that is clearly not in its best interests. In the typical case, the events leading to a lease arrangement follow the sequence described next.

- The business decides to acquire a particular building or piece of equipment; this decision is based on the standard capital budgeting procedures discussed in Chapters 12 and 13. The decision to acquire the asset is not at issue in the typical lease analysis; this decision was made previously as part of the capital budgeting process. In lease analysis, we are concerned simply with whether to obtain the use of the property by lease or by purchase.
- Once the business has decided to acquire the asset, the next question is how to finance its acquisition. A well-run business does not have excess cash lying around and, even if it does, there are opportunity costs associated with its use.
- Funds to purchase the asset could be obtained by borrowing, by retaining earnings, or, if the business is investor-owned, by selling new equity. If the firm is not-for-profit, perhaps the funds could be raised by soliciting contributions for the project. Or, some combination of these sources could be used. Alternatively, the asset could be leased. Because of the capitalization/disclosure provisions for leases, leasing is assumed to have the same impact on a firm's financial condition as debt financing (borrowing).

As indicated earlier, a lease is comparable to a loan in the sense that the business is required to make a specified series of payments, and that failure to meet these payments could result in bankruptcy. Thus, the most appropriate comparison when making lease decisions is the cost of lease financing versus the cost of debt financing, **regardless of how the asset actually would be financed if it were not leased.** The asset may be purchased with available cash if not leased or financed by a new equity sale or a cash contribution; but because leasing is a substitute for debt financing, the appropriate comparison would still be to debt financing.

To illustrate the basic elements of lease analysis, consider this simplified example. Nashville Radiology Group (the Group) requires the use of a piece of diagnostic equipment for two years that costs $100, and the Group must choose between leasing and buying the machine. (The actual cost is $100,000, but let's keep the numbers simple.) If the machine is purchased, the bank would lend the Group the needed $100 at a rate of 10 percent on a two-year, simple interest loan. Thus, the Group would have to pay the bank $10 in interest at the end of each year, plus return the $100 in principal at the end of Year 2. For simplicity, assume that the Group could depreciate the entire cost of the machine over two years for tax purposes by the straight-line method if it were purchased, resulting in tax depreciation of $50 in each year. Furthermore, the Group's tax rate is 40 percent. Thus, the depreciation expense produces a tax savings, or *tax shield*, of $50 × 0.40 = $20 in each year. Also for simplicity, assume the machine's value at the end of two years (its residual value) is estimated to be $0.

Alternatively, the Group could lease the asset under a guideline lease for two years for a payment of $55 at the end of each year. The analysis for the lease-versus-buy decision consists of (1) estimating the cash flows associated with borrowing and buying the asset—that is, the flows associated with debt financing; (2) estimating the cash flows associated with leasing the asset; and (3) comparing the two financing methods to determine which has the lower cost. Here are the borrow-and-buy flows:

Cash Flows if the Group Buys	Year 0	Year 1	Year 2
Equipment cost	($100)		
Loan amount	100		
Interest expense		($10)	($ 10)
Tax savings from interest		4	4
Principal repayment			(100)
Tax savings from depreciation		20	20
Net cash flow	$ 0	$14	($ 86)

The net cash flow is zero in Year 0, positive in Year 1, and negative in Year 2. Because the operating cash flows (the revenues and operating costs) will be the same regardless of whether the machine is leased or purchased, they can be ignored. Cash flows that are not affected by the decision at hand are said to be *nonincremental* to the decision.

Here are the cash flows associated with the lease:

Cash Flows if the Group Leases	Year 0	Year 1	Year 2
Lease payment		($55)	($55)
Tax savings from payments		22	22
Net cash flow	$0	($33)	($33)

Note that the two sets of cash flows reflect the tax savings associated with interest expense, depreciation, and lease payments, as appropriate. If the lease had not met IRS guidelines, then ownership would effectively reside with the lessee, and the Group would depreciate the asset for tax purposes whether it was "leased" or purchased. Furthermore, only the implied interest portion of the lease payment would be tax deductible. Thus, the analysis for a nonguideline lease would consist of simply comparing the after-tax financing flows on the loan with the after-tax lease-payment stream.

To compare the cost streams of buying and leasing, we must put them on a present value basis. As we explain later, the correct discount rate is the after-tax cost of debt, which for the Group is $10\% \times (1-T) = 10\% \times (1-0.4) = 6.0\%$. Applying this rate, we find the present value cost of buying to be $63.33, and the present value cost of leasing to be $60.50. Because leasing has the lower present value of costs, it is the less-costly financing alternative, and the Group should lease the asset.

This simplified example shows the general approach used in lease analysis, and it also illustrates a concept that can simplify the cash flow estimation process. Look back at the loan-related cash flows if the Group buys the machine. The after-tax loan-related flows are −$6 in Year 1 and −$106 in Year 2. When these flows are discounted to Year 0 at the 6.0 percent after-tax cost of debt, their present value is −$100, which is the negative of the loan amount shown in Year 0. This equality results because we first used the cost of debt to estimate the future financing flows, and we then used this same rate to discount the flows back to Year 0, all on an after-tax basis. In effect, the loan amount positive cash flow and the loan cost negative cash flows cancel one another out. Here is the cash flow stream associated with buying the asset after the Year 0 loan amount and the related Year 1 and Year 2 flows have been removed:

Cash Flows if the Group Buys	Year 0	Year 1	Year 2
Cost of asset	($100)		
Tax savings from depreciation		$20	$20
Net cash flow	($100)	$20	$20

The present value cost of buying here is, of course, $63.33, which is the same number we found earlier. The consistency between the two approaches will always occur regardless of the specific terms of the debt financing—as long as the discount rate is the after-tax cost of debt, the cash flows associated with the loan can be ignored.

To examine a more realistic example of lease analysis, consider the following lease-versus-buy decision facing the Nashville Radiology Group:

- The Group plans to acquire a new computer system that will automate the Group's clinical records as well as its accounting, billing, and collection process. The computer has an economic life of eight years and costs $200,000, delivered and installed. However, the Group plans to lease the equipment for only four years because it believes that computer technology is changing rapidly, and it wants the opportunity to reevaluate the situation at that time.
- The Group can borrow the required $200,000 from its bank at a before-tax cost of 10 percent.
- The computer's estimated scrap value is $5,000 after eight years of use; but its estimated residual value when the lease expires after four years of use is

$20,000. Thus, if the Group buys the equipment, it would expect to receive $20,000 before taxes when the equipment is sold in four years.

- The Group can lease the equipment for four years at a rental charge of $57,000, payable at the beginning of each year; but the lessor will own the equipment upon the expiration of the lease. (The lease payment schedule is established by the potential lessor, as described in a later section, and the Group can accept it, reject it, or negotiate.)
- The lease contract stipulates that the lessor will maintain the computer at no additional charge to the Group. However, if the Group borrows and buys the computer, it will have to bear the cost of maintenance, which would be performed by the equipment manufacturer at a fixed contract rate of $2,500 per year, payable at the beginning of each year.
- The computer falls in the MACRS five-year class life, the group's marginal tax rate is 40 percent, and the lease qualifies as a guideline lease under a special IRS ruling. (Refer to Chapter 2 to review tax depreciation if necessary.)

Dollar Cost Analysis

Table 9.2 shows the steps involved in a complete dollar cost analysis. Again, our approach here is to compare the cost of owning (borrowing and buying) the computer to the cost of leasing the computer. All else the same, the lower cost alternative is preferable. Part I of the table is devoted to the costs of borrowing and buying. Here, Line 1 gives the equipment's cost and Line 2 shows the maintenance expense; both are cash costs, or outflows. Note that whenever an analyst is setting up cash flows on a time line, one of the first decisions to be made is what time interval will be used—that is, months, quarters, years, or some other period. As a starting point, we generally assume that all cash flows occur at the end of each year. If, at some point later in the analysis, we conclude that another interval is better, we will change. Longer intervals, such as years, simplify the analysis, but introduce some inaccuracies because all cash flows do not actually occur at year end. For example, tax benefits occur quarterly because businesses pay taxes on a quarterly basis. On the other hand, shorter intervals, such as months, often are used for lease analyses because lease payments typically occur monthly. For ease of illustration, we are using annual flows in this example.

Line 3 gives the maintenance tax savings, and because maintenance expense is tax deductible, the Group saves $0.40 \times \$2,500 = \$1,000$ in taxes by virtue of paying the maintenance fee. Line 4 contains the depreciation tax savings, which is the depreciation expense times the tax rate. For example, the MACRS allowance for the first year is 20 percent, so the depreciation expense is $0.20 \times \$200,000 = \$40,000$ and the depreciation tax savings is $0.40 \times \$20,000 = \$16,000$.

Lines 5 and 6 contain the residual value cash flows: the residual value is estimated to be $20,000, but the tax book value after four years of depreciation

TABLE
9.2
Lessee's
Dollar
Cost
Analysis

	Year 0	Year 1	Year 2	Year 3	Year 4
I. Cost of Owning (Borrowing and Buying)					
1. Net purchase price	($200,000)				
2. Maintenance cost	(2,500)	($ 2,500)	($ 2,500)	($ 2,500)	
3. Maintenance tax savings	1,000	1,000	1,000	1,000	
4. Depreciation tax savings		16,000	25,600	15,200	$ 9,600
5. Residual value					20,000
6. Residual value tax					5,600
7. Net cash flow	($201,500)	$ 14,500	$ 24,100	$ 13,700	$ 35,200
8. PV cost of owning =	($126,987)				
II. Cost of Leasing					
9. Lease payment	($ 57,000)	($ 57,000)	($ 57,000)	($ 57,000)	
10. Tax savings	22,800	22,800	22,800	22,800	
11. Net cash flow	($ 34,200)	($ 34,200)	($ 34,200)	($ 34,200)	$ 0
12. PV cost of leasing =	($ 125,617)				
III. Cost Comparison					
13. Net advantage to leasing (NAL)	= PV cost of leasing − PV cost of owning				
	= −$125,617 − (−$126,987) = $1,370.				

Notes:
a. The MACRS depreciation allowances are 0.20, 0.32, 0.19, and 0.12 in Years 1 through 4, respectively.
b. In practice, a lease analysis, such as this, would be done on a monthly basis using a spreadsheet program.

is $34,000. Thus, the Group is losing $14,000 for tax purposes, which results in the $0.4 \times \$14,000 = \$5,600$ tax savings shown as an inflow on Line 6. Line 7, which sums the component cash flows, contains the net cash flows associated with borrowing and buying.

Part II of Table 9.2 contains an analysis of the cost of leasing. The lease payments, shown on Line 9, are $57,000 per year; this rate, which includes maintenance, was established by the prospective lessor and offered to the Group. If the Group accepts the lease, the full amount will be a deductible expense, so the tax savings, shown on Line 10, is $0.40 \times$ Lease payment $= 0.40 \times \$57,000 = \$22,800$. The net cash flows associated with leasing are shown on Line 11.

The final step is to compare the net cost of owning with the net cost of leasing. However, we must first put the annual cash flows associated with owning and leasing on a common basis. This requires converting them to present values, which brings up the question of the proper rate at which to discount the net cash flows. We know that the riskier the cash flows, the higher will be the discount rate used to find the present value. This same principle was observed in our discussion of security valuation, and it applies to all discounted cash flow analyses, including lease analysis. Just how risky are the cash flows under consideration here? Most of them are relatively certain, at least when compared with the types of cash flow estimates associated with stock investments or with the Group's operating cash flows. For example, the loan payment schedule is set by contract, as is the lease payment schedule. The depreciation expenses are also established by law and not subject to change, and the annual maintenance fee is fixed by contract as well. The tax savings are somewhat uncertain, but they will be as projected as long as the Group's marginal tax rate remains at 40 percent. The residual value is the least certain of the cash flows; but, even here, the Group's management is fairly confident because the estimated residual value distribution is relatively tight.

Because the cash flows under the lease and under the borrow-and-purchase alternatives are both relatively certain, they should be discounted at a relatively low rate. Most analysts recommend that the firm's cost of debt financing be used, and this rate seems reasonable in our example. However, the Group's cost of debt—10 percent—must be adjusted to reflect the tax deductibility of interest payments because this benefit of borrowing and buying is not accounted for in the cash flows. Thus, the Group's effective cost of debt becomes Before-tax cost × (1 − Tax rate) = 10% × 0.6 = 6.0%. Accordingly, the cash flows in Lines 7 and 11 are discounted at a 6.0 percent rate. The resulting present values are $126,987 for the cost of owning and $125,617 for the cost of leasing, as shown on Lines 8 and 12. Leasing is the lower cost-financing alternative, so the Group should lease, rather than buy, the computer.

The cost comparison can be formalized by defining the *net advantage to leasing (NAL)* as follows:

$$\text{NAL} = \text{PV cost of leasing} - \text{PV cost of owning}$$

$$= -\$125,617 - (-\$126,987) = \$1,370.$$

The positive NAL shows that leasing creates more value than buying, so the Group should lease the equipment. Indeed, the value of the Group is increased by $1,370 if it leases, rather than buys, the computer.

Percentage Cost Analysis

The Group's lease-versus-buy decision can also be analyzed by looking at the effective cost rate on the lease and comparing it to the effective cost rate on the loan. Here, we know the after-tax cost of debt—6.0 percent—so we must find the after-tax cost rate implied in the lease contract and compare it with the cost of the loan. Signing a lease is similar to signing a loan contract—the firm has the use of equipment, but must make a series of payments under either type of contract. We know the cost rate built into the loan: It is 6.0 percent interest rate. If the after-tax cost rate in the lease is less than 6.0 percent, then there is an advantage to leasing.

Table 9.3 sets forth the cash flows needed to determine the percentage cost of the lease. Here is an explanation of the table:

- The first step is to calculate the lease-versus-owning cash flows. To calculate, we merely subtract the owning cash flows, Line 7 from Table 9.2, from the leasing cash flows shown on Line 11. The differences are the incremental cash flows that the Group would obtain if it leases rather than buys the computer.
- Note that Table 9.3 consolidates the analysis shown in Table 9.2 into a single set of cash flows. At this point, we can discount the consolidated cash flows shown on Line 3 by 6.0 percent to obtain the NAL, $1,370. In Table 9.2, we discounted the owning and leasing cash flows separately, and then subtracted their present values to obtain the NAL. In Table 9.3, we subtracted the cash flows first to obtain a single set of flows, and then found their present value. The end result is the same.
- The consolidated cash flows provide a good insight into the economics of leasing. If the Group leases the computer, it avoids the Year 0 cash outlay required to buy the equipment; but it is then obligated to a series of cash outflows for four years.
- By inputting the leasing-versus-owning cash flows listed in Table 9.3 into the cash flow registers of a calculator and solving for IRR, or by using a spreadsheet's IRR function, we can find the cost rate inherent in the cash flow stream: It is 5.6 percent. This is the equivalent after-tax cost rate implied in the lease contract. Because this cost rate is less than the 6.0 percent after-tax cost of a regular loan, leasing is cheaper than borrowing and buying. Thus, the percentage cost analysis confirms the NAL analysis.

Some Additional Points

So far, we have discussed the main features of a lessee's analysis. However, before we move on to the lessor, note the following points:

- The dollar cost and percentage cost approaches will always lead to the same decision. Thus, one method is as good as the other from a decision standpoint.
- If the net residual value cash flow (residual value and tax effect) is considered to be riskier than the other cash flows in the analysis, it is possible to account for this differential risk by applying a higher discount

TABLE 9.3 Lessee's Percentage Cost Analysis

	Year 0	Year 1	Year 2	Year 3	Year 4
1. Leasing cash flow	($ 34,200)	($34,200)	($34,200)	($34,200)	$ 0
2. Less: Owning cash flow	(201,500)	14,500	24,100	13,700	35,200
3. Leasing-versus-owning CF	$167,300	($48,700)	($58,300)	($47,900)	($35,200)

NAL = $1,370.
IRR = 5.6%.

rate to this flow, which results in a lower present value. Because the net residual value flow is an inflow in the cost of owning analysis, a lower present value leads to a higher present value cost of owning. Thus, increasing residual value risk decreases the attractiveness of owning an asset. To illustrate the concept, assume that the Group's managers believe that the computer's residual value is much riskier than the other flows in Table 9.2. Furthermore, they believe that 10.0 percent, rather than 6.0 percent, is the appropriate discount rate to apply to the residual value flows. When the Table 9.2 analysis is modified to reflect this risk, the present value cost of owning increases to $129,780, while the NAL increases to $4,163. The riskier the residual value, all else the same, the more favorable leasing becomes, because residual value risk is borne by the lessor.

• As we will discuss in Chapter 12, net present value (NPV) is the dollar value of a project, assuming that it is financed using debt and equity financing. In lease analysis, the NAL is the additional dollar value of a project attributable to leasing, as opposed to conventional financing. Thus, as an approximation of the value of a leased asset to the firm, the project's NPV can be increased by the amount of NAL:

$$\text{Adjusted NPV} = \text{NPV} + \text{NAL}.$$

The value added through leasing, in some cases, can turn unprofitable (negative NPV) projects into profitable (positive adjusted NPV) projects.

Self-Test Questions

1. Explain how the cash flows are structured in conducting a dollar-based (NAL) analysis.
2. What discount rate should be used when lessees perform lease analyses?
3. What is the economic interpretation of the net advantage to leasing?
4. What is the economic interpretation of a lease's IRR?

Evaluation by the Lessor

Thus far, we have considered lease analysis from the lessee's viewpoint. It is also useful to analyze the transaction as the lessor sees it: Is the lease a good investment for the party that *writes* the lease (i.e., the party that must put up the money to buy the asset)? The lessor will generally be a specialized leasing firm, a bank or bank affiliate, or a manufacturer, such as General Electric Medical Systems, that uses leasing as a marketing tool.

Any potential lessor needs to know the rate of return on the capital invested in the lease, and this information is also useful to the prospective lessee because lease terms on large leases are generally negotiated; so, the lessor and the lessee should know one another's position. The lessor's analysis involves (1) determining the net cash outlay, which is usually the invoice price of the leased equipment less any lease payments made in advance; (2) determining the periodic cash inflows, which consist of the lease payments minus both income taxes and any maintenance expenses the lessor must bear; (3) estimating the after-tax residual value of the property when the lease expires; and (4) determining whether the rate of return on the lease is adequate for the risk of the investment.

To illustrate the lessor's analysis, we assume the same facts as for the Nashville Radiology Group lease as well as this situation: (1) The potential lessor is Medicomp, Inc., a commercial leasing company that specializes in leasing computers to healthcare providers. Medicomp's marginal federal-plus-state tax rate is 40 percent. (2) To provide maintenance to the Group, Medicomp must contract with the computer manufacturer under the same terms available to the Group—that is, $2,500 at the beginning of each year. (3) Medicomp views computer lease arrangements as relatively low risk investments. There is, however, some small chance of default on the lease, so Medicomp typically assumes that a lease investment is about as risky as buying AA-rated corporate bonds. Because four-year, AA-rated bonds are yielding about 9 percent, Medicomp could earn an after-tax yield of $9.0\% \times (1 - T) = 9.0\% \times 0.6 = 5.4\%$ on such investments. This is the after-tax return that Medicomp can obtain on alternative investments of similar risk.

The lease analysis from the lessor's standpoint is developed in Table 9.4. Here, we see that the cash flows to the lessor are similar to those for the lessee shown in Table 9.2. Line 1 contains the purchase price of the computer—$200,000. Line 2 contains the maintenance costs, while Line 3 lists the tax savings attributable to these costs. Line 4 contains the depreciation tax savings, or tax shields, that accrue to the owner of the computer. On Line 5, we show the annual lease rental payment as an inflow, while the taxes that must be paid on the rental payments are shown in Line 6. Lines 7 and 8 contain the residual value and resulting taxes (tax savings in this case). Finally, the cash flows are summed in Line 9.

The net present value (NPV) of the lease to Medicomp can be easily found by discounting the Line 9 cash flows at the firm's after-tax opportunity cost of capital—5.4 percent—and then summing the resultant present values. For Medicomp, the NPV of the lease investment is $815, which means that the firm is somewhat better off, on a present value basis, if it writes the lease rather than invests in comparable-risk AA-rated bonds. Conversely, if the NPV of the lease were negative, Medicomp would be better off investing in the bonds. Because we saw earlier that the lease is also advantageous to the Group, the transaction is beneficial to both the lessee and lessor.

We can also calculate Medicomp's expected percentage rate of return on the lease by finding the IRR of the net cash flows shown on Line 9 of Table 9.4. Simply use the IRR function on a financial calculator or spreadsheet. The answer is 5.6 percent. Thus, the lease provides a 5.6 after-tax return to Medicomp, which exceeds the 5.4 percent after-tax return available on alternative investments of similar risk, AA-rated, four-year bonds. So, using either the dollar-rate-of-return (NPV) method or the percentage-rate-of-

TABLE 9.4
Lessor's
Analysis

	Year 0	Year 1	Year 2	Year 3	Year 4
1. Net purchase price	($200,000)				
2. Maintenance cost	(2,500)	($ 2,500)	($ 2,500)	($ 2,500)	
3. Maintenance tax savings	1,000	1,000	1,000	1,000	
4. Depreciation tax savings		16,000	25,600	15,200	$ 9,600
5. Lease payment	57,000	57,000	57,000	57,000	
6. Tax on lease payment	(22,800)	(22,800)	(22,800)	(22,800)	
7. Residual value					20,000
8. Tax on residual value					5,600
9. Net cash flow	($167,300)	$48,700	$58,300	$47,900	$35,200

NPV = $815.
IRR = 5.6%.

return (IRR) method gives us the same result: The lease appears to be a satisfactory investment for Medicomp.

Note, however, that the lease investment is actually slightly more risky than the alternative bond investment because the residual value cash flow is less certain than a principal repayment. Thus, Medicomp would probably require a rate of return somewhat above the 5.4 percent promised on the bond investment; and the higher the risk of the residual value, the higher the required return. Also, note that the lessor's NPV analysis could be extended by using a higher discount rate on the residual value cash flows than used on the other flows. This would lower the NPV, and hence make the lease investment look less attractive vis-a-vis the bond investment.

Self-Test Questions
1. What discount rate is used in a lessor's NPV analysis?
2. What is the economic interpretation of the lessor's NPV? The lessor's IRR?

Lease Analysis Symmetry

Stop for a moment and compare the cash flows in Tables 9.3 and 9.4. Upon examination, we find that the cash flows to the lessee and lessor are symmetrical. They differ in sign, but their values are the same. This symmetry occurs because there are only two parties to a lease transaction, and our example assumed that the parties would pay the same amount for the computer, paid taxes at the same rate, forecasted the same residual value, and so on. Thus, a cash inflow to one party becomes a cash outflow to the other. Taken one step further, if the cost of debt to the lessee in our example had equaled the opportunity cost to the lessor, then the NAL to the lessee would be equal, but opposite in sign, to the lessor's NPV.

The conclusion of this simple observation is that when there is symmetry between the lessor and the lessee—same tax rates, costs, and so on—leasing is a *zero-sum game*.[4] If the lease is attractive to the lessee, the lease is unattractive to the lessor, and vice versa. However, conditions often are such that leasing can be of benefit to both parties. This situation arises because of asymmetries, generally in taxes, estimated residual values, or the ability to bear residual value risk. We will explore this issue in detail in a later section.

1. What is "lease analysis symmetry"?

2. What impact does this symmetry have on the economic viability of leasing?

Self-Test Questions

Setting the Lease Payment

In the preceding sections, we evaluated the lease assuming that the lease payments had already been specified. However, as a general rule, in large leases, the parties will sit down and work out the terms of the lease, including the size of the lease payments. In situations where the lease terms are not negotiable, which is often the case for small leases, the lessor must still go through the same type of analysis, setting terms, which provide a target rate of return, and then offering these terms to the potential lessee on a take-it-or-leave-it basis.

Competition in the leasing industry will force lessors to build market-related returns into their lease payment schedules. To illustrate all this, suppose Medicomp, after examining other alternative investment opportunities, decides that the 5.4 percent return on the Nashville Radiology Group lease is too low, and that the lease should provide an after-tax return of 6.0 percent. What lease payment schedule would provide this return?

To answer this question, note again that Table 9.4 contains the lessor's cash flow analysis. If the basic analysis is computerized, it is very easy to change the lease payment until the lease's NPV = $0 at a 6.0 percent discount rate or, equivalently, its IRR = 6.0 percent. We did this with our spreadsheet lease evaluation model, and we found that the lessor must set the lease payment at $57,622 to obtain an expected after-tax rate of return of 6.0 percent. However, if this lease payment is not acceptable to the Group, then it may not be possible to strike a deal.

1. How do lessors set the lease payment amount?

Self-Test Question

Leveraged Leases

In the early days of lease transactions, only two parties were involved: (1) the lessor, who put up the front money; and (2) the lessee, who used the asset. In recent years, however, a new type of lease—the *leveraged lease*—has come into widespread use. Under a leveraged lease, the lessor arranges to borrow all or part of the required funds, generally giving the lender a lien on the property being leased, or a first mortgage if the lease is for real estate. The lessor still receives the tax benefits associated with depreciation. However, the lessor now has a riskier position because of its use of debt financing. Incidentally, whether or not a lease is leveraged is not important to the lessee; from the lessee's standpoint, the method of analyzing a proposed lease is unaffected by whether or not the lessor borrows part of the required capital.

The analysis in Table 9.4 can be easily modified if the lessor borrows all or part of the required $200,000, making the transaction a leveraged lease. First, we would add a set of lines to Table 9.4 to show the financing cash flows. The interest component would represent another tax deduction, while the loan repayment would constitute an additional cash outlay. The "initial cost" would be reduced by the amount of the loan. With these changes made, a new NPV and IRR could be calculated and used to evaluate whether or not the lease represents a good investment.

To illustrate the concept, assume that Medicomp can borrow $100,000 of the $200,000 purchase price at a rate of 9 percent on a four-year, simple interest loan. Table 9.5 contains the lessor's leveraged lease analysis. Line 1 contains the unleveraged lease cash flows from Table 9.4, while the leveraging cash flows are shown on Lines 2 through 5. The net cash flows to Medicomp are shown on Line 6. The NPV of the leveraged lease is $815, which is the same as for the unleveraged lease.[5] Note, though, that the lessor has a net investment of only $67,300 on the leveraged lease compared to a net investment of $167,300 on the unleveraged lease. Therefore, the lessor could invest in a total of $167,300/$67,300 = 2.5 identical leveraged leases for the same $167,300 investment required to finance a single unleveraged lease, producing a total net present value of 2.5 × $815 = $2,038. The effect of leverage on the lessor's return is also reflected in the leveraged lease's IRR. The IRR of the leveraged lease is 9.1 percent, which is substantially higher than the 5.6 percent after-tax return on the unleveraged lease.

Typically, leveraged leases provide lessors with higher expected rates of return (IRRs) and higher NPVs per dollar of invested capital than unleveraged

TABLE 9.5
Leveraged
Lease Analysis

	Year 0	Year 1	Year 2	Year 3	Year 4
1. Unleveraged cash flow	($167,300)	$48,700	$58,300	$47,900	$35,200
2. Loan amount	100,000				
3. Interest	(9,000)		(9,000)	(9,000)	(9,000)
4. Interest tax savings		3,600	3,600	3,600	3,600
5. Principal repayment					(100,000)
6. Net cash flow	($ 67,300)	$43,300	$52,900	$42,500	($70,200)

NPV = $815.
IRR = 9.1%.

leases. However, such leases are also riskier for the same reason that any leveraged investment is riskier. Sophisticated lessors use simulations similar to those described in Chapter 13 to assess the riskiness associated with leveraged leases. Then, given the apparent riskiness of the lease investment, the lessor can decide whether the returns built into the contract are sufficient to compensate for the risks involved.

1. What is a leveraged lease?
2. How does leveraging affect the lessee's analysis?
3. What is the usual impact of lease leveraging on the lessor's expected rate of return and risk?

Self-Test Questions

Motivations for Leasing

We noted earlier that leasing is a zero-sum game unless there are differentials between the lessee and the lessor. In this section, we discuss some of the differentials that motivate lease agreements.

Tax Differentials

Many leases are driven by tax differentials. Historically, the typical tax asymmetry arose between highly taxed lessors and lessees with sufficient tax shields (primarily depreciation) to drive their tax rates very low, even to zero. In these situations, the asset's depreciation tax benefits could be taken by the lessor, and then this value is shared with the lessee. However, many other possible tax motivations exist including tax differentials between not-for-profit providers and investor-owned lessors as well as the alternative minimum tax, which we discuss next.

Taxable corporations are permitted to use accelerated depreciation and other tax shelters to reduce taxable income, but then to use straight-line depreciation for stockholder reporting, and hence to report higher profits to shareholders than to the IRS. Thus, under the normal procedure for determining federal income taxes, many very profitable businesses pay little or no federal income taxes. The *alternative minimum tax (AMT)*, which roughly amounts to 24 percent of profits as **reported to shareholders**, is designed to force profitable firms to pay at least some taxes.

Those firms that are exposed to heavy tax liabilities under the AMT naturally seek ways to reduce reported income. Leasing can be beneficial here—because firms can use a relatively short period for the lease and consequently have a high annual payment, resulting in lower reported profits and a lower AMT liability. Note that the lease payments do not have to qualify as a deductible expense for regular tax purposes; all that is needed is that they reduce reported income shown on a firm's income statement.

Lessors have designed spreadsheet models to deal with AMT considerations, and they are generating a substantial amount of leasing business as a direct result of the alternative minimum tax. Thus, one of the important motivations for leasing is tax differentials.

Ability to Bear Obsolescence (Residual Value) Risk

Leasing is an attractive financing alternative for many high-tech items that are subject to rapid and unpredictable technological obsolescence. For example, assume that a small, rural hospital wants to acquire a magnetic resonance imaging (MRI) device. If it buys the MRI equipment, it is exposed to the risk of technological obsolescence. In a relatively short time, some new technology might be developed which makes the current system almost worthless, and this large economic depreciation could create a severe financial burden on the hospital. Because it does not use much equipment of this nature, the hospital would bear a great deal of risk if it buys the MRI device.

Conversely, a lessor that specializes in state-of-the-art medical equipment might be exposed to significantly less risk. By purchasing and then leasing many different high-tech items, the lessor benefits from portfolio diversification; over time, some items will lose more value than the lessor expected, but these losses will be offset by other items that retain more value than expected. Also, because lessors are especially familiar with the markets for used medical equipment, they can both estimate residual values better and negotiate better prices when the asset is resold than can a hospital. Because the lessor is better able to bear residual value risk than the hospital, the lessor could charge a premium for bearing this risk that is less than the premium inherent in ownership.

Some lessors also offer programs that guarantee that the leased asset is modified as necessary to keep it abreast of technological advancements. For an increased rental fee, lessors will provide upgrades to keep the leased equipment current regardless of the cost. To the extent that lessors are better able to forecast such upgrades; negotiate better terms from manufacturers; and, by greater diversification, control the risks involved with such upgrades, it may be cheaper for lessees to ensure state-of-the art equipment by leasing than by buying.

Ability to Bear Utilization Risk

A type of lease that is gaining popularity among healthcare providers is the *per procedure lease*. In this type of lease, instead of a fixed annual or monthly payment, the lessor charges the lessee a fixed amount for each procedure performed. For example, the lessor may charge the hospital $300 for every scan performed using a leased MRI device. Or it may charge $400 per scan for the first 100 scans in each month and $200 for each scan above 100. Because the hospital's reimbursement for MRI scans often depends on the amount of utilization, and because the per procedure lease changes the hospital's costs for the MRI from a fixed payment to a variable payment, the hospital's risk is reduced.

However, the conversion of the payment to the lessor from a known amount to an uncertain stream increases the lessor's risk. Although the passing of risk often produces no net benefit, a per procedure lease can be beneficial to both parties if the lessor is better able to bear the utilization risk than is the lessee. As before, if the lessor has written a large number of per procedure leases, then some of the leases will be more profitable than expected and some will be less profitable than expected, but if the lessor's expectations are unbiased, the aggregate return on all the leases will be quite close to that expected.

Ability to Bear Project Life Risk

Leasing can also be attractive when a business is uncertain about how long an asset will be needed. To illustrate the concept, consider the following example. Hospitals sometimes offer services that are dependent on a single staff member—for example, a physician who does liver transplants. To support the physician's practice, the hospital might have to invest millions of dollars in equipment that can be used only for this particular procedure. The hospital will charge for the use of the equipment, and if things go as expected, the investment will be profitable. However, if the physician dies or leaves the hospital staff, and if no other qualified physician can be recruited to fill the void, then the project is dead and the equipment becomes useless to the hospital. In this situation, the annual usage may be quite predictable; but the need for the asset could suddenly cease. A lease with a cancellation clause would permit the hospital to simply return the equipment to the lessor. The lessor would charge something for the cancellation clause because such clauses increase the riskiness of the lease to the lessor. The increased lease cost would lower the expected profitability of the project, but it would provide the hospital with an option to abandon the equipment, and such an option could have a value that exceeds the incremental cost of the cancellation clause. The leasing company would be willing to write this option because it is in a better position to remarket the equipment, either by writing another lease or by selling it outright.

Maintenance Services

Some businesses find leasing attractive because the lessor is able to provide maintenance services on favorable terms. For example, MEDTRANS, Inc., a for-profit ambulance and medical transfer service that operates in Pennsylvania, recently leased 25 ambulances and transfer vans. The lease agreement, with a lessor that specializes in purchasing, maintaining, and then reselling automobiles and trucks, permitted the replacement of an aging fleet that MEDTRANS had built up over seven years. "We are pretty good at providing emergency services and moving sick people from one facility to another, but we aren't very good at maintaining an automotive fleet," said MED-TRANS's CEO.

Lower Information Costs

Leasing may be financially attractive for smaller businesses that have limited access to debt markets. For example, a small, recently formed physician group practice may need to finance one or more diagnostic devices such as an EKG machine. The group has no credit history, so it would be relatively difficult, and hence costly, for a bank to assess the group's credit risk. Some banks might think the loan is not even worth the effort. Others might be willing to make the loan, but only after building the high cost of credit assessment into the cost of the loan. On the other hand, some lessors specialize in leasing to group practices, so their analysts have assessed the financial worthiness of hundreds, or even thousands, of group practices. Thus, it would be relatively easy for them to make the credit judgment, and hence they might be more willing to provide the financing, and charge lower rates, than conventional lenders.

Lower Risk in Bankruptcy

Finally, leasing may be less expensive than buying to firms that are poor credit risks. As discussed earlier, in the event of financial distress leading to reorganization or liquidation, lessors generally have more secure claims than do lenders. Thus, lessors may be willing to write leases to firms with poor financial characteristics, which are less costly than loans offered by lenders, if such loans are even available.

There are other reasons that might motivate firms to lease an asset rather than buy it. Often, these reasons are difficult to quantify, so they cannot be easily incorporated into a numerical analysis. Nevertheless, a sound lease analysis must begin with a quantitative analysis, and then qualitative factors can be considered before making the final lease-or-buy decision.

Self-Test Questions

1. What are some economic factors that motivate leasing; that is, what asymmetries might exist that make leasing beneficial to both lessors and lessees?
2. Would it ever make sense to lease an asset that has a negative NAL when evaluated by a conventional lease analysis? Explain.

Additional Issues

Before we close our discussion of leasing, we present some additional issues associated with leasing that warrant discussion.

Residual Value Levels

It is important to note that the lessor owns the property upon expiration of a lease, so the lessor has claim to the asset's residual value. Superficially, it would appear that if residual values were expected to be large, owning would have an advantage over leasing. However, this apparent advantage is usually eliminated by market forces. If expected residual values are large, as they may be under inflation for certain types of equipment and also if real estate is involved, competition among leasing firms will force lease rental rates down to the point where potential residual values are fully recognized in the lease payment. Thus, the existence of large residual values is not likely to create a bias in favor of owning.

Credit Availability

There are those who argue that leasing has an advantage for businesses that are seeking the maximum degree of financial leverage. First, it is sometimes argued that firms can obtain more money, and for longer terms, under a lease arrangement than under a loan secured by a specific piece of property. Second, because some leases do not appear on the balance sheet, lease financing has been said to give the business a stronger appearance in a *superficial* credit analysis, and thus it permits the firm to use more, or cheaper, debt financing than would otherwise be possible.

As discussed previously, there may be some truth to these claims for smaller businesses or for businesses facing financial distress. However, because businesses are required to capitalize financial leases and to report them on their balance sheets, and to disclose operating leases in the footnotes to the financial statements, this point is of questionable validity for any financially sound business large enough to have audited financial statements.

Liquidity Preservation

Most of the promotional material prepared by lessors states that the biggest advantage of leasing is that it preserves liquidity; that is, by leasing, a business avoids using cash resources to make the initial outlay required to purchase the asset. Although the statement is true, it ignores the fact that the lessee becomes contractually obligated to make a series of payments to the lessor. The alternative to leasing—borrowing and buying—also avoids using current cash to buy the asset because the loan amount is used to make the purchase. Under the borrow-and-buy scenario, the potential lessee again is obligated to make a series of payments, but this time to the lender. When one carefully considers the situation, it is obvious that leasing is advantageous only when it costs less than borrowing and buying.

Computer Models

Lease analysis is particularly well suited for computer analysis. Both the lessee and lessor can create computer models for their analyses. Setting the analysis up on a computer is especially useful when negotiations are under way. When investment banking houses, such as Merrill Lynch, are working out a leasing deal between a group of investors and a firm, the analysis is always computerized.

1. Does leasing lead to increased credit availability?
2. Do larger residual values favor owning over leasing? Explain.

Self-Test Questions

3. What is your reaction to this statement: "Leasing is preferable to buying because it preserves the business's liquidity."

Key Concepts

In this chapter, we discussed the leasing decision from the standpoints of both the lessee and lessor. Here are its key concepts:

- Lease agreements often are categorized as (1) *operating leases*; (2) *financial*, or *capital*, *leases*; and (3) *combination leases*.
- The IRS has specific guidelines that apply to lease arrangements. A lease that meets these guidelines is called a *guideline*, or *tax-oriented*, *lease* because the IRS permits the lessee to deduct the lease payments. A lease that does not meet IRS guidelines is called a *non-tax-oriented lease*. In such leases, ownership effectively resides with the lessee rather than the lessor.
- *FASB Statement 13* spells out the conditions under which a lease must be *capitalized* (shown directly on the balance sheet), as opposed to being shown only in the notes to the financial statements. Generally, leases that run for a period equal to or greater than 75 percent of the asset's life must be capitalized.
- The lessee's analysis consists of a comparison of the costs and benefits associated with leasing the asset and the costs and benefits associated with owning the asset. There are two analytical techniques that can be used: (1) the *dollar-cost (NAL) method* and (2) the *percentage-cost (IRR) method*.
- One of the key issues in the lessee's analysis is the appropriate discount rate. Because the cash flows in a lease analysis are known with relative certainty, the appropriate discount rate is the *lessee's after-tax cost of debt*. A higher discount rate may be used on the *residual value* if it is substantially riskier than the other flows.
- In a *lessor's analysis*, the return on a lease investment is compared with the return available on alternative investments of similar risk.
- In a *leveraged lease*, the lessor borrows part of the funds required to buy the asset. Generally, the asset is pledged as collateral for the loan.
- Leasing is motivated by differentials between lessees and lessors. Some of the more common reasons for leasing are (1) *tax rate differentials*, (2) *alternative minimum taxes*, (3) *residual risk bearing*, and (4) *lack of access* to conventional debt markets.

This chapter concludes our discussion of capital acquisition. In the next chapter, we begin our coverage of cost of capital and capital structure decisions.

Selected References

Beggan, John F., and Lauren K. McNulty. 1991. "Restrictions on Depreciation Where Tax-Exempt Entities are Involved." *Topics in Health Care Financing* (Fall): 62–69.

Berg, Ian J., and Alan N. Frankel. 1988. "Equipment Leasing: How, When, and If." *Health Progress* (November 15): 22–26.

Conbeer, George P. 1990. "Leasing Can Add Flexibility to High-Tech Asset Management." *Healthcare Financial Management* (July): 26–34.

Dine, Deborah Denaro. 1988. "Equipment Leasing Firms Offer Deals to Hospitals." *Modern Healthcare* (November 18): 50–51.

Grant, Larry and Diane O'Donnell. 1990. "Watch for Pitfalls When Analyzing Lease Options." *Healthcare Financial Management* (July): 36–43.

"Leasing: Three Experts Discuss the Advantages of Equipment Leasing." 1989. *HealthWeek* (November): 51–53.

Meyers, Stewart C., David A. Dill, and Alberto J. Bautista. 1976. "Valuation of Financial Lease Contracts." *Journal of Finance* (June): 799–819.

Rosenthal, Robert A. 1992. "Creative Leasing Strategies for Medical Office Buildings." *Healthcare Financial Management* (December): 30–34.

Selected Web Sites

To obtain information about leasing from the Equipment Leasing Association (an association of equipment lessors), see *www.leaseassistant.org*.

For one example of a leasing company web site, see the PMC Asset Corporation site at *www.financingfordocs.com*.

The following site contains a glossary of leasing terminology: *www.lease-one.com/glossary.htm*.

Although not directly related to healthcare equipment leasing, the following site has a wealth of information on automobile leases: *www.leasesource.com*.

Selected Cases

There is one case in *Cases in Healthcare Finance* that is applicable to this chapter:

Case 15: Texas Medical Center, which focuses on leasing decisions from the perspectives of both the lessee and lessor.

Notes

1. For more information about the motivating forces and extent of leasing in the hospital industry, see Louis C. Gapenski and Barbara Langland-Orban, "Leasing Capital Assets and Durable Goods: Opinions and Practices in Florida Hospitals," *Health Care Management Review*, Summer 1991, 73–81.

2. In fact, General Electric has a subsidiary, GE Capital Corporation, which is one of the largest lessors in the world. The subsidiary was originally set up to finance consumers' purchases of GE's durable goods, such as refrigerators and wash machines, but it has become a major player in the commercial loan and leasing markets.

3. Financial Accounting Standards Board (FASB) Statement 13, "Accounting for Leases," spells out in detail both the conditions under which the lease must be capitalized and the procedures for capitalizing it. FASB is the primary

organization that promulgates the rules that form the basis of generally accepted accounting principles (GAAP), which in turn guide the preparation of financial statements.

4. The zero-sum game feature of leasing can be useful in debugging lease analysis models. Whenever we build a new spreadsheet model that contains both lessee's and lessor's analyses, we test it by trying symmetrical input values for the lessee and lessor. If the lessee's NAL and lessor's NPV are not equal, but opposite in sign, there is something wrong with the model!

5. In this situation, leveraging had no impact on the lessor's per lease NPV. This result occurred because the cost of the loan to the lessor—5.4 percent after taxes—equals the discount rate, and thus the leveraging cash flows are netted out on a present value basis.

Cost of Capital and Capital Structure

COST OF CAPITAL

Learning Objectives

After studying this chapter, readers should be able to:

- Describe the general process for estimating a business's corporate cost of capital.
- Estimate the component costs of debt and equity as well as the overall (corporate) cost of capital for any healthcare business.
- Describe the uncertainties inherent in the cost of capital estimation process.
- Explain the economic meaning of the corporate cost of capital and how it is used in capital investment decisions.

Introduction

The cost of capital is an extremely important concept in healthcare financial management. All businesses, whether investor-owned or not-for-profit, have to raise funds to buy the assets required to meet their strategic objectives. Hospitals, nursing homes, clinics, group practices, and so on all need assets to provide services. The funds to acquire the assets come in many shapes and forms, including contributions, profit retention, equity sales to stockholders, and debt capital supplied by creditors such as banks, bondholders, lessors, and suppliers. Most of the capital raised by organizations has a cost that is either explicit, such as the interest payments on debt, or implicit, such as the opportunity cost associated with equity (fund) capital. Because many business decisions require the cost of capital as an input, it is necessary for managers to both understand the cost of capital concept and to know how to estimate the costs of capital for their own firms.

Overview of the Cost of Capital Estimation Process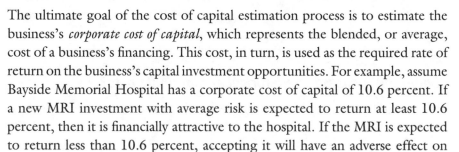

The ultimate goal of the cost of capital estimation process is to estimate the business's *corporate cost of capital*, which represents the blended, or average, cost of a business's financing. This cost, in turn, is used as the required rate of return on the business's capital investment opportunities. For example, assume Bayside Memorial Hospital has a corporate cost of capital of 10.6 percent. If a new MRI investment with average risk is expected to return at least 10.6 percent, then it is financially attractive to the hospital. If the MRI is expected to return less than 10.6 percent, accepting it will have an adverse effect on the hospital's financial soundness. Here, we assumed that the project under consideration has average risk. As we will discuss in Chapter 13, the corporate cost of capital must be adjusted to reflect project risk when it differs from the overall risk of the business.

The corporate cost of capital is a weighted average of the *component* (i.e., debt and equity) *costs*, adjusted for tax effects. After the component costs have been estimated, they are combined to form the corporate cost of capital. Thus, the first step in the cost of capital estimation process is to estimate both the cost of debt and the cost of equity. However, before the mechanics of cost estimation are discussed, some other points regarding the estimation process should be mentioned.

What Capital Components Should Be Included?

The first task in estimating a business's corporate cost of capital is to determine which sources of capital, shown on the right side of the business's balance sheet, should be included in the estimate. In general, the corporate cost of capital focuses on the cost of *permanent capital* (long-term capital) because these are the sources used to finance capital asset acquisitions. Thus, for most firms, the capital components included in the corporate cost of capital estimate are equity and long-term debt. Typically, short-term debt is used only as temporary financing to support seasonal or cyclical fluctuations in volume, so it is not included in the cost of capital estimate. However, if a firm does use short-term debt as part of its permanent financing mix, then such debt should be included in the cost of capital estimate. (We will discuss why short-term debt is not well suited for financing permanent assets in Chapter 11.)

Do Taxes Need to Be Considered?

In developing component costs, the issue of taxes arises for investor-owned businesses. Should the component costs be estimated on a before- or after-tax basis? As we will discuss in the next chapter, the use of debt financing creates a tax benefit because interest expense is tax deductible, while the use of equity financing has no impact on taxes. This tax benefit can be handled in several ways when working with capital costs; but the most common way is to include it in the cost of capital estimate. Thus, the tax benefit associated with debt financing will be recognized in the component cost of debt estimate, resulting in an after-tax cost of debt. For not-for-profit businesses, the benefit that arises from the issuance of tax-exempt debt will be incorporated directly in the cost estimate because investors require a lower interest rate on tax-exempt (i.e., municipal) debt.

Should the Focus Be on Historical or Marginal Costs?

Two very different sets of capital costs can be measured: (1) *historical*, or *embedded*, *costs*, which reflect the cost of funds raised in the past; and (2) *new*, or *marginal*, *costs*, which measure the cost of funds to be raised in the future. Historical costs are important for many purposes. For example, payers that reimburse on a cost basis are concerned with embedded costs. However, the primary purpose in developing a business's corporate cost of capital is to use it in making capital investment decisions, which involve future asset acquisitions and future financing. Thus, for these purposes, the relevant costs are the marginal costs of new funds to be raised during some future planning period—say, a year—and not the cost of funds raised in the past.

1. What is the basic concept of the corporate cost of capital?
2. What financing sources are typically included in a firm's cost of capital estimate?
3. Should the component costs be estimated on a before-tax or an after-tax basis?
4. Should the component costs reflect historical or marginal costs?

Self-Test Questions

Estimating the Cost of Debt

It is unlikely that a business's managers will know at the start of a planning period the exact types and amounts of debt that will be issued in the future; the type of debt actually used will depend on the specific assets to be financed and on market conditions as they develop over time. However, a business's managers do know what types of debt the firm usually issues. For example, Bayside Memorial Hospital typically uses bank debt to raise short-term funds to finance seasonal or cyclical working capital needs, and it uses 30-year tax-exempt bonds to raise long-term debt capital.[1] Because Bayside does not use short-term debt to finance permanent assets, its managers include only long-term debt in their corporate cost of capital estimate, and they assume that this debt will consist solely of 30-year tax-exempt bonds.

Suppose that Bayside's managers are developing the hospital's corporate cost of capital estimate for the coming year. How should they estimate the hospital's *cost of debt*? Most managers would begin by discussing current and prospective interest rates with their firms' investment bankers, which are the institutions that help firms bring security issues to market. Assume that the municipal bond analyst at Suncoast Securities, Inc., Bayside's investment banker, stated that a new 30-year tax-exempt healthcare issue would require semiannual interest payments of $30.50 ($61 annually) for each $1,000 par value bond issued. Thus, municipal bond investors currently require a $61/$1,000 = 0.061 = 6.1% return on Bayside's 30-year bonds. This required rate of return by investors (the interest rate) establishes the cost of debt to Bayside.

The true cost of debt to Bayside would be somewhat higher than 6.1 percent because the hospital must incur issuance expenses, called *flotation costs*, to sell the bonds. However, such expenses are typically small, so their impact on the cost of debt estimate is inconsequential, especially when the uncertainty inherent in the entire cost of capital estimation process is considered. Therefore, as we will discuss later in the chapter, it is common practice to ignore flotation costs when estimating a business's cost of capital. Bayside follows this practice, so its managers would estimate the component cost of debt as 6.1 percent:

$$\text{Tax-exempt component cost of debt} = R(R_d) = 6.1\%.$$

If Bayside's currently outstanding debt was actively traded, then the current **yield to maturity (YTM)** on this debt could be used to estimate the cost of new debt. For example, assume that Bayside has an actively traded issue outstanding that has a 7 percent coupon rate with semiannual payments, currently sells for $1,114.69, and has 25 years remaining to maturity. Using a financial calculator, the semiannual yield to maturity on this bond is found to be 3.05 percent:

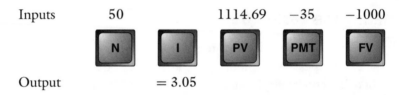

Because this is a semiannual rate, the resulting solution, 3.05 percent, must be multiplied by two to get the annual yield to maturity, resulting in a cost of debt estimate of 6.1 percent.[2]

Using the yield to maturity on an outstanding issue to estimate the cost of new debt works reasonably well when the remaining life of the old issue approximates the anticipated maturity of the new issue. If this is not the case, then yield curve differentials may cause the estimate to be biased. For example, if the yield curve were upward sloping in the 25- to 30-year range, the yield to maturity on a 25-year outstanding issue would understate the actual cost of a new 30-year issue. If material, an adjustment could be made on the basis of the current yield curve on Treasury securities.

A taxable healthcare provider would use one or more of the techniques described here to estimate its before-tax cost of debt. However, the tax benefits of interest payments must then be incorporated into the estimate. To illustrate, consider Ann Arbor Health Systems, Inc., an investor-owned firm that operates 16 acute care hospitals in Michigan, Indiana, and Ohio. The firm's investment bankers indicate that a new 30-year corporate bond issue that has Ann Arbor's BBB rating would require an interest rate of 10.0 percent. Because the firm's federal-plus-state tax rate is 40 percent, its after-tax cost of debt estimate is lowered to 6.0 percent:

$$\text{After-tax cost of debt} = R(R_d) \times (1 - T)$$
$$= 10.0\% \times (1 - 0.40) = 10.0\% \times 0.60 = 6.0\%.$$

By reducing Ann Arbor's component cost of debt from 10.0 percent to 6.0 percent, the cost of debt estimate has incorporated the benefit associated with interest payment tax deductibility.

In general, the **effective** cost of debt is roughly comparable between investor-owned and not-for-profit firms of similar risk. Investor-owned firms have the benefit of tax deductibility of interest payments, while not-for-profit firms have the benefit of being able to issue tax-exempt debt. Under normal economic conditions, these two benefits are roughly the same, resulting in a similar cost of debt. In our illustrations, the effective cost of debt is 6.1 percent for Ann Arbor Health Systems, an investor-owned firm, and 6.0 percent for Bayside Memorial Hospital, a similar not-for-profit business.

1. What are some methods used to estimate a business's cost of debt?
2. For investor-owned firms, how is the before-tax cost of debt converted to an after-tax cost?
3. Does the cost of debt differ materially between businesses that are similar in all respects except ownership?

Self-Test Questions

Estimating the Cost of Equity to Investor-Owned Businesses

Investor-owned businesses raise equity capital by selling new common stock and by retaining earnings for use by the firm rather than paying them out as dividends to shareholders. Not-for-profit firms raise equity capital through contributions and grants, and by generating an excess of revenues over expenses, none of which can be paid out as dividends. This section describes how to estimate the cost of equity capital within investor-owned businesses.[3] The next major section focuses on not-for-profit businesses.

The cost of debt is based on the return that investors require on debt securities, and the *cost of equity* to investor-owned firms can be defined similarly: It is the rate of return that investors require on the firm's common stock. At first glance, it may appear that equity raised through **retained earnings** is a costless source of capital to investor-owned businesses. After all, dividend payments must be paid at some point in time on any new shares of stock that are issued; but no such payments are required on funds that are obtained by retaining earnings. The reason why a cost of capital must be assigned to all forms of equity financing involves the *opportunity cost principle*. An investor-owned firm's net income literally belongs to its common stockholders. Employees are compensated by wages, suppliers are compensated by cash payments for supplies, bondholders are compensated by interest payments, governments are compensated by tax payments, and so on. The residual earnings of a firm, its net income, belongs to the stockholders and serves to "pay the rent" on stockholder-supplied capital.

Management can either pay out earnings in the form of dividends or retain earnings for reinvestment in the business. If part of the earnings is retained, an opportunity cost is incurred: Stockholders could have received these earnings as dividends and then invested this money in stocks, bonds, real estate, commodity futures, or any other investment. Thus, the firm should earn on its retained earnings at least as much as its stockholders themselves could earn on alternative investments of similar risk. If the firm cannot earn as much as stockholders can in similar risk investments, then the firm's net income should be paid out as dividends rather than retained for reinvestment within the firm. What rate of return can stockholders expect to earn on other investments of equivalent risk? The answer is $R(R_e)$, the required rate of return on equity. Investors can earn this return either by buying more shares of the firm in question or by buying the stock of similar businesses.

Whereas debt is a contractual obligation with an easily estimated cost, it is not nearly as easy to estimate the cost of equity. Three primary methods are used in the estimation process: (1) the Capital Asset Pricing Model (CAPM), (2) the discounted cash flow (DCF) model, and (3) the debt cost plus risk premium method. These methods should not be regarded as mutually exclusive, for no single approach dominates the estimation process. In practice, all approaches should be used to estimate the cost of equity, and then the final value should be chosen on the basis of the managers' confidence in the data at hand.

Capital Asset Pricing Model (CAPM) Approach

The *Capital Asset Pricing Model (CAPM)*, which was first discussed in Chapter 5, is a widely accepted finance model that specifies the equilibrium risk/return relationship on common stocks. Basically, the model assumes that investors consider only one risk factor when setting required rates of returns: the volatility of returns on the stock relative to the volatility of returns on a well-diversified portfolio called the *market portfolio*, or just the *market*. The measure of risk in the CAPM is the stock's *market beta*. The market, which is a large collection of stocks such as the S&P 500 Index, has a beta of 1.0. A stock with a beta of 2.0 has twice the volatility of returns as the market, while a stock with a beta of 0.5 has only half the volatility of returns as the market. Because relative volatility measures market risk, a low beta stock—which has a beta less than 1.0—is less risky than the market; while a high beta stock—which has a beta greater than 1.0—is more risky than the market.

Within the CAPM, the actual equation that relates risk to return is called the *Security Market Line (SML)*:

$$R(R_e) = RF + [R(R_M) - RF] \times b_i$$
$$= RF + (RP_M \times b_i).$$

Here,

$$RF = \text{risk-free rate.}$$

$$R(R_M) = \text{required rate of return on the market.}$$

$$b_i = \text{beta coefficient of the stock in question.}$$

$$[R(R_M) - RF)] = RP_M = \text{market risk premium, the premium}$$

above the risk-free rate that investors require

to buy a stock with average risk.

$$(RP_M) \times b_i = \text{stock risk premium, the premium above the risk-free rate}$$

that investors require to buy the stock in question.

Managers can calculate the required rate of return on a firm's stock given estimates of the risk-free rate, RF; the beta of the firm's stock, b_i; and the required rate of return on the market, $R(R_M)$. This result in turn, can be used as one estimate for the firm's cost of equity.

The starting point for the CAPM cost of equity estimate is RF, the risk-free **Estimating the** rate. Unfortunately, there is no unambiguous proxy for this rate. Treasury **Risk-Free Rate** securities are essentially free of default risk; but long-term T-bonds will suffer capital losses if interest rates rise, and a portfolio invested in short-term T-bills will provide a volatile earnings stream because the rate paid on T-bills varies over time.

Because we cannot, in practice, find a truly riskless rate on which to base the CAPM, what rate should we use? In recent years, most analysts have used the rate on long-term Treasury bonds, where "long-term" usually denotes 20–30 year maturities. There were many reasons for favoring the T-bond rate, including the fact that T-bill rates are very volatile because they are directly affected by actions taken by the Federal Reserve Board. Perhaps the most persuasive argument is that common stocks have traditionally been viewed as long-term securities, so stock returns should embody the long-term inflation expectations embodied in bonds, rather than the short-term inflation expectations embodied in bills. On this account, the cost of equity should be more highly correlated with T-bond rates than with T-bill rates.

However, some recent events have shaken the position that the CAPM risk-free rate should be based on long-term T-bonds. First, there is no doubt that many investors view common stocks not as long-term investments but rather as short-term trading vehicles. This view is clearly espoused by day traders, but what about other investors such as fund managers? Until the mid-1960s, stock-fund managers bought and sold about 15 percent of their portfolios each year, which implies a holding period of about 7 years. Since then, however, managers have been trading with ever increasing frequency, with turnover rates today at about 90 percent, which translates into a holding period of just over a year.

Second, U.S. Treasury surpluses have resulted in a major government buyback program of Treasury securities. This program has focused on 30-year bonds, which have higher interest payments than shorter-term securities because of yield curve effects. The end result is a downward bias on 30-year rates as well as decreasing liquidity in the market for long-term Treasuries. The destabilization of the long-term T-bond market has even caused the *Wall Street Journal* to change its "benchmark" long-term interest rate from 30-year Treasuries to 10-year Treasuries.

Whether or not these changes will cause analysts to begin using the 10-year note as the basis for the CAPM risk-free rate has not yet been determined. However, we are not going to agonize over the issue because typically there is little difference in the yields on the two securities. Still, we feel strongly that the risk-free rate should not be based on the T-bill rate, which is subject to many influences that are not related to stock returns.

Estimating the Market Risk Premium

The market risk premium, $RP_M = [R(R_M) - RF)]$, can be estimated on the basis of historical returns or expected returns.

The most complete, accurate, and up-to-date historical returns study is published annually by Ibbotson Associates. It examines market data over long periods of time to determine the average annual rates of return and standard deviations of various classes of securities.[4] To illustrate the concept, consider Table 10.1, which presents selected historical average returns and volatility from 1926–1999.

Note that common stocks provided the highest average return over the period studied, while Treasury bills gave the lowest. In fact, T-bills barely covered inflation over the period; but common stocks provided a substantial real (inflation adjusted) return. However, the superior returns on stock investments had its cost—stocks were by far the riskiest of the investments listed as judged by standard deviation, which measures dispersion about the mean, and they would also rank as riskiest within a market-risk framework. To further illustrate the risk differentials, the range on annual returns on stocks was from −43.3 to 54.0 percent, while the range on T-bills was only 0.0 to 14.7 percent. These data provide strong empirical support for the basic

TABLE 10.1
Selected Historical Total Returns Data, 1926–1999

	Annual Average	Standard Deviation
Common stocks	13.3%	20.1%
Long-term corporate bonds	5.9	8.7
Long-term Treasury bonds	5.5	9.3
Treasury bills	3.8	3.2
Inflation rate	3.2	4.5

Note: The listed return on common stocks is the return on large company stocks.

premise that we discussed in Chapter 8—namely, in efficient markets, higher returns can be obtained only by bearing greater risk.

By examining the spread between the historical rates on stocks and Treasury bonds, it is possible to obtain the historical risk premium of stocks over T-bonds. The data in Table 10.1 suggest that this risk premium is 7.8 percentage points. However, the basic returns data have large standard deviations, so one must use them with caution. Also, the abnormally high returns on stocks in the 1990s has tended to push the premium calculated in this way to new highs. Finally, it should be noted that the choice of the beginning and ending periods can have a major impact on the calculated risk premiums. Indeed, in many years, historical returns data indicate **negative** risk premiums, which would lead to the conclusion that Treasury securities have a higher required return than common stocks—a conclusion contrary to both financial theory and common sense. All of this suggests that the historical risk premium should be used with caution, although in some situations it may be the only measure available. As one businessman muttered after listening to a professor give a lecture on the CAPM: "Beware of academics bearing gifts!"

The historical approach to risk premiums assumes that investors expect future results, on average, to equal past results. However, as we noted, the historical risk premium varies greatly depending on the period selected; and, in any event, investors today probably expect results in the future to be different from those achieved during the Great Depression of the 1930s, during the World War II years of the 1940s, and during the peaceful boom years of the 1950s and 1990s, all of which are included, and given equal weight, in the historical returns data. The questionable assumption that future expectations are equal to past realizations, together with the sometimes nonsensical results obtained when calculating historical risk premiums, has led to the search for expected (forward looking) risk premiums.

The most common approach used to estimate expected market risk premiums uses the Discounted Cash Flow (DCF) model to estimate the expected market rate of return, $E(R_M)$. Then, assuming market equilibrium, the expected rate of return is used as proxy for the required rate of return, $R(R_M)$. Finally, RF is subtracted to obtain the estimate for the expected market risk premium. Many financial services firms publish forecasts for the expected rate of return on the market, and these values can be used as inputs into the CAPM.

Estimating Beta

The last parameter needed for a CAPM cost of equity estimate is the beta coefficient. Recall from Chapter 5 that a stock's beta is a measure of its volatility relative to that of an average stock, and that betas are generally estimated from the stock's characteristic line, which is estimated by running a linear regression between past returns on the stock in question and past returns on some market index. We will define betas developed in this manner as *historical betas*.

Unfortunately, historical betas show how risky a stock was *in the past,* whereas investors are interested in *future* risk. It may be that a given firm appeared to be quite safe in the past, but that things have changed and its future risk is judged to be higher than its past risk, or vice versa. The hospital industry presents a good example. Prior to 1983, when the industry operated on a cost-plus basis, investor-owned hospitals were among the bluest of the blue chips. However, when prospective payment began, the industry became riskier. The increasing market power of managed care plans has further added to hospitals' risk.

Now, consider the use of beta as a measure of a firm's equity risk. If we use a historical beta in a CAPM framework to measure the firm's cost of equity, we are implicitly assuming that future risk is the same as past risk. This would be a troublesome assumption for a hospital in 1983. But what about most firms in most years? As a general rule, is future risk sufficiently similar to past risk to warrant the use of historical betas in a CAPM framework? For individual firms, historical betas are often not very stable, so past risk is often *not* a good predictor of future risk.

Because historical betas may not be good predictors of future risk, researchers have sought ways to improve them. This has led to the development of two other types of betas: (1) adjusted betas and (2) fundamental betas. *Adjusted betas* recognize the fact that true betas tend to move toward 1.0 over time.[5] Therefore, one can begin with a firm's pure historical statistical beta; make an adjustment for the expected future movement toward 1.0; and produce an adjusted beta that, on average, will be a better predictor of the future beta than would the unadjusted historical beta.

Finally, *fundamental betas* extend the adjustment process to include such fundamental risk variables as the use of debt financing, sales volatility, and the like. These betas are constantly adjusted to reflect changes in a firm's operations and capital structure, whereas with historical betas, including adjusted ones, such changes might not be fully reflected until several years after the firm's "true" beta has changed.

Adjusted betas are obviously heavily dependent on unadjusted historical betas, and so are fundamental betas as they are actually calculated. Therefore, the "regular" historical beta, calculated as the slope of the characteristic line, is important even if one goes on to develop a more exotic version. With this in mind, it should be noted that several different sets of data can be used to calculate historical betas, and the different data sets produce different results. Here are some points to note:

- Betas can be based on historical periods of different lengths. For example, data for the past one, two, three, and so on, years may be used. Most analysts who calculate betas today use five years of data, but this choice is arbitrary, and different lengths of time usually alter significantly the calculated beta for a given firm.[6]

- Returns may be calculated on holding periods of different lengths—a day, a week, a month, a quarter, a year, and so on. For example, if it has been decided to analyze data on NYSE stocks over a five-year period, then we might obtain $52 \times 5 = 260$ weekly returns, or $1 \times 5 = 5$ annual returns. The set of returns on each stock, however large it turns out to be, would then be regressed on the corresponding market returns to obtain the stock's beta. In statistical analysis, it is generally better to have more, rather then fewer, observations because using more observations generally leads to greater statistical confidence. This suggests the use of weekly returns and, say, five years of data, for a sample size of 260, or even daily returns for an even larger sample size. However, the shorter the holding period, the more likely the data are to exhibit random "noise;" and the greater the number of years of data, the more likely it is that the firm's market risk will have changed. Thus, the choice of both the number of years of data and the length of the holding period involves a trade-off between a desire to have many observations versus a desire to have recent and consequently more relevant data.
- The value used to represent "the market" is also an important consideration, and one that can have a significant effect on the calculated beta. Most beta calculators today use the New York Stock Exchange Composite Index, which is based on over 2,000 stocks, weighted by the value of each firm; but others use the S&P 500 Index or some other group, including one—the Wilshire Index—with over 8,000 stocks. In theory, the broader the index, the better the beta; indeed, the index should really include returns on all risky assets including stocks, bonds, leases, private businesses, real estate, and even "human capital." As a practical matter, however, we cannot get accurate returns data on most types of assets, so measurement problems dictate the use of stock indexes to measure market returns.

The bottom line of all of this is that one can calculate betas in many different ways; and, depending on the methods used, different betas, and hence different cost of equity estimates, will result. Where does this leave managers regarding the proper beta? The choice is a matter of judgment and data availability because there is no "right" beta. With luck, the betas derived from different sources will, for a given firm, be close together. If they are not, then the confidence in the CAPM cost of equity estimate will be diminished.

Table 10.2 contains the betas of some representative investor-owned healthcare businesses as provided by *Market Guide*, an online Financial information service. *Market Guide* uses 60 monthly returns along with the S&P 500 Index as its proxy for the market. It does not adjust the betas for their tendency to move toward 1.0 over time. On the basis of this very limited selection, it appears that healthcare businesses carry above-average market risk for stockholders. Drug producers carry the lowest market risk, while practice management firms carry the highest.

Illustration of the CAPM Approach 🖬

To illustrate the CAPM approach, consider Ann Arbor Health Systems, which has a beta coefficient, b, of 1.10. Furthermore, assume that the current yield on T-bonds, RF, is 7.0 percent, and that the best estimate for the current market risk premium, RP_M, is 7 percentage points. In other words, the current required rate of return on the market, $R(R_M)$, is 14.0 percent. All the required input parameters have been estimated, and the SML equation can be completed as follows:

$$R(R_e) = RF + [R(R_M) - RF] \times b_{AAHS}$$
$$= 7.0\% + (14.0\% - 7.0\%) \times 1.10$$
$$= 7.0\% + (7.0\% \times 1.10)$$
$$= 7.0\% + 7.7\% = 14.7\%.$$

Thus, according to the CAPM, Ann Arbor's required rate of return on equity is 14.7 percent.

What does the 14.7 percent estimate for $R(R_e)$ imply? In essence, equity investors believe that Ann Arbor's stock, with a beta of 1.10, is slightly more risky than the average stock with a beta of 1.00. With a risk-free rate of 7.0 percent, and a market risk premium of 7 percentage points, an average firm, with b = 1.0, has a required rate of return on equity of $7.0\% + (7.0\% \times 1.00) = 7.0\% + 7.0\% = 14.0\%$. Thus, according to the CAPM,

TABLE 10.2

Beta Coefficients for Selected Healthcare Businesses

Company	Symbol	Primary Line of Business	Beta
Aetna	AET	Managed care	1.40
Ann Arbor Health Systems	AAHS	Acute care hospitals	1.10
Beverly Enterprises	BEV	Long-term care	1.31
HCA	HCA	Acute care hospitals	1.00
Guidant	GCT	Medical devices	0.69
HEALTHSOUTH	HRC	Outpatient/rehabilitative care	1.40
Humana	HUM	Managed care	1.83
Manor Care	HCR	Long-term care	1.20
Medtronic	MDT	Medical devices	0.86
Merck	MRK	Major pharmaceutical	0.93
Phycor	PHYC	Practice management	1.75
Pfizer	PFE	Major pharmaceutical	0.86
Tenet Healthcare	THC	Acute care hospitals	0.86
United Healthcare	UNH	Managed care	1.77
US Oncology	USON	Practice Management	1.98

Note: Historically, finding the market betas of firms meant obtaining hardcopy reports from investment bankers or investment advisory firms. Now, there are numerous web sites that supply such information in a matter of seconds.
Source: www.marketguide.com, 2000.

equity investors require 70 basis points more return for investing in Ann Arbor Health Systems, with b = 1.10, rather than an average stock, with b = 1.00.

There is a great deal of uncertainty in the CAPM estimate of the cost of equity. Some of this uncertainty stems from the fact that there is no assurance that the CAPM is correct (i.e., the CAPM accurately describes the risk/return preference of stock investors). Additionally, there is a great deal of uncertainty in the input parameter estimates, especially the beta coefficient. Because of these uncertainties, it is highly unlikely that Ann Arbor's true, but unobservable, cost of equity is 14.7 percent. Thus, instead of picking single values for each parameter, it may be better to develop high and low estimates, and then to combine all of the high estimates and all of the low estimates to develop a range, rather than a point estimate, for the CAPM cost of equity.

Discounted Cash Flow (DCF) Approach

The second procedure for estimating the cost of equity is the *discounted cash flow (DCF) method*. As we discussed in Chapter 8, the value of a stock with a predictable dividend stream can be found as the present value of that expected dividend stream. Furthermore, if the dividend is expected to grow each year at a constant rate, $E(g)$, then the *constant growth model* can be used to estimate the expected rate of return on equity, $E(R_e)$:

$$E(R_e) = \frac{D_0 \times [1 + E(g)]}{P_0} + E(g) = \frac{E(D_1)}{P_0} + E(g) = R(R_e).$$

Because stock prices typically are in equilibrium, the expected rate of return, $E(R_e)$, is also the required rate of return, $R(R_e)$.

As in the CAPM approach, there are three input parameters in the DCF model. **Estimating the** Current stock price is readily available for firms that are actively traded. Ann **Current Stock** Arbor Health Systems' stock is traded in the over-the-counter (OTC) market, **Price** so its stock price generally can be found in the *Wall Street Journal*. At the time of the analysis, Ann Arbor's stock price was $35, so $P_0 = \$35$.

Next year's dividend payment is also relatively easy to estimate. If you are **Estimating the** one of Ann Arbor's managers, you can look in the firm's five-year financial **Next Dividend** plan for the dividend estimate. If you are an outsider, dividend data on larger **Payment** publicly traded firms are available from brokerage houses and investment advisory firms. Also, current dividend information is published in the *Wall Street Journal*, and it can be used as a basis for estimating next year's dividend. Ann Arbor Health Systems is followed by several analysts at major brokerage houses, and their consensus estimate for next year's dividend payment is $2.50, so for purposes of this analysis, $E(D_1) = \$2.50$.

The expected growth rate, $E(g)$, is the most difficult of the DCF model **Estimating the** parameters to estimate. Here, we discuss several methods for estimating $E(g)$. **Expected Growth Rate**

- **Using historical growth rates to forecast future growth.** If growth rates in earnings and dividends have been relatively stable in the past, and if investors expect these trends to continue, then the past realized growth rate may be used as an estimate of the expected future growth rate. To illustrate the concept, consider Table 10.3, which gives earnings per share (EPS) and dividends per share (DPS) data from 1991 to 2000 for Ann Arbor Health Systems. Ten years (nine growth periods) of data are shown in the table; but we could have used 15 years or five years, or some other historical time period. There is no rule about the appropriate number of years to analyze when calculating historical growth rates. However, the period chosen should reflect, to the extent possible, the longest period that replicates conditions expected in the future.

    The easiest historical growth rate to calculate is the compound rate between two dates, called the *point-to-point rate*. For example, EPS grew at an annual rate of 6.8 percent from 1991 to 2000, and DPS grew at a 7.2 percent rate during this same period. (To obtain the EPS growth rate using a financial calculator, enter 2.95 [or −2.95] as PV, 5.35 as FV, 9 as N because with ten data points we have nine growth periods; then, press I to obtain the growth rate, 6.8 percent.) Note that the point-to-point growth rate could change radically if we used two other points. For example, if we calculate the five-year EPS growth rate from 1995 to 2000, we would obtain only 2.8 percent. This radical change occurs because the point-to-point rate is extremely sensitive to the beginning and ending years chosen.

    To alleviate the problem of beginning and ending year sensitivity, some analysts use the *average-to-average method*, which reduces the sensitivity of the growth rate to beginning and ending year values. The 1991–1993 average EPS is ($2.95 + $3.07 + $3.22)/3 = $3.08, the average 1998–2000 EPS is ($5.20 + $5.12 + $5.35)/3 = $5.22, and the number of years of growth between the two averages is 1992 to 1999 = 7.

TABLE 10.3
Ann Arbor Health Systems: Historical EPS and DPS Data

Year	EPS	DPS
1991	$2.95	$1.24
1992	3.07	1.32
1993	3.22	1.32
1994	3.40	1.52
1995	4.65	1.72
1996	5.12	1.92
1997	5.25	2.00
1998	5.20	2.20
1999	5.12	2.20
2000	5.35	2.32

The average-to-average DPS growth rate is 8.2 percent, and the average-to-average EPS growth rate is 7.8 percent. Note that we are calculating compound annual growth rates, which are much easier to interpret than a single growth rate over the entire period.

A third way, and in our view the best way, to estimate historical growth rates is by *log-linear least squares regression.*[7] The regression method gives consideration to all data points in the series; thus, it is the least likely to be biased by a randomly high or low beginning or ending year. The only practical way to estimate a least squares growth rate is to use a computer or a financial calculator. Using a spreadsheet's data regression capability, we find the growth rate in earnings to be 7.9 percent, while the growth rate in dividends is 7.7 percent.

When earnings and dividends are growing at approximately the same rate, there is more confidence in the resultant growth rate forecast. However, if EPS and DPS historically have grown at different rates, something is going to have to change in the future because these two series cannot grow at different rates indefinitely. There is no rule for handling differences in historical earnings and dividend growth rates, and when they differ, this simply demonstrates in yet another way the problems with using historical growth as a proxy for expected future growth. Like many aspects of healthcare finance, judgment is required when estimating growth rates.

Table 10.4 summarizes the historical growth rates that were just discussed. It is obvious that one can take a given set of historical data and, depending on the years and the calculation method used, obtain a large number of quite different growth rates. If past growth rates have been stable, then investors might base future expectations on past trends. This is a reasonable proposition; but, unfortunately, one rarely finds much historical stability. Therefore, the use of historical growth rates in a DCF analysis must be applied with judgment and also used, if at all, in conjunction with the estimation methods discussed next.

- **Retention growth model.** The *retention growth method* is another method for estimating the expected growth rate in dividends:

$$E(g) = \text{Retention ratio} \times \text{Expected ROE.}$$

This model produces a constant growth rate, and when we use it we

Method	EPS	DPS	Average
Point-to-point	6.8%	7.2%	7.0%
Average-to average	7.8	8.2	8.0
Log-linear regression	7.9	7.7	7.8

TABLE 10.4
Ann Arbor Health Systems Historical Growth Rates, 1991–2000

are, by implication, making four important assumptions: (1) We expect the payout ratio, and thus the retention ratio, to remain constant; (2) we expect the return on equity on new investment to equal the firm's current ROE, which implies that we expect the return on equity to remain constant; (3) the firm is not expected to issue new common stock or, if it does, we expect this new stock to be sold at a price equal to its book value; and (4) future projects are expected to have the same degree of risk as the firm's existing assets.

Ann Arbor Health Systems has had an average return on equity of about 14 percent over the past ten years. The ROE has been relatively steady, but even so, it has ranged from a low of 8.9 percent to a high of 17.6 percent during this period. In addition, the firm's dividend payout ratio has averaged 0.45 over the past ten years, so its retention ratio has averaged $1.0 - 0.45 = 0.55$. Using these data, the retention growth method gives a divided growth estimate of 7.7 percent:

$$E(g_{AAHS}) = 0.55 \times 14\% = 7.7\%.$$

This figure, together with the historical EPS and DPS growth rates summarized in Table 10.4, might lead us to conclude that Ann Arbor Health System's expected dividend growth rate is in the range of 7.0 to 8.0 percent.

- **Analysts' forecasts.** A third growth-rate estimation technique calls for using security analysts' forecasts. Analysts forecast and then publish growth rate estimates for most of the larger publicly owned businesses. For example, *Value Line* provides such forecasts on about 1,700 firms, and all of the larger brokerage houses provide similar forecasts. Also, many online sites provide dividend forecast data. Finally, several data collection firms compile analysts' forecasts on a regular basis and provide summary information, such as the median and range of forecasts, on widely followed businesses. These growth-rate summaries, such as the one compiled by Lynch, Jones & Ryan in its *Institutional Brokers Estimate System (I/B/E/S)* and by Zacks Investment Research, can be ordered for a fee and obtained either in hard-copy format or as online computer data. In addition, some data are available free on the web.

The problem for our purposes is that most analysts' forecasts correctly assume nonconstant growth. For example, some analysts that follow Ann Arbor Health Systems are forecasting a 12.0 percent annual growth rate in earnings and dividends over the next five years, followed by a steady-state (constant) growth rate of 6.5 percent. A simple way to handle this situation is to use the nonconstant growth forecast to develop a proxy constant growth rate. Computer simulations indicate that dividends beyond Year 50 contribute very little to the value of any stock—the present value of dividends beyond Year 50 is virtually zero, so for practical purposes, anything beyond that point can be ignored. If we consider only a 50-year horizon, we can develop a weighted-average growth rate and use it as a constant growth rate for cost of capital purposes. For Ann Arbor Health Systems, we assumed a growth rate of 12.0 percent for five years followed by a growth rate of 6.5 percent for 45 years, which produced an arithmetic average annual growth rate of $(0.10 \times 12.0\%) + (0.90 \times 6.5\%) = 7.2\%$.[8]

To illustrate the DCF approach, consider the data developed thus far for Ann Arbor Health Systems. The firm's current stock price, P_0, is \$35, and its next expected annual dividend, $E(D_1)$, is \$2.50. Thus, the firm's DCF estimate of $E(R_e) = R(R_e)$, according to the DCF model is:

Illustration of the DCF Approach

$$E(R_e) = \frac{E(D_1)}{P_0} + E(g)$$

$$= \frac{\$2.50}{\$35} + E(g) = 7.14\% + E(g).$$

With an $E(g)$ estimate range of 7 to 8 percent, the midpoint—7.5 percent—will be used as the final estimate. Thus, the DCF estimate for Ann Arbor Health System's cost of equity is $7.14\% + 7.5\% = 14.64\% \approx 14.6\%$.

Debt Cost Plus Risk Premium Approach

The *debt cost plus risk premium approach* relies on the assumption that stock investments are riskier than debt investments; hence the cost of equity for any business can be thought of as the cost of debt to **that business** plus a risk premium:

$$R(R_e) = R(R_d) + \text{Risk premium}.$$

The cost of debt is relatively easy to estimate, so the key input to this model is the risk premium.

Note that the risk premium used here is **not** the same as the market risk premium used in the Capital Asset Pricing Model. The market risk premium is the amount that investors require above the **risk-free rate** to invest in average risk common stocks. Here, we need the risk premium above the **cost of debt**. How might this new risk premium be estimated? Using the data from above, we know that the cost of equity for an average risk (b = 1.0) stock is 14.0 percent. Furthermore, the cost of debt for an average firm, which has roughly an A rating, is 9.0 percent. Thus, for an average firm, the risk premium of the cost of equity over the cost of debt is $14.0\% - 9.0\% = 5.0$ percentage points.

Empirical work suggests that the risk premium for use in the debt cost plus risk premium model has ranged from 4 to 7 percentage points. When interest rates are high in the economy, this risk premium tends to be at the lower end of the range, while lower interest rates often lead to higher risk premiums. Perhaps the biggest weakness of this approach is that there is no assurance that the risk premium for the average firm is the same as the risk premium for the firm in question, which in this case is Ann Arbor Health Systems. Thus, the risk premium method does not have the theoretical precision that the other models do. On the other hand, the input values required by the debt cost plus risk premium model are fewer and easier to estimate than in the other models.

With a cost of debt estimate of 10.0 percent and a current risk premium estimate of 5.0 percentage points, the debt cost plus risk premium estimate for Ann Arbor's cost of equity is 15.0 percent:

$$R(R_e) = R(R_d) + \text{Risk premium}$$

$$= 10.0\% + 5.0\% = 15.0\%.$$

Comparison of the CAPM, DCF, and Debt Cost Plus Risk Premium Methods

We have discussed three methods for estimating the cost of equity. The CAPM estimate was 14.7 percent, the DCF estimate was 14.6 percent, and the debt cost plus risk premium estimate was 15.0 percent. At this point, most analysts would conclude that there is sufficient consistency in the results to warrant the use of 14.8 percent, or thereabouts, as the final estimate of the cost of equity for Ann Arbor Health Systems. If the three methods had produced widely different estimates, then Ann Arbor's managers would have to use their judgment regarding the relative merits of each estimate and then choose the estimate, or some average of the estimates, that seemed most reasonable under the circumstances. In general, this choice would be made on the basis of the managers' confidence in the input parameters of each approach.

Self-Test Questions

1. Briefly, describe the CAPM approach to estimating a business's cost of equity.
2. What is the best proxy for the risk-free rate in the CAPM? Why?
3. What are the three types of beta that can be used in the CAPM?
4. Briefly describe the DCF approach to estimating a business's cost of equity.
5. What are three common methods for estimating the future dividend growth rate for use in the DCF model?
6. Briefly, describe the debt cost plus risk premium approach to estimating a business's cost of equity.
7. Is there a difference between the risk premium used in the CAPM and the one used in the debt cost plus risk premium model?
8. How would you choose among widely different estimates of $R(R_e)$?

Estimating the Cost of Equity to Not-for-Profit Businesses

Not-for-profit firms raise equity (fund) capital in two basic ways: (1) by receiving contributions and grants and (2) by earning an excess of revenues over expenses (retained earnings). In this section we first discuss some views regarding the cost of fund capital, and then we illustrate how this cost might be estimated.

Is There a Cost to Fund Capital?

Our primary purpose in this chapter is to develop a corporate cost of capital estimate that can be used in capital budgeting decisions. Thus, the estimated "costs" represent the cost of using capital to purchase fixed assets, rather than for alternative uses. What is the cost of using equity capital for real-asset investments within not-for-profit businesses? There are at least four positions that can be taken on this question.[9]

1. **Fund capital has a zero cost**. The rationale here is that (1) contributors do not expect a monetary return on their contributions; and that (2) the firm's stakeholders, especially the patients who pay more for services than warranted by the firm's tangible costs, do not require an explicit return on the capital retained by the firm.

2. **Fund capital has a cost equal to the return forgone on marketable securities investments**. When a not-for-profit firm receives contributions or retains earnings, it can always invest these funds in marketable securities (highly liquid, safe securities) rather than purchase real assets. Thus, fund capital has a relatively low opportunity cost that should be acknowledged; this cost is roughly equal to the return available on a portfolio of short-term, low-risk securities such as T-bills.

3. **Fund capital has a cost equal to the expected growth rate of the business's assets**.[10] To better understand the logic here, assume that a hospital in a growing city must increase services and, because it does not have excess capacity, its total assets must increase by 8 percent per year to keep pace with the increasing patient load. To purchase the required assets without increasing the proportion of debt used to finance its assets, the hospital must grow its fund capital at an 8 percent rate. In this way, it can finance asset growth by growing both debt and equity at the same 8 percent rate, and hence can hold the relative amount of debt constant. If the hospital earned zero return on its fund capital, its equity base would remain constant over time; and the only way it could add new assets would be to take on additional debt without matching equity, and hence drive up its debt ratio, or to rely solely on contributions to provide the needed equity. In general, reliance on contribution capital is quite risky, and, at some point, lenders would be unwilling to provide additional debt financing, so it would be difficult to support the desired growth without a return on the equity invested.

   Even if no volume growth is expected, a not-for-profit business must earn a return on its fund capital just to replace its existing asset base as assets wear out or become obsolete. The return on the equity invested is required because new assets will cost more than the old ones being replaced because of inflation, so depreciation cash flow in itself will not be sufficient to replace assets as needed. The bottom line here is that not-for-profit firms must earn a return on equity merely to support dollar growth in assets; and the greater the growth rate, including that caused by inflation, the greater the return that must be earned.

4. **Fund capital has a cost equal to the cost of equity to similar for-profit businesses**. The rationale here also rests on the opportunity cost concept as discussed in the second argument, but the opportunity cost is now defined as the return available from investing fund capital in alternative investments of **similar risk**.

To illustrate this position, suppose Bayside Memorial Hospital, a not-for-profit corporation, receives $500,000 in contributions in 2001 and also retains $4.5 million in earnings, so it has $5 million of new fund capital available for investment. The $5 million could be (1) used to purchase assets related to its core business, such as an outpatient clinic or diagnostic equipment; (2) temporarily invested in securities with the intent of purchasing healthcare assets some time in the future; (3) used to retire debt; (4) used to pay management bonuses; or (5) placed in a non-interest-bearing account at the bank; and on and on. By using this capital to invest in real assets, Bayside is deprived of the opportunity to use this capital for other purposes, so an opportunity cost must be assigned that reflects the riskiness associated with an equity investment in hospital assets. What return is available on securities with similar risk to hospital assets? The answer is the return that is expected from investing in the stock of an investor-owned hospital business, such as Ann Arbor Health Systems. Instead of using fund capital to purchase real healthcare assets, Bayside could always use the funds to buy the stock of a hospital business, such as Ann Arbor Health Systems, and delay the real-asset purchase until some time in the future.

With these four positions in mind, which one should prevail in practice? Unfortunately, the answer is not clear cut. Here are our views on this issue. At a minimum, a not-for-profit business should require a return on its equity investments in real assets that is at least as large as its projected asset growth rate. In that way, the business is setting the minimum rate of return that will, if it is actually achieved, ensure the financial stability of the organization. Thus, the expected growth rate sets the minimum required rate of return, and hence the minimum cost of equity, for not-for-profit businesses.

However, to fully recover **all opportunity costs**, including the opportunity cost of employing equity capital in real assets, the real-asset investments must offer an expected return equal to the return expected on similar-risk securities investments. Thus, the "true" economic cost of equity to a not-for-profit healthcare provider is the rate that could be earned on stock investments in similar investor-owned firms. Using this cost of equity, a not-for-profit business is requiring that all costs, including opportunity costs, be considered in the cost of capital estimate.

Although we believe the "full opportunity cost" approach to be most correct, many would argue that the unique mission of not-for-profit businesses precludes securities investments as realistic alternatives to healthcare plant and equipment because securities investments do not contribute directly to the mission of providing healthcare services. On the other hand, full opportunity costs do not have to be recovered on every new capital investment. Not-for-profit firms do invest in negative profit projects that benefit its stakeholders; but we believe that managers should be aware of the financial opportunity costs inherent in such investments. We will have more to say about this issue in Chapter 12.

In closing, note that there is one exception to the rule. If contributions are made for a specific purpose, such as a children's wing to a hospital, then those funds do indeed have zero cost. Because their use is restricted to a particular project, the firm does not have the opportunity to invest the funds in other alternatives. Furthermore, if the contribution is dependent upon a particular project being initiated, it makes no sense to charge the minimum "growth rate" cost.

Measuring the Cost of Fund Capital

We have defined the appropriate cost of equity capital to not-for-profit firms as the return available on the stocks of similar investor-owned firms. Thus, if Bayside Memorial Hospital and Ann Arbor Health Systems were equivalent in all respects, then we could use the 14.8 percent estimate for Ann Arbor's cost of equity as our estimate for Bayside's cost of fund capital. However, it is impossible to find identical investor-owned and not-for-profit firms because even when they are in the same line of business and about the same size, they will often use different amounts of debt financing and one is taxable and the other is not. Because of these dissimilarities, most theorists would argue that it is necessary to adjust the cost estimate before it can be used by not-for-profit businesses.

The adjustment is accomplished by using *Hamada's equation*, which was developed by Robert Hamada in 1969. Hamada combined the CAPM with Modigliani and Miller's capital structure model, which we will discuss in the next chapter, to obtain the following equation:[11]

$$b_{Equity} = b_{Assets} \times [1 + (1 - T) \times (D/E)].$$

Here, b_{Equity} is the market beta of the business's stock, b_{Assets} is the inherent market beta of the assets, assuming that the business uses no debt financing; T is the tax rate; D is the market value of the business's debt; and E is the market value of the business's equity. In essence, b_{Assets} measures the inherent market risk of the assets, and b_{Equity} measures the market risk of the assets when operated by a business with a given capital structure and tax rate.

To illustrate the use of Hamada's equation, remember that the market beta of Ann Arbor's stock is 1.10 and its tax rate is 40 percent. Also, Ann Arbor's target capital structure consists of 60 percent debt and 40 percent equity. Assuming that the firm is at, or close to, its target capital structure, then these weights represent the firm's current market value structure. To begin the adjustment, use Hamada's equation to obtain the beta for hospital assets:

$$b_{AAHS} = b_{Assets} \times [1 + [(1 - T) \times (D/E)]]$$

$$1.10 = b_{Assets} \times [1 + [(1 - 0.40) \times (0.60/0.40)]]$$

$$1.10 = b_{Assets} \times 1.90$$

$$b_{Assets} = 1.10/1.90 = 0.58.$$

Now, if 0.58 is the inherent market beta of hospital assets, what is the implied beta of such assets when they are **employed by Bayside Memorial Hospital**, which uses 50 percent debt financing and is tax exempt? To find the answer, we must again use Hamada's equation; but this time, we know the asset beta and are solving for the Bayside's implied equity beta:

$$b_{BMH} = b_{Assets} \times [1 + [(1 - T) \times (D/E)]]$$

$$= 0.58 \times [1 + [(1 - 0) \times (0.50/0.50)]]$$

$$= 0.58 \times 2.0 = 1.16.$$

Finally, remembering that the risk-free rate is 7.0 percent and the required rate of return on the market is 14.0 percent, we use the SML to estimate Bayside's cost of equity capital:

$$R(R_e) = RF + [R(R_M) - RF] \times b_{BMH}$$

$$= 7.0\% + [(14.0\% - 7.0\%) \times 1.16]$$

$$= 7.0\% + (7.0\% \times 1.16) = 15.12\% \approx 15.1\%.$$

Because the tax rate difference is greater than the debt financing difference, Bayside's 15.1 percent cost of equity is slightly greater than Ann Arbor's 14.8 percent cost of equity.

Before closing this section, a few words of caution are in order. There are a lot of issues that cast doubt not only on the accuracy of the adjustment process just described, but also on the entire concept of looking to a for-profit firm's cost of equity to set the opportunity cost inherent in the use of fund capital. Here are just a few:

• The risk to an investor-owned firm's stockholders is not the same as the risk to a not-for-profit business's stakeholders. Stockholders are well-diversified investors regarding stock ownership; but stakeholders may not be so well diversified regarding their "investment" in not-for-profit businesses. The point here is that failure of one stock in a well-diversified investment portfolio has minimal impact on a typical equity investor; but the failure of a not-for-profit business has a catastrophic impact on its stakeholders.

• In general, stock betas, and hence required rates of return on equity, are available only for very large firms, and the risk inherent in the stock ownership of a large, well-diversified firm typically is less than the riskiness of the equity capital of a smaller, less-diversified business. For example, stock ownership of HEALTHSOUTH, which has over 1,000 locations across the United States, even if held in isolation, is less risky than a stakeholder's position in a single outpatient rehabilitation center. In effect, corporate diversification lowers risk, so the comparison of a widely diversified firm with a single enterprise is suspect.

• The use of Hamada's equation is suspect because (1) there is no market value of a not-for-profit firm's fund capital, so the market value of equity is not really defined for not-for-profit firms; and (2) the derivation of Hamada's equation requires many unrealistic assumptions.

The bottom line here is that the entire process of estimating the cost of equity for not-for-profit businesses must be viewed with some skepticism. Nevertheless, the full opportunity cost estimate is the best that finance theory can muster; and a corporate cost of capital developed in this way is better, at least in our view, than ignoring the fact that there is an opportunity cost inherent in fund capital. One reaction to all the uncertainty involved in the estimation process might be to not use Hamada's equation to refine the estimate. Rather, just use Ann Arbor's cost of equity, without adjustment, as a proxy for Bayside's cost of fund capital. This simpler approach would result in an estimate for Bayside's cost of fund capital that is almost identical to the more complicated Hamada-adjusted estimate. Alternatively, if the entire opportunity cost process appears to be flawed, the growth rate cost could be assigned.

1. Is there a cost of equity for not-for-profit businesses?

2. How can this cost be estimated?

3. What does Hamada's equation attempt to do when it is used in the cost of equity estimation process?

Self-Test Questions

Estimating the Corporate Cost of Capital (CCC)

The final step in the cost of capital estimation process is to combine the debt and equity cost estimates to form the *corporate cost of capital (CCC)*. As we will discuss in the next chapter, each business has a target capital structure in mind, which is defined as the particular mix of debt and equity that causes its overall cost of capital to be minimized. Furthermore, when a business raises new capital, it generally tries to finance in a way that will keep the actual capital structure reasonably close to its target over time. The corporate cost of capital for any business, regardless of ownership, is calculated using the following equation:

$$CCC = [w_d \times R(R_d) \times (1 - T)] + [w_e \times R(R_e)].$$

Here, w_d and w_e are the target weights for debt and equity, respectively. The cost of the debt component, $R(R_d)$, will be an average if the firm uses several types of debt for its permanent financing. Alternatively, the above equation could be expanded to include multiple debt terms. Investor-owned businesses would use their marginal tax rate for T, while T would be zero for not-for-profit firms.

      The corporate cost of capital represents the cost of each new dollar of capital raised at the margin. It is **not** the average cost of all the dollars that the firm has raised in the past. Our primary interest is in obtaining a cost of capital for use in capital investment analysis; for such purposes, a *marginal cost* is required. The corporate cost of capital formula implies that each new dollar of capital will consist of both debt and equity that is raised, at least conceptually, in proportion to the firm's target capital structure.

Investor-Owned Businesses

To illustrate the corporate cost of capital calculation for investor-owned businesses, consider Ann Arbor Health Systems, which has a target capital structure of 60 percent debt and 40 percent equity. As previously estimated, the firm's before-tax cost of debt, $R(R_d)$, is 10.0 percent; its tax rate, T, is 40 percent; and its cost of equity, $R(R_e)$ is 14.8 percent. Using these data, Ann Arbor's corporate cost of capital is estimated to be 9.5 percent:

$$
\begin{aligned}
CCC_{AAHS} &= [w_d \times R(R_d) \times (1 - T)] + [w_e \times R(R_e)] \\
&= [0.60 \times 10.0\% \times (1 - 0.40)] + [0.40 \times 14.8\%] \\
&= 9.5\%.
\end{aligned}
$$

      Conceptually, every dollar of new capital that Ann Arbor obtains consists of 60 cents of debt, with an after-tax cost of 6.0 percent, and 40 cents of equity, with a cost of 14.8 percent. The average cost of each new dollar is 9.5 percent. In any one year, Ann Arbor may raise all its required new capital by issuing debt, by retaining earnings, or by selling new common stock. But over the long run, Ann Arbor plans to use 60 percent debt financing and 40 percent equity financing, so these are the appropriate weights for the cost of capital calculation.

Not-for-Profit Firms

The corporate cost of capital for not-for-profit firms is developed in the same way as for investor-owned businesses. To illustrate the concept, consider the following example. The corporate cost of capital for Bayside Memorial Hospital, assuming a target capital structure of 50 percent debt and 50 percent equity and using the estimates for the component costs that were developed earlier, is 10.6 percent:

$$CCC_{BMH} = [w_d \times R(R_d) \times (1 - T)] + [w_e \times R(R_e)]$$
$$= [0.50 \times 6.1\% \times (1 - 0)] + [0.50 \times 15.1\%]$$
$$= 10.6\%.$$

The primary reason that Bayside's corporate cost of capital estimate is greater than Ann Arbor's is that Ann Arbor uses more debt financing in its target mix, and hence uses more of the lower cost-financing component. Perhaps Ann Arbor, as a hospital system, has lower business risk, and hence can carry more debt in its optimal financing structure. (This issue will be pursued in the next chapter.)

Businesses, regardless of ownership, cannot raise unlimited amounts of new capital in any given year at a constant cost. Eventually, as more new capital is raised, investors will require higher returns on debt and equity capital, even though the capital is raised in accordance with the firm's target structure. Thus, the corporate costs of capital, as estimated here for Ann Arbor and Bayside, are only valid when the amount required for capital investment falls within each business's normal range. If capital is required in amounts that far exceed those normally raised, the corporate cost of capital must be subjectively adjusted upward to reflect the higher costs involved.

1. What is the general formula for the corporate cost of capital?
2. What weights should be used in the formula? Why?
3. What is the primary difference between the corporate costs of capital for investor-owned and not-for-profit firms?
4. Is the corporate cost of capital constant regardless of the amount of new capital required? Explain your answer.

Self-Test Questions

An Economic Interpretation of the Corporate Cost of Capital

Thus far, the focus of the cost of capital discussion has been on the mechanics of the estimation process. Now, it is worthwhile to step back from the mathematics of the process and to examine the corporate cost of capital's economic interpretation.

The component cost estimates (the costs of debt and equity) that make up a business's corporate cost of capital are based on the returns that investors require to supply capital to the firm. In turn, investors' required rates of return are based on the opportunity costs borne by investing in the debt and equity of the business in question, rather than in alternative investments of similar risk. These opportunity costs to investors, when combined into the corporate cost of capital, establish the **opportunity cost** to the business; that is, the corporate cost of capital is the return that the business could earn by investing in alternative investments that have the same risk as its own real assets. From a pure financial perspective, if a business cannot earn its corporate cost of capital on new capital investments, no new investments should be made and no new capital should be raised. If existing investments are not earning the corporate cost of capital, they should be terminated, the assets liquidated, and the proceeds returned to investors for reinvestment elsewhere.

Note that the corporate cost of capital sets the minimum return required on real-asset investments **regardless of the actual financing anticipated during the planning period**; that is, even if Ann Arbor planned to finance all new capital investments with debt financing, which has an estimated after-tax cost of 6.0 percent, the appropriate cost of capital to the firm is 9.5 percent. The rationale is that the debt financing could not be obtained at the current cost rate without Ann Arbor's equity base; so, in reality, the new capital investments are constructively being financed at the firm's target capital structure.

However, the corporate cost of capital is not the appropriate minimum rate of return for all new real-asset investments. The required rates of return set by investors on the business's debt and equity are based on perceptions regarding the riskiness of their investments, which, in turn, are based on two factors: (1) the inherent riskiness of the business and (2) the amount of debt financing used. Thus, the firm's inherent business risk and capital structure are embedded in its corporate cost of capital estimate.

Because different firms have different business risk and use different proportions of debt financing, different firms have different corporate costs of capital. Differential capital costs are most pronounced for firms in different industries, as evidenced by the wide variation in beta values contained in Table 10.3. Still, even firms in the same industry can have different business risk, and capital structure differences among such firms can compound corporate cost of capital differences.

The primary purpose of estimating a business's corporate cost of capital is to help make capital budgeting decisions; that is, the cost of capital will be used as the benchmark capital budgeting *hurdle rate* or the minimum return necessary for a project to be attractive financially. The firm can always earn its cost of capital by investing in securities that in the aggregate have the same risk as the firm's assets, so it should not invest in real assets unless it can earn at least as much. However, remember that the corporate cost of capital reflects opportunity costs based on the aggregate risk of the firm (i.e., the riskiness of the firm's average project). Thus, the corporate cost of capital can be applied without modification only to those projects under consideration that have average risk, where average is defined as that applicable to the firm's currently held assets in the aggregate. If a project under consideration has risk that differs significantly from that of the firm's average asset, then the corporate cost of capital must be adjusted to account for the differential risk when the project is being evaluated.[12]

To illustrate the concept, Ann Arbor Health System's corporate cost of capital, 9.5 percent, is probably appropriate for use in evaluating a new outpatient clinic that has risk similar to the hospital's average project, which involves the provision of both inpatient and outpatient services. Clearly, it would **not** be appropriate to apply Ann Arbor's 9.5 percent corporate cost of capital without adjustment to a new project that involves establishing a managed care subsidiary; this project does not have the same risk as the hospital's average asset. (To confirm the risk differential, refer to Table 10.3. Managed care plans have higher betas, and hence greater risk, than do hospitals.)

As discussed in Chapter 5, investors require higher returns for riskier investments. Thus, a high-risk project must have a higher *project cost of capital* than a low-risk project. Figure 10.1 illustrates the relationship between project risk, the corporate cost of capital, and project costs of capital. The figure illustrates that Ann Arbor's 9.5 percent corporate cost of capital is the appropriate hurdle rate **only** for an **average risk** project, Project A, where average means a project that has the same risk as the aggregate business. Project L, which has less risk than Ann Arbor's average project has a project cost of capital, 7.5 percent, that is less than the corporate cost of capital. Conversely, Project H, with more risk than the average project, has a higher project cost of capital, 11.5 percent.

The key point here is that the corporate cost of capital is merely a **benchmark** that will be used as the basis for estimating project costs of capital. It is not a one-size-fits-all rate that can be used with abandon whenever an opportunity cost is needed in a financial analysis. This point will be revisited in Chapter 13 when capital investment risk considerations are addressed.

1. Explain the economic interpretation of the corporate cost of capital.	**Self-Test**
2. Is the corporate cost of capital affected by short-term financing plans? Explain your answer.	**Questions**
3. Is the corporate cost of capital the appropriate opportunity cost for all projects that a business evaluates?	
4. Draw a graph similar to the one shown in Figure 10.1 and explain its implications.	

Flotation Costs

In our discussion of the corporate cost of capital, we have ignored flotation (issuance) costs. Under some circumstances, such costs can be large, especially for equity issues. One way of handling flotation costs is to incorporate them into the corporate cost of capital estimate, which has the effect of increasing the corporate cost of capital. Here are some points to consider regarding flotation costs.

FIGURE 10.1
Ann Arbor
Health Systems:
Corporate and
Project Costs of
Capital

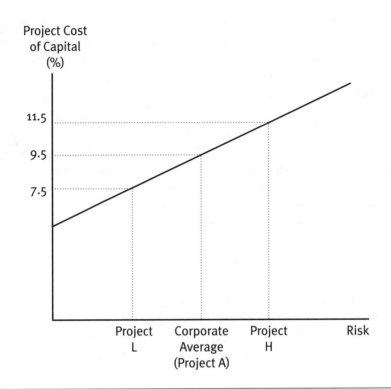

- For-profit businesses rarely issue new common stock. Rather, it is cheaper to obtain equity capital by earnings retention, which avoids flotation costs. Furthermore, flotation costs on public debt issues are relatively small, while such costs on private placements are near zero. Thus, only businesses that must go to the equity markets frequently bear substantial flotation costs.
- There is considerable uncertainty inherent in the cost of capital estimation process. Thus, attempting to "fine tune" the resulting estimate by incorporating flotation costs may be an exercise in futility.
- When flotation costs are significant, they can be incorporated into the decision process by adding them to the cost of the capital investments under consideration. Thus, if new capital to fund a business's new investments requires $2 million in flotation costs, this dollar cost can be assigned directly to the projects under consideration.

    For these reasons, and the fact that flotation costs do not play a major role in the corporate cost of capital of not-for-profit businesses, we have chosen not to incorporate flotation costs into the estimation process.[13]

Self-Test Question

1. Are flotation costs relevant to the corporate cost of capital estimate? Explain your answer.

Divisional Costs of Capital

The corporate cost of capital reflects the riskiness of the overall business in the aggregate. If the firm has only one line of business, then the corporate cost of capital can be used, with appropriate risk adjustments, on most projects under consideration by the firm. However, the corporate cost of capital may not be the appropriate benchmark (starting point) for projects that are in a line of business that differs from the overall firm.

When a firm has multiple divisions that operate in different business lines, it may be best to estimate a *divisional cost of capital* for each division and to use these estimates as the benchmarks for all capital project evaluations. The assumption here is that capital budgeting analyses will be conducted at the divisional level, so the best benchmark for such analyses is the one that reflects the riskiness of each division's business line.

To illustrate the concept, consider the following example. A for-profit healthcare system might, along with its provider network, have one subsidiary that invests primarily in real estate for medical uses and another subsidiary that runs an HMO. Clearly, each of these subsidiaries has its own unique business risk and optimal capital structure. The low-risk, high debt capacity real-estate subsidiary might have a divisional cost of capital of 10 percent, while the high-risk, low debt capacity HMO subsidiary might have a cost of capital of 14 percent. The health system, which consists of these two divisions plus provider assets, would likely have a cost of capital that falls between 10 and 14 percent, say, 12 percent.

If all capital budgeting decisions within the system were made on the basis of the system's 12 percent corporate cost of capital, the process would be biased in favor of the higher-risk HMO subsidiary. The cost of capital would be too low for the HMO subsidiary and too high for the real-estate subsidiary. Over time, this cost of capital bias would result in too many HMO projects being accepted and too few real-estate projects, which would skew the business line mix toward HMO assets, and hence increase the overall riskiness of the system. Of course, the answer to this problem is to use subsidiary costs of capital, rather than the corporate cost of capital, in the capital budgeting decision process.

Unlike individual project costs of capital, subsidiary costs of capital often can be estimated with some confidence because it is usually possible to identify publicly traded firms that are predominantly in the same line of business as the subsidiary. For example, the cost of capital for the HMO subsidiary could be estimated by looking at the debt and equity costs of the major for-profit HMOs, such as Humana and Aetna. This approach, in which a publicly traded firm in the same line of business is used as a proxy for a non-publicly traded business is called the *pure play* approach. If market data are at hand for pure play firms, it is relatively easy to develop subsidiary costs of capital.

As a final check in the process of estimating divisional costs of capital, note that the corporate cost of capital must equal the weighted average—say, by proportion of assets—of all of the subsidiary costs of capital. If this is not the case, then there are problems in the estimation process that must be resolved.

Self-Test Question
1. Explain the concept of divisional costs of capital.

Cost of Capital Estimation for Small Businesses

The guidance given thus far in the chapter focuses on the cost of capital estimation process for large healthcare businesses. But what if the business is small, such as a solo practice or small group practice? The estimation process is the same as described, but the manner in which the component costs are estimated must be handled differently.

Estimating the Cost of Debt

Small businesses typically obtain the bulk of their debt financing from commercial banks; so a business's bankers will be able to provide some insights on the cost of future debt financing. Alternatively, managers of small businesses can look to marketplace activity for guidance; that is, the interest rate currently being set on the debt issues of similar-risk firms can be used as an estimate of the cost of debt. Here, similar risk can be judged by subjective analysis (same industry, similar size, similar use of debt, and so on). Alternatively, the prime rate gives small businesses a benchmark for bank loan rates. If the business has borrowed from commercial banks in the past, its managers will know the historical premium charged above the prime rate for the business's bank debt. An awareness of the current interest rate environment generally permits managers to make a reasonable estimate for their own business's cost of debt, even when the business is quite small.

Estimating the Cost of Equity

Although estimating the cost of debt for a small business is relatively easy, the cost of equity estimate is more problematic.

Debt Cost plus Risk Premium Approach   Perhaps the easiest way to estimate the cost of equity of a small business is to use the debt cost plus risk premium method. Because the cost of debt is easy to estimate, it is equally easy to add some risk premium—say, 5 percentage points—to the business's cost of debt to obtain its cost of equity estimate. However, this can only be considered a "ballpark" estimate because the risk premiums that are applicable to small businesses may not be the same as those estimated for large firms.

Pure Play Approach   As an alternative, a proxy publicly traded firm in the same line of business can be identified, and its beta used to estimate the equity risk of the small business. This is the pure play approach introduced in the last major section. For example, consider the market betas given in Table 10.2. Here, we see that the betas for the two practice management firms listed are 1.75 and 1.98, for an average of roughly 1.85. **If the riskiness inherent in practice management is the same as the risk involved in the ownership of a small group practice**, then a beta of 1.85 can be used to proxy such ownership risk. Then, the CAPM approach can be used to estimate the small business's cost of equity. As in our previous discussions, Hamada's equation could be applied to refine the beta estimate.

To use the pure play approach for a small business, the assumption must be made that the risk to the owners of the publicly traded proxy firm is the same as the risk to the owners of the small business. However, there are several important differences between the ownership of stock in a large corporation and the ownership of, say, a small group practice. First, the geographic and business line diversification of a large business typically makes ownership less risky than a similar position in a small, localized single-line business. Second, most stockholders of large businesses hold that stock as part of a well-diversified investment portfolio that has returns that are not highly correlated with the stockholders' employment earnings. With a small group practice, the employment returns and equity returns typically are one and the same. Third, stock owned in an investment portfolio is highly liquid—the owner can sell it quickly at a fair market price with a single phone call. Conversely, an ownership position in a group practice is very difficult to sell.

All of these factors suggest that the cost of equity to a small owner-managed business is higher than that calculated using the CAPM and a proxy company. Unfortunately, finance theory cannot tell us how much higher. Finally, owners of small firms have a controlling interest in their businesses, while stockholders of large corporations do not. Control reduces risk, so this factor tends to reduce the cost of equity for small businesses as compared with large firms.

The Size Premium

Although returns data on businesses as small as a group practice are not readily available, studies using historical returns data indicate that the cost of equity for the smallest stocks—those in the bottom decile of market value—listed on the New York Stock Exchange is about 6 percentage points higher than the cost of equity for large businesses—those in the S&P500. This added premium to compensate for the additional risk inherent in the ownership of small, as opposed to large, businesses is called the *size premium*. It could be argued that the size premium is even larger than 6 percentage points for firms so small that their equity is not publicly traded. The bottom line here is when the cost of equity of a small business is estimated on the basis of equity costs to similar large businesses, an additional premium must be added just to account for size differences.

Final Thoughts on the Cost of Capital to Small Businesses

Although the estimation process clearly is more difficult, it may be even more important for small businesses to recognize their corporate costs of capital than it is for large businesses. The reason is that in small businesses, owners often have their livelihoods, as well as their equity investment, tied to the business. With the techniques described in this section, even a small business owner can "make a stab" at estimating his or her business's corporate cost of capital.

Self-Test Questions

1. What are the problems faced by small businesses when estimating the corporate cost of capital?
2. What is the size premium and how is it used?

Factors That Influence a Business's Cost of Capital

The corporate cost of capital estimate for any business is influenced by several factors. Some are external to the business, but some can be influenced by managerial actions.

Factors That Cannot Be Influenced

- **The level of interest rates.** Perhaps the factor that has the greatest impact on the cost of capital estimate is the general level of interest rates, which typically is a function of inflation expectations. In the early 1980s, interest rates were very high, and hence corporate costs of capital were very high. In such circumstances, only very high return projects are acceptable, and hence capital investment is low. Conversely, during the 1990s, interest rates in the United States were low, especially in comparison with other industrialized countries. The resulting relatively low cost of capital created an economic, and stock market, boom in the United States.
- **Tax rates.** High corporate tax rates lead to a lower cost of capital because the cost of debt is reduced by one minus the tax rate. At the same time, differential personal taxes encourage the use of one form of capital over another. For example, a capital gains tax rate that is lower than the ordinary tax rate lowers the cost of equity to taxable businesses relative to the cost of debt, and hence encourages the use of equity financing. High personal tax rates also affect the cost of debt to not-for-profit businesses because high tax rates makes tax-exempt debt more attractive to investors, and hence lowers the cost of tax-exempt (municipal) debt capital.

Factors That Can Be Influenced

- **Capital structure policy.** As we will discuss in the next chapter, the optimal capital structure is the structure that produces the lowest cost of capital to the business. Thus, businesses that are not using the optimal proportion of debt financing have a corporate cost of capital that is higher than necessary.

- **Capital investment policy.** A business's capital investment policy defines its line of business, which establishes the basic risk of the business. If a business adds more and more risky assets to its fixed asset portfolio, its corporate cost of capital will increase. Likewise, the addition of low risk assets will lower the cost of capital. Don't forget, however, that the corporate cost of capital is merely a benchmark, and new projects that have differential risk as compared to the business as a whole must use a cost of capital that differs from the corporate cost of capital.

1. What are the factors that affect the corporate cost of capital estimate?

Self-Test Question

Key Concepts

This chapter discusses the corporate cost of capital, which is a very important concept to the financial well-being of healthcare businesses. Here are its key concepts:

- The cost of capital to be used in capital budgeting decisions is the *weighted average* of the various types of permanent capital the firm uses, typically debt and common equity.
- The *component cost of debt* is the *after-tax* cost of new debt. For taxable businesses, it is found by multiplying the before-tax cost of new debt by $(1 - T)$, where T is the firm's marginal tax rate, so the component cost of debt is $R(R_d) \times (1 - T)$. For not-for-profit businesses, the debt is often tax-exempt, but no other tax effects apply, so the component cost of debt is merely the tax-exempt $R(R_d)$.
- The *cost of equity* for an investor-owned business is the rate of return investors require on the firm's common stock, and it is usually estimated by three methods: (1) the Capital Asset Pricing Model (CAPM) approach, (2) the discounted cash flow (DCF) approach, and (3) the debt cost plus risk premium approach.
- In the *CAPM approach*, the firm's beta coefficient is multiplied by the market risk premium to determine the firm's risk premium, and this risk premium is added to the risk-free rate to obtain the firm's cost of equity estimate.
- The best proxy for the *risk-free rate* is the yield on long-term T-bonds.
- There are three types of betas that can be used in the CAPM: (1) *historical,* (2) *adjusted,* and (3) *fundamental.*
- The market risk premium can be estimated either *historically* or *prospectively.*
- The *DCF approach* uses the dividend valuation model, which requires the current stock price, last dividend paid, and dividend growth rate to estimate the cost of equity.

- The growth rate can be estimated from historical dividend data, by using the *retention growth model,* or from securities analysts' forecasts.
- The *debt cost plus risk premium model* adds a risk premium to the firm's cost of debt estimate to obtain the cost of equity estimate.
- For not-for-profit businesses, the *cost of equity (fund capital)* can be approximated by the cost of equity of similar investor-owned firms. This approach considers the opportunity costs associated with the use of equity capital.
- Alternatively, the cost of equity to not-for-profit businesses can be set at the expected asset growth rate. This approach does not consider opportunity costs, but it does recognize that a return on equity is required if the business is to maintain a sound financial posture.
- Each firm has a *target capital structure,* and the target weights are used to estimate the firm's *corporate cost of capital (CCC)*:

$$CCC = [w_d \times R(R_d) \times (1 - T)] + [w_e \times R(R_e)].$$

- When making *capital investment decisions,* the firm will use the corporate cost of capital as the *hurdle rate* for **average-risk** projects.
- If a business has multiple divisions that operate in different business lines, then it is best to estimate a *divisional cost of capital* for each division.
- The corporate cost of capital for small businesses is estimated using the same techniques as for large businesses. However, the estimation of the component costs, particularly the cost of equity, becomes more difficult.
- There are several factors that influence the cost of capital estimate for any business including (1) the *current level of interest rates,* (2) *tax rates,* (3) *capital structure policy,* and (4) *capital investment policy.*

The concepts developed here will be used extensively throughout the text, especially in capital structure decisions—Chapter 11—and in capital budgeting decisions—Chapters 12 and 13.

Selected References

Boles, Keith E. 1986. "Implications of the Method of Capital Cost Payment on the Weighted Average Cost of Capital." *Health Services Research* (June): 191–211.

Sloan, Frank A., Joseph Valvona, and Mahmud Hassan. 1988. "Cost of Capital to the Hospital Sector." *Journal of Health Economics* (March): 25–45.

Smith, Dean G., and John R. C. Wheeler. 1989. "Accounting Based Risk Measures for Not-for-Profit Hospitals." *Health Services Management Research* (November): 221–226.

Wheeler, John R. C., and Dean G. Smith. 1988. "The Discount Rate for Capital Expenditure Analysis in Health Care." *Health Care Management Review* (Spring): 43–51.

Selected Web Sites

Selected web sites listed in Chapter 7 are applicable to cost of capital estimation.

To see some interesting articles related to cost of capital estimation, see the Ibbotson Associates site at *www.ibbotson.com*. When there, click on the button labeled Research at the top of the page and then click on Cost of Capital along the left side. You will then see a list of available articles.

Ibbotson Associates has another web site that gives some sample cost of capital estimate data, including a sample for the hospital industry. However, most of the data at this web site must be purchased; see *valuation.ibbotson.com*.

To access a "calculator" that can be used to estimate the corporate cost of capital for any business, see the Valuation Technologies site at *www.valtechs.com*. Then, click on the valuation methods button that refers to cost of capital calculation.

To access I/B/E/S EPS growth rate estimates, see the Market Guide site at *www.marketguide.com*. Then, enter the stock symbol for a firm (for example, HCA) in the Search For box, and click on Go. Finally, click on Earnings Estimates on the left side of the page to see the EPS forecasts.

The TeachMeFinance web site has several tutorial-type discussions that cover various aspects of financial management. For a cost of capital tutorial, see *teachmefinance.com*. Then, click on Cost of Capital in the list along the left side of the page.

Selected Cases

There is one case in *Cases in Healthcare Finance* that is applicable to this chapter:

Case 13: Bay Area Homecare, which focuses on the cost of capital estimation process for both investor-owned and not-for-profit businesses.

Notes

1. In our initial discussion of the cost of capital, we focus on large businesses. In a later section, we will discuss the estimation process for small businesses.

2. A question arises here as to whether the stated rate or the effective annual rate should be used in the cost of debt estimate. In general, the difference will be inconsequential, so most analysts opt for the easier approach, which is simply to use the stated rate. (The effective annual rate in this example is $[1.0305]^2 - 1.0 = 6.19\%$ versus a 6.1 percent stated rate.) More importantly, most capital budgeting analyses use end-of-year cash flows to approximate cash flows that occur throughout the year; in effect creating stated, as opposed to effective, cash flows. For consistency, we prefer to use a cost of capital that does not recognize intra-year compounding—the cash flows will be understated, but so will the cost of capital.

3. Only a few firms in the health services industry use preferred stock financing, so we will not include preferred stock in our cost of capital examples. If preferred stock is used as a source of permanent financing, then it should be included in the cost of capital estimate, and its cost would be estimated using procedures like those discussed for the cost of debt.

4. See *Stocks, Bonds, Bills and Inflation: 2000 Yearbook* (Chicago: Ibbotson Associates, 2000). Also, note that Ibbotson Associates now recommends using the T-bond rate as the proxy for the risk-free rate when using the CAPM. Before 1988, Ibbotson Associates recommended that the T-bill rate be used.

5. See Marshall E. Blume, "Betas and Their Regression Tendencies," *Journal of Finance,* June 1973, 785–796.

6. A commercial provider of betas once admitted that his firm, and others, did not know what the right period was to use, but that they decided to use five years to reduce the apparent differences between various services' betas—large differences reduced everyone's credibility!

7. Log-linear regression is a standard time-series linear regression in which the data points are plotted as natural logarithms. The advantage of a log-linear regression is that the slope of the regression line is the average annual growth rate, assuming continuous compounding. In a standard time-series linear regression of EPS or DPS, the slope of the regression line is the average annual dollar change.

8. The calculation given in the text produces an *arithmetic average* growth rate. A better measure of average growth is the *geometric average* growth rate, which is calculated as follows to be 7.0 percent:

$$(1.12)^5 \times (1.065)^{45} = (1+x)^{50}$$

$$1.76234 \times 17.01110 = (1+x)^{50}$$

$$29.97934 = (1+x)^{50}$$

$$1+x = (29.97934)^{1/50}$$

$$1+x = 1.070$$

$$x = 0.070 = 7.0\%.$$

The equation is asking: What annual growth rate in dividends over the entire 50 year period is equivalent to growth at 12 percent for 5 years, followed by growth at 6.5 percent for 45 years? The answer is an annual growth rate of 7.0 percent.

9. For one of the classic works on this topic, see Douglas A. Conrad, "Returns on Equity to Not-For-Profit Hospitals: Theory and Implementation," *Health Services Research,* April 1984, 41–63. Also, see the follow-up articles by Pauly; Conrad; and Silvers and Kauer in the April 1986 issue of *Health Services Research.*

10. For an excellent discussion of this issue, see William O. Cleverley, "Return on Equity in the Hospital Industry: Requirement or Windfall?" *Inquiry,* Summer 1982, 150–159.

11. For more information on Hamada's equation, see Robert S. Hamada, "Portfolio Analysis, Market Equilibrium, and Corporation Finance," *Journal of Finance,* March 1969, 13–31; or Eugene F. Brigham, Louis C. Gapenski, and Phillip R. Daves, *Intermediate Financial Management* (Fort Worth, TX: Dryden Press, 2000), Chapter 8.

12. In theory, the cost of capital should also be adjusted when projects under evaluation have optimal capital structures that differ from the business's target mix. Thus, if a project under evaluation by Ann Arbor had a *debt capacity* of 80 percent, versus 60 percent debt for the average project, this differential should

be considered when evaluating the project. However, in reality, debt capacities for individual projects typically are impossible to estimate; so the adjustments made to the corporate cost of capital usually are confined to risk differentials.

13. For more information on flotation cost adjustments, see Eugene F. Brigham, Louis C. Gapenski, and Phillip R. Daves, *Intermediate Financial Management* (Fort Worth, TX: Dryden Press, 2000), Chapter 5.

CAPITAL STRUCTURE DECISIONS

Learning Objectives

After studying this chapter, readers should be able to:

- Explain the effects of debt financing on a business's risk and return.
- Briefly describe the primary capital structure theories and their implications for managers.
- Discuss the factors that influence the choice between debt and equity financing.
- Explain how businesses choose debt maturities.

Introduction

In Chapter 10, when we discussed a business's corporate cost of capital, we noted that the weights used in the calculation represent the optimal, or target, mix of debt and equity financing. These weights are defined by the *capital structure* decision. We will see in this chapter that managers analyze a number of quantitative and qualitative factors, and then establish the *optimal*, or *target*, *capital structure* for the business. Often, because of uncertainties in the estimation process, the target is expressed as a range rather than as a point value. The target will undoubtedly change over time as conditions that are both internal and external to the business change; but at any given moment, managers have a specific capital structure in mind.

The target structure plays a major role in financing decisions for the business. If too little debt is actually on hand, new financings will be biased toward the use of debt. Conversely, if too much debt is on the books, equity would be the first choice for new capital. The key here is that one of the most important factors that influence financing decisions is the target capital structure. Managers prefer to finance in a way that keeps the business on target. Once the choice of optimal capital structure is made, managers must consider the maturity structure of the debt component. Should the debt be all long term, all short term, or some combination of the two? This chapter addresses both decisions in detail.

Impact of Debt Financing on Risk and Return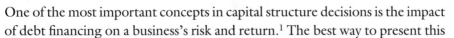

One of the most important concepts in capital structure decisions is the impact of debt financing on a business's risk and return.[1] The best way to present this concept is by illustration. Assume that a new business, Super Health, Inc., is being formed. The business requires $200,000 in assets to get into operation, and there are only two financing alternatives available to it: (1) all equity and (2) 50 percent equity and 50 percent debt.

Table 11.1 contains the business's projected starting balance sheet and first year's income statement under the two financing alternatives. To begin, consider the balance sheets shown in the top portion of the table. The business will require $100,000 in current assets and $100,000 in fixed assets to begin operations. Because asset requirements depend on the nature and size of the business rather than on how the business will be financed, the asset side of the balance sheet is unaffected by the financing scheme. However, the capital, or claims, side of the balance sheet is influenced by the type of financing. Under the all-equity alternative, the owners must put up the entire $200,000 needed to purchase the assets. If 50 percent debt financing is used, the owners will contribute only $100,000, with the remaining $100,000 to be obtained from creditors—say, a bank loan with a 10 percent interest rate.

Now, consider the impact of the two financing alternatives on Super Health's projected income statement. First-year revenues are projected to be $150,000 and operating costs are forecasted at $100,000, so the business's operating income—earnings before interest and taxes (EBIT)—is expected to be $50,000. Because the method of financing does not affect revenues

TABLE 11.1
Super Health, Inc.: Projected Financial Statements Under Two Financing Alternatives

Balance Sheets

	Equity	Debt/Equity
Current assets	$ 100,000	$ 100,000
Fixed assets	100,000	100,000
Total assets	$ 200,000	$ 200,000
Bank loan (10% cost)	$ 0	$ 100,000
Total equity	200,000	100,000
Total claims	$ 200,000	$ 200,000

Income Statements

	Equity	Debt/Equity
Revenues	$ 150,000	$ 150,000
Operating costs	100,000	100,000
Operating income (EBIT)	$ 50,000	$ 50,000
Interest expense	0	10,000
Taxable income	$ 50,000	$ 40,000
Taxes (40%)	20,000	16,000
Net income	$ 30,000	$ 24,000
ROE	15%	24%
Total dollar return to investors	$ 30,000	$ 34,000

and operating costs, the operating income projection is the same under both financing alternatives. However, interest expense must be paid if debt financing is used, so the debt/equity alternative results in a $0.10 \times \$100,000 = \$10,000$ annual interest charge, while no interest expense occurs if the business is entirely equity financed. The result is taxable income of $50,000 under the all-equity alternative, and lower taxable income of $40,000 under the 50 percent debt alternative. Because the business anticipates being taxed at a 40 percent federal-plus-state rate, the expected tax liability is $0.40 \times \$50,000 = \$20,000$ under the all-equity alternative and $0.40 \times \$40,000 = \$16,000$ for the debt/equity alternative. Finally, when taxes are deducted from the income stream, Super Health projects a net income of $30,000 if all-equity financed and $24,000 if 50 percent debt financing is used.

At first glance, all-equity financing appears to be the best strategy. After all, if the business uses 50 percent debt financing, its projected net income will fall by $\$30,000 - \$24,000 = \$6,000$. But the conclusion that debt financing is bad requires closer examination. Business owners are less concerned with net income than with the return that is expected on their equity investment. Perhaps the most meaningful measure of return to a business's owners is the rate of return on equity, or just return on equity (ROE), which is defined as Net income / Total equity. Under all-equity financing, the projected ROE is $\$30,000 / \$200,000 = 0.15 = 15\%$; but with 50 percent debt financing, projected ROE increases to $\$24,000 / \$100,000 = 24\%$. The key here is that although net income decreases with debt financing, so does the amount of owner-supplied capital, and the capital requirement decreases proportionally more than does net income.

The end result is that the use of debt financing increases the expected rate of return on equity capital. Why does this positive result happen? There is no magic here. The key is in the tax code—Interest expense is tax-deductible for investor-owned businesses while dividend distributions are not. To understand the impact of the tax deductibility of interest, take another look at the Table 11.1 income statements. The total dollar return to all investors, including both owners and creditors, is $30,000 in net income if all-equity financed, but $24,000 in net income plus $10,000 of interest, for a total of $34,000, when 50 percent debt financing is used. Where did the "extra" $4,000 come from? The answer is "from the tax man." Taxes are $20,000 if Super Health is all-equity financed, but only $16,000 when debt financing is used; and $4,000 less in taxes means $4,000 more for investors. Because debt financing reduces taxes, more of a business's operating income (EBIT) is available for distribution to investors, including both owners and creditors.

It now appears that Super Health's financing decision is clear. Given only the two alternatives, Super Health should use the 50 percent debt alternative because it provides the owners with the higher return on investment. Unfortunately, like the proverbial no free lunch, there is a catch. The use of debt financing not only increases owners' return, it also increases their risk.

To demonstrate the risk-increasing characteristics of debt financing, consider Table 11.2. Here we recognize that Super Health, like all businesses, is risky. The owners do not know precisely what the first year's revenues and operating costs will be. Assume, for illustrative purposes, that Revenues − Operating costs = Operating income could be as low as $0 or as high as $100,000 in the business's first year of operations. Furthermore, assume that there is a 25 percent chance of the worst and the best cases occurring, and a 50 percent chance that the Table 11.1 forecast, with an operating income of $50,000, will be realized.

The assumptions regarding uncertainty in the future profitability of the business lead to three different ROEs for each financing alternative. The expected ROEs—the sum of the probability-outcome products—are the same as when we ignored uncertainty; that is, 15 percent if Super Health is all-equity financed and 24 percent when 50 percent debt financing is used. However, the uncertainty in operating income produces uncertainty, and hence risk, in owners' returns. If we measure owners' risk by the standard deviation of ROE, we see that the return is more risky when 50 percent debt financing is used. To be precise, owners' risk is twice as much in the 50 percent debt financing alternative: 21.2 percent standard deviation of ROE versus 10.6 percent standard deviation in the zero-debt alternative.

Intuitively, this risk increase occurs because the use of debt financing imposes a fixed cost—the $10,000 interest expense—into an uncertain income stream; that is, the fixed interest payment must be made regardless of the level of operating income. The insertion of the fixed interest expense magnifies the variability of all values below the insertion point. Note that the increased risk is apparent without performing any calculations. Under all-equity financing, the worst result is an ROE of zero. However, with 50 percent debt financing,

	Equity			Debt/Equity		
TABLE 11.2 Super Health, Inc.: Partial Income Statements in an Uncertain World						
Probability	0.25	0.50	0.25	0.25	0.50	0.25
Operating income (EBIT)	$0	$50,000	$100,000	$0	$50,000	$100,000
Interest expense	0	0	0	10,000	10,000	10,000
Taxable income	$0	$50,000	$100,000	($10,000)	$40,000	$90,000
Taxes (40%)	0	20,000	40,000	(4,000)	16,000	36,000
Net income	$0	$30,000	$60,000	($6,000)	$24,000	$54,000
ROE	0%	15%	30%	−6%	24%	54%
Expected ROE		15%			24%	
Standard deviation of ROE		10.6%			21.2%	

the owners could realize a ROE of −6 percent. (Here the assumption is made that the business's $10,000 loss could be used to offset the owners' personal income, resulting in a $4,000 tax savings. If this were not the case, the loss would be even worse.) In fact, with no operating income to pay the $10,000 interest due if the worst case scenario occurs, the owners would either have to put up additional personal funds or declare the business bankrupt. Clearly, the use of 50 percent debt financing has increased the riskiness of the equity investment in the business.

This simple example illustrates two key points about the use of debt financing:

1. The use of debt financing increases the percentage return (ROE) to a business's owners. Note, however, that for the use of debt financing to increase owners' returns, the basic (inherent) return on the business must be greater than the interest rate on the debt. The basic return on the business in the Super Health illustration is 25 percent ($50 in operating income divided by $200 in assets), and debt financing costs only 10 percent, so the use of debt financing increases ROE.
2. At the same time that return is increased, the use of debt financing also increases owners' risk. In the Super Health example, we saw that 50 percent debt financing doubled the risk to owners (as measured by standard deviation of ROE).

Super Health's ultimate decision regarding financial structure is not clear-cut. One alternative—no debt—has a lower expected ROE, but also lower risk. The second alternative—50 percent debt—offers a higher expected ROE, but only at the price of higher risk. To complicate matters even more, there is actually an almost unlimited number of debt level choices available to the business, not just the 50/50 mix used in the illustration. Later sections will try to resolve the dilemma facing Super Health; but first we need to introduce some other concepts.

Self-Test Questions

1. What is the impact of debt financing on a business's risk and return?
2. Why does the use of debt financing leverage up (increase) the return to stockholders?

Business and Financial Risk

In Chapter 5, we discussed several different dimensions of risk, including stand-alone risk and portfolio (corporate and market) risk. Now, we introduce two new dimensions: (1) business risk and (2) financial risk. Here, the term "financial risk" has a very specific connotation, as opposed to its use in Chapter 5 where the term was used generically to mean the risk arising from business transactions as opposed to other types of risk such as risk to life and limb. Note that the concepts of business and financial risk apply just as much to not-for-profit businesses as they do to for-profit businesses; but in not-for-profits the risk concepts apply to the business's noncreditor stakeholders, rather than to the business's owners.

Business Risk

Business risk is the inherent riskiness of a business as seen by its owners, and it is measured by the uncertainty inherent in the business's ROE **assuming that no debt financing is used**. To illustrate the concept of business risk, consider Santa Fe Healthcare, Inc., a **debt-free** investor-owned hospital chain that operates in the Southwestern United States. Figure 11.1 provides some insights into the firm's business risk.

The top graph gives both security analysts and Santa Fe's management an idea of the historical variability of ROE, and consequently how the firm's ROE might vary in the future. This graph also shows that Santa Fe's ROE is growing slowly; so the relevant variability of ROE is the dispersion about the trend line rather than the overall standard deviation of historical ROE. The lower graph shows the beginning-of-year subjectively estimated probability distribution of Santa Fe's ROE for 2000, based on the trend line in the top section of Figure 11.1. As both graphs indicate, Santa Fe's actual ROE in 2000 was only 8 percent, well below the expected value of 12 percent.

Santa Fe's past fluctuations in ROE were caused by many factors—changes in the economy, actions by competing hospitals, changes in payer mix, payment policies of third-party payers, changing labor costs, and so on. Similar events will undoubtedly occur in the future and because they do, Santa Fe's realized ROE will almost always be higher or lower than the projected level. Furthermore, there is always the possibility that some event that permanently depresses the company's earning power might occur. For example, the federal government could move to a single-payer system with dramatically reduced hospital reimbursement rates.

Because Santa Fe uses no debt financing, the uncertainty regarding its future ROE defines the firm's business risk. The key point here is that we are trying to measure the riskiness of the business before it is influenced by the use of debt financing. Business risk varies not only from industry to industry, but also among firms in a given industry. Furthermore, business risk can change over time. As mentioned in the previous chapter, hospitals were regarded for years as having little business risk, but events in the 1980s and 1990s—primarily the move of governmental payers to prospective payment and the increasing bargaining power of managed care plans—greatly increased the industry's business risk.

Business risk depends on a number of factors, including the following:

• **Demand variability.** The more stable the demand for a business's products or services, other things held constant, the lower its business risk.

FIGURE 11.1

Sante Fe
Healthcare:
Trend in ROE,
1990–2000,
and Subjective
ROE
Distribution,
2000

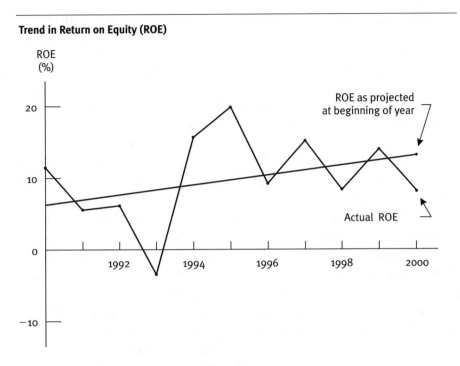

Trend in Return on Equity (ROE)

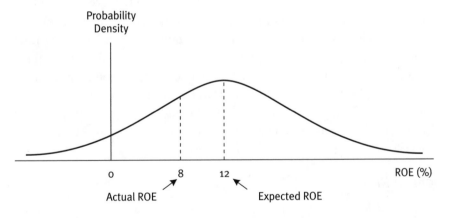

Subjective Probability Distribution of (ROE)

- **Sales price variability.** Businesses whose products or services are sold in markets with highly volatile prices are exposed to more business risk than firms whose sales prices are more stable.
- **Input cost variability.** Businesses whose input costs—labor, materials, and capital—are highly uncertain are exposed to a high degree of business risk.
- **Ability to raise output prices.** Some businesses are better able than others to raise their own prices when input costs rise. The greater the ability to adjust prices to reflect cost conditions, the lower the degree of business risk, other things held constant.
- **Operating leverage.** *Operating leverage* measures the proportion of fixed

costs, as opposed to variable costs, in a business's cost structure. If a high percentage of a business's costs are fixed, and hence do not decline when demand falls off, then the business is exposed to a relatively high degree of business risk.

Each of the factors that influence business risk is determined partly by industry characteristics; but each of them also can be influenced to some extent by managerial decisions. For example, consider operating leverage. Higher fixed costs generally are associated with more highly technical, capital-intensive businesses and industries. Thus, hospitals have higher fixed costs, relative to total costs, than do home health care agencies. Also, healthcare providers that employ highly skilled workers who must be retained and paid even during periods of low utilization have a relatively high proportion of fixed costs.

To what extent can businesses control their operating leverage? Operating leverage is determined by industry characteristics to a large extent. Firms such as drug manufacturers, hospitals, and ambulatory care clinics simply must have heavy investments in fixed assets and labor, which results in a high proportion of fixed costs and, hence, high operating leverage. On the other hand, firms such as home health agencies generally have significantly lower fixed cost proportions and, hence, lower operating leverage. Still, although industry factors do exert a major influence, all businesses do have some control over their operating leverage. For example, a hospital can expand its diagnostic imaging capability by either buying a new imaging device or by leasing it on a per procedure basis.[2] If the device were purchased, the hospital would incur fixed costs, but the device's per procedure operating costs would be relatively low. If leased, the hospital would have lower fixed costs, but the variable—per procedure—costs for the device would be higher. Thus, by its financing decisions, and also by its capital investment decisions, a business can influence its operating leverage, and hence its basic business risk.

Financial Risk

Financial risk is the additional risk placed on owners as a result of the decision to use debt financing. Conceptually, a business has a certain amount of risk inherent in its operations—this is its business risk. However, the use of debt financing, or *financial leverage*, concentrates (increases) the risk seen by the business's owners. Because the return to debt suppliers is fixed by contract and is independent of fluctuations in the business's revenues and costs, creditors bear a fixed amount of the firm's business risk. To illustrate the concept, consider the Super Health illustration. The business could be financed either by $200,000 of equity or $100,000 of equity and $100,000 of debt. Using debt financing concentrates the business risk of the enterprise, which is fixed, on a smaller equity base, and hence increases owner's risk.

Business and financial risk can be easily measured. Refer again to Table 11.2. The standard deviation of ROE to Super Health if it uses no debt financing, $\sigma_{ROE(U)}$, where U stands for unleveraged (no debt), measures its business risk. The standard deviation of ROE at any positive debt level, $\sigma_{ROE(L)}$, where L stands for leveraged (some debt), measures the risk borne by owners. Because the use of debt financing increases the risk to owners, $\sigma_{ROE(L)}$ is always greater than $\sigma_{ROE(U)}$. Financial risk is the difference between the actual risk seen by owners and the inherent business risk of the enterprise, or $\sigma_{ROE(L)} - \sigma_{ROE(U)}$. Applying these measures to Super Health, we see that its business risk is $\sigma_{ROE(U)} = 10.6\%$ and its risk under 50 percent debt financing is $\sigma_{ROE(L)} = 21.2\%$, so the financial risk at that level of debt is $\sigma_{ROE(L)} - \sigma_{ROE(U)} = 21.2\% - 10.6\% = 10.6\%$.

Operating leverage and financial leverage normally work in the same way; they both increase expected ROE, but they also increase the risk borne by owners. Operating leverage affects the business risk of the enterprise, while financial leverage affects its financial risk.

1. What is business risk? How can it be measured?
2. What are some determinants of business risk?
3. What is operating leverage?
4. What is financial risk? How can it be measured?
5. What are the similarities between operating leverage and financial leverage?

Self-Test Questions

Capital Structure Theory

The preceding discussion points out the fact that the use of debt financing increases the expected return on equity capital, but it also increases the overall risk of the business. The obvious question now is whether the benefit of debt financing—increased expected return—exceeds the cost of debt financing—increased risk. *Capital structure theory* attempts to determine the relationship between the amount of debt financing and the value of a business; thus, its goal is to determine, after risk is considered, whether the use of financial leverage is beneficial or not. Although capital structure theory does not provide a complete answer to the optimal capital structure question, it does provide many insights into the value of debt financing versus equity (or fund) financing. Thus, an understanding of capital structure theory will aid managers in making capital structure decisions.

The Modigliani-Miller Models

Until 1958, capital structure theories were little more than loose assertions about investor behavior rather than carefully constructed models that could be tested by formal statistical studies. In what has been called the most influential set of financial papers ever published, *Franco Modigliani and Merton Miller (MM)* addressed the capital structure issue in a rigorous, scientific fashion, and set off a chain of research that continues to this day.[3]

Assumptions

To begin, Modigliani and Miller made the following assumptions, some of which were later relaxed.

- The business risk of an enterprise can be measured by the standard deviation of earnings before interest and taxes (σ_{EBIT}). Firms with the same degree of business risk are said to be in a *homogeneous risk class*.
- All present and prospective investors have identical estimates of each firm's future EBIT; that is, investors have *homogeneous expectations* about expected future corporate earnings and the riskiness of those earnings.
- Stocks and bonds are traded in *perfect capital markets*. This assumption implies, among other things, that there are no brokerage costs and that investors—both individual and institutions—can borrow at the same rate as corporations.
- The debt of businesses and individuals is *riskless*, so the interest rate on debt is the risk-free rate. Furthermore, this situation holds regardless of how much debt a business, or an individual, uses.
- All cash flows are perpetuities; that is, businesses are assumed to have *zero growth* with an "expectationally constant" EBIT, and its bonds are perpetuities. "Expectationally constant" means that investors expect EBIT to be constant; but the realized, or after the fact, value in any year could be different from the expected level.

MM Without Taxes

Modigliani and Miller first performed their analysis under the assumption that there are no corporate or personal income taxes. On the basis of the preceding assumptions, and in the absence of taxes, they proposed and then algebraically proved two propositions:[4]

Proposition I   The value of any business, V, is established by discounting its expected net operating income (EBIT when T = 0) at a constant rate that is appropriate for its risk class, regardless of the amount of debt financing used:

$$V_L = V_U = \frac{EBIT}{CCC} = \frac{EBIT}{R(R_{eU})}.$$

Here, the subscripts L and U designate levered—with debt financing—and unlevered—without debt financing—businesses in a given risk class; CCC is the corporate cost of capital; and $R(R_{eU})$ is the required rate of return on equity for an unlevered (zero debt) business. The key point here is that the discount rate used to determine the value of the business is a constant, $CCC = R(R_{eU})$, regardless of the amount of debt financing used, and because EBIT is unaffected by debt financing, the value of the business also is a constant.

Since V, as established by Proposition I, is a constant regardless of the level of debt financing, then **under the MM model with no taxes, the value**

of a business is independent of its leverage. This also implies (1) that the CCC to any business is completely independent of its capital structure; and (2) that the CCC for all businesses with the same business risk (in the same risk class) is equal to the cost of equity to an unlevered firm in that same risk class, regardless of the amount of debt financing used.

The cost of equity to a levered firm, $R(R_{eL})$, is equal to (1) the cost of equity **Proposition II** to an unlevered firm in the same risk class, $R(R_{eU})$, plus (2) a risk premium that depends both on the differential between the costs of equity and debt to an unlevered firm and the amount of leverage used:

$$R(R_{eL}) = R(R_{eU}) + \text{Risk Premium} = R(R_{eU}) + \{[R(R_{eU}) - R(R_d)] \times (D/E)\}.$$

Here, D = market value of the business's debt; E = market value of the business's equity; and $R(R_d)$ = constant cost of debt. Proposition II states that **as a business's use of debt increases, its cost of equity also rises, and in a mathematically precise manner.**

Taken together, the two MM propositions imply that the inclusion of debt in a business's capital structure will not increase its value because the benefits of the less costly, as compared to equity, debt financing will be exactly offset by an increase in the riskiness, and hence in the cost, of the business's equity. Thus, MM theory implies that **in a world without taxes, both the value of a firm and its corporate cost of capital are unaffected by its capital structure.**

MM used an *arbitrage proof* to support their propositions.[5] They showed that, under their assumptions, if two firms differed only (1) in the way they are financed and (2) in their total market values, then investors would sell shares of the higher-valued firm, buy those of the lower-valued firm, and continue this process until the firms had exactly the same market value. Thus, the actions of investors would ensure that the two firms had identical market values, and hence stock prices. Once the values are proved to be equal, the two MM propositions are the logical result.[6]

Note that each of the assumptions listed in the beginning of this section is necessary for the arbitrage proof to work. For example, if the firms are not identical in business risk, then the arbitrage process could not be invoked. We will discuss further implications of the assumptions later in the chapter.

MM with Corporate Taxes

Modigliani and Miller's original work, published in 1958, assumed zero taxes. In 1963, MM published a second article that includes corporate tax effects. With corporate income taxes, the authors concluded that the use of financial leverage will increase a business's value. When businesses are subject to income taxes, the Modigliani and Miller propositions are as follows.

Proposition I   The value of a levered firm is equal to (1) the value of an unlevered firm in the same risk class plus (2) the gain from leverage, which is the present value of the tax savings and which equals the corporate tax rate, T, times the amount of debt the firm uses, D:[7]

$$V_L = V_U + (T \times D).$$

The important point here is that when corporate taxes are introduced, the value of a levered business exceeds that of a similar unlevered business by the amount $T \times D$. Note also that the differential increases as the use of debt increases, so a business's value is maximized at virtually 100 percent debt financing.

To find the value for V_U for any business, recognize that all businesses are assumed to have zero growth, a constant EBIT, and all earnings are paid out as dividends. Thus, the total market value of a business's equity, E, can be found using perpetuity valuation techniques as follows:

$$E = \frac{\text{Dividends}}{R(R_e)} = \frac{\text{Net income}}{R(R_e)} = \frac{\{\text{EBIT} - [R(R_d) \times D]\} \times (1-T)}{R(R_e)}.$$

With zero debt, $D = \$0$ and the total value of the firm is its equity value, so

$$E = V_U = \frac{\text{EBIT} \times (1-T)}{R(R_{eU})}.$$

Proposition II   The cost of equity to a levered firm is equal to (1) the cost of equity to an unlevered firm in the same risk class (equal business risk); plus (2) a risk premium that depends on the differential between the costs of equity and debt to an unlevered firm, the amount of financial leverage used, **and the corporate tax rate**:

$$R(R_{eL}) = R(R_{eU}) + \text{Risk Premium}$$

$$= R(R_{eU}) + \{[R(R_{eU}) - R(R_d)] \times (1-T) \times (D/E)\}.$$

Notice that Proposition II here is identical to the corresponding without-tax equation, **except for the term $(1-T)$**. Because $(1-T)$ is less than 1.0 for any positive tax rate, the imposition of corporate taxes causes the cost of equity to rise at a slower rate when debt is used than it did in the absence of taxes. It is this characteristic, along with the fact that the effective cost of debt is reduced because of the tax deductibility of interest, that produces the Proposition I result—namely, the increase in firm value as leverage increases.

Illustration of the MM models

To illustrate the Modigliani and Miller models, assume that the following data and conditions hold for New England Clinical Laboratories, Inc., an old, established firm that operates in several no-growth areas in rural Maine, New Hampshire, and Vermont:

- New England currently has no debt; it is an all-equity firm.
- Expected EBIT = $2,400,000. EBIT is not expected to increase over time, so New England is in a no-growth situation.
- New England pays out all of its income as dividends because no retained earnings are required to finance growth. (Worn-out assets are replaced using depreciation cash flow.)
- If New England begins to use debt, it can borrow at a rate $R(R_d)$ = 8%. This borrowing rate is constant, and it is independent of the amount of debt used. Any money raised by selling debt would be used to retire common stock, so New England's assets and EBIT would remain constant.
- The risk of New England's assets, and thus its EBIT, is such that its shareholders require a rate of return, $R(R_{eU})$, of 12 percent if no debt is used.

To begin, assume that there are no taxes, so T = 0%. At any level of debt, **With Zero** Proposition I can be used to find New England's value, $20 million: **Taxes**

$$V_L = V_U = \frac{EBIT}{R(R_{eU})} = \frac{\$2.4 \text{ million}}{0.12} = \$20.0 \text{ million}.$$

With zero debt, the $20 million represents all-equity value. Now, assume that New England decides to use $10 million of debt financing. According to Proposition I, its total value will not change, so the business's equity value must fall to $10 million:

$$E = V - D = \$20 \text{ million} - \$10 \text{ million} = \$10 \text{ million}.$$

This decrease occurs because the $10 million of new debt financing is used to repurchase $10 million of existing equity.

We can also find New England's cost of equity, $R(R_{eL})$, and its corporate cost of capital (CCC) at a debt level of $10 million. First, we use Proposition II to find $R(R_{eL})$, New England's levered cost of equity:

$$R(R_{eL}) = R(R_{eU}) + \{[R(R_{eU}) - R(R_d)] \times (D/E)\}$$
$$= 12\% + \{[12\% - 8\%] \times (\$10\text{million}/\$10\text{million})\}$$
$$= 12\% + 4.0\% = 16.0\%.$$

Now, we can find the firm's corporate cost of capital:

$$CCC = [w_d \times R(R_d) \times (1 - T)] + [w_e \times R(R_{eL})]$$
$$= [(\$10/\$20) \times 8\% \times 1.0] + [(\$10/\$20) \times 16.0\%] = 12.0\%.$$

We could easily expand the illustration to show New England's value and corporate cost of capital at various debt levels. We would see that in a MM world without taxes, financial leverage does not matter: The value of the firm and its overall cost of capital are independent of the amount of debt financing. The key to this result is that the additional risk imposed by the use of debt financing increases the cost of equity just enough to counteract any benefit that results from the fact that debt costs are lower than equity costs. In essence, each of these security classes is priced—has a required rate of return—such that the business is indifferent to the choice. Debt costs less than equity, but it is a riskier form of financing than equity. Thus, each type of capital is priced correctly on the basis of the risk that it brings to a business.

With Corporate Taxes
To illustrate the MM model with corporate taxes, assume that all of the previous assumptions hold except these two:

1. Expected EBIT = $4,000,000.
2. New England has a 40 percent federal-plus-state tax rate, so T = 40%.

Note that we increased New England's EBIT from $2.4 million to $4 million to make the numerical comparison between the two models easier. If we had not, **the introduction of corporate taxes would lower New England's value by Expected EBIT × (1 − T) = $2.4 million × 0.6 = $1.44 million.**

When New England has zero debt but pays taxes, and its expected EBIT is increased to $4 million, its value with zero debt financing is $20 million:

$$V_U = \frac{EBIT \times (1-T)}{R(R_{eU})} = \frac{\$4 \text{ million} \times 0.6}{0.12} = \$20.0 \text{ million.}$$

With $10 million of debt in a world with taxes, Proposition I indicates that New England's total market value rises to $24 million.

$$V_L = V_U + (T \times D) = \$20 \text{ million} + (0.4 \times \$10 \text{ million}) = \$24 \text{ million.}$$

Therefore, the value of New England's equity must be $14 million:

$$E = V_L - D = \$24 \text{ million} - \$10 \text{ million} = \$14 \text{ million.}$$

We can also find New England's cost of equity and its corporate cost of capital at a debt level of $10 million. First, we use Proposition II to find the levered cost of equity:

$$R(R_{eL}) = R(R_{eU}) + \{[R(R_{eU}) - R(R_d)] \times (1-T) \times (D/E)\}$$
$$= 12\% + [(12\% - 8\%) \times 0.6 \times (\$10 \text{ million}/\$14 \text{ million})]$$
$$= 12\% + 1.71\% = 13.71\%.$$

Now, we can find the firm's weighted average cost of capital:

$$CCC = [w_d \times R(R_d) \times (1-T)] + [w_e \times R(R_{eL})]$$
$$= [(\$10/\$24) \times 8\% \times 0.6] + [(\$14/\$24) \times 13.71\%] = 10.0\%.$$

Again, we could easily expand the illustration to include additional debt levels. We see that in a MM world with corporate taxes, financial leverage does matter: The value of the firm is maximized and its overall cost of capital is minimized if it uses virtually 100 percent debt financing. Furthermore, we know that the increase in value solely results from the tax deductibility of interest payments, which causes both the cost of debt and the increase in the cost of equity with leverage to be reduced by $(1 - T)$. With tax deductibility of interest payments, the cost of debt is now less than that warranted by the risk that it bring to a business, and hence businesses prefer debt to equity, which remains fairly priced in relationship to the risk that it brings to a business.

1. What is the single most important conclusion of the MM zero-tax model?
2. What is the single most important conclusion of the MM model with corporate taxes?
3. What is the underlying cause of the "gain from leverage" in the MM model with corporate taxes?

The Miller Model

Although Modigliani and Miller included **corporate** taxes in the second version of their model, they did not extend the model to analyze the effects of **personal** taxes. However, Merton Miller later introduced a model designed to show how leverage affects firms' values when both personal and corporate taxes are taken into account.[8] To explain Miller's model, let us begin by defining T_c as the corporate tax rate, T_e as the personal tax rate on equity returns, and T_d as the personal tax rate on debt returns. Note that equity returns typically come partly as dividends and partly as capital gains, so T_e is a weighted average of the effective tax rates on dividends and capital gains, while essentially all debt income comes from interest, which is taxed at investors' top rates.

With personal taxes included, **and under the remaining assumptions used in the earlier MM models,** the value of an unlevered firm is found by the following equation:

$$V_U = \frac{EBIT \times (1 - T_c) \times (1 - T_e)}{R(R_{eU})}.$$

Note that this is the same equation as used in the previous examples, except for the addition of the $(1 - T_e)$ term, which adjusts for personal taxes. Now, the numerator shows how much of a business's operating cash flow is available to investors after the unlevered firm itself pays corporate income taxes and the equityholders subsequently pay personal taxes on the equity income. In effect, the numerator is the perpetual after-all-taxes cash flow stream to equity investors. Because the introduction of personal taxes lowers the usable income to equityholders, personal taxes reduce the value of the unlevered firm, other things held constant.

The Miller model, which can be derived using an arbitrage proof similar to the one used to prove the MM models, is as follows.

$$V_L = V_U + \left\{ \left[1 - \frac{(1 - T_c) \times (1 - T_e)}{1 - T_d} \right] \times D \right\}.$$

Here are some relevant points about the Miller Model:

- The term bracketed by [ ] , when multiplied by D, is the new gain from leverage. It replaces $T = T_c$ in the earlier MM model with corporate taxes.
- If we ignore all taxes—that is, if $T_c = T_e = T_d = 0$—then the bracketed term reduces to zero; so, in that case, the Miller model is the same as the original MM model without taxes.
- If we ignore personal taxes—that is, if $T_e = T_d = 0$—then the bracketed term reduces to T_c; so the Miller model reduces to the MM model with corporate taxes.
- If the effective personal tax rates on stock and bond incomes were equal—that is, if $T_e = T_d$—then the bracketed term would again reduce to T_c.
- If $(1 - T_c) \times (1 - T_e) = 1 - T_d$, then the bracketed term would go to zero, and the value of using leverage would also be zero. This implies that the tax advantage of debt to the firm would be exactly offset by the personal tax advantage of equity. Under this condition, capital structure would have no effect on a firm's value or its cost of capital, so we would be back to Modigliani and Miller's original zero-tax theory.
- Because the capital gains tax rate in all brackets is less than the tax rate on ordinary income (i.e., 20 percent versus 36 percent in one bracket), and because taxes on capital gains are deferred, the effective tax rate on equity income is normally less than the effective tax rate on debt income. This being the case, what would the Miller model predict as the gain from leverage? To answer this question, assume that the tax rate on corporate income is $T_c = 34\%$, the effective rate on bond income is $T_d = 36\%$, and the effective rate on stock income is $T_e = 25\%$. Using these values in the Miller model, we find that a levered firm's value increases over that of an unlevered firm by 23 percent of the market value of corporate debt:

$$\text{Gain from leverage} = \left[1 - \frac{(1 - T_c) \times (1 - T_e)}{1 - T_d} \right] \times D$$

$$= \left[1 - \frac{(1 - 0.34) \times (1 - 0.25)}{1 - 0.36} \right] \times D$$

$$= [1 - 0.77] \times D = 0.23 \times D.$$

Note that with these data the MM model with corporate taxes would indicate a gain from leverage of $T_c \times D = 0.34 \times D$, or 34 percent of the amount of corporate debt. Thus, with these assumed tax rates, adding personal taxes to the model lowers the benefit derived from corporate debt financing. In general, whenever the effective tax rate on equity income is less than the effective rate on debt income, the Miller model produces a lower gain from leverage than is produced by the MM with corporate taxes model.

In his paper, Miller argued that firms in the aggregate would issue a mix of debt and equity securities such that the before-tax yields on corporate securities and the personal tax rates of the investors who bought these securities would adjust until equilibrium was reached. At the equilibrium, $(1-T_d)$ would equal $(1 - T_c) \times (1 - T_e)$; so, as we noted earlier, the tax advantage of debt to the firm would be exactly offset by personal taxation, and capital structure would have no effect on a firm's value or its cost of capital. Thus, according to Miller, the conclusions derived from the original Modigliani-Miller zero-tax model are correct!

Others have extended and tested Miller's analysis. Generally, these extensions disagree with Miller's conclusion that there is no advantage to the use of corporate debt. In the United States, the effective tax rate on equity income probably is less than the effective tax rate on debt income, so it appears that there is an advantage to the corporate use of debt financing. However, Miller's work does show that personal taxes offset some of the benefits of corporate debt; so the tax advantages of corporate debt probably are less than were implied by the earlier MM model that considered only corporate taxes.

1. How does the Miller model differ from the MM model with corporate taxes?
2. What are the implications of the Miller model under various tax assumptions?
3. What is the primary implication of the Miller model given the current tax situation in the United States?

Self-Test Questions

Criticisms of the MM and Miller Models

The conclusions of each of the three models follow logically from their initial assumptions: If the assumptions are correct, then the resulting conclusions must be reached. However, both academics and managers have voiced concern over the validity of these models, and virtually no businesses follow the recommendations of any of the models. The MM zero-tax model leads to the conclusion that capital structure does not matter, but we observe some regularities in structure within industries. Furthermore, when used with "reasonable" tax rates, both the MM model with corporate taxes and the Miller model lead to the conclusion that firms should use 100 percent debt financing. That situation is not observed in practice except by firms whose equity has been eroded by operating losses. Those who disagree with the MM and Miller models and their suggestions for financial policy generally attack the models on the grounds that their assumptions do not reflect real-world conditions. Some of the main objections include the following:

- Modigliani and Miller and, later, Miller assume that personal and corporate leverage are perfect substitutes. However, an individual investing in a levered firm has less loss exposure, and hence more limited liability, than if he or she used "homemade" leverage by taking on personal debt. This increased personal risk exposure would tend to restrain investors from engaging in the type of arbitrage required to derive the models, and that could cause the models to be incorrect.
- Brokerage costs were assumed away in the MM and Miller models. However, brokerage and other transaction costs do exist, and they too impede the arbitrage process.
- MM initially assumed that both businesses and individual investors can borrow at the risk-free rate. Although risky debt has been introduced into the analysis by others with no significant change in results, it is still necessary to assume that both corporations and investors can borrow at the same rate to reach the MM and Miller conclusions. Although major institutional investors probably can borrow at the corporate rate, many institutions are not allowed to borrow to buy securities. Furthermore, most individual investors must borrow at higher rates than those paid by large corporations.
- The MM and Miller models assume that there are no costs associated with financial distress. These costs are discussed in the next section.

Self-Test Questions

1. Should we accept one of the models presented thus far as being correct? Why or why not?
2. In your view, which of the assumptions used in the models is most likely to cause the models to be invalid?

Financial Distress Costs

Some of the assumptions inherent in the MM and Miller models can be relaxed, and when this is done, their basic conclusions remain unchanged. However, as we discuss next, when financial distress costs are added, the MM and Miller results are altered significantly.[9]

A number of firms experience *financial distress* each year, and some of them are forced into bankruptcy. Financial distress includes, but is not restricted to, bankruptcy, and when it occurs, several things can happen including:

- Arguments between claimants often delay the liquidation of assets. Bankruptcy cases can take many years to settle, and during this time equipment loses value, buildings are vandalized, inventories become obsolete, and so on.
- Lawyer's fees, court costs, and administrative expenses can absorb a large part of a business's value. Together, the costs of physical deterioration plus

legal fees and administrative expenses are called the *direct costs of bankruptcy*.

- Managers generally lose their jobs when a firm fails. Knowing this, the managers of a business that is in financial distress often take actions that keep it alive in the short run, but that dilute its long-run value. For example, a hospital in financial distress may fail to modernize, or may sell off valuable nonessential assets at bargain prices to raise cash or cut costs so much that the quality of its services is impaired and the firm's long-run market position is eroded.
- Stakeholders of organizations that are experiencing financial difficulties are aware of the problems, and often take actions that further damage troubled firms. For example, patients may go elsewhere, suppliers may be reluctant to sell on credit, and it may be difficult to recruit and retain medical staff. Suboptimal managerial actions associated with financial distress, as well as the costs imposed by stakeholders, are called the *indirect costs of financial distress*. Of course, a business in financial distress may incur these costs even if it does not go into bankruptcy; bankruptcy is just one point on the continuum of financial distress.

All things considered, the direct and indirect costs associated with financial distress are high; but financial distress typically occurs only if a firm uses debt financing because debt-free businesses rarely experience financial distress. Therefore, the greater the use of debt financing, and the larger the fixed interest charges, the greater the probability that a decline in earnings will lead to financial distress, and hence the higher the probability that the costs of financial distress will be incurred.

An increase in the probability of financial distress raises a firm's cost of equity capital and, hence, lowers the current value of the firm's equity. Furthermore, the probability of financial distress increases with leverage, causing the expected present value cost of financial distress to rise as more and more debt financing is used. A firm's creditors also feel the effects of financial distress. Businesses that experience financial distress have a higher probability of defaulting on debt payments, so the expectation of financial distress influences creditors' required rates of return: The higher the probability of financial distress, the higher the required return on debt. Thus, as a firm uses more and more debt financing, and hence increases the probability of financial distress, its cost of debt also increases.

1. Describe some types of financial distress costs.
2. How are financial distress costs related to the use of financial leverage?

Self-Test Questions

Trade-off Models

Both the MM with corporate taxes and Miller models as modified to reflect financial distress costs are described as *trade-off models*; that is, the optimal capital structure is found, at least conceptually, by balancing the tax shield benefits of leverage against the financial distress costs of leverage, so the costs and benefits are "traded off" against one another.

Model Structure

If the MM model with corporate taxes were correct, a firm's value would rise continuously as it moved from zero debt toward 100 percent debt: The equation $V_L = V_U + (T \times D)$ shows that $T \times D$, and hence V_L, is maximized if D is at a maximum. Recall that the rising component of value, $T \times D$, results directly from the tax shelter provided by interest on the debt. However, the present value of the costs associated with potential future financial distress could cause V_L to decline as the level of debt increases. Therefore, the MM with corporate taxes model's relationship between a firm's value and its use of leverage should look like this when financial distress costs are added:

$$V_L = V_U + (T \times D) - \text{PV of expected financial distress costs.}$$

The relationship expressed in this equation is graphed in Figure 11.2. The tax shelter effect totally dominates until the amount of debt reaches Point A. After Point A, financial distress costs become increasingly important, offsetting some of the tax advantages. At Point B, the marginal tax shelter benefits of additional debt are exactly offset by the marginal disadvantages of debt, and beyond Point B, the marginal disadvantages outweigh the marginal benefits.

The Miller model can also be modified to reflect financial distress costs. The equation would be identical to that developed above for the MM with corporate taxes model, except that the gain-from-leverage term, $T \times D$, would be adjusted to reflect the addition of personal taxes. In either the MM or Miller models, the gain from leverage can at least be roughly estimated, but the value reduction resulting from potential financial distress costs is almost entirely subjective. We know that these costs must increase as the use of debt financing rises, but we simply do not know the specific functional relationships.

Model Implications

The trade-off models are not capable of specifying precise optimal capital structures, but they do enable us to make three statements about debt usage:

1. Higher-risk businesses, as measured by the variability of returns on the business's assets, ought to borrow less than lower-risk firms, with other things being equal. The greater this variability, the greater the probability of financial distress at any level of debt, and hence the greater the expected costs of distress. Thus, firms with lower business risk can borrow more before the expected costs of distress offset the tax advantages of borrowing.
2. Businesses that employ tangible assets, such as real estate and standardized equipment, should borrow more than firms whose value is derived either

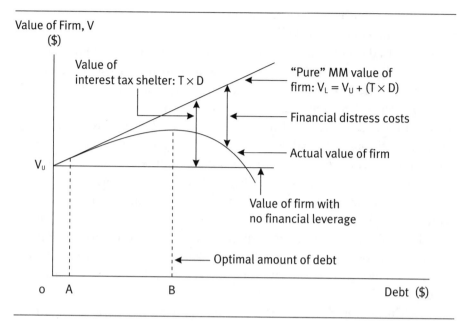

FIGURE 11.2

Net Effect of Financial Leverage on the Value of the Firm

from intangible assets, such as patents and goodwill, or from growth opportunities. The costs of financial distress depend not only on the probability of incurring distress, but also on what happens if distress occurs. Specialized assets, intangible assets, and growth opportunities are more likely to lose value if financial distress occurs than are standardized, tangible assets.

3. Businesses that are currently paying taxes at the highest rate, and that are likely to continue to do so in the future, should carry more debt than firms with current and/or prospectively lower tax rates should. High corporate tax rates lead to greater benefits from debt financing, and hence high-tax rate firms can carry more debt, other factors held constant, before the tax shield is offset by financial distress costs.

According to the trade-off models, each business should set its target capital structure such that its costs and benefits of leverage are balanced at the margin because such a structure will maximize its value. We would expect to find actual target structures that are consistent with the three points just noted. Furthermore, we would generally expect to find that firms within an industry have similar capital structures because such firms have roughly the same types of assets, business risk, and profitability.

The Empirical Evidence

The trade-off models have intuitive appeal because they lead to the conclusion that both no debt and all debt are bad, while a "moderate" debt level is good. However, we must ask ourselves whether these models explain actual behavior. If they do not, then we must search for other explanations or else assume that managers, and hence investors, are acting irrationally, which is an assumption that we are unwilling to make.

The trade-off models do have some empirical support.[10] For example, businesses that have primarily tangible assets tend to borrow more heavily than firms whose value stems from intangibles and/or growth opportunities do. However, other empirical evidence refutes the trade-off models. First, several studies have examined models of financing behavior to see if firms' financing decisions reflect adjustment toward a target capital structure. These studies provide some evidence that this occurs; but the explanatory power of the models is very low, suggesting that trade-off models capture only a part of actual behavior. Second, no study has clearly demonstrated that a firm's tax rate has a predictable, material effect on its capital structure. In fact, firms used debt financing long before corporate income taxes even existed. Finally, actual debt ratios tend to vary widely across apparently similar firms, whereas the trade-off models suggest that the use of debt should be relatively consistent within industries.

All in all, empirical support for the trade-off models is not strong, which suggests that other factors not incorporated into these models are also at work. In other words, the trade-off models do not tell the full story.

Self-Test Questions
1. What is a trade-off model of capital structure?
2. What are the implications of the trade-off models?
3. Does the empirical evidence support the trade-off models?

Asymmetric Information Model of Capital Structure

The asymmetric information model of capital structure traces its roots back to the work done in the 1960s by Gordon Donaldson.[11] Donaldson conducted an extensive survey of investor-owned corporations to find out how managers make financing decisions, and reached the following conclusions:

- Businesses prefer to finance with internally generated funds—that is, with retained earnings and depreciation cash flow.
- Businesses set target dividend payout ratios on the basis of their expected future investment opportunities and their expected future cash flows. The target payout ratio is set at a level such that expected retentions plus depreciation cash flow will meet expected capital expenditure requirements.
- Dividends are "sticky" in the short run because firms are reluctant to make major changes in the dollar dividend, and they are especially reluctant to cut the dividend. Thus, in any given year, depending on realized cash flows and actual investment opportunities, a business may or may not have sufficient internally generated funds to cover its capital expenditures.
- If a business has more internal cash flow than is needed for capital investment, then it will invest the excess in marketable securities or else use the funds to retire debt.

- If a business has insufficient internal cash flow to finance its capital investments, then it will first draw down its marketable securities portfolio, then issue debt, then issue convertible bonds—bonds that can be exchanged in the future for common stock—and only as a last resort will it sell new equity.

Thus, Donaldson observed a "pecking order" of financing, and not the balanced approach that is called for by the trade-off models. Indeed, the pecking order causes firms to move away from rather than toward a well-defined capital structure because equity funds are raised in two forms: (1) retained earnings at the top of the pecking order and (2) new common stock sales at the bottom.

Until recently, no theoretical model was available to explain this observed behavior of firms, so Donaldson's survey results were not given much credence by academics. Then, Stewart C. Myers proposed the *asymmetric information model* of capital structure.[12] The model is based on two assumptions: (1) Managers know more about their firms' future prospects than do investors; and (2) managers are motivated to maximize the wealth of their firms' current shareholders.

If managers think that their firm's equity is undervalued, they will be motivated to use debt financing because selling stock at a "bargain" price is detrimental to the firm's existing shareholders. However, if managers think that their firm's equity is overvalued, they will be motivated to issue new common stock. By issuing stock for more than it is actually worth, value is transferred from the buyers of the new stock to the existing shareholders. Thus, managers are motivated to issue new stock only when they believe that the stock is overvalued. Because equity investors are rational, they treat new common stock issues as "signals" that management considers the stock to be overvalued. Thus, investors revise downward their expectations for the firm and the stock price falls.[13]

Because new equity issues have an adverse effect on stock price, managers are reluctant to issue new stock. Although large amounts of new stock are issued each year, the vast majority is issued by small, rapidly growing firms that have large capital needs and, hence, little choice. Equity issues by mature firms are relatively rare. If external financing is required, debt is the first choice, and new common stock will be used only in unusual circumstances. Thus, the asymmetric information model leads managers to act in accordance with Donaldson's pecking order.

Because managers want to avoid new stock issues, especially when they might be least advantageous, it becomes prudent for firms to maintain a *reserve borrowing capacity* that can be used whenever capital investments require an unusually large amount of external capital. By maintaining a reserve borrowing capacity, and then tapping it when necessary, managers can avoid issuing new common stock under unfavorable conditions.

Note that the degree of information asymmetry and its impact on investors' perceptions differ substantially across firms. To illustrate the concept, consider that the degree of asymmetry is typically much greater in the drug industry than in the hospital industry because success in the drug industry depends on secretive proprietary research and development. Thus, managers in the drug industry hold significantly more information about their firms' prospects than do outside analysts and investors. Also, start-up businesses with limited capital and good growth opportunities are recognized as having to use external financing, so new stock offerings by such firms are not viewed with as much concern by investors as are new offerings by mature firms with limited growth opportunities. Thus, although the asymmetric information theory is applicable to all investor-owned firms, its influence on managerial decisions varies from firm to firm and over time.

Self-Test Questions

1. Briefly, explain the asymmetric information model of capital structure.
2. What does the model suggest about capital structure decisions?

A Summary of the Capital Structure Models

The great contribution of the trade-off models of MM, Miller, and their followers is that these models identify the specific benefits and costs of using debt—the tax effects, financial distress costs, and so on. Prior to these models, no capital structure theory existed and we had no systematic way of analyzing the effects of debt financing.

The trade-off model is summarized in Figure 11.3. The top graph shows the relationships between the debt ratio and the cost of debt, cost of equity, and the corporate cost of capital. Both the cost of equity and the effective (after-tax) cost of debt rise steadily with increases in leverage, but the rate of increase accelerates at higher debt levels, reflecting the increased probability of financial distress and its attendant costs. The corporate cost of capital first declines, then hits a minimum, and then begins to rise. Note that a business's corporate cost of capital is minimized and its value is maximized **at the same capital structure**. Also note that the general shapes of the curves apply once we consider the effects of financial distress costs, regardless of whether we are using the MM with corporate taxes model or the Miller model.

The fact that the same capital structure both minimizes the cost of capital and maximizes value should be no surprise. The value of any business is nothing more than the present value of its expected after-tax operating income stream. What discount rate is used to find the present value? It is the corporate cost of capital. Therefore, by minimizing its corporate cost of capital, a business is automatically creating the greatest value.

Unfortunately, it is extremely difficult for financial managers to actually quantify the costs and benefits of debt financing to their firms; so it is virtually impossible to pinpoint the capital structure that truly maximizes a business's

FIGURE 11.3

Summary of the
Trade-Off
Models

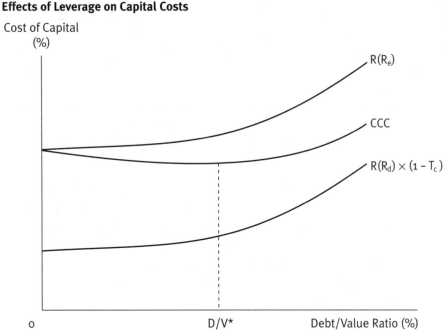

Effects of Leverage on Capital Costs

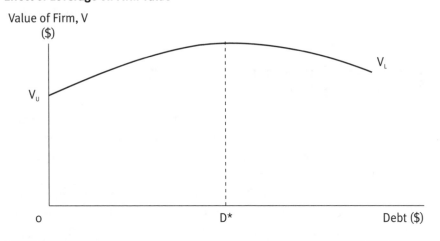

Effect of Leverage on Firm Value

value. Most experts believe that such a structure exists for every taxable business, but that it changes substantially over time as the nature of the business and the capital markets changes. Most experts also believe that, as shown in the lower portion of Figure 11.3, the relationship between firm value and leverage is relatively flat; thus, relatively large deviations from the optimal structure can occur without materially affecting a business's value.

Now, consider the asymmetric information model. Because of asymmetric information, investors know less about a firm's prospects than do its managers. Furthermore, managers try to maximize value for current stockholders, not new ones; so if the firm has excellent prospects, management will not want to issue new shares, but if things look bleak, then a new stock offering may be sold. Therefore, investors take a stock offering to be a signal of bad news, so stock prices tend to decline when new issues are announced. As a result, new equity financing can be very expensive, and this fact must be incorporated into the capital structure decision. Its effect is to motivate firms to maintain a reserve borrowing capacity, which permits future investment opportunities to be financed by debt when internal funds are insufficient.

By combining the two theories, we obtain this possible explanation for the capital structure decisions of taxable firms:

- Debt financing provides benefits because of the tax deductibility of interest. Hence, firms should have some debt in their capital structures.
- However, financial distress costs place limits on debt usage—beyond some point, these costs offset the tax advantage of debt.
- Finally, because of asymmetric information, businesses maintain a reserve borrowing capacity to take advantage of good investment opportunities and, at the same time, avoid having to issue stock at distressed prices.

Self-Test Questions
1. Do the capital structure models provide managers with specific quantifiable guidance regarding optimal capital structures?
2. Summarize the information that capital structure models provide to decision makers.

Application of Capital Structure Theory to Not-for-Profit Firms

So far, the discussion of capital structure theory has focused on investor-owned businesses. Do the models presented in this chapter apply to not-for-profit firms? No rigorous research has been conducted into the optimal capital structures of not-for-profit firms, but some loose analogies can be drawn. Although not-for-profit firms do not receive a direct tax subsidy when debt financing is used, they do have access to the tax-exempt debt market, which provides an indirect tax subsidy. (If not-for-profits had to issue taxable debt, their costs of debt would be higher.) Thus, not-for-profit firms receive about the same benefits from the use of debt financing as do investor-owned firms.

What about the costs associated with debt financing? As discussed in Chapter 10, from a pure opportunity cost perspective, a not-for-profit firm's fund capital has a cost that is roughly equivalent to the cost of equity of a similar investor-owned firm. Thus, we would expect the opportunity cost of fund capital to rise as more and more debt financing is used, just as for an investor-owned firm. After all, the use of debt financing increases the risk to the stakeholders of the organization. Furthermore, not-for-profit firms are subject to the same types of financial distress costs that are borne by investor-owned firms, so these costs are equally applicable. Thus, we would expect the trade-off models to be roughly applicable to not-for-profit firms, and hence for such firms to have optimal capital structures defined, at least in theory, as a trade-off between the costs and benefits of debt financing. Note, however, that the asymmetric information model is not applicable to not-for-profit firms because such firms do not sell common stock.

Although the trade-off models may be partially applicable for not-for-profit firms, a problem arises because for-profit firms have more-or-less unlimited access to equity capital. Thus, if they have more capital investment opportunities than they can finance with retained earnings and debt financing, investor-owned firms can always raise the needed funds by a new stock issue. (According to the asymmetric information theory, managers may not want to issue new stock, but the opportunity still exists.) Additionally, it is quite easy for investor-owned firms to alter their capital structures. If they are financially underleveraged—using too little debt—they can simply issue more debt and use the proceeds to repurchase stock. On the other hand, if they are financially overleveraged—using too much debt—they can issue additional shares and use the proceeds to refund debt.

Not-for-profit firms do not have access to the equity markets; their sole source of "equity" capital is through governmental grants, private contributions, and excess revenues (retained earnings). Managers of not-for-profit organizations do not have the same degree of flexibility in either capital investment or capital structure decisions as do their proprietary counterparts. Thus, it is often necessary for not-for-profit firms to (1) delay new projects, even profitable ones, because of funding insufficiencies; and (2) use more than the theoretically optimal amount of debt because that is the only way that needed services can be financed. Although these actions may be required in certain situations, not-for-profit managers must recognize that such strategies increase costs. Project delays mean that needed services are not being provided on a timely basis. Using more debt than optimal pushes the firm beyond the point of the greatest net benefit of debt financing, and hence capital costs are increased above the minimum. If a not-for-profit firm is forced into a situation where it is using more than the optimal amount of debt financing, its managers should plan to reduce the firm's level of debt as soon as the situation permits.

The ability of a not-for-profit firm to garner governmental grants, attract private contributions, and generate excess revenues plays an important role in establishing its competitive position. A firm that has an adequate amount of fund capital can operate at its optimal capital structure, and thus minimize capital costs. If insufficient fund capital is available, too much financial leverage is then used, and the result is higher capital costs. Consider two not-for-profit hospitals that are similar in all respects, except that one has more fund capital and can operate at its optimal structure, while the other has insufficient fund capital and, thus, must use more debt financing than optimal. In effect, the hospital with insufficient fund capital must operate at an inefficient capital structure. The former has a significant competitive advantage because it can either offer more services at the same cost by using additional (suboptimal) debt financing, or it can offer matching services at lower costs. Thus, sufficient fund capital provides the flexibility to offer all of the necessary services and still operate at the lowest capital cost structure. Like firms that have low operating cost structures, firms that are at their optimal capital structures, and hence have a low capital cost structure, have an advantage over their competitors that have higher capital cost structures.

Any business that is forced to use more than the optimal amount of debt financing is operating inefficiently, and hence has an economic incentive to obtain more fund capital. As in any competitive industry, not-for-profit healthcare managers have limited control over their firms' abilities to generate excess revenues. On the other hand, managers have much greater control over the amount of effort applied to public and private fundraising. Thus, not-for-profit firms that require fund capital to operate efficiently must emphasize fundraising. Years ago, public and private contributions were a critical source of funds for not-for-profit providers, but many firms de-emphasized this source of capital during the cost-plus era of the 1970s and early 1980s. It might be time for many not-for-profit managers to reevaluate their fundraising efforts.

Self-Test Questions
1. Do the capital structure models apply to not-for-profit firms?
2. Why is capital structure important to not-for-profit firms?

Making the Capital Structure Decision

Because one cannot determine precisely the optimal capital structure, managers must apply judgment along with quantitative analysis. The judgmental analysis involves several different factors, and in one situation a particular factor might have great importance, while the same factor might be relatively unimportant in another situation. This section discusses some of the more important judgmental issues that should be taken into account.

Long-Run Viability

Managers of large businesses, especially those providing vital healthcare services, have a responsibility to provide continuous service, so they must refrain from using leverage to the point where the firm's long-run viability is endangered.

Managerial Conservatism

Well-diversified investors have eliminated most, if not all, of the diversifiable risk from their portfolios. Therefore, the typical investor can tolerate some chance of financial distress because a loss on one stock will probably be offset by random gains on other stocks in the investor's portfolio. However, managers of investor-owned firms often view financial distress with more concern because they are typically not well diversified in their careers, and thus the present value of their expected earnings can be seriously affected by the onset of financial distress. Therefore, it is not difficult to imagine that managers might be more "conservative" in their use of leverage than the average stockholder would desire. If this were true, then managers would set somewhat lower target capital structures than the ones that maximize firm value.

For not-for-profit firms, one could argue that managerial conservatism is appropriate. Not-for-profit firms have no shareholders, and many of the stakeholders are typically not well diversified in regard to their relationships with the firm. Thus, these stakeholders have much more to lose if the firm fails than do well-diversified shareholders of investor-owned firms. However, the managers of not-for-profit firms can adopt a conservative approach to capital structure only if the firm has sufficient fund capital.

Lender and Rating Agency Attitudes

Regardless of a manager's own analysis of the proper leverage for his or her firm, there is no question that lenders' and rating agencies' attitudes are frequently important determinants of financial structures. In the majority of cases, corporate managers discuss the firm's financial structure with lenders and rating agencies and give much weight to their advice. Typically, managers want to maintain some target debt rating—say, single-A. Also, if a particular firm's management is so confident of the future that it seeks to use leverage beyond the norms for its industry, its lenders may be unwilling to accept such debt increases, or may do so only at a high price.

Rating agencies publish data that give managers the rough relationship between the use of debt financing and debt rating. For example, Table 11.3 lists the relationship between financial leverage and debt rating for not-for-profit hospitals as provided by Standard & Poor's. In general, the greater the use of debt, the lower the debt rating. Note, however, that factors other than financial leverage affect debt ratings because the relationship is not precise.

TABLE 11.3 Relationship Between Financial Leverage and Debt Rating for Not-for-Profit Hospitals

Debt Rating	Long-Term Debt to Capital Ratio
AA+	29.2%
AA	27.1
A+	32.3
A	33.2
BBB+	36.8
BBB	43.5
BBB-	50.7
Speculative	62.7

Notes: (1) Data are for 1998.
  (2) Capital is defined as long-term debt plus equity.
Source: Standard & Poor's Health Care Rating Lists, August 16, 1999.

Reserve Borrowing Capacity

Under the asymmetric information model, businesses should maintain a re-serve borrowing capacity that preserves the ability to issue debt at favorable terms. For example, suppose Merck had just successfully completed an R&D program on a new drug, and its internal projections forecast much higher earnings in the future. However, the new earnings are not yet anticipated by investors, and hence are not reflected in the price of its stock. Merck's managers would not want to issue stock; they would prefer to finance with debt until the higher earnings materialized and were reflected in the stock price, at which time the firm could sell an issue of common stock, retire the debt, and return to its target capital structure. To maintain a reserve borrowing capacity, firms generally use less debt under "normal" conditions, and hence present a stronger financial picture than they otherwise would. This is not suboptimal from a long-run standpoint, although it might appear so if viewed strictly on a short-run basis.

Industry Averages

Presumably, managers act rationally, so the capital structures of other firms in the industry, particularly the industry leaders, should provide insights as to the optimal structure. In general, there is no reason to believe that the managers of one firm are better than the managers of any other firm. Thus, if one firm has a capital structure that is significantly different from other firms in its industry, the managers of that firm should identify the unique circumstances that contribute to the anomaly. If unique circumstances cannot be identified, then it is doubtful that the firm has identified the correct target structure.

Control of Investor-Owned Corporations

The effect that a firm's choice of securities has on a management's control position may also influence its capital structure decision. If a firm's manage-ment just barely has majority control—just over 50 percent of the stock—but is not in a position to buy any more stock, debt may be the choice for new financing. On the other hand, a management group that is not concerned about voting control may decide to use equity rather than debt if the firm's financial situation is so weak that the use of debt might subject the firm to serious risk of default.

Asset Structure

Firms whose assets are suitable as security for loans tend to use debt rather heavily. Thus, hospitals tend to be highly leveraged; but firms involved in technological research employ relatively little debt. Also, if the firm's assets carry high business risk, then it will be less able to use financial leverage than a firm with low business risk will. Accordingly, factors such as sales stability and operating leverage, which influence business risk, also influence firms' optimal capital structure.

Growth Rate

Other factors the same, faster-growing firms must rely more heavily on external capital—slow growth can be financed with retained earnings, but rapid growth generally requires the use of external funds. As postulated in the information asymmetry theory, businesses first use debt financing to meet external funding needs. Furthermore, the flotation costs involved in selling common stock exceed those incurred when selling debt. Thus, rapidly growing firms tend to use somewhat more debt than do slower-growth firms.

Profitability

Firms with very high rates of return on investment tend to use relatively little debt. This behavior is consistent with the asymmetric information theory, and the practical reason seems to be that highly profitable firms simply do not need to use much debt financing because their high rates of return enable them to use retained earnings for the bulk of their financing.

Taxes

Interest is a deductible expense, while dividends are not deductible; so the higher a firm's corporate tax rate, the greater the advantage of using corporate debt.

It is clear that some of the considerations that go into the decision are quantitative and some are qualitative. Thus, in practice, the capital structure decision requires a great deal of judgment. Often, businesses use forecasting models to help assess the impact of alternative capital structures, but the final decision is always somewhat judgmental.

1. Is the capital structure decision mostly objective or subjective?
2. What are some of the factors that managers must consider when setting a business's optimal capital structure?

Self-Test Questions

Capital Structure Decisions for Small Investor-Owned Businesses

Capital structure theory, and hence its prescriptions for business behavior, is based on large corporations, in which owners and managers are separate groups and the securities issued are publicly traded. Thus, like its application to not-for-profit businesses, the application of capital structure theory to small investor-owned businesses raises more questions than it provides answers.

In small businesses—say, a medical practice of one or just a few physicians—the situation changes dramatically. Now, it is common to distribute returns to the owner/managers through salary bonuses, as opposed to dividends. What makes this situation different? The key to the value of debt financing is that interest on debt financing is tax deductible to a business, while dividends on equity financing are not. In other words, interest is paid from pretax income, while dividends are paid from after-tax income. It is the asymmetric tax deductibility of interest that creates the value inherent in the use of debt. As proved by Modigliani and Miller (MM), if there were no differential tax effects (the zero-tax case), the increase in riskiness to owners would exactly offset the benefits associated with a cost of debt that is lower than the cost of equity. The tax impact makes the effective cost of debt lower than that appropriate for the risk that it brings to the business, and it is this "externality" that drives the value of debt financing.

When "dividends" to equityholders are paid in the form of bonuses, they too are tax deductible. Thus, we are in a situation in which there are tax advantages inherent in both debt and equity financing. Debt financing still leverages up owners' return, but the increase in risk that debt financing brings to owners either partially or fully offsets the increase in ROE. Thus, there is no clear value-increasing benefit to debt financing. Should such small businesses use debt? The answer is probably yes because owner/managers often cannot provide the amount of equity capital needed by the business. If owners do not have the capital needed by the business, and control considerations preclude bringing in outside equity, debt financing is the only choice.

Interestingly, the debt could be obtained either by the business or by the owners as personal debt, which would then be contributed to the business as equity. This amounts to the "homemade" leverage argument made by MM in their proofs. In general, if the business can borrow at a lower interest rate than can the individual owners, then business debt makes sense, and vice versa. However, the issue becomes cloudy because, under many forms of organization, personal debt has different liability characteristics than does business debt. To add to the complexity, the owners of small businesses typically have to sign personal guarantees on business debt, which further blurs the line between business and personal debt. The end result is that each small business situation is somewhat unique, and it is impossible to give guidance for capital structure decision making that is applicable in all situations.

Self-Test Question

1. Do the general prescriptions for capital structure decisions apply to small businesses? Explain your answer.

The Debt Maturity Decision

Thus far, we have focused on the primary capital structure decision, which is identifying the optimal mix of debt and equity financing. Once this is done, a secondary decision arises: What is the optimal mix of debt maturities? In other words, what is the optimal debt *maturity structure*? The answer, like the optimal capital structure, involves a trade-off between risk and return.

The Concept of Temporary and Permanent Assets

Most businesses experience seasonal and/or cyclical fluctuations in demand. Typically, businesses respond to such fluctuations by having a sufficient level of fixed assets on hand to meet peak demand needs, but allowing current assets to fluctuate as necessary to match rising and falling demand conditions. Still, current assets **never** drop to zero, and this realization has led to the concept of permanent versus temporary assets.

To illustrate the situation, consider Sun Coast Clinics, a for-profit operator of four ambulatory care clinics in South Florida. Table 11.4 contains the business's December 2000 and April 2001 balance sheets. Sun Coast's optimal, or target, capital structure is 40–45 percent debt financing, and its current structure falls within this range. The question at hand now is what maturity structure should Sun Coast use for its 55–60 percent debt financing.

Note that the provision of ambulatory care services in this part of Florida is a seasonal business. The peak season for Sun Coast is December through April, when the population of the area soars because of tourism. Even more important to Sun Coast's peak level of operations is the arrival of the "snow birds" (i.e., retirees who typically live in the north during the summer and fall months, but move to residences in Florida for the winter).

In December of each year, Sun Coast has just finished its slow season and is preparing for its busy season. Thus, the firm's accounts receivables are relatively low, but its cash and marketable securities and inventories are relatively high. By the end of April, Sun Coast has completed its busy season, so its accounts receivable are relatively high, but its cash and marketable

	December 2000	April 2001
TABLE 11.4 Sun Coast Clinics, Inc.: End-of-Month Balance Sheets (thousands of dollars)		
Cash and marketable securities	$ 30	$ 20
Accounts receivable	155	210
Inventories	15	10
Total current assets	$200	$240
Net fixed assets	500	500
Total assets	$700	$740
Accounts payable	$ 30	$ 40
Accruals	15	25
Short-term debt	85	105
Total current liabilities	$130	$170
Long-term debt	170	170
Common equity	400	400
Total liabilities and equity	$700	$740

Note: These statements have been simplified for ease of illustration.

securities and inventories are relatively low in preparation for the slow summer season. On the current liabilities side, Sun Coast's accounts payable and accruals are relatively high at the end of April, just after the busy season. Sun Coast's fluctuations in assets and liabilities result from seasonal factors. Similar fluctuations in current asset requirements, and hence in financing needs, can occur because of business cycles; typically, current asset requirements and financing needs contract during recessions and expand during good times.

Note that at this stage in its life cycle, Sun Coast's total assets fluctuate between $700,000 and $740,000. The minimum amount of total assets required to sustain operations during seasonal, or cyclical, lows is defined as a firm's *permanent assets*. Thus, Sun Coast has $700,000 of permanent assets, which are composed of $500,000 of fixed assets and $200,000 of *permanent current assets*. By their nature, fixed assets are always considered as permanent, so temporary assets arise solely from current assets. Sun Coast carries *temporary current assets* that fluctuate seasonally from zero to a maximum of $40,000. The manner in which the permanent and temporary current assets are financed defines the business's debt maturity mix.

Alternative Debt Maturity Policies

There are three basic debt maturity policies: (1) maturity matching, (2) aggressive, and (3) conservative.

Maturity Matching *Maturity matching*, which represents a moderate approach to the debt maturity decision, calls for the business to match asset and liability maturities **in the financial sense**; that is, permanent assets are financed with permanent capital (i.e., equity and long-term debt) and temporary assets are financed with temporary capital (i.e., short-term debt). To illustrate maturity matching, consider that if Sun Coast were using this strategy, it would have $700,000 of permanent financing. Because it has $400,000 in equity, this would suggest $300,000 in long-term debt. However, Sun Coast would take all the free financing it can get, so it will use the Accounts payable + Accruals = $30,000 + $15,000 = $45,000 in spontaneous (free) current liabilities available during the slow season to replace long-term debt. Thus, maturity matching would call for $400,000 in equity, $255,000 in long-term debt, and $45,000 in free current liabilities for a total of $700,000 in financing. This is all the financing that would be on the books in December 2000. But, to get to April 2001, Sun Coast would use $20,000 of short-term debt. Although total assets increase by $40,000, the business gets the benefit of an additional $20,000 of free current liabilities, so only $20,000 of short-term debt is needed.

The maturity matching strategy limits the risk that a business will be unable to pay off its maturing obligations. To see this point, suppose Sun Coast borrows on a one-year basis and uses the funds obtained to build and equip a new clinic. Cash flows from the clinic (i.e., profits plus depreciation) would almost never be sufficient to pay off the loan at the end of only one year, so the loan must be renewed at that time. If interest rates increase during the year, Sun Coast's new debt would cost more. Even worse, if the lender refused to renew the loan, Sun Coast would have problems. Had the clinic been financed with long-term financing, however, the required loan payments would have been better matched with cash flows from profits and depreciation, and the problem of loan renewal would not have arisen.

At the limit, a business could attempt to match exactly the maturity structure of its assets and liabilities. Inventory expected to be sold in 30 days could be financed with a 30-day bank loan, a machine expected to last for five years could be financed by a five-year loan, a 20-year building could be financed by a 20-year mortgage bond, and so forth. Actually, three factors make this exact maturity matching strategy both unpractical and wrong: (1) uncertainty about the lives of assets; (2) some common equity, or fund capital, must be used, and this capital has no maturity; and (3) to develop a sound current asset financing policy it is necessary to consider whether an asset is permanent or temporary.

In the *aggressive approach,* a business finances part of its permanent current **Aggressive** assets with short-term debt. A look back at Table 11.4 will show that Sun **Approach** Coast actually follows this strategy. Sun Coast has $500,000 in net fixed assets and $570,000 of long-term capital, leaving only $70,000 of long-term capital to finance $200,000 in permanent current assets. Additionally, Sun Coast has a minimum of $45,000 of free short-term liabilities. Thus, Sun Coast must use $200,000 − $70,000 − $45,000 = $85,000 of short-term debt to help finance its permanent level of current assets.

Note that there are an almost infinite number of degrees of aggressiveness. For example, at the extreme, Sun Coast could replace the $170,000 of long-term debt with short-term debt, and hence have only $400,000 of permanent capital—its equity. Such a policy would be a highly aggressive, extremely unconservative position, and Sun Coast would be very much subject to dangers from rising interest rates as well as to loan-renewal problems. However, short-term debt is often cheaper than long-term debt, and some businesses are willing to take on additional financial risk for the chance of higher profits.

In the *conservative approach,* the level of permanent financing exceeds the level **Conservative** of permanent assets. For Sun Coast, the conservative approach would call for **Approach** say, $400,000 in equity plus $300,000 in long-term debt for total permanent financing of $700,000. Then, $45,000 of marketable securities would be held at the end of December 2000, and $65,000 would be held at the end of April 2001. The conservative approach provides Sun Coast with a "safety" reserve of liquid assets that could be tapped at any time to cover unexpected operating losses or for other purposes.

Conclusions Regarding Debt Maturities

The proper framework for evaluating debt maturity policies requires the use of the concept of permanent and temporary assets. Thus, for financing purposes, assets are **not** classified by their accounting definitions of current and long-term, but rather as either permanent or temporary. In this framework, maturity matching calls for the permanent portion of cash, receivables, and inventories (i.e., permanent current assets) to be financed with *permanent capital* (i.e., long-term debt and equity). The key is that each dollar of cash, each individual receivable, and each dollar of inventory may well be short-term in that these items will be quickly turned over or converted to cash. However, as each individual current asset item is converted, it will be replaced by a like item if it is permanent in nature, and hence such short-term assets are actually carried permanently over the long term. The implication is that the accounting definition of current assets, although useful for many purposes, does not provide managers with the correct guidance regarding the financing of such assets.

The choice among alternative financing policies involves a risk/return trade-off. The aggressive policy, with its high use of generally lower cost short-term debt, has the highest expected return but the highest risk, while the conservative policy has the lowest expected return and lowest risk. The maturity matching policy falls between the extremes. Unfortunately, there is no underlying finance theory that managers can use to pick the "correct" debt maturity policy. Often, firms that have low business risk elect to take on higher-than-average financial risk. Thus, such firms tend to have more debt in their target capital structures and are more likely to use an aggressive debt maturity policy. Conversely, firms with high business risk usually take a conservative view regarding added financial risk, whether that risk arises from a high level of debt or an aggressive debt maturity policy.

Self-Test Questions

1. Explain the difference between permanent and temporary assets.
2. What are the three strategies for choosing debt maturities?
3. How is the choice made?

Key Concepts

This chapter presented a variety of topics related to capital structure decisions. Here are its key concepts:

- The use of debt financing increases the *rate of return* to owners, but it also increases their *risk*.
- *Business risk* is the inherent riskiness in a firm's operations if it uses no debt financing. *Financial risk* is the additional risk that is concentrated on the business's owners when debt financing is used.

- In 1958, Franco Modigliani and Merton Miller (MM) startled the academic community by proving, under a very restrictive set of assumptions including *zero taxes*, that capital structure is irrelevant because a business's value is not affected by its financing mix.
- Modigliani and Miller later added *corporate taxes* to their model, leading to the conclusion that capital structure does matter, and that businesses should use almost 100 percent debt financing to maximize value.
- The MM model with corporate taxes illustrates that the benefits of debt financing stem solely from the *tax deductibility of interest payments.*
- Much later, Miller extended the model to include *personal taxes.* The introduction of personal taxes reduces, but does not eliminate, the benefits of debt financing. Thus, the *Miller model* also prescribes 100 percent debt financing.
- The addition of *financial distress costs* to either the MM corporate tax model or the Miller model results in a *trade-off model.* Here the marginal costs and benefits of debt financing are balanced against one another, and the result is an optimal capital structure that falls somewhere between zero and 100 percent debt.
- *Not-for-profit firms* face a set of benefits and costs associated with debt financing similar to those faced by investor-owned firms, so the trade-off model is at least partially applicable to such firms. However, the inability to sell equity may keep a not-for-profit firm's capital structure above the optimal point, at least temporarily.
- The *asymmetric information model*, which is based on the assumption that managers have better information than investors, postulates that there is a preferred order to financing: First, retained earnings (and depreciation); then, debt; and finally, as a last resort only, new common stock.
- The asymmetric information model prescribes that businesses maintain a *reserve borrowing capacity* so that they can always issue debt on reasonable terms rather than forced into a new equity issue at the wrong time.
- Unfortunately, capital structure theory does not provide neat, clean answers to the question of the optimal capital structure. Thus, many factors must be considered when actually choosing a firm's target capital structure, and the final decision will be based on both analysis and judgment.
- The second decision regarding capital structure is the selection of *debt maturities.*
- There are three general approaches to debt maturities: (1) *maturity matching*, (2) *conservative*, and (3) *aggressive.*
- The debt maturity choice is a classic *risk/return trade-off.*

This chapter concludes our discussion of cost of capital and capital structure. In the next two chapters, we discuss capital budgeting decisions.

Selected References

Boles, Keith E. 1986. "What Accounting Leaves Out of Hospital Financial Management." *Hospital & Health Services Administration* (March/April): 8–27.

Gapenski, Louis C. 1993. "Hospital Capital Structure Decisions: Theory and Practice." *Health Services Management Research* (November): 237–247.

———. 1999. "Debt Maturity Structures Should Match Risk Preferences." *Healthcare Financial Management* (December): 56–59.

Harris, John P., and Victor E. Schimmel. 1987. "Market Value: An Underused Financial Planning Tool." *Healthcare Financial Management* (April): 40–46.

McCue, Michael J., and Yazar A. Ozcan. 1992. "Determinants of Capital Structure." *Hospital & Health Services Administration* (Fall): 333–346.

Messinger, Stephen F., and Paul B. Stevenson. 1999. "Practice Financing Strategies Should Match Investors' Objectives." *Healthcare Financial Management* (May): 72–76.

Sterns, Jay B., and Todd K. Majidzadeh. 1995. "A Framework for Evaluating Capital Structure." *Journal of Health Care Finance* (Winter): 80–85.

Valvona, Joseph and Frank A. Sloan. 1988. "Hospital Profitability and Capital Structure: A Comparative Analysis." *Health Services Research* (August): 343–357.

Vaughan, Jim and Joan Wise. 1996. "How to Choose the Right Capitalization Option." *Healthcare Financial Management* (December): 72–74.

Wedig, Gerald J., Frank A. Sloan, Mahmud Hassan, and Michael A. Morrisey. 1988. "Capital Structure, Ownership, and Capital Payment Policy: The Case of Hospitals." *Journal of Finance* (March): 1–40.

Selected Web Sites

Ohio State University maintains a web site with video clips by various finance professionals briefly discussing topics of relevance to this course. Unfortunately, the clips do not include healthcare executives. To access the clips, go to *www.cob.ohio-state.edu/fin/clips.htm*. Then, click on the clip of interest. For this chapter, try the clips by Steve Walsh titled "On the Cost of Capital and Debt" and "What We Think of Modigliani/Miller Around Here." Note that video clips are large files that are best accessed using a fast Internet link. Furthermore, player software is required to see the clips.

Selected Cases

There is one case in *Cases in Healthcare Finance* that is applicable to this chapter:
Case 14: Nurses Unlimited, which focuses on the choice between debt and equity financing for a for-profit business.

Notes

1. The use of preferred stock has roughly the same effect on a business's risk and return, and hence capital structure decision, as does debt financing. However,

because most businesses in the health services industry do not use preferred stock, we will confine our discussion to debt financing.

2. Per procedure leases are discussed in Chapter 9.

3. See Franco Modigliani and Merton H. Miller (MM), "The Cost of Capital, Corporation Finance and the Theory of Investment," *American Economic Review*, June 1958, 261–297; "The Cost of Capital, Corporation Finance and the Theory of Investment: Reply," *American Economic Review*, September 1958, 655–669; "Taxes and the Cost of Capital: A Correction," *American Economic Review*, June 1963, 433–443; and "Reply," *American Economic Review*, June 1965, 524–527. In a 1979 survey of Financial Management Association members, the original MM article was judged to have had the greatest impact on the field of finance of any work ever published. See Philip L. Cooley and J. Louis Heck, "Significant Contributions to Finance Literature," *Financial Management*, Tenth Anniversary Issue 1981, 23–33.

4. MM actually developed three propositions, but the third one is not material to our discussion.

5. *Arbitrage* means the simultaneous buying and selling of essentially identical assets at different prices. The buying increases the price of the undervalued asset, and the selling decreases the price of the overvalued asset. Arbitrage operations will continue until prices have been adjusted to the point where the arbitrager can no longer earn a profit. At this point, the prices are in equilibrium.

6. For an illustration of MM's arbitrage proof, see Eugene F. Brigham, Louis C. Gapenski, and Phillip R. Daves, *Intermediate Financial Management* (Fort Worth, TX: Dryden Press, 2000), Chapter 11.

7. The annual interest expense associated with D dollars of debt financing is $R(R_d) \times D$, and the resulting tax savings is $T \times R(R_d) \times D$. Because MM assumed that all cash flows are perpetuities, the present value of the tax savings stream is $[T \times R(R_d) \times D]/R(R_d) = T \times D$.

8. See Merton H. Miller, "Debt and Taxes," *Journal of Finance*, May 1977, 261–275. The paper was first presented as the Presidential Address at the 1976 meeting of the American Finance Association.

9. The recognition of *agency costs*, which we introduced in Chapter 2, also affects the MM and Miller results. However, this impact is secondary in importance to financial distress costs, and hence we will not include agency costs in our discussion.

10. For examples of the empirical research in this area, see Robert Taggart, "A Model of Corporate Financing Decisions," *Journal of Finance*, December 1977, 1467–1484; and Paul Marsh, "The Choice Between Equity and Debt: An Empirical Study," *Journal of Finance*, March 1982, 121–144.

11. See Gordon Donaldson, *Corporate Debt Capacity: A Study of Corporate Debt Policy and the Determination of Corporate Debt Capacity* (Boston: Harvard Graduate School of Business Administration, 1961).

12. See Stewart C. Myers, "The Capital Structure Puzzle," *Journal of Finance*, July 1984, 575–592. It is interesting to note that, like the Miller model, Myers' paper was presented as a Presidential Address to the American Finance Association.

13. Many studies support the contention that the announcement of a new stock issue results in a decrease in stock price. For example, one study found that stock prices decline about 3 percent following the announcement of a new stock issue. See Paul Asquith and David W. Mullins, Jr., "Equity Issues and Offering Dilution," *Journal of Financial Economics*," June 1986, 61–89.

Capital Allocation

THE BASICS OF CAPITAL BUDGETING

Learning Objectives

After studying this chapter, readers should be able to:

- Explain how managers use project classifications and post-audits in the capital budgeting process.
- Discuss the role of financial analysis in health services capital budgeting decisions.
- Discuss the key elements of cash flow estimation, breakeven analysis, and profitability analysis.
- Conduct basic capital budgeting analyses.

Introduction

Chapters 10 and 11 described how healthcare managers estimate their business's corporate costs of capital and make capital structure decisions. Now, we change our focus to fixed asset acquisition decisions. Although some investment decisions, such as the decision to expand the operating hours of a walk-in clinic, involve only the expenditure of operating funds, most investment decisions entail the acquisition of new facilities or equipment. Thus, decisions of this type often are called *capital investment*, or *capital budgeting*, *decisions*. The term "capital budgeting" is used because the listing of projects to be undertaken in the future, along with their total dollar cost, is called the *capital budget*. Capital budgeting decisions are of fundamental importance to the success or failure of any business because a firm's capital budgeting decisions, more than anything else, shape its future.

The discussion of capital budgeting is divided into two chapters. Chapter 12 provides an overview of the capital budgeting process, a discussion of the key elements of project cash flow estimation, and an explanation of the basic techniques used to assess a project's breakeven characteristics and profitability. In Chapter 13, capital budgeting risk analysis and the optimal capital budget are considered.

Importance of Capital Budgeting

Capital budgeting decisions are among the most critical ones that healthcare managers must make. First, and most importantly, the results of capital budgeting decisions generally affect the business for an extended period. If a business invests too heavily in fixed assets, it will have too much capacity and its costs will necessarily be too high. On the other hand, a business that invests too little in fixed assets may face two problems: (1) technological obsolescence and (2) inadequate capacity. A healthcare provider without the latest in technology will lose patients to its more up-to-date competitors and, further, will deprive its patients of the best healthcare diagnostics and treatments available. A provider with inadequate capacity may lose a portion of its market share to competitors, which would then require it to increase its marketing costs or aggressively reduce prices to regain the lost share.

Effective capital budgeting procedures provide several benefits to businesses. A business that forecasts its needs for capital assets well in advance will have the opportunity to plan the purchases carefully, and thus will be able to negotiate the highest quality assets at the best prices. Additionally, asset expansion typically involves substantial expenditures, and because large amounts of funds are not usually at hand, they must be raised externally. Good capital budgeting practices permit a business to identify its financing needs and sources well in advance, which ensures both the lowest possible procurement costs and the availability of funds as they are needed.

Self-Test Questions
1. Why are capital budgeting decisions so crucial to the success of a business?
2. What are the benefits of effective capital budgeting procedures?

Project Classifications

Although benefits can be gained from the careful analysis of capital investment proposals, such efforts can be costly. For certain types of projects, a relatively detailed analysis may be warranted; for others, cost/benefit studies suggest that simpler procedures should be used. Accordingly, healthcare businesses generally classify projects into categories, and then analyze those in each category differently. For example, Ridgeland Community Hospital uses the following classifications:

- **Category 1: Mandatory replacement.** This category consists of expenditures necessary to replace worn-out or damaged equipment necessary to the operations of the hospital. In general, these expenditures are mandatory, so they are usually made without going through an elaborate decision process.
- **Category 2: Discretionary replacement.** This category includes expenditures to replace serviceable, but obsolete, equipment. The purpose of these projects generally is to lower costs or to provide more clinically effective services. Because Category 2 projects are not mandatory, a more detailed analysis is generally required to support the expenditure than that needed for Category 1 projects.
- **Category 3: Expansion of existing products, services, or markets.** This category includes expenditures to increase capacity, or to expand within

markets currently being served by the hospital. These decisions are more complex, so still more detailed analysis is required, and the final decision is made at a higher level within the organization.

- **Category 4: Expansion into new products, services, or markets.** This category consists of projects necessary to provide new products or services, or to expand into geographical areas not currently being served. Such projects involve strategic decisions that could change the fundamental nature of the hospital, and they normally require the expenditure of large sums of money over long periods. Invariably, a particularly detailed analysis is required, and the board of trustees generally makes the final decision as part of the hospital's strategic planning process.
- **Category 5: Safety/Environmental projects.** This category consists of expenditures necessary to comply with government orders, labor agreements, accreditation requirements, and so on. Unless the expenditures are large, Category 5 expenditures are treated like Category 1 expenditures.
- **Category 6: Other.** This category is a catchall for projects that do not fit neatly into another category. The primary determinant of how Category 6 projects are evaluated is their size.

1. What is the advantage of classifying capital projects?
2. What are some typical classifications?

Self-Test Questions

The Role of Financial Analysis in Health Services Capital Budgeting

For investor-owned businesses, with shareholder wealth maximization as the primary goal, the role of financial analysis in investment decisions is clear. Those projects that contribute to shareholder wealth should be undertaken, while those that do not should be ignored. However, what about not-for-profit firms that do not have shareholder wealth maximization as a goal? In such firms, the appropriate goal is providing quality, cost-effective service to the communities served. (A strong argument could be made that this should also be the goal of investor-owned firms in the health services industry.) In this situation, capital budgeting decisions must consider many factors besides a project's financial implications. For example, the needs of the medical staff and the good of the community must be taken into account. Indeed, in some instances, these noneconomic factors will outweigh financial considerations.

Nevertheless, good decision making, and hence the future viability of health services organizations, requires that the financial impact of capital investments be fully recognized. If a business takes on a series of highly unprofitable projects that meet nonfinancial goals, and such projects are not offset by other profitable projects, the business's financial condition will deteriorate. If this situation persists over time, the business will eventually lose its financial viability and may even be forced into bankruptcy and closure.

Because bankrupt businesses obviously cannot meet a community's needs, even managers of not-for-profit businesses must consider a project's potential impact on the firm's financial condition. Managers may make a conscious decision to accept a project with a poor financial prognosis because of its nonfinancial virtues, but it is important that managers know the financial impact up front, rather than be surprised when the project drains the firm's financial resources. Financial analysis provides managers with the relevant information about a project's financial impact, and hence helps managers make better decisions, including those decisions based primarily on nonfinancial considerations.

Self-Test Questions

1. What is the role of financial analysis in capital budgeting decision making within for-profit firms?
2. Why is project financial analysis important in not-for-profit businesses?

Overview of Capital Budgeting Financial Analysis

The financial analysis of capital investment proposals typically involves the following five steps:

1. The capital outlay, or cost, of the project must be estimated.
2. The operating and terminal cash flows of the project must be forecasted. The first two steps constitute the cash flow estimation phase, which is discussed in the next section.
3. The riskiness of the estimated cash flows must be assessed. Risk assessment will be discussed in Chapter 13.
4. Given the riskiness of the project, the project's cost of capital is estimated. As discussed in Chapter 10, a business's corporate cost of capital reflects the aggregate risk of the business's assets—that is, the riskiness inherent in the average project. If the project being evaluated does not have average risk, the corporate cost of capital must be adjusted.
5. Finally, the financial impact of the project is assessed, including profitability. Several measures can be used for this purpose; we will discuss five in this chapter.

Self-Test Question

1. Describe the five steps in capital budgeting financial analysis.

Cash Flow Estimation

The most important, but also the most difficult, step in evaluating capital investment proposals is cash flow estimation: The investment outlays, the annual net operating flows expected when the project goes into operation, and the cash flows associated with project termination. Many variables are involved in cash flow forecasting and many individuals and departments participate in the process. It is difficult to make accurate projections of the revenues and costs associated with a large, complex project, so forecast errors can be quite large. Thus, it is essential that risk analyses be performed on prospective projects. One manager with a good sense of humor developed the following five principles of capital budgeting cash flow estimation:

1. It is very difficult to forecast cash flows, especially those that occur in the future.
2. Those who live by the crystal ball soon learn how to eat ground glass.
3. The moment you forecast cash flows, you know that you are wrong; you just don't know by how much and in what direction.
4. If you are right, never let your bosses forget.
5. An expert is someone who has been right at least once.

It is hard to overstate either the difficulty or the importance of correctly forecasting a project's cash flows. However, if the principles discussed in the next sections are observed, errors that often arise in the process can be minimized.

Identifying the Relevant Cash Flows

The relevant cash flows to consider when evaluating a new capital investment are the project's *incremental cash flows*, which are defined as the difference in the firm's cash flows in each period if the project is undertaken versus the firm's cash flows if the project is not undertaken:

$$\text{Incremental } CF_t = CF_{t(\text{Firm with project})} - CF_{t(\text{Firm without project})}.$$

Here, the subscript t specifies a time period, normally years, so CF_0 is the cash flow during Year 0, which is generally assumed to end today; CF_1 is the cash flow during the first year; CF_2 is the cash flow during Year 2; and so on. In practice, the early cash flows, and Year 0 in particular, are usually cash outflows—the costs associated with getting the project "up and running." Then, as the project begins to generate revenues, the cash flows normally turn positve.

Cash Flow Versus Accounting Income

Accounting income statements prepared in accordance with generally accepted accounting principles are in some respects a mix of apples and oranges. For example, accountants deduct labor costs, which are cash outflows, from revenues, which may not be entirely cash. (For healthcare providers most of the collections are from third-party payers, and payment may not be received until several months after the service is provided.) At the same time, the income statement does not recognize capital outlays, which are cash flows, but it does deduct depreciation expense, which is not a cash flow. In capital investment decisions, it is critical that the decision be based on the actual dollars that flow into and out of the firm because a firm's true profitability, and hence its ability to provide healthcare services, depends on its cash flows and not on income as reported in accordance with generally accepted accounting principles. Note, however, that accounting items can influence cash flows because items like depreciation can affect tax or reimbursement cash flows.

Cash Flow Timing

Financial analysts must be careful to account properly for the timing of cash flows. Accounting income statements are for periods, such as years or quarters, so they do not reflect exactly when, during the period, revenues and expenses occur. In theory, capital budgeting cash flows should be analyzed exactly as they occur. Of course, there must be a compromise between accuracy and simplicity. A time line with daily cash flows would, in theory, provide the most accuracy, but daily cash flow estimates would be costly to construct, unwieldy to use, and probably no more accurate than annual cash flow estimates. Thus, in most cases, analysts simply assume that all cash flows occur at the end of every year. However, for some projects, it may be useful to assume that cash flows occur every six months, or even to forecast quarterly or monthly cash flows.

Project Life

One of the first decisions that must be made in forecasting a project's cash flows is the life of the project: Do we need to forecast cash flows for 20 years, or is five years sufficient? Many projects, such as a new hospital wing or an ambulatory care clinic, potentially have very long lives, perhaps as long as 50 years. In theory, a cash flow forecast should extend for the full life of a project, yet most managers would have very little confidence in any cash flow forecasts beyond the near term. Thus, most organizations set an arbitrary limit on the project life assumed in capital budgeting analyses, often five or ten years. If the forecasted life is less than the arbitrary limit, the forecasted life is used to develop the cash flows, but if the forecasted life exceeds the limit, project life is truncated and the operating cash flows beyond the limit are ignored in the analysis.

Although cash flow truncation is a practical solution to a difficult problem, it does create another problem—the value inherent in the cash flows beyond the truncation point is lost to the project. This problem can be addressed either objectively or subjectively. The standard procedure at some organizations is to estimate the project's *terminal value*, which is a proxy for the value of the cash flows beyond the truncation point. Often, the terminal value is estimated as the liquidation value of the project at that point in time. If the terminal value is too difficult to estimate, the fact that some portion of the project's cash flow stream is being ignored should, at a minimum, be subjectively recognized by decision makers. The saving grace in all of this is that cash flows well into the future typically contribute a relatively small amount to a project's profitability. For example, a $100,000 terminal value projected ten years in the future contributes only about $38,500 to the project's value when the cost of capital is 10 percent.

Sunk Costs

A *sunk cost* refers to an outlay that has already occurred, or has been irrevocably committed, so it is an outlay that is unaffected by the current decision to accept or reject the project. To illustrate the concept, suppose that it is the year 2001 and Ridgeland Community Hospital is evaluating the purchase of a lithotripter system. To help in the decision, the hospital hired and paid $10,000 to a consultant in 2000 to conduct a marketing study. Is this 2000 cash flow relevant to the 2001 capital investment decision? The answer is no. The $10,000 is a sunk cost; Ridgeland cannot recover it whether or not the lithotripter is purchased. Sometimes a project appears to be unprofitable when all of the associated costs, including sunk costs, are considered. However, on an *incremental* basis, the project may be profitable and should be undertaken. Thus, the correct treatment of sunk costs may be critical to the decision.

Assume for a moment that Ridgeland goes ahead with the lithotripter project. Then, in 2002, when conducting a periodic analysis of the **historical** profitability of the project, the $10,000 cost of the consultant's report might be included because it was part of the total cash flows attributable to the project. However, when making the 2001 decision regarding whether or not to go ahead with the project, the $10,000 is *nonincremental*, and hence not relevant to the decision.

Opportunity Costs

All relevant *opportunity costs* must be included in a capital investment analysis. To illustrate the concept, note that one opportunity cost involves the use of the capital. When Ridgeland uses its capital to invest in a lithotripter system, it cannot use the same capital to invest in—say, a new surgical suite. The opportunity cost associated with capital use is accounted for in the project's cost of capital, which is used to discount the project's expected cash flows and represents the return that the business could earn by investing in alternative investments of similar risk.

There are other types of opportunity costs, and all such costs should be built into a project's cash flows. For example, assume that Ridgeland's lithotripter would be installed in a freestanding facility, and that the hospital currently owns the land on which the facility would be constructed. In fact, the hospital purchased the land ten years ago at a cost of $50,000, but the current market value of the property is $130,000, net of (if applicable) taxes and fees. When evaluating the lithotripter, should the value of the land be disregarded because no cash outlay is necessary? The answer is no because there is an opportunity cost inherent in the use of the property. Using the property for the lithotripter facility deprives Ridgeland of its use for anything else. The property might be used for a walk-in clinic or ambulatory surgery center or parking garage rather than sold, but the best measure of its value to Ridgeland, and hence the opportunity cost inherent in its use, is the cash flow that could be realized from selling the property. By considering the property's current market value, Ridgeland is letting market forces assign the value for the land's best alternative use. Thus, the lithotripter project should have a $130,000 opportunity cost charged against it. Note that the opportunity cost is the property's $130,000 net market value, irrespective of whether the property was acquired for $50,000 or $200,000.

Effect on the Business's Other Projects

Capital budgeting analyses must consider the effect of the project under consideration on the business's other projects. When the effect is negative, it is often called *cannibalization*. To illustrate the concept, assume that some of the patients that are expected to use Ridgeland's new lithotripter would have been treated surgically at Ridgeland, so these surgical revenues will be lost if the lithotripter facility goes into operation. Thus, the incremental revenues to Ridgeland are the revenues attributable to the lithotripter, less the revenues lost from forgone surgery services. Of course, the costs saved by virtue of losing these surgery patients would be a benefit to the lithotripter project. Note, however, that if the surgical patients would be lost to **other providers** that are buying lithotripters, then the loss of these patients does not impact the lithotripter project at all because these losses would occur whether or not the lithotripter project is accepted.

Thus far we have focused on the negative impact of a new project on other services. The impact could be positive. To illustrate the concept, note that new patients that use the lithotripter may utilize other services provided by the hospital. In this situation, the incremental cash flows generated by the lithotripter patients' utilization of other services should be credited to the lithotripter project. If possible, both positive and negative effects on other projects should be quantified, but, at a minimum, they should be noted so that the final decision maker will be aware of their existence.

Shipping and Installation Costs

When a firm acquires fixed assets, it often incurs substantial costs for shipping and installing the equipment. These charges are added to the invoice price of the equipment to determine the overall cost of the project. Also, the full cost of the equipment, including shipping and installation charges, is used as the basis for calculating depreciation charges. Thus, if Ridgeland Community Hospital purchases intensive care monitoring equipment that costs $200,000, but another $20,000 is required for shipping and installation, then the full cost of the equipment would be $220,000, and this amount would be the starting point for all depreciation calculations.

Changes in Net Working Capital

Normally, expansion projects require additional inventories, and added patient services also lead to additional accounts receivable. The increase in these current asset accounts must be financed, just as an increase in fixed assets must be financed. However, accounts payable and accruals will probably also increase as a result of the expansion, and these current liability additions will reduce the cash needed to finance the increase in inventories and receivables. The difference between the increase in current assets and the increase in current liabilities that result from a new project is called a *change in net working capital*. If this change is positive—that is, if the increase in current assets exceeds the increase in current liabilities—then this amount is as much a cash cost to the project as is the cost of the asset itself. Such projects must be charged an additional amount above the cost of the new asset to reflect the net financing needed for the current asset accounts. Similarly, if the change in net working capital is negative, the project is generating a working capital cash inflow because the increase in liabilities exceeds the project's current asset requirements, and this cash flow partially offsets the cost of the asset being acquired.

As the project approaches termination, inventories will be sold off and not replaced, and receivables will be converted to cash without new receivables being created. In effect, the business will recover its investment in net working capital when the project is terminated. This will result in a cash flow that is equal, but opposite in sign, to the change in net working capital cash flow that arises at the beginning of a project.

For healthcare providers, the change in net working capital often can be ignored without materially affecting the results of the analysis. However, when a project results in a large change in net working capital, failure to consider the net investment in current assets will result in an overstatement of the project's profitability.

Inflation Effects

Because inflation is a fact of life, and because inflation effects can have a considerable influence on a project's profitability, it must be considered in any sound capital budgeting analysis. As we discussed in Chapter 10, a business's corporate cost of capital is based on its costs of debt and equity, which in turn are estimated on the basis of investors' required rates of return. Because investors must protect themselves against the loss of purchasing power as a result of inflation, they incorporate an inflation premium into their required returns. For example, a debt investor might require a 5 percent return on a ten-year bond in the absence of inflation. However, if inflation is expected to average 4 percent over the coming ten years, then the investor would require a 9 percent return.

Because inflation effects are already embedded in the corporate cost of capital, and because this rate is the benchmark used to discount the cash flows in our profitability measures, it is necessary to ensure that inflation effects are also built into the project's estimated cash flows. If cash flow estimates do not include inflation effects (*real* cash flows), and then a discount rate is used that does include inflation effects (*nominal* discount rate), then the profitability of the project will be understated.

The most effective way to deal with inflation is to build inflation effects into each cash flow component using the best available information about how each component will be affected. For example, per procedure revenues may be expected to increase at a 4 percent rate, labor costs could be expected to increase at an 8 percent rate, supplies costs might be expected to increase at a 2 percent rate, and so on. Because it is impossible to estimate future inflation rates with much precision, errors are bound to be made. For simplicity, inflation sometimes is assumed to be neutral; that is, it is assumed to affect all revenues and costs, except depreciation, equally. However, such an assumption rarely reflects the actual situation facing healthcare businesses, so, in general, different inflation rates should be applied to each cash flow component. Inflation adds to the uncertainty, or riskiness, of capital budgeting, as well as to its complexity. Fortunately, computers and spreadsheet programs are available to help with inflation analysis, so the mechanics of inflation adjustments are not difficult.

Cash Flow Estimation Bias

As stated previously, cash flow estimation is the most critical, and the most difficult, part of the capital budgeting process. Cash flow components, such as volume and charges, often must be forecasted many years into the future, and estimation errors are bound to occur, some of which can be quite large.[1] However, large firms evaluate and accept many projects every year, and as long as cash flow estimates are unbiased and the errors are random, the estimation errors will tend to offset one another; that is, some cash flow estimates will be too high and some will be too low, but, in the aggregate for all projects, the realized cash flows will be very close to the estimates, and hence realized total profitability will be close to that expected.

Unfortunately, there are strong indications that capital budgeting cash flow forecasts are not unbiased; rather, managers tend to be overly optimistic in their forecasts and, as a result, revenues tend to be overstated and costs tend to be understated.[2] The result is an upward bias in estimated profitability. This bias may result because managers are often rewarded on the basis of the size of their divisions or departments, so they have an incentive to maximize the number of projects accepted rather than the profitability of the projects. Or, managers may be emotionally attached to their projects and become unable to objectively assess a project's potential.

Top management can use two procedures to identify cash flow estimation bias. First, if a project is judged to be highly profitable, this question should be asked: "What is the underlying cause of this project's high profitability?" If the business has some underlying advantage, such as a monopoly position in a managed care market, or a superior reputation in providing a specific service, such as organ transplants, then there may be a logical rationale supporting the high profitability. If no such unique factor can be identified, then senior management should be concerned about the possibility of estimation bias. Even when these unique factors exist, it is likely that the project's profitability, at some point in the future, will be eroded by competitive pressure from other businesses seeking to capture the high profitability inherent in the project.

Second, the post-audit process, which we discuss later in this chapter, will help to identify divisions and departments that habitually overstate or understate project profitability. (It is difficult to identify projects whose cash flows are understated because many of those projects will be rejected, and hence no cash flow comparisons can be made. Perhaps the best indicator of underestimation bias is when competing firms undertake projects of the type that are being rejected.) Many firms are now identifying managers and divisions that typically submit biased cash flow estimates, and are compensating for this bias in the decision process by reducing cash inflows that are thought to be too rosy or by increasing the cost of capital to such projects.

Strategic Value

In the previous section, we discussed the problem of cash flow estimation bias, which can result in overstating a project's profitability. Another problem that can occur in cash flow estimation is underestimating a project's true profitability by not recognizing its *strategic value*, which is the value of future investment opportunities that can be undertaken only if the project currently under consideration is accepted.

To illustrate this concept, consider a hospital management company that is analyzing a management contract for a hospital in Hungary, which is its first move into Eastern Europe. On a stand-alone basis this project might be unprofitable, but the project might provide entry into the Eastern European market, which would unlock the door to a whole range of highly profitable new projects. Or consider Ridgeland Community Hospital's decision to start a kidney transplant program. The financial analysis of this project showed the program to be unprofitable, but Ridgeland's managers considered kidney transplants to be the first step in an aggressive transplant program that would not only be profitable in itself, but would enhance the hospital's reputation for technological and clinical excellence, and thus would contribute to the hospital's overall profitability.

In theory, the best approach to dealing with strategic value is to forecast the cash flows from the follow-on projects, estimate their probabilities of occurrence, and then add the expected cash flows from the follow-on projects to the cash flows of the project under consideration. In practice, this is usually impossible to do—either the follow-on cash flows are too nebulous to forecast or the potential follow-on projects are too numerous to quantify. In most situations, the strategic value of a project stems from managerial options that arise by virtue of the project being undertaken. Thus, at a minimum, decision makers must recognize that some projects have strategic value, and this value should be qualitatively considered when making capital budgeting decisions.

Strategic value is but one type of "added" value that arises when projects have embedded in them options that managers may or may not exercise (take advantage of) in the future. Options that are inherent in projects, as opposed to options on securities, are called *real options*. In the next chapter, we will discuss other types of real options and their implications for a project's risk and value.

Self-Test Question

1. Briefly, discuss the following concepts associated with cash flow estimation:
   a. Incremental cash flow
   b. Cash flow versus accounting income
   c. Cash flow timing
   d. Project life
   e. Sunk costs
   f. Opportunity costs
   g. Effects on other projects
   h. Shipping and installation costs
   i. Changes in net working capital
   j. Inflation effects
   k. Cash flow estimation bias
   l. Strategic value

Cash Flow Estimation Example

Up to this point, we have discussed a number of key concepts related to cash flow estimation. In this section, we present an example that illustrates some of the concepts already covered, and introduces several others that are important to good cash flow estimation.

The Basic Data

Consider the situation facing Ridgeland Community Hospital, a not-for-profit hospital, in its evaluation of a new magnetic resonance imaging (MRI) system. The system costs $ 1.5 million, and the hospital would have to spend another $1 million for shipping, site preparation, and installation. Because the system would be installed in the hospital, the space to be used has a very low, or zero, market value to outsiders, and thus no opportunity cost has been assigned to account for the value of the space.

The MRI site is estimated to generate weekly usage (volume) of 40 scans, and each scan would, on average, cost the hospital $15 in supplies. The site is expected to operate 50 weeks a year, with the remaining two weeks devoted to maintenance. The estimated average charge per scan is $500, but 25 percent of this amount, on average, is expected to be lost to indigent patients, contractual allowances, and bad debt losses. Ridgeland's managers developed the project's forecasted revenues by conducting the revenue analysis contained in Table 12.1.

The MRI site would require two technicians, resulting in an incremental increase in annual labor costs of $50,000, including fringe benefits. Cash overhead costs would increase by $10,000 annually if the MRI site is activated. The equipment would require maintenance, which would be furnished by the manufacturer for an annual fee of $150,000, which is payable at the end of each year of operation. For book (financial statement) purposes, the MRI site will be depreciated by the straight-line method over a five-year life.

The MRI site is expected to be in operation for five years, at which time the hospital's master plan calls for a brand-new imaging facility. The hospital plans to sell the MRI system at that time for an estimated $750,000 salvage value, net of removal costs. The inflation rate is estimated to average 5 percent over the period, and this rate is expected to apply to all revenues and costs except depreciation. Ridgeland's managers initially assume that projects under evaluation have average risk, and thus the hospital's 10 percent cost of capital is the appropriate project cost of capital. Later, in Chapter 13, a risk assessment of the project may indicate that a different cost of capital is appropriate.

Although the MRI project is expected to take away some patients from the hospital's other imaging systems, the new MRI patients are expected to generate revenues for some of the hospital's other departments. On net, the two effects are expected to balance out; that is, the cash flow loss from other imaging systems is expected to be offset by the cash flow gain from other services utilized by the new MRI patients.

Cash Flow Analysis

The first step in the financial analysis is to estimate the MRI site's net cash flows. This analysis is presented in Table 12.2. Here are the key points of the analysis by line number:

- **Line 1.** Line 1 contains the estimated cost of the MRI system. In general, capital budgeting analyses assume that the first cash flow, normally an outflow, occurs today or at the end of Year 0. Note that expenses, or cash outflows, are shown in parentheses.
- **Line 2.** The related shipping, site preparation, and installation expense—$1 million—is also assumed to occur at Year 0.
- **Line 3.** Gross revenues = Weekly volume × Weeks of operation × Charge per scan = 40 × 50 × $500 = $1,000,000 in the first year. The 5 percent inflation rate is applied to all charges and costs that would likely be affected by inflation, so the gross revenue amount shown on Line 3 increases by 5 percent over time. Although most of the operating revenues and costs

TABLE 12.1
Ridgeland Community Hospital: MRI Site Revenue Analysis

Payer	Number of Scans per Week	Charge per Scan	Total Charges	Basis of Payment	Net Payment per Scan	Total Payments
Medicare	10	$500	$ 5,000	Fixed fee	$370*	$ 3,700
Medicaid	5	500	2,500	Fixed fee	350*	1,750
Private insurance	9	500	4,500	Full charge	500	4,500
Blue Cross	5	500	2,500	Percent of charge	420*	2,100
Managed care	7	500	3,500	Percent of charge	390*	2,730
Self-pay	4	500	2,000	Full charge	55**	220
Total	40		$20,000			$15,000
Average			$ 500			$ 375

*Net of contractual allowances.
**Net of bad debt losses.

TABLE 12.2
Ridgeland Community Hospital: MRI Site Cash Flow Analysis

			Annual Cash Flows, Years 0–5			
	0	1	2	3	4	5
1. System cost	($1,500,000)					
2. Related expenses	(1,000,000)					
3. Gross revenues		$1,000,000	$1,050,000	$1,102,500	$1,157,625	$1,215,506
4. Deductions		250,000	262,500	275,625	289,406	303,877
5. Net revenues		$ 750,000	$ 787,500	$ 826,875	$ 868,219	$ 911,630
6. Labor costs		50,000	52,500	55,125	57,881	60,775
7. Maintenance costs		150,000	157,500	165,375	173,644	182,326
8. Supplies		30,000	31,500	33,075	34,729	36,465
9. Incremental overhead		10,000	10,500	11,025	11,576	12,155
10. Depreciation		350,000	350,000	350,000	350,000	350,000
11. Operating cash flow		$ 160,000	$ 185,500	$ 212,275	$ 240,389	$ 269,908
12. Taxes		0	0	0	0	0
13. Net operating cash flow		$ 160,000	$ 185,500	$ 212,275	$ 240,389	$ 269,908
14. Depreciation		350,000	350,000	350,000	350,000	350,000
15. Net salvage value						750,000
16. Net cash flow	($2,500,000)	$ 510,000	$ 535,500	$ 562,275	$ 590,389	$1,369,908

Note: Calculations are rounded.

would occur more or less evenly over the year, it is very difficult to forecast exactly when most of the flows would occur. Furthermore, there is significant potential for large errors in cash flow estimation. For these reasons, operating cash flows are often assumed to occur at the end of each year. Also, we assume that the MRI system could be placed in operation quickly. If this were not the case, then the first year's operating flows would be reduced because it would be a partial year of operations. In some situations, it might take several years from the first cash outflow to the point when the project is operational and begins to generate operating cash inflows.

- **Line 4.** Deductions from charges are estimated to average 25 percent of gross revenues, so in Year 1, $0.25 \times \$1,000,000 = \$250,000$ of gross revenues would be uncollected. This amount increases each year by the 5 percent inflation rate.
- **Line 5.** Line 5 contains the net revenues in each year, Line 3–Line 4.
- **Line 6.** Labor costs are forecasted to be $50,000 during the first year, but increase over time at the 5 percent inflation rate.
- **Line 7.** Maintenance fees must be paid to the manufacturer at the end of each year of operation. These fees are assumed to increase at the 5 percent inflation rate.
- **Line 8.** Each scan uses $15 of supplies, so supply costs in the first year total $40 \times 50 \times \$15 = \$30,000$, which are expected to increase each year by the inflation rate.
- **Line 9.** If the project is accepted, overhead cash costs will increase by $10,000 in the first year. Note that the $10,000 are cash costs that are related directly to the acceptance of the MRI project. Existing overhead costs that are arbitrarily allocated to the MRI site are not incremental cash flows, and thus should not be included in the analysis. Overhead costs are also assumed to increase over time at the inflation rate.
- **Line 10.** For book purposes, depreciation in each year is calculated by the straight-line method, assuming a five-year depreciable life. The depreciable basis is equal to the capitalized cost of the project, which includes the cost of the asset and related expenses, less the estimated salvage value. Thus, the depreciable basis is $(\$1,500,000 + \$1,000,000) - \$750,000 = \$1,750,000$. Then, the straight-line depreciation in each year of the project's five-year depreciable life is $(1 / 5) \times \$1,750,000 = \$350,000$. Note that depreciation is based solely on acquisition costs, so it is unaffected by inflation. Also, note that the Table 12.2 cash flows are presented in a generic format that can be used by both investor-owned and not-for-profit hospitals. Depreciation expense is not a cash flow, but an accounting convention that prorates the cost of a long-term asset over its productive life. Because Ridgeland Community Hospital is tax exempt, and hence depreciation will not affect taxes, and because depreciation is added back to the cash flows on Line 14, depreciation could be totally

omitted from the cash flow analysis.

- **Line 11.** Line 11 shows the project's operating cash flow in each year, which is merely net revenues less all operating expenses.
- **Line 12.** Line 12 contains zeros because Ridgeland is not-for-profit, and hence does not pay taxes.
- **Line 13.** Ridgeland pays no taxes, so the project's net operating cash flow equals its operating cash flow.
- **Line 14.** Because depreciation, a noncash expense, was deducted on Line 10, it must be added back to the project's net operating cash flow in each year to obtain each year's net cash flow.
- **Line 15.** Finally, the project is expected to be terminated after five years, at which time the MRI system would be sold for an estimated $750,000. This salvage value cash flow is shown as an inflow at the end of Year 5 on Line 15.
- **Line 16.** The project's net cash flows are shown on Line 16. The project requires a $2.5 million investment at Year 0, but then generates cash inflows over its five-year operating life.

Note that the Table 12.2 cash flows do not include any allowance for interest expense. On average, Ridgeland hospital will finance new projects in accordance with its target capital structure, which consists of 50 percent debt financing and 50 percent equity (fund) financing. The costs associated with this financing mix, including interest costs, are incorporated into Ridgeland's corporate cost of capital of 10.0 percent. Because the cost of debt financing is included in the discount rate that will be applied to the cash flows, recognition of interest expense in the cash flows would be double counting.

Taxable Organizations

The Table 12.2 cash flow analysis can be easily modified to reflect tax implications if the analyzing firm is taxable. For example, assume that the MRI project is being evaluated by Ann Arbor Health Systems, an investor-owned hospital chain. Furthermore, assume that all of the project data presented earlier apply to Ann Arbor, except that (1) the MRI falls into the MACRS five-year class for tax depreciation and (2) the firm has a 40 percent tax rate. Table 12.3 contains Ann Arbor's cash flow analysis. Note the following differences:

- **Line 10.** First, depreciation expense must be modified to reflect tax depreciation rather than book depreciation. As we discussed in Chapter 2, tax depreciation is calculated using the Modified Accelerated Cost Recovery System (MACRS). Table 2.9 in Chapter 2 gives the MACRS depreciation factors for several different class lives. To determine the MACRS depreciation allowance in any year, multiply the asset's depreciable basis, without considering its estimated salvage value, by the appropriate depreciation factor. In the MRI illustration, the depreciable basis is $2,500,000, and the MACRS factors for the five-year class are

TABLE 12.3
Ann Arbor Health Systems: MRI Site Cash Flow Analysis

		Annual Cash Flows, Years 0–5				
	0	1	2	3	4	5
1. System cost	($1,500,000)					
2. Related expenses	(1,000,000)					
3. Gross revenues		$1,000,000	$1,050,000	$1,102,500	$1,157,625	$1,215,506
4. Deductions		250,000	262,500	275,625	289,406	303,877
5. Net revenues		$ 750,000	$ 787,500	$ 826,875	$ 868,219	$ 911,630
6. Labor costs		50,000	52,500	55,125	57,881	60,775
7. Maintenance costs		150,000	157,500	165,375	173,644	182,326
8. Supplies		30,000	31,500	33,075	34,729	36,465
9. Incremental overhead		10,000	10,500	11,025	11,576	12,155
10. Depreciation		500,000	800,000	475,000	300,000	275,000
11. Operating cash flow		$ 10,000	($ 264,500)	$ 87,275	$ 290,389	$ 344,908
12. Taxes		4,000	(105,800)	34,910	116,156	137,963
13. Net operating cash flow		$ 6,000	$ 158,700	$ 52,365	$ 174,233	$ 206,945
14. Depreciation		500,000	800,000	475,000	300,000	275,000
15. Net salvage value						510,000
16. Net cash flow	($2,500,000)	$ 506,000	$ 641,300	$ 527,365	$ 474,233	$ 991,945

Note: Calculations are rounded.

0.20, 0.32, 0.19, 0.12, 0.11, and 0.06 in Years 1 to 6, respectively. Thus, the tax depreciation in Year 1 is 0.20 × $2,500,000 = $500,000; in Year 2 the depreciation is 0.32 × $2,500,000 = $800,000; and so on.

- **Line 12.** Taxable businesses must reduce the operating cash flow on Line 11 by the amount of taxes. Taxes, which appear on Line 12, are computed by multiplying the Line 12 pretax operating cash flow by the business's marginal tax rate. For example, the project's taxes for Year 1 are 0.40 × $10,000 = $4,000. Note that the taxes shown for Year 2 are a negative $105,800. In this year, the project is expected to lose $264,500, and hence Ann Arbor's taxable income, assuming its existing projects are profitable, will be reduced by this amount if the project is undertaken. This reduction in taxable income would lower the firm's tax bill by T × Taxable income reduction = 0.40 × $264,500 = $105,800.[3]

- **Line 14.** The MACRS depreciation, because it is a noncash expense, is added back in Line 14.

- **Line 15.** Investor-owned firms will normally incur a tax liability on the sale of a capital asset at the end of the project's life. According to the IRS, the value of the MRI system at the end of Year 5 is the *tax book value*, which is the depreciation that remains on the tax books. In the illustration, five years worth of depreciation would be taken, so only one year of depreciation remains. The MACRS factor for Year 6 is 0.06, so by the end of Year 5, Ann Arbor has expensed 0.94 of the MRI's depreciable basis and the remaining tax book value is 0.06 × $2,500,000 = $150,000. Thus, according to the IRS, the value of the MRI system is $150,000. When Ann Arbor sells the system for its estimated salvage value of $750,000, it realizes a "profit" of $750,000 − $150,000 = $600,000, and it must repay the IRS an amount equal to 0.4 × $600,000 = $240,000. The $240,000 tax bill recognizes that Ann Arbor took too much depreciation on the MRI system, so it represents a *recapture* of the excess tax benefit taken over the five-year life of the system. The $240,000 in taxes reduces the cash received from the sale of the MRI equipment, so the salvage value net of taxes is $750,000 − $240,000 = $510,000.

As can be seen by comparing Line 16 in Tables 12.1 and 12.2, all else the same, the taxes paid by investor-owned firms tend to reduce a project's net operating cash flows and net salvage value, and hence reduce the project's profitability.

Replacement Analysis

Ridgeland Community Hospital's MRI project was used to illustrate how the cash flows from an *expansion project* are analyzed. All businesses, including Ridgeland Community Hospital, also make *replacement decisions*, in which a new asset is being considered to replace an existing asset that could, if not replaced, continue in operation. The cash flow analysis for a replacement decision is somewhat more complex than for an expansion decision because the cash flows from the existing asset must be considered.

Again, the key to cash flow estimation is to focus on the incremental cash flows. If the new asset is acquired, the existing asset can be sold, so the current market value of the existing asset is a cash inflow at Time 0 in the analysis. When considering the operating flows, the incremental flows are the cash flows expected from the replacement asset less the flows that the existing asset produces. By applying the incremental cash flow concept, the correct cash flows can be estimated for replacement decisions.[4]

Self-Test Questions

1. Briefly, describe how a project cash flow analysis is constructed.
2. Is it necessary to include depreciation expense in a cash flow analysis by a not-for-profit provider? Explain your answer.
3. What are the key differences in cash flow analyses performed by investor-owned and not-for-profit organizations?
4. How do expansion and replacement project analyses differ?

Breakeven Analysis

Breakeven analysis is used to gain insights into the potential profitability and risk of a project. Furthermore, breakeven analysis often is useful in evaluating projects that do not require an initial capital investment, such as expanding the hours of operation of a clinic. Although breakeven analysis can be applied in many different ways, we will focus here on two types of breakeven: (1) utilization (volume) breakeven and (2) time breakeven.

Utilization (Volume) Breakeven

To illustrate utilization breakeven, first consider how it can be applied to operating cash flows. Specifically, let's examine operating breakeven in Year 1. From Table 12.2, we know that 40 scans a week would produce a net cash flow in Year 1 of $510,000. But, a logical question to ask would be how many scans per week would be necessary to reach operating breakeven in Year 1? That is, how many scans per week are required to generate a positive net cash flow in Year 1? With the basic analysis performed using a spreadsheet program, it is very easy to do breakeven analysis. Table 12.4 contains the Year 1 net cash flow at different utilization levels and, as indicated by the data, the project breaks even in Year 1 if the hospital performs 12 scans per week.

Utilization breakeven can also be applied to the entire project. Here, we want to know the answer to this question: What weekly utilization would allow the hospital to breakeven economically—that is, to recover all of the costs associated with the project, including capital costs? Again, if the analysis is modeled on a spreadsheet, answers to these types of questions are easy to

Number of Scans per Week	Year 1 Net Cash Flow
0	($210,000)
5	(120,000)
10	(30,000)
11	(12,000)
12	6,000
13	24,000
14	42,000
15	60,000
20	150,000
30	330,000
40	510,000

TABLE 12.4
Ridgeland
Community
Hospital: MRI
Site Year 1
Breakeven
Analysis

develop. As we discuss in a later section, economic breakeven occurs for a project when its net present value (NPV) equals zero or just turns positive. In Ridgeland's MRI project, this occurs at a weekly usage of 39 scans, so the project in its entirety just breaks even when the hospital averages 39 scans per week over the five-year forecasted life of the project. Such information is clearly useful to Ridgeland's managers. If they feel strongly that utilization will exceed 39 scans per week, then it is highly likely that the project will be economically profitable. Conversely, if they believe that utilization will be less than the breakeven level, then the project will probably be unprofitable. Also, if, as in this situation, the projected volume is just above breakeven, a small forecasting error can result in a project that appears profitable on paper, but actually is unprofitable if undertaken.

Time Breakeven (Payback)

The *payback*, or *payback period*, measures time breakeven. Payback is defined as the expected number of years required to recover the investment in the project. To illustrate the concept, consider the net cash flows for the MRI project contained in Table 12.2. The best way to determine the project's payback is to construct the project's cumulative cash flows as shown in Table 12.5. Here, the cumulative cash flow in each year is the sum of the annual cash flows up to and including that year. For example, the cumulative cash flow in Year 2 is −$2,500,000 + $510,000 + $535,000 = −$1,454,500.

Because the cumulative cash flows turn positive in Year 5, the $2.5 million investment in the MRI site would be recovered some time during Year 5. If the project's cash flows are assumed to come in evenly during the year, then breakeven would occur $301,836 / $1,369,908 = 0.22 of the way through Year 5, so the payback is 4.22 years.

TABLE 12.5
Ridgeland
Community
Hospital: MRI
Site Cumulative
Cash Flows

Year	Annual Cash Flow	Cumulative Cash Flow
0	($2,500,000)	($2,500,000)
1	510,000	(1,990,000)
2	535,500	(1,454,500)
3	562,275	(892,225)
4	590,389	(301,836)
5	1,369,908	1,068,072

Payback = 4 + $301,836 / $1,369,908 = 4.22 years.

Initially, payback was used by managers as the primary financial evaluation tool in project analyses. For example, a business might accept all projects with paybacks less than five years. However, payback has two serious deficiencies when it is used as a project selection criterion. First, payback ignores all cash flows that occur after the payback period. For example, assume that Ridgeland is evaluating a competing project that has the same cash flows as the MRI project in Years 0 through 5. However, the alternative project has a cash inflow of $2 million in Year 6. Both projects would have the same payback, 4.22 years, and hence be ranked the same, even though the alternative project clearly is better from a financial perspective. Second, payback ignores the opportunity costs associated with the capital employed. For these reasons, payback generally is no longer used as the primary evaluation tool.

However, payback is useful in capital investment analysis. The shorter the payback, the more quickly the funds invested in a project will become available for other purposes, and hence the more liquid the project. Also, cash flows expected in the distant future are generally regarded as being riskier than near-term cash flows, so shorter payback projects generally are less risky than those with longer paybacks. Therefore, payback is often used as a rough measure of a project's *liquidity* and *risk*.

Another measure, the *discounted payback*, is similar to the straight payback, except that the cash flows in each year are discounted by the project's cost of capital prior to calculating the payback. Thus, discounted payback solves the straight payback's problem of not considering the project's cost of capital in the payback calculation. To illustrate discounted payback, consider Table 12.6. Here, we have created a new column labeled "Discounted Cash Flow." Each entry in this column is the matching annual cash flow discounted at the 10 percent cost of capital for the number of years that it occurs into the future. For example, the discounted Year 2 cash flow is $535,500 / (1.10)^2 = $442,562. The discounted payback is 4 + 768,112 / 850,605 = 4.90 years. Because time value is recognized in the discounted payback, it is longer than the regular payback of 4.22 years.

Year	Annual Cash Flow	Discounted Cash Flow	Cumulative Discounted Cash Flow
0	($2,500,000)	($2,500,000)	($2,500,000)
1	510,000	463,636	(2,036,364)
2	535,500	442,562	(1,593,802)
3	562,275	422,446	(1,171,356)
4	590,389	403,244	(768,112)
5	1,369,908	850,605	82,493

Discounted payback = 4 + 768,112 / 850,605 = 4.90 years.

TABLE 12.6
Ridgeland Community Hospital: MRI Site Cumulative Discounted Cash Flows

1. Why is breakeven information valuable to decision makers?
2. Describe several types of breakeven analysis.
3. What is the difference between "regular" payback and discounted payback?

Self-Test Questions

Profitability Analysis

Up to this point, the chapter has focused on cash flow estimation and break-even analysis. Perhaps the most important element in a project's financial analysis is expected profitability. In general, the expected profitability of capital investments can be measured either in dollars or in percentage rate of return. In the next sections, we present one dollar measure—net present value—and two rate of return measures—(1) internal rate of return and (2) modified internal rate of return.

Net Present Value (NPV)

Net present value (NPV) is a profitability measure that uses the discounted cash flow (DCF) techniques discussed in Chapter 4, so it is often referred to as a *DCF measure*. To apply the NPV method, we proceed as follows:

- Find the present (Time 0) value of each net cash flow, including both inflows and outflows, discounted at the project cost of capital.
- Sum the present values. This sum is defined as the project's net present value.
- If the NPV is positive, the project is profitable, and the higher the NPV the more profitable the project. If the NPV is zero, the project just breaks even in profitability. If the NPV is negative, the project is unprofitable.

Assuming a project cost of capital of 10 percent, the NPV of Ridgeland's MRI project is calculated as follows:

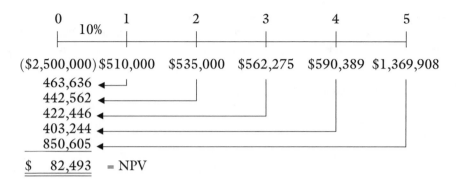

$$ \$ \quad 82,493 \quad = NPV $$

Financial calculators and spreadsheets have NPV functions that easily perform the mathematics given the cash flows and cost of capital.[5]

The rationale behind the NPV method is straightforward. An NPV of zero signifies that the project's cash inflows are just sufficient to (1) return the capital invested in the project and (2) provide the required rate of return on that invested capital. In other words, the project just breaks even in an economic sense, which considers **all costs** associated with the employment of capital. If a project has a positive NPV, then it is generating excess cash flows, and these excess cash flows are available to management to reinvest in the firm and, for investor-owned firms, to pay dividends. For investor-owned firms, NPV is a direct measure of the contribution of the project to shareholder wealth. If a project has a negative NPV, its cash inflows are insufficient to compensate the business for the capital invested, or perhaps will not ever recover the invested capital, so the project is unprofitable, and acceptance would cause the financial condition of the business to deteriorate.

The NPV of the MRI project is $82,493, so on a present value basis the project is projected to generate a cash flow excess of over $80,000. Thus, the project is profitable, and its acceptance would have a positive impact on Ridgeland's financial condition.

Internal Rate of Return (IRR)

Whereas NPV measures a project's dollar profitability, *internal rate of return (IRR)*, which is another DCF profitability measure, measures a project's percentage profitability or expected rate of return. Mathematically, the IRR is defined as the discount rate that equates the present value of the project's expected cash inflows to the present value of the project's expected cash outflows, so the IRR is simply that discount rate which forces the NPV of the project to equal zero. Financial calculators and spreadsheets have IRR functions that calculate IRRs very rapidly. Simply input the project's cash flows, and the computer or calculator computes the IRR.

For Ridgeland's MRI project, the IRR is that discount rate that causes the sum of the present values of the cash inflows to equal the $2.5 million cost of the project:

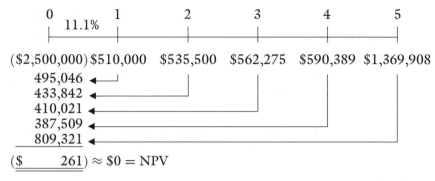

When all of the MRI project's cash flows are discounted at 11.1 percent, the NPV of the project is approximately zero. Thus, the MRI project's IRR is 11.1 percent. Put another way, the project is expected to generate an 11.1 percent rate of return on its $2.5 million investment.

If the IRR exceeds the project cost of capital, a surplus remains after recovering the invested capital and paying for its use, and this surplus accrues to the firm's stockholders (in Ridgeland's case, to its stakeholders). On the other hand, if the IRR is less than the project cost of capital, then taking on the project imposes a cost on the firm's stockholders, or stakeholders. The MRI project's 11.1 percent IRR exceeds the project's 10.0 percent cost of capital. Thus, as measured by the IRR, the MRI project is profitable and its acceptance would enhance Ridgeland's financial condition.

Comparison of the NPV and IRR Methods

Consider a project with a zero NPV. In this situation, the project's IRR must equal its cost of capital. The project has zero profitability, and acceptance would neither enhance nor diminish the firm's financial condition. To have a positive NPV, the project's IRR must be greater than its cost of capital, and a negative NPV signifies a project with an IRR less than its cost of capital. Thus, projects that are deemed profitable by the NPV method will also be deemed profitable by the IRR method. In the MRI example, the project would have a positive NPV for all costs of capital less than 11.1 percent. If the cost of capital is greater than 11.1 percent, the project would have a negative NPV. In effect, the NPV and IRR are perfect substitutes for one another in measuring whether a project is profitable or not.

Modified Internal Rate of Return (MIRR)

In general, academics prefer the NPV profitability measure. This preference stems from two factors: (1) NPV measures profitability in dollars, which is a direct measure of the contribution of the project to the value of the business; and (2) both the NPV and the IRR, because they are discounted cash flow techniques, require an assumption about the rate at which project cash flows can be reinvested, and the NPV method has the better assumption.

To further explain the second point, consider the MRI project's Year 2 net cash flow of $535,500 as shown in Table 12.2. In effect, the discounting process inherent in the NPV and IRR methods automatically assigns a reinvestment rate to this cash flow; that is, both the NPV and IRR methods assume that Ridgeland has the opportunity to reinvest the $535,500 Year 2 cash flow in other projects, and each method automatically assigns a reinvestment rate to this flow for Years 3, 4, and 5. The NPV method assumes reinvestment at the project cost of capital, 10 percent, while the IRR method assumes reinvestment at the IRR rate, 11.1 percent. Which is the better assumption— reinvestment at the cost of capital or reinvestment at the IRR rate? In general, businesses will take on all projects that exceed their cost of capital. Thus, at the margin, the returns from capital reinvested within the firm are more likely to be at, or close to, the cost of capital than at the project's IRR, especially for projects with exceptionally high or low IRRs. Furthermore, businesses can obtain outside capital at a cost roughly equal to the cost of capital, so project cash flows can be replaced by capital having this cost. Thus, in general, reinvestment at the cost of capital is a better assumption than reinvestment at the IRR rate, so NPV is a theoretically better measure of profitability than IRR.[6]

Even though academics strongly favor the NPV method, practicing managers prefer the IRR method by a margin of three to one. Apparently, managers find it intuitively more appealing to analyze investments in terms of percentage rates of return than dollars of NPV. Thus, an alternative rate of return measure has been developed that eliminates the primary problem with IRR. This method is the *modified IRR (MIRR)*, and it is calculated as follows:

• Discount all the project's net cash outflows back to Year 0 at the project cost of capital.
• Compound all the project's net cash inflows forward to the last (terminal) year of the project, at the project cost of capital. This value is called the *inflow terminal value.*
• The discount rate that forces the present value of the inflow terminal value to equal the present value of costs is defined as the MIRR.

Applying these steps to Ridgeland's MRI project produces a MIRR of about 10.7 percent:

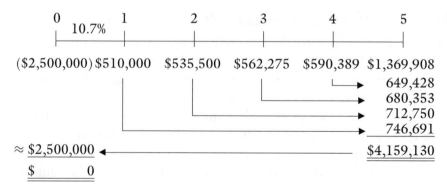

The MIRR method, by compounding the cash inflows forward at 10 percent, forces the reinvestment rate to equal 10 percent, which is the project cost of capital. Note that the MIRR for the MRI project is less than the project's IRR because the cash inflows are reinvested at only 10 percent rather than the project's 11.1 percent IRR. In general, the MIRR is less than the IRR when the IRR is greater than the cost of capital, but greater than the IRR when the IRR is less than the cost of capital. In effect, the IRR overstates the profitability of profitable projects and understates the profitability of unprofitable projects. By forcing the correct reinvestment rate, the MIRR method provides decision makers with a theoretically better measure of a project's expected rate of return than does the IRR.

Self-Test Questions

1. Briefly, describe net present value (NPV), internal rate of return (IRR), and modified IRR (MIRR).
2. Explain the rationale behind each method.
3. Why is MIRR a better rate of return measure than IRR?

Some Final Thoughts on Breakeven and Profitability Analysis

We have presented several approaches to breakeven analysis and three profitability measures. In the course of our discussion, we purposely compared the methods against one another to highlight their relative strengths and weaknesses, but, in the process, we may have created the impression that businesses would use only one method in the decision process. Today, virtually all capital budgeting decisions of financial consequence are analyzed by computer, and hence it is easy to calculate and list numerous breakeven measures along with NPV, IRR, and MIRR. Because each measure contributes slightly different information about the financial consequences of a project, it would be foolish for decision makers to focus on a single financial measure. Thus, we believe that a thorough financial analysis of a new project should include numerous financial measures, and that capital budgeting decisions are enhanced if all the information inherent in all of the measures is considered.

Self-Test Question

1. Should capital budgeting analyses look at only one breakeven or profitability measure? Explain.

Evaluating Projects with Unequal Lives

Occasionally, businesses must choose between two mutually exclusive projects that have unequal lives. (Two projects are *mutually exclusive* when acceptance of one implies rejection of the other.) When this situation arises, if the shorter-life project will be replicated, then an adjustment to the normal capital budgeting process is necessary. We now discuss two procedures—(1) the replacement chain method and (2) the equivalent annual annuity method—to both illustrate the problem and to show how to deal with it.

Suppose American Dental Equipment Corporation is planning to modernize its production facilities, and as part of the process, it is considering either a conveyor system (Project C) or forklift trucks (Project F) for moving materials from the parts department to the main assembly line. Table 12.7 shows both the expected net cash flows and the NPVs for these two mutually exclusive alternatives. We see that Project C, when discounted at the firm's 11.5 percent corporate cost of capital, has the higher NPV and, thus, appears to be the more profitable project.

Replacement Chain (Common Life) Analysis

Although the analysis in Table 12.7 suggests that Project C is the more profitable project, the analysis is incomplete and this conclusion is actually incorrect. If the firm chooses Project F, it will have the opportunity to make a similar investment in three years, and if cost and revenue conditions continue at the Table 12.7 levels, this second, or replication, investment will also be profitable. However, if the firm chooses Project C, it will not have this second investment opportunity. Therefore, to make a proper comparison between the three-year and six-year projects, we could apply the *replacement chain (common life)* approach; that is, we could find the extended NPV of Project F over a six-year period by assuming the project is replicated, and then compare this extended NPV with the NPV of Project C over the same period.

The NPV for Project C, as calculated in Table 12.7, is already over the six-year common life. For Project F, however, we must take three additional steps: (1) determine the NPV of the replication project three years hence, (2) discount this NPV back to the present, and (3) sum the two components to obtain the project's extended NPV. If we assume that the replication project will have the same cash flows as the original project, then Project F's extended NPV is $9,280:

TABLE 12.7
Expected Net Cash Flows for Projects C and F

Year	Project C	Project F
0	($40,000)	($20,000)
1	8,000	7,000
2	14,000	13,000
3	13,000	12,000
4	12,000	—
5	11,000	—
6	10,000	—
NPV @ 11.5%	($ 7,165)	($ 5,391)

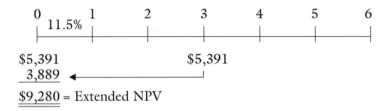

$5,391
 3,889
$9,280 = Extended NPV

Because Project F's six-year (extended) NPV is greater than Project C's six-year NPV, Project F is more profitable when the opportunity to replicate the project is considered.

Note that the time line analysis above uses NPVs to summarize Project F's estimated cash flows. An alternative approach to the analysis is to place the individual cash flows on the time line:

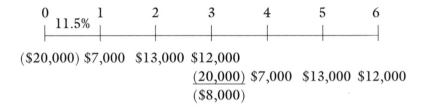

NPV ≈ $9,280.

Clearly, the former method is simpler. However, if the cash flows for the replicated project are not the same as the cash flows for the initial project, then the more complex individual cash flow method must be used. By showing each cash flow, the analysis can accommodate changes in project cash flows that occur when the project is replicated.

Equivalent Annual Annuity Approach

Although the preceding example illustrates why an extended analysis is necessary if two mutually exclusive projects with different lives are being analyzed, the analysis is generally more complex in practice. For example, one project might have a six-year life versus a ten-year life for the other. This would require a replacement chain analysis over 30 years, which is the lowest common multiple of the two lives. In such a situation, it is simpler to use the *equivalent annual annuity (EAA)* approach.

The EAA approach involves three steps:

1. Find each project's NPV over its original life. In Table 12.7, we see that $NPV_C = \$7,165$ and $NPV_F = \$5,391$.
2. For each project, find the annuity (constant value) cash flow over the project's original life that has the same present value as the project's NPV. This cash flow is called the *equivalent annual annuity*. Here is the concept on a time line for Project F:

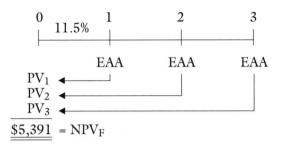

To find the value of EAA$_F$ on a financial calculator, enter 5,391 (or −5,391) as the PV, I = 11.5, and N = 3. Then, solve for PMT = 2,225. Thus, the equivalent annual annuity for Project F is $2,225. This is the annuity stream over the original life of the project—three years—that when discounted at the project cost of capital—11.5 percent—has a present value equal to Project F's NPV, $5,391. The EAA for Project C is found in a like manner, and it is $1,718. Thus, Project C has an NPV that is equivalent to an annuity of $1,718 per year for six years, while Project F's NPV is equivalent to an annuity of $2,225 for three years.

3. Now, when projects are replicated, assuming that the cash flows remain the same, they earn the same NPV over and over, which is equivalent to replicating the project's EAA over time. Thus, over any common life, whether six years or 30 years, the project with the higher EAA will have the higher NPV because its equivalent cash flow will be higher in every year. Because Project F has the higher EAA, under the assumption of constant cash flow replication, it is more profitable than Project C.

The EAA method is generally easier to apply, but the replacement chain method is often easier to explain to decision makers. Still, the two methods always lead to the same results if consistent assumptions are used. When should managers worry about unequal life analysis? As a general rule, the unequal life issue does not arise for independent projects; it is only an issue when mutually exclusive projects are being analyzed. However, even for mutually exclusive projects, it is not always appropriate to extend the analysis to a common life. This should only be done if there is a high probability that the projects will actually be replicated beyond their original lives.

There are several weaknesses inherent in the types of analysis just described. First, if inflation is expected, then replacement cost will probably be higher than the initial cost, both revenues and operating costs will probably rise, and hence the static conditions built into the example would not be appropriate. Second, future replacements may use different technologies, which might also change the project's cash flows. Third, it is difficult enough to estimate the lives of most projects, so estimating the lives of a future series of projects is often just speculation.

In view of these problems, no experienced manager would be too concerned about comparing mutually exclusive projects with lives of, say, eight years and ten years. Given all of the uncertainties in the estimation process, such projects could, for all practical purposes, be assumed to have the same life. Still, it is important to recognize that a problem does exist if mutually exclusive projects that will be replicated have substantially different lives. When the managers of Ann Arbor Health Systems encounter such problems, they build expected inflation or possible efficiency gains, or both, directly into the cash flow estimates, and then use the replacement chain approach to estimate the projects' extended NPVs. The cash flow estimation is more complicated than in our example, but the concepts involved are exactly the same.

1. Is it always necessary to adjust project cash flows to account for unequal lives?
2. Briefly, describe the two methods for adjusting for unequal lives.

Self-Test Questions

Abandonment Value

Customarily, projects are analyzed as though the business will operate the project over its full *physical*, or *engineering, life*. However, this may not be the best course of action financially; it may be best to abandon a project prior to the end of its potential life, and this possibility can materially affect a project's estimated profitability. To illustrate the concept of *abandonment value* and its effects on capital budgeting decisions, consider Ridgeland Community Hospital's proposal to establish a taxable medical transportation division that would offer specialized medical transportation services to Ridgeland's patients and others in the community. The project's cash flows are contained in Table 12.8. For simplicity, we have shortened the physical life of the project to three years. The project's investment and operating cash flows are shown in the second column, while the third column contains the project's *abandonment values*. Abandonment values are equivalent to net salvage values, except that they have been estimated for each year of the project's physical life.

Using a 10 percent cost of capital, the NPV over the project's three-year physical life, with zero abandonment value, is −$11,743. Thus, the project is unprofitable when the single alternative of a three-year life with a zero salvage value is considered. However, what would its NPV be if the project

Year	Initial Investment and Operating Cash Flows	End of Year Net Abandonment Value	NPV If Abandoned at the End of the Year Listed
0	($480,000)	$ 480,000	$ 0
1	200,000	300,000	(25,455)
2	187,500	190,000	13,802
3	175,000	0	(11,743)

Note: The project cost of capital is 10 percent.

TABLE 12.8
Medical Transportation Division's Projected Cash Flows

were abandoned after two years? In this situation, Ridgeland would receive operating cash flows for two years, plus the $190,000 abandonment value at the end of Year 2, and the project's NPV would be $13,802. Thus, the project is profitable if Ridgeland operates it for only two years and then sells it. To complete the abandonment analysis, note that if the project were abandoned after one year, its NPV would be −$25,455.

The *economic life* of the project, which is the life that produces the highest NPV, is two years. As a general rule, if profitability were the sole criterion in capital budgeting decisions, a project should be abandoned when the net abandonment value is greater than the present value of all cash flows beyond the abandonment point, discounted to the abandonment point. For example, if Ridgeland were to operate the division for one year, the abandonment value at that point is $300,000, but the present value at Year 1 of the cash flows beyond Year 1 would be $187,500 / (1.10)^1 + $190,000 / (1.10)^1 = $343,182, assuming abandonment at the end of Year 2. Thus, the Year 1 abandonment value is less than the Year 1 present value of continuing the project, so the project should not be abandoned at this point. However, a similar analysis at the end of Year 2 would show that the abandonment value is greater than the discounted value of future cash flows, so abandonment at Year 2 would produce the greater profitability. This is, of course, the same conclusion that we reached when calculating the NPVs of each possible project life. In essence, the abandonment decision examines the incremental cash flows to the firm at the abandonment point—the abandonment cash flows versus the cash flows associated with continuing the project—to determine the most profitable course of action.

In this illustration, we examined the concept of abandonment by looking at a project initially being evaluated. However, project performance should be examined on a regular basis, and those that are not meeting financial goals should, if feasible, be abandoned. (Project performance is reviewed in the post-audit process, which we discuss in a later section.) Once a project is up and running, two very different types of abandonment can occur: (1) sale by a business of a still-valuable product or service line because some other party can operate the line more efficiently and (2) abandonment of a product or service line because it is losing money. The first type of situation is illustrated by Ridgeland Community Hospital's sale of its two walk-in clinics to a physician group. Although the clinics were profitable to Ridgeland, the physician group could presumably operate them more efficiently, and hence were willing to pay Ridgeland a premium over the value the clinics would have if they remained under hospital control. The second type of abandonment is illustrated by Northeast Medical's decision to discontinue its HMO operation in Boston. Although Northeast's GoodHealth plan had proved profitable in several areas, competition in the Boston market proved destructive, so the firm made the decision to cut its losses.

1. Define economic life, as opposed to physical life.
2. Should projects be viewed as having one fixed life, or should they be considered as having alternative lives?

Capital Budgeting by Not-for-Profit Businesses

Although the capital budgeting techniques discussed up to this point are appropriate for use by both investor-owned and not-for-profit businesses, a not-for-profit firm has the additional consideration of meeting its charitable mission. In this section, we discuss two models that extend the capital budgeting decision to not-for-profit firms.

Net Present Social Value (NPSV) Model[7]

Except for the discussion of strategic value, the financial analysis techniques discussed so far have focused exclusively on the cash flow implications of a proposed project. Some healthcare businesses, particularly not-for-profit providers, have the goal of producing social services along with commercial services. For such firms, the proper analysis of proposed projects must systematically consider the *social value* of a project along with its pure financial, or cash flow, value.

When social value is considered, the *total net present value* (*TNPV*) of a project can be expressed as follows:

$$TNPV = NPV + NPSV.$$

Here, NPV represents the conventional NPV of the project's cash flow stream and *NPSV* is the *net present social value* of the project. The NPSV term, which represents managers' assessment of the social value of the project in dollar terms, clearly differentiates capital budgeting in not-for-profit firms from that in investor-owned firms.

In evaluating each project, a project is acceptable if its TNPV is greater than or equal to zero. This means that the sum of the project's financial and social values is at least zero, so when both facets of value are considered, the project has positive, or at least nonnegative, worth. Probably not all projects will have social value, but if a project does, it is considered formally in this decision model. However, no project should be accepted if its NPSV is negative, even if its TNPV is positive. Furthermore, to ensure the financial viability of the business, the sum of the NPVs of all projects initiated in a planning period must equal or exceed zero. If this restriction were not imposed, social value could displace financial value over time, and a firm cannot continue to provide social value without financial integrity.

NPSV is the sum of the present (Year 0) values of each year's social value. In essence, the suppliers of fund capital to a not-for-profit firm never receive a cash return on their investment. Instead, they receive a return on their investment in the form of social dividends. These dividends take the form of services with social value to the community such as charity care, medical research and education, and a myriad of other services that, for one reason or another, do not pay their own way. A service provided to a patient at a price equal to or greater than its cost does not create social value. Similarly, if governmental entities purchase care directly for beneficiaries of a program or support research, the resulting social value is created by the payer, and not by the provider of the services.

In estimating a project's NPSV, it is necessary to estimate the social value of the services provided by the project in each year, and determine the discount rate to apply to those services. When a project produces services to individuals who are willing and able to pay for those services, the value of those services is captured by the amount that they actually pay. Thus, the value of the services provided to those who cannot pay, or to those who cannot pay the full amount, can be estimated by the average net price paid by those individuals who are able to pay.

This approach to valuing social services has intuitive appeal, but certain points merit further discussion.

• Price is a fair measure of value only if the payer has the capacity to judge the true value of the service provided. Many observers of the health services industry would argue that information asymmetries between the provider and the purchaser inhibit the ability of the purchaser to judge true value.
• The fact that most payments for healthcare services are made by third-party payers may result in price distortions. For example, insurers may be willing to pay more for services than an individual would pay in the absence of insurance, or the existence of monopsony power by Medicare may result in a net price that is less than individuals would be willing to pay.
• A great deal of controversy exists over the true value of treatment in many situations. Suppose that some people are entitled to whatever healthcare is available, regardless of cost, and are not required to personally pay for the care. Even though society as a whole must cover the bill, people may demand a level of care that is of questionable value. For example, should $500,000 be spent to keep a comatose 92-year old alive for a few more days? If the true value of such an expenditure is zero, assigning a $500,000 value just because that is its cost makes little sense.

In spite of the potential problems, it still seems reasonable to assign a social value to many, but not all, healthcare services on the basis of the price that others are willing to pay for those services.

The second element required to estimate the NPSV of a project is the discount rate to apply to the annual social value stream. Like the required rate of return on equity for not-for-profit firms, there has been considerable controversy over the proper discount rate to apply to future social values. However, contributors of fund capital clearly can capture social value two ways. First, as is commonly done, contributions can be made directly to not-for-profit organizations. Second, contributors could always invest the funds in a portfolio of securities, and then use the proceeds to purchase the healthcare services directly. In the second situation, there would be no tax consequences on the portfolio's return because the contributed proceeds would qualify for tax exemption, but the contributor would lose the tax exemption on the full amount of the funds placed in the portfolio. Because the second alternative exists, providers should require a return on their social value stream that approximates the return available on the equity investment in for-profit firms that offer the same services.

The NPSV model formalizes the capital budgeting decision process applicable to not-for-profit healthcare businesses. Although few organizations actually attempt to quantify NPSV, not-for-profit providers should, at a minimum, subjectively consider the social value inherent in projects under consideration.

Project Scoring Approach

Managers of not-for-profit firms, as well as most managers of investor-owned businesses, recognize that nonfinancial factors should be considered in any capital budgeting analysis. The NPSV model examines only one other factor, and it is difficult to implement in practice. Thus, many firms use a quasi-subjective project scoring approach to capital budgeting decisions that attempts to capture both financial and nonfinancial factors. Table 12.9, the *project scoring matrix* used by Ridgeland Community Hospital, illustrates one such approach.

Ridgeland ranks projects on three dimensions: (1) stakeholder factors, (2) operational factors, and (3) financial factors. Within each dimension, multiple factors are examined and assigned scores that range from two points for very favorable impact, to minus one point for negative impact. The scores within each dimension are added to obtain scores for stakeholder, operational, and financial factors, and then the dimension scores are aggregated to obtain a total score for the project. The total score gives Ridgeland's managers a feel for the relative values of projects under consideration when all factors, including financial, are taken into account.

Ridgeland's managers recognize that the scoring system is completely arbitrary, so a project with a score of 16, for example, may be more or less than twice as good as a project with a score of 8. Nevertheless, use of the project scoring matrix forces managers to address multiple issues when making capital budgeting decisions. Although Ridgeland's approach should not be used at other organizations without modification for firm- and industry-unique circumstances, it does provide insight into how a firm-unique matrix might be developed.

TABLE 12.9
Project Scoring Matrix

Criteria	Relative Score			
	2	1	0	−1
Stakeholder Factors:				
Physicians	Strongly support	Support	Neutral	Opposed
Employees	Helps morale a lot	Helps morale a little	No effect	Hurts morale
Visitors	Greatly enhances visit	Enhances visit	No effect	Hurts image
Social value	High	Moderate	None	Negative
Operational Factors:				
Outcomes	Greatly improves	Improves	No effect	Hurts outcomes
Length of stay	Documented decrease	Anecdotal decrease	No effect	Increases
Technology	Breakthrough	Improves current	Adds to current	Lowers
Productivity	Large decrease in FTEs	Decrease in FTEs	No change in FTEs	Adds FTEs
Financial Factors:				
Life cycle	Innovation	Growth	Stabilization	Decline
Payback	Less than 2 years	2–4 years	4–6 years	Over 6 years
IRR	Over 20 %	15–20%	10–15%	Less than 10%
Correlation	Negative	Uncorrelated	Somewhat positive	Highly positive
Stakeholder factor score	_____			
Service factor score	_____			
Financial factor score	_____			
Total score	_____			

**Self-Test
Questions**

1. Describe the net present social value model of capital budgeting.
2. Describe the construction and use of a project-scoring matrix.

The Post-Audit

Capital budgeting is not a static process. If there is a long lag between a project's acceptance and its implementation, any new information concerning either capital costs or the project's cash flows should be analyzed before the actual start-up occurs. Furthermore, the performance of each project should be monitored throughout the project's life. The process of formally monitoring project performance over time is called the *post-audit*. It involves comparing actual results with those projected by the project's sponsors, explaining why differences occur, and analyzing potential changes to the project's operations including replacement or termination.

The post-audit has several purposes:

- **Improve forecasts.** When managers systematically compare their projections to actual outcomes, there is a tendency for estimates to improve. Conscious or unconscious biases that occur can be identified and, one hopes, eliminated; new forecasting methods are sought as the need for them becomes apparent; and managers tend to do everything better, including forecasting, if they know that their actions are being monitored.
- **Develop historical risk data.** Post-audits permit managers to develop historical data on new project analyses regarding risk and expected rates of return. These data can then be used to make judgments about the relative risk of future projects as they are evaluated.
- **Improve operations.** Businesses are run by managers, and they can perform at higher or lower levels of efficiency. When a forecast is made, for example, by the surgery department, the department director and medical staff is, in a sense, putting their reputations on the line. If costs are above predicted levels and utilization is below expectations, the people involved will strive, within ethical bounds, to improve the situation and to bring results into line with forecasts. As one hospital CEO put it: "You academics worry only about making good decisions. In the health services industry, we also have to worry about making decisions good."
- **Reduce losses.** Post-audits monitor the performance of projects over time, so the first indication that termination or replacement should be considered often arises when the post-audit indicates that a project is performing poorly.

1. What is a post-audit?
2. Why are post-audits important to the efficiency of a business?

**Self-Test
Questions**

Using Capital Budgeting Techniques in Other Contexts

The techniques developed in this chapter can help healthcare managers make a number of different types of decisions in addition to project selection. One example is the use of NPV and IRR to evaluate corporate merger opportunities. Healthcare businesses often acquire other firms to increase capacity, to expand into other service areas, or for other reasons. A key element of any merger analysis is the valuation of the target firm. Although the cash flows in such an analysis typically are structured differently than in project analysis, the same evaluation tools are applied. We will demonstrate the use of these techniques in the business valuation section of Chapter 18.

Managers also use capital budgeting techniques when deciding whether or not to divest assets or reduce staffing. Like capital budgeting, these actions require an analysis of the impact of the decision on the business's cash flows. When cutting personnel, businesses typically spend money up-front in severance payments, but then receive benefits in the form of lower wages and benefits in the future. When assets are sold, the pattern of cash flows is reversed. That is, cash inflows occur when the asset is sold, but any future cash inflows associated with the asset are sacrificed. (If future cash flows are negative, the decision, at least from a financial perspective, should be easy.) In both situations, the techniques discussed here, perhaps with modifications, can be applied to assess the financial consequences of the action.

Self-Test Question

1. Can capital budgeting tools be used in different settings? Explain your answer.

Key Concepts

This chapter discussed the basic capital budgeting process. Here are its key concepts:

- *Capital budgeting* is the process of analyzing potential expenditures on fixed assets and deciding whether the firm should undertake those investments.
- The *capital budgeting* process requires the firm to (1) estimate the investment outlay on the project, (2) estimate the expected cash inflows from the project, (3) assess the riskiness of those flows, (4) determine the appropriate cost of capital at which to discount those flows, and (5) determine the project's profitability and breakeven characteristics.
- The most important, but also the most difficult, step in analyzing a project is estimating the *incremental cash flows* that the project will generate.
- In determining incremental cash flows, *opportunity costs*—the cash flows forgone by using an asset—must be considered, but *sunk costs*—cash

outlays that cannot be recouped—are not included. Further, any impact of the project on the firm's *other cash flows* must be included in the analysis.

- *Tax laws* generally affect investor-owned firms in three ways: (1) taxes reduce a project's operating cash flows, (2) tax laws prescribe the depreciation expense that can be taken in any year, and (3) taxes affect a project's salvage value cash flow.

- Capital projects often require an investment in *net working capital* in addition to the investment in fixed assets. Such increases represent a cash outlay that, if material, must be included in the analysis. This investment is recovered when the project is terminated.

- *Cash flow estimation bias* can result if managers are overly optimistic in their forecasts. Estimation bias should be identified and dealt with in the decision process.

- A project may have some *strategic value* that is not accounted for in the estimated cash flows. At a minimum, strategic value should be noted and considered qualitatively in the analysis.

- The *effects of inflation* must be considered in project analyses. The best procedure is to build inflation effects directly into the component cash flow estimates.

- *Breakeven analysis* provides decision makers with insights concerning a project's profitability, liquidity, and risk. Intertemporal (time) breakeven is measured by the *payback period*.

- The *net present value (NPV)*, which is simply the sum of the present values of all the project's net cash flows when discounted at the project cost of capital, measures a project's dollar profitability. An NPV greater than $0 indicates that the project is profitable, and the higher the NPV, the more profitable the project.

- The *internal rate of return (IRR)*, which is that discount rate that forces a project's NPV to equal zero, measures a project's percentage rate of return profitability. If a project's IRR is greater than its cost of capital, the project is profitable, and the higher the IRR, the more profitable the project.

- The NPV and IRR profitability measures provide identical indications of profitability; that is, a project that is judged to be profitable by its NPV will also be profitable by its IRR. However, when mutually exclusive projects are being evaluated, NPV might rank a different project higher than IRR. This difference can occur because the two measures have different *reinvestment rate assumptions*—IRR assumes that cash flows can be reinvested at the project's IRR, while NPV assumes that cash flows can be reinvested at the project's cost of capital.

- The *modified internal rate of return (MIRR)*, which forces a project's cash flows to be reinvested at the project's cost of capital, is a better measure of a project's percentage rate of return than the IRR.

- If mutually exclusive projects have *unequal lives*, it may be necessary to adjust the analysis to place the projects on an equal life basis. This can be done using either the *replacement chain* approach or the *equivalent annual annuity (EAA)* approach.

- A project's profitability may be enhanced if it can be *abandoned* before the end of its physical life.
- The *net present social value (NPSV) model* formalizes the capital budgeting decision process for not-for-profit firms.
- Businesses often use *project scoring matrixes* to subjectively incorporate a large number of factors, including financial and nonfinancial, into the capital budgeting decision process.
- The *post-audit* is a key element in capital budgeting. By comparing actual results with predicted results, decision makers can improve both their operations and their cash flow estimation process.

This concludes our discussion of the basics of capital budgeting. In the next chapter, we will discuss risk assessment and incorporation, key issues in capital budgeting analysis.

Selected References

Allen, Robert J. 1989. "Proper Planning Reduces Risk in New Technology Acquisitions." *Healthcare Financial Management* (December): 48–56.

Bergman, Judson T., and Brett J. McIntyre. 1989. "Valuation Analysis." *Topics in Health Care Financing* (Summer): 32–40.

Campbell, Claudia.1994. "Hospital Plant and Equipment Replacement Decisions: A Survey of Hospital Financial Managers." *Hospital & Health Services Administration* (Winter): 538–556.

"Capital Management." J. Bruce Ryan and Matthews E. Ward, editors. 1992. *Topics in Health Care Financing (Fall)*.

Chow, Chee W., and Alan H. McNamee. 1991. "Watch for Pitfalls of Discounted Cash Flow Techniques." *Healthcare Financial Management* (April): 34–43.

Chow, Chee W., Kamal M. Haddad, and Adrien Wong-Boren.1991. "Improving Subjective Decision Making in Health Care Administration." *Hospital & Health Services Administration* (Summer): 191–210.

Cleverley, William O., and Joseph G. Felkner.1984. "The Association of Capital Budgeting Techniques with Hospital Financial Performance." *Health Care Management Review* (Summer): 45–55.

Gapenski, Louis C. 1989a. "A Better Approach to Internal Rate of Return." *Healthcare Financial Management* (April): 93–99.

———. 1989b. "Analysis Provides Test for Profitability of New Services." *Healthcare Financial Management* (November): 48–58.

———. 1993. "Capital Investment Analysis: Three Methods." *Healthcare Financial Management* (August): 60–66.

Gordon, David C., and Douglas F. Londal. 1989. "Guidelines to Capital Investment." *Topics in Health Care Financing* (Summer): 9–17.

Horowitz, Judith L. 1993. "Contribution Margin Analysis: A Case Study." *Healthcare Financial Management* (June): 129–133.

Horowitz, Judith L., and Peter F. Straley. 1988. "Developing Investment Criteria: There Is More To It Than Financial Criteria Alone." *Topics in Health Care Financing* (Fall): 23–31.

Kamath, Ravindra R., and Julie Elmer. 1989. "Capital Investment Decisions in Hospitals: Survey Results." *Health Care Management Review* (Spring): 45–56.

Kennedy, William F., and D. Anthony Plath. 1994. "A Return-Based Alternative to IRR Evaluations." *Healthcare Financial Management* (March): 38–49.

Magiera, Frank T., and Robert A. McLean. 1996. "Strategic Options in Capital Budgeting and Program Selection." *Health Care Management Review* (Fall): 7–17.

Manecke, Stephen R. 1993. "Practice Acquisition: Buy or Build." *Healthcare Financial Management* (December): 33–41.

Mellen, Chris M. 1992. "Valuing a Long-Term Care Facility." *Healthcare Financial Management* (October): 20–25.

Meyer, Alan D. 1985. "Hospital Capital Budgeting: Fusion of Rationality, Politics and Ceremony." *Health Care Management Review* (Spring): 17–27.

Ryan, J. Bruce, Mathews E. Ward, and Deborah S. Kolb. 1990. "Capital Management Balances Charitable, Financial Goals." *Healthcare Financial Management* (March): 32–40.

Schramm, Carl J., and George D. Pillari. 1987. "Investing in the Wrong Future for Hospitals." *Health Care Management Review* (Fall): 31–37.

Singhvi, Suren. 1996. "Using an Affordability Analysis to Budget Capital Expenditures." *Healthcare Financial Management* (June): 70–75.

Straley, Peter F., and Carol R. Swaim. 1993. "Financial Analysis of Medical Office Buildings." *Topics in Health Care Financing* (Spring): 76–85.

Vanden Brink, John, and Steve Gray. 1997. "Cost Modeling to Justify Acquisitions." *Healthcare Financial Management* (June): 72–76.

Watts, Dave, Donna L. Finney, and Brian Louie. 1993. "Integrating Technology Assessment into the Capital Budgeting Process." *Healthcare Financial Management* (February): 21–29.

Wedig, Gerald J., Mahmud Hassan, and Frank A. Sloan. 1989. "Hospital Investment Decisions and the Cost of Capital." *Journal of Business*, 517–537.

Selected Web Sites

The TeachMeFinance web site has several tutorial-type discussions that cover various aspects of financial management. For a capital budgeting tutorial, go to *teachmefinance.com*. Then, click on Capital Budgeting in the list along the left side of the page.

Selected Cases

Because Chapters 12 and 13 contain related material, most of the applicable cases require material from both chapters and, hence, are listed at the end of the next chapter. However, there is one case in *Cases in Healthcare Finance* that is applicable solely to this chapter:

Case 6: Surf City Medical Center, which focuses on estimating the breakeven utilization of a walk-in clinic.

Notes

1. For a discussion of the cash flow estimation practices of some large firms, as well as some estimates of the inaccuracies involved, see Randolph A. Pohlman, Emmanual S. Santiago, and F. Lynn Markel, "Cash Flow Estimation Practices of Large Firms," *Financial Management*, Summer 1988, 71–79.

2. For more on cash flow estimation bias, see Stephen W. Pruitt and Lawrence J. Gitman, "Capital Budgeting Forecast Biases: Evidence from the *Fortune* 500," *Financial Management*, Spring 1987, 46–51.

3. If Ann Arbor did not have taxable income to offset in Year 2, and had had no taxable income to offset in the three previous years, then the loss would have to be carried forward, and hence the tax benefit would not be immediately realized. In this situation, the tax shield value of the loss would be reduced because it would be pushed into the future rather than recognized immediately.

4. For a more complete discussion of replacement analysis, see Eugene F. Brigham, Louis C. Gapenski, and Phillip R. Daves, *Intermediate Financial Management* (Fort Worth, TX: Dryden Press, 2000), Chapter 7.

5. Note that the NPV is the same as the cumulative discounted cash flow shown for Year 5 in Table 12.6. In essence, NPV can be thought of as the total cumulative discounted cash flow of the project.

6. One could argue that not-for-profit firms do not have unlimited access to capital, and thus such firms cannot replace project cash flows with external capital. Furthermore, not-for-profit firms usually do not have sufficient capital to accept all projects that have positive NPVs, so the return on a not-for-profit firm's marginal project may not equal the firm's cost of capital. Nevertheless, for not-for-profit firms, the average aggregate return on projects will usually be close to the firm's cost of capital, so the cost of capital is still a better reinvestment rate than the project's IRR, especially when projects with exceptionally high or low IRRs are being evaluated.

7. This section is drawn primarily from an article by John R. C. Wheeler and Jan P. Clement. See "Capital Expenditure Decisions and the Role of the Not-for-Profit Hospital: An Application of the Social Goods Model," *Medical Care Review*, Winter 1990, 467–486.

PROJECT RISK ANALYSIS

Learning Objectives

After studying this chapter, readers should be able to:

- Describe the three types of risk relevant to capital budgeting decisions.
- Discuss the techniques used in project risk assessment.
- Conduct a project risk assessment.
- Discuss several types of real options and their impact on a project's value.
- Explain how risk is incorporated into the capital budgeting process.

Introduction

Chapter 12 covered the basics of capital budgeting, including cash flow estimation, breakeven analysis, and profitability measures. This chapter extends the discussion of capital budgeting to include risk analysis, which is composed of three elements: (1) defining the type of risk relevant to the project, (2) measuring the project's risk, and (3) incorporating that risk assessment into the capital budgeting decision process. Although risk analysis is a key element in all financial decisions, the importance of capital investment decisions to a healthcare provider's success or failure makes risk analysis vital in such decisions.

The higher the risk associated with an investment, the higher its required rate of return. This principle is just as valid for healthcare businesses that make capital expenditure decisions as it is for individuals who make personal investment decisions. Thus, the ultimate goal in project risk analysis is to ensure that the cost of capital used as the discount rate in a project's profitability analysis properly reflects the riskiness of that project. The corporate cost of capital, which was covered in detail in Chapter 10, reflects the cost of capital to the organization based on its aggregate risk—that is, based on the riskiness of the business's average project. In project risk analysis, a project's risk is assessed relative to the firm's average project: Does the project have average risk, below-average risk, or above-average risk? The corporate cost of capital is then adjusted to reflect any differential risk, resulting in a *project cost of capital*. In general, high-risk projects are assigned a project cost of capital that is higher than the corporate cost of capital, average risk projects are evaluated at the corporate cost of capital, and low-risk projects are assigned a discount rate that is less than the corporate cost of capital.

Types of Project Risk

Three separate and distinct types of project risk can be defined and, at least in theory, measured:

1. Stand-alone risk, which views the risk of a project as if it were held in isolation and, hence, ignores portfolio effects both within the firm and among equity investors.
2. Corporate risk, which views the risk of a project within the context of the business's portfolio of projects.
3. Market risk, which views a project's risk from the perspective of the business's owners who are assumed to hold a well-diversified portfolio of stocks.[1]

The type of risk that is most relevant to a particular capital budgeting decision depends on the number of projects that the firm holds and the business's form of ownership.

Stand-Alone Risk

Stand-alone risk is present in a project whenever there is a chance of a return that is less than the expected return. In effect, **a project is risky whenever its cash flows are not known with certainty**. Furthermore, the greater the probability of a return far below the expected return, the greater the risk. In this context, stand-alone risk can be measured by the *standard deviation* of the project's profitability, as measured typically by net present value (NPV) or internal rate of return (IRR). Because standard deviation measures the dispersion of a distribution about its expected value, the larger the standard deviation, the greater the dispersion, and hence the greater the probability of the project's profitability (NPV or IRR) being far below that expected.

Conceptually, *stand-alone risk* is only relevant in one situation: when a not-for-profit firm is evaluating its first project. In this situation, the project will be operated in isolation, so no portfolio diversification is present—the business does not have a collection of different projects, nor does the firm have stockholders who hold diversified portfolios of stocks. Although stand-alone risk is generally not relevant in real-world decision making, the other types of risk, which are more relevant, are very difficult, if not impossible, to measure. In practice, most project risk analyses measure stand-alone risk, and then subjective adjustments are applied to convert the project's assessed stand-alone risk to either corporate risk or market risk.

Corporate Risk

In reality, businesses usually offer a myriad of different products or services, and thus can be thought of as having a large number (perhaps even hundreds or thousands) of individual projects. For example, MinuteMan Healthcare, a

New England HMO, offers healthcare services to a large number of diverse employee groups in numerous service areas, and each different group could be considered to be a separate project. In this situation, the stand-alone risk of a project under consideration by MinuteMan is not relevant because the project will not be held in isolation. The relevant risk of a new project to MinuteMan is its contribution to the HMO's overall risk or the impact of the project on the variability of the overall profitability of the business. This type of risk, which is relevant when the project is part of a not-for-profit business's portfolio of projects, is called *corporate risk*.

Conceptually, a project's corporate risk is measured by its *corporate beta*, which reflects the volatility of the project's profitability relative to that of the firm as a whole, which has a corporate (aggregate) beta of 1.0. A project with a corporate beta of 1.5 has returns that are more volatile than the firm's average project, and hence has high corporate risk. Similarly, a project with a corporate beta of 0.5 has returns that are less volatile than the aggregate business, and hence has low corporate risk. A project's corporate risk depends on the context (i.e., the firm's other projects); so a project may have high corporate risk to one business, but low corporate risk to another, particularly when the two businesses operate in widely different industries.

Market Risk

Market risk is generally viewed as the relevant risk for projects being evaluated by investor-owned businesses. The goal of shareholder (owner) wealth maximization implies that a project's returns, as well as its risk, should be defined and measured from the shareholders' perspective. The riskiness of an individual project, as seen by a well-diversified shareholder, is not the riskiness of the project as if it were owned and operated in isolation, which is defined as stand-alone risk, nor is it the contribution of the project to the riskiness of the business, which is defined as corporate risk. Most shareholders hold a large diversified portfolio of stocks of many firms, which can be thought of as a very large diversified portfolio of individual projects. Thus, the risk of any single project as seen by a business's stockholders is its contribution to the riskiness of a well-diversified stock portfolio, which is measured by the project's *market beta*.

A project's market beta measures the volatility of the project's returns relative to the returns on a well-diversified portfolio of stocks. To managers of investor-owned businesses, a project's market risk relative to the market risk of the firm's other projects is measured by comparing the project's market beta to the firm's market beta. A project with a market beta higher than the business's market beta has higher-than-average market risk, where average is defined as the market risk of the firm's stock. Note that a project's absolute market risk, as measured by its market beta, is independent of the context; that is, a project's market beta does not depend on the characteristics of the business, assuming the project's cash flows are the same to all firms. However, the market risk of a project, **relative to the market risk of the firm's other projects**, depends on the aggregate market risk of the firm.

1. What are the three types of project risk?
2. How is each type of project risk measured, both in absolute and relative terms?

Relationships Among Stand-Alone, Corporate, and Market Risks

After discussing the three different types of project risk, and the situations in which each is relevant, it is tempting to say that stand-alone risk is almost never important because not-for-profit businesses should focus on a project's corporate risk and investor-owned businesses should focus on a project's market risk. Unfortunately, the situation is not that simple.

First, it is almost impossible in practice to quantify a project's corporate or market risk because it is extremely difficult—some practitioners would say impossible—to estimate the prospective returns distributions for given economic states for either the project, the firm as a whole, or for the market. If these return distributions cannot be estimated, then it is impossible to precisely quantify a project's corporate or market risk.

Fortunately, as will be demonstrated in the next section, it is possible to get a rough idea of the relative stand-alone risk of a project. Thus, managers can make statements such as Project A has above-average risk, Project B has below-average risk, or Project C has average risk, all in the stand-alone sense. After a project's stand-alone risk has been assessed, the primary factor in converting stand-alone risk to either corporate or market risk is correlation. If a project's returns are expected to be highly positively correlated with the firm's returns, high stand-alone risk translates to high corporate risk. Similarly, if the firm's returns are expected to be highly correlated with the stock market's returns, high corporate risk translates to high market risk. The same analogies hold when the project is judged to have average or low stand-alone risk.

Most projects will be in a firm's primary line of business, and hence will be in the same line of business as the firm's average project. Because all projects in the same line of business are generally affected by the same economic factors, such projects' returns are usually highly correlated. When this situation exists, a project's stand-alone risk is a good proxy for its corporate risk. Furthermore, most projects' returns are also positively correlated with the returns on other assets in the economy—most assets have high returns when the economy is strong, and low returns when the economy is weak. When this situation holds, a project's stand-alone risk is a good proxy for its market risk.

Thus, for most projects, the stand-alone risk assessment also gives good insights into a project's corporate and market risk. The only exception is when a project's returns are expected to be independent of or negatively correlated to the business as a whole. In these situations, considerable judgment is required because the stand-alone risk assessment will overstate the project's corporate risk. Similarly, if a project's returns are expected to be independent of or negatively correlated to the market's returns, the project's stand-alone risk overstates its market risk.

An additional problem arises with investor-owned healthcare businesses. Finance theory specifies that investor-owned businesses should focus on market risk when making capital budgeting decisions. However, most healthcare businesses, even proprietary ones, have corporate goals that focus on the provision of quality healthcare services in addition to shareholder wealth maximization. Furthermore, a proprietary healthcare business's stability and financial condition, which primarily depend on corporate risk, is important to all the firm's other stakeholders: its managers, physicians, patients, community, and so on. Some financial theorists even argue that stockholders, including those that are well diversified, consider factors other than market risk when setting required returns. This point is especially meaningful for small businesses, where the owner/managers are not well diversified in regards to their relationship to the business. Considering all the factors, it may be reasonable for managers of investor-owned healthcare businesses to be just as concerned about corporate risk as are managers of not-for-profit businesses. Fortunately, in most real-world situations, a project's risk in the corporate sense will be the same as its risk in the market sense.[2]

1. Name and define the three types of risk relevant to capital budgeting.
2. How are these risks related?
3. Should managers of investor-owned providers focus exclusively on a project's market risk?

**Self-Test
Questions**

Risk Analysis Illustration

To illustrate project risk analysis, consider Ridgeland Community Hospital's evaluation of a new MRI system presented in Chapter 12. Table 13.1 contains the project's cash flow analysis. If all of the project's component cash flows were known with certainty, the project's projected profitability would be known with certainty, and hence the project would have no risk. However, in most project analyses, future cash flows, and hence profitability are uncertain and, in many cases, highly uncertain, so risk is present.

The starting point for analyzing a project's risk involves estimating the uncertainty inherent in the project's cash flows. Most of the individual cash flows in Table 13.1 are subject to uncertainty. For example, volume was projected at 40 scans per week. However, utilization would almost certainly be higher or lower than the 40 scan forecast. In effect, the volume estimate is really an expected value taken from some probability distribution of potential utilization, as are many of the other values listed in Table 13.1. The

TABLE 13.1
Ridgeland Community Hospital: MRI Site Cash Flow Analysis

	0	1	2	3	4	5
			Annual Cash Flows, Years 0–5			
1. System cost	($1,500,000)					
2. Related expenses	(1,000,000)					
3. Gross revenues		$1,000,000	$1,050,000	$1,102,500	$1,157,625	$1,215,506
4. Deductions		250,000	262,500	275,625	289,406	303,877
5. Net revenues		$ 750,000	$ 787,500	$ 826,875	$ 868,219	$ 911,630
6. Labor costs		50,000	52,500	55,125	57,881	60,775
7. Maintenance costs		150,000	157,500	165,375	173,644	182,326
8. Supplies		30,000	31,500	33,075	34,729	36,465
9. Incremental overhead		10,000	10,500	11,025	11,576	12,155
10. Depreciation		350,000	350,000	350,000	350,000	350,000
11. Operating cash flow		$ 160,000	$ 185,500	$ 212,275	$ 240,389	$ 269,908
12. Taxes		0	0	0	0	0
13. Net operating cash flow		$ 160,000	$ 185,500	$ 212,275	$ 240,389	$ 269,908
14. Depreciation		350,000	350,000	350,000	350,000	350,000
15. Net salvage value						750,000
16. Net cash flow	($2,500,000)	$ 510,000	$ 535,500	$ 562,275	$ 590,389	$1,369,908

Profitability measures:
Net present value (NPV) = $82,493.
Internal rate of return (IRR) = 11.1%.

distributions of the variables could be relatively tight, reflecting small standard deviations and low risk, or they could be relatively flat, denoting a great deal of uncertainty about the variable in question, and hence a high degree of risk.

The nature of the component cash flow distributions and their correlations with one another determine the nature of the project's profitability distribution, and thus the project's risk. In the following sections, three techniques for assessing a project's risk are discussed: (1) sensitivity analysis, (2) scenario analysis, and (3) Monte Carlo simulation.

1. What condition creates project risk?
2. What makes one project riskier than another?

Self-Test Questions

Sensitivity Analysis

Many of the variables that determine a project's cash flows are subject to some type of probability distribution rather than known with certainty. If the realized value of such a variable is different from its expected value, the project's profitability will differ from its expected value. *Sensitivity analysis* is a technique that indicates exactly how much a project's profitability (NPV or IRR) will change in response to a given change in a single input variable, with other things held constant.

Sensitivity analysis begins with a *base case* developed using **expected values** (in the statistical sense) for all uncertain variables. To illustrate the concept, assume that Ridgeland's managers believe that all of the MRI project's component cash flows, except for weekly volume and salvage value, are known with certainty. The expected values for these variables (volume = 40 and salvage value = $750,000) were used in Table 13.1 to obtain the base case NPV of $82,493. Sensitivity analysis is designed to provide managers the answers to such questions as these: What if volume is more or less than the expected level? What if salvage value is more or less than expected?

In a sensitivity analysis, each uncertain input variable is usually changed by a fixed percentage amount above and below its expected value, while all other variables are held constant at their expected values. Thus, all input variables except one are held at their base case values. The resulting NPVs, or IRRs, are recorded and plotted. Table 13.2 contains the NPV sensitivity analysis for the MRI project, assuming that there are two uncertain variables: (1) volume and (2) salvage value.

Note that the NPV is a constant $82,493 when there is no change in either of the uncertain variables. This situation occurs because a zero percent change recreates the base case. Also, managers can examine the Table 13.2 values to get a feel for which input variable has the greatest impact on the MRI project's NPV—the larger the NPV change for a given percentage input change, the greater the impact. Considering only these two variables, the MRI

TABLE 13.2
MRI Project
Sensitivity
Analyses

Change from Base Case Level	Net Present Value (NPV)	
	Volume	Salvage Value
−30%	($814,053)	($ 57,215)
−20	(515,193)	(10,646)
−10	(216,350)	35,923
0	82,493	82,493
+10	381,335	129,062
+20	680,178	175,631
+30	979,020	222,200

project's NPV is affected by changes in volume to a much greater degree than it is by changes in salvage value.

Often, the results of sensitivity analyses are shown in graphical form. For example, the Table 13.2 sensitivity analysis is graphed in Figure 13.1. Here, the slopes of the lines show how sensitive the MRI project's NPV is to changes in each of the uncertain input variables—the steeper the slope, the more sensitive NPV is to a change in the variable. Note that the sensitivity lines intersect at the base case values—0 percent change from base case level and $82,493. Also, spreadsheet models are ideally suited for performing sensitivity analyses because such models both automatically recalculate NPV when an input value is changed and facilitate graphing.[3]

Figure 13.1 vividly illustrates that the MRI project's NPV is very sensitive to volume and only mildly sensitive to changes in salvage value. If a sensitivity plot has a negative slope, it indicates that **increases** in the value of that variable **decrease** the project's NPV. If two projects were being compared, the one with the steeper sensitivity lines would be regarded as riskier because a relatively small error in estimating a variable—for example, volume—would produce a large error in the project's projected NPV. If information was available on the sensitivity of NPV to input changes for Ridgeland's average project, similar judgments regarding the riskiness of the MRI project could be made, but now relative to the firm's average project.

Although sensitivity analysis is widely used in project risk analysis, it does have severe limitations. For example, suppose that Ridgeland Community Hospital had a contract with an HMO that guaranteed a minimum MRI utilization at a fixed reimbursement rate. In that situation, the project would not be very risky at all, in spite of the fact that the sensitivity analysis showed NPV to be highly sensitive to changes in volume. In general, a project's **stand-alone** risk, which is what is being measured by sensitivity analysis, depends on both the sensitivity of its profitability to changes in key input variables as well as the ranges of likely values of these variables. Because sensitivity analysis considers only the first factor, it can give misleading results.

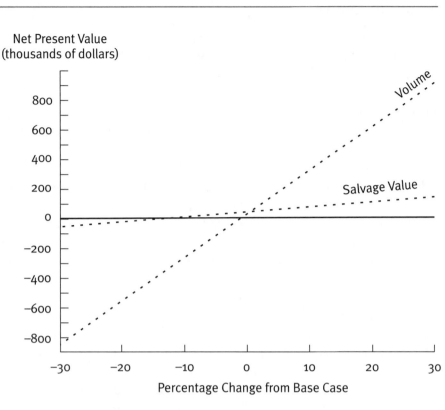

FIGURE 13.1
Sensitivity
Analysis Graphs

Furthermore, sensitivity analysis does not consider any interactions among the uncertain input variables; it considers each variable independently of the others.

In spite of its shortcomings, sensitivity analysis does provide managers with valuable information. First, it provides profitability breakeven information for the project's uncertain variables. For example, Table 13.2 and Figure 13.1 show that just a few percent decrease in expected volume makes the project unprofitable, whereas the project remains profitable even if salvage value falls by more than 10 percent. Although somewhat rough, this breakeven information is clearly of value to Ridgeland's managers.

Second, sensitivity analysis tells managers which input variables are most critical to the project's profitability, and hence to the project's financial success. In this MRI example, volume is clearly the key input variable of the two that were examined, so Ridgeland's managers should ensure that the volume estimate is the best possible. The concept here is that Ridgeland's managers have a limited amount of time to spend on analyzing the MRI project, so the resources expended should be as productive as possible.

1. Briefly, describe sensitivity analysis?
2. What type of risk does it attempt to measure?
3. What are its strengths and weaknesses?

**Self-Test
Questions**

Scenario Analysis

Scenario analysis is a stand-alone risk analysis technique that considers the sensitivity of NPV to changes in key variables, the likely range of variable values, and the interactions among variables. To conduct a scenario analysis, managers pick a "bad" set of circumstances (i.e., low volume, low salvage value, and so on), an average or "most likely" set, and a "good" set (i.e., high volume, high salvage value, and so on). The resulting input values are then used to create a probability distribution of NPV.

To illustrate scenario analysis, assume that Ridgeland's managers regard a drop in weekly volume below 30 scans as very unlikely, and a volume above 50 is also improbable. On the other hand, salvage value could be as low as $500,000 or as high as $1 million. The *most likely* values are 40 scans per week for volume and $750,000 for salvage value. Thus, volume of 30 and a $500,000 salvage value define the lower bound or *worst case* scenario, while volume of 50 and a salvage value of $1 million define the upper bound or *best case* scenario.

Ridgeland can now use the worst, most likely, and best case values for the input variables to obtain the NPV corresponding to each scenario. Ridgeland's managers used a spreadsheet model to conduct the analysis, and Table 13.3 summarizes the results. The most likely case results in a positive NPV; the worst case produces a large negative NPV; and the best case results in an even larger positive NPV. These results, along with the probability of occurrence of each scenario, can now be used to determine the expected NPV and standard deviation of NPV. Suppose that Ridgeland's managers estimate that there is a 20 percent chance of the worst case occurring, a 60 percent chance of the most likely case, and a 20 percent chance of the best case. Of course, it is difficult to estimate scenario probabilities with any confidence, and, in most situations, the probabilities used will not be symmetric. For example, in an environment of increasing managed care penetration and increasing competition among providers, the probability may be higher for the worst case scenario than for the best case scenario.

Table 13.3 contains a discrete distribution of returns, so the expected NPV can be found as follows:

TABLE 13.3
MRI Project
Scenario
Analysis

Scenario	Probability of Outcome	Volume	Salvage Value	NPV
Worst case	0.20	30	$ 500,000	($819,844)
Most likely case	0.60	40	750,000	82,493
Best case	0.20	50	1,000,000	984,829
Expected value		40	$ 750,000	$ 82,493
Standard deviation				$ 570,688

$$\text{Expected NPV} = (0.20 \times [-\$819{,}844]) + (0.60 \times \$82{,}493)$$
$$+ (0.20 \times \$984{,}829)$$
$$= \$82{,}493.$$

The expected NPV in the scenario analysis is the same as the base case NPV, $82,493. The consistency of results occurs because the values of the uncertain variables used in the scenario analysis—30, 40, and 50 scans for volume and $500,000, $750,000, and $1 million for salvage value—produce the same expected values that were used in the Table 13.1 base case analysis. If inconsistencies exist between the base case NPV and the expected NPV in the scenario analysis, the two analyses have inconsistent input assumptions. In general, such inconsistencies should be identified and removed to ensure that common assumptions are used throughout the project risk analysis. However, remember that our purpose here is to conduct a risk assessment, not to measure profitability. Ultimately, we will use the base case (expected value) cash flows to reassess the project's profitability when the risk assessment has been completed.

The standard deviation of NPV, as shown here, is $570,688:

$$\sigma_{\text{NPV}} = [0.20 \times (-\$819{,}844 - \$82{,}493)^2$$
$$+ 0.60 \times (\$82{,}493 - \$82{,}493)^2$$
$$+ 0.20 \times (\$984{,}829 - \$82{,}493)^2]^{1/2}$$
$$= \$570{,}688,$$

while the coefficient of variation (CV) of NPV is 6.9:

$$CV = \frac{\sigma_{\text{NPV}}}{\text{Expected NPV}} = \frac{\$570{,}688}{\$82{,}493} = 6.9.$$

The MRI project's standard deviation and coefficient of variation measure its stand-alone risk. Suppose that when a similar scenario analysis is applied to Ridgeland's aggregate cash flows (average project), the result is a coefficient of variation of NPV in the range of 1.5 to 2.5. Then, on the basis of its stand-alone risk measured by coefficient of variation, along with subjective judgments, Ridgeland's managers might conclude that the MRI project is riskier than the firm's average project, so it would be classified as a high-risk project.

Scenario analysis can also be interpreted in a less mathematical way. The worst case NPV, a loss of about $800,000 for the MRI project, represents an estimate of the worst possible financial consequences of the project. If Ridgeland can absorb such a loss in value without much impact on its financial condition, the project does not represent a significant financial danger to the hospital. Conversely, if such a loss would mean financial ruin for the hospital, its managers might be unwilling to undertake the project, regardless of its profitability under the most likely and best case scenarios.

While scenario analysis provides useful information about a project's stand-alone risk, it is limited in two ways. First, it only considers a few discrete states of the economy, and hence provides information on only a few potential profitability outcomes for the project. In reality, an almost infinite number of possibilities exist. Although the illustrative scenario analysis contained only three scenarios, it could be expanded to include more states of the economy, say five or seven. However, there is a practical limit on how many scenarios can be included in a scenario analysis.

Second, scenario analysis, at least as normally conducted, implies a very definite relationship among the uncertain variables; that is, the analysis assumed that the worst value for volume (30 scans per week) would occur at the same time as the worst value for salvage value ($500,000) because the worst case scenario is defined by combining the worst possible value of each uncertain variable. Although this relationship (all worst values occurring together) may hold in some situations, it may not hold in others. For example, if volume is low, maybe the MRI will have less wear and tear, and hence be worth more after five years of use. The worst value for volume, then, should be coupled with the best salvage value. Conversely, poor volume may be symptomatic of poor medical effectiveness of the MRI, and hence lead to limited demand for used equipment and a low salvage value. Scenario analysis tends to create extreme profitability values for the worst and best cases because it automatically combines all worst and best input values, even if these values actually have only a remote chance of occurring together. The next section describes a method of assessing a project's stand-alone risk that deals with these two problems.

Self-Test Questions

1. Briefly, describe scenario analysis.
2. What type of risk does it attempt to measure?
3. What are its strengths and weaknesses?

Monte Carlo Simulation

Monte Carlo simulation, so named because it grew out of work on the mathematics of casino gambling, describes uncertainty in terms of *continuous* probability distributions, which have an infinite number of outcomes rather than just a few *discrete* values. Thus, Monte Carlo simulation provides a more realistic view of a project's risk than does scenario analysis.

Although the use of Monte Carlo simulation in capital investment decisions was first proposed over 25 years ago, it had not been used extensively in practice primarily because it required a mainframe computer along with relatively powerful financial planning or statistical software. Recently, however, Monte Carlo simulation software has become available for personal computers as an add-in to spreadsheet software. Because most financial analysis today is being done with spreadsheets, Monte Carlo simulation is now accessible to virtually all health services organizations.

The first step in a Monte Carlo simulation is to create a model that calculates the project's net cash flows and profitability measures, just as was done for Ridgeland's MRI project. The relatively certain variables are estimated as single, or point, values in the model, while continuous probability distributions are used to specify the uncertain cash flow variables. After the model has been created, the simulation software automatically executes the following steps:

1. The Monte Carlo program chooses a single random value for each uncertain variable on the basis of its specified probability distribution.
2. The value selected for each uncertain variable, along with the point values for the relatively certain variables, are combined in the model to estimate the net cash flow for each year.
3. Using the net cash flow data, the model calculates the project's profitability, say, as measured by NPV. A single completion of these three steps constitutes one iteration, or "run," in the Monte Carlo simulation.
4. The Monte Carlo software repeats the above steps many times, say, 5,000. Because each run is based on different input values, each run produces a different NPV.

The ultimate result of the simulation is an NPV probability distribution based on 5,000 individual scenarios, and hence which encompasses almost all of the likely financial outcomes. Monte Carlo software usually displays the results of the simulation in both tabular and graphical forms, and automatically calculates summary statistical data such as expected value, standard deviation, and skewness.[4]

To illustrate Monte Carlo simulation, again consider Ridgeland Hospital's MRI project. As in the scenario analysis, the illustration has been simplified by specifying the distributions for only two key variables: (1) weekly volume and (2) salvage value. Weekly volume is not expected to vary by more than +/−10 scans from its expected value of 40 scans. Because this is a symmetrical situation, the normal (bell-shaped) distribution can be used to represent the uncertainty inherent in volume. In a normal distribution, the expected value plus or minus three standard deviations will encompass almost the entire distribution. Thus, a normal distribution with an expected value of 40 scans and a standard deviation of $10 / 3 = 3.33$ scans is a reasonable description of the uncertainty inherent in weekly volume.

A triangular distribution was chosen for salvage value because it specifically fixes the upper and lower bounds, whereas the tails of a normal distribution are, in theory, limitless. The triangular distribution is also used extensively when the input distribution is nonsymmetrical because it can easily accommodate skewness. Salvage value uncertainty was specified by a triangular distribution with a lower limit of $500,000, a most likely value of $750,000, and an upper limit of $1 million.

The basic MRI model containing these two continuous distributions was used, plus a Monte Carlo add-in to the spreadsheet program, to conduct a simulation with 5,000 iterations. The output is summarized in Table 13.4, and the resulting probability distribution of NPV is plotted in Figure 13.2. The mean, or expected, NPV, $82,498, is about the same as the base case NPV and expected NPV indicated in the scenario analysis, $82,493. In theory, all three results should be the same because the expected values for all input variables are the same in the three analyses. However, there is some randomness in the Monte Carlo simulation, which leads to an expected NPV that is slightly different from the others. The more iterations that are run, the more likely the Monte Carlo NPV will be the same as the base case NPV, assuming that the assumptions are consistent.

The standard deviation of NPV is lower in the simulation analysis because the NPV distribution in the simulation contains values within the entire range of possible outcomes, while the NPV distribution in the scenario analysis contains only the most likely value and best and worst case extremes.

In this illustration, one value for volume uncertainty was specified for all five years; that is, the value chosen by the Monte Carlo software for volume in Year 1—for example, 40 scans—was used as the volume input for the remaining four years in that iteration of the simulation analysis. As an

FIGURE 13.2
NPV
Probability
Distribution

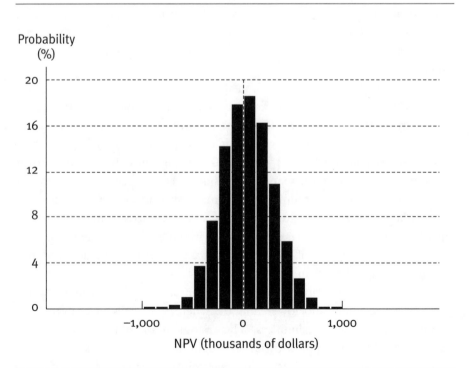

		TABLE 13.4
Expected NPV	$ 82,498	Simulation
Minimum NPV	($ 951,760)	Results
Maximum NPV	$ 970,191	Summary
Probability of a positive NPV	62.8%	
Standard deviation	$ 256,212	
Skewness	0.002	

alternative, the normal distribution for Year 1 could be applied to each year separately, and hence specify individual volumes for each year. Then, the Monte Carlo software might choose 35 as the value for Year 1, 43 as the Year 2 input, 32 for Year 3, and so on. This approach, however, probably does not do a good job of describing real-world behavior—high usage in the first year presumably means strong acceptance of the MRI system, and hence high usage in the remaining years. Similarly, low usage in the first year probably portends low usage in future years.

The volume and salvage value variables were treated as independent in the simulation; that is, the value chosen by the Monte Carlo software from the salvage value distribution was not related to the value chosen from the volume distribution. Thus, in any run, a low volume could be coupled with a high salvage value, and vice versa. If Ridgeland's managers believed that high usage at the hospital indicates a strong national demand for MRI systems, they could specify a positive correlation between these variables. This would tend to increase the riskiness of the project because a low volume pick in one iteration could not be offset by a high salvage value pick. Conversely, if the salvage value is more a function of the technological advances that occur over the next five years than local usage, then it may be best to specify the variables as being independent, as was done.

As in scenario analysis, the project's simulation results must be compared with a similar analysis of the firm's average project. If Ridgeland's average project was considered to have less stand-alone risk when a Monte Carlo simulation was conducted, then the MRI project would be judged to have above-average (i.e., high) stand-alone risk.

Monte Carlo simulation has two primary advantages over scenario analysis: (1) all possible input variable values are considered, and (2) correlations among the uncertain inputs can be incorporated in the analysis. However, these two advantages lead to the primary disadvantage: Although it is mechanically easy to input the probability distributions for the uncertain variables as well as their correlations into a Monte Carlo simulation, it is much more difficult to determine what those distributions and correlations are. The problem is that the more information a risk analysis technique requires, the harder it is to develop the data with any confidence, and hence managers can be left with a very elegant result of questionable value.

1. Briefly, what is Monte Carlo simulation?
2. What type of risk does it attempt to measure?
3. What are its strengths and weaknesses?

Incorporating Risk into the Decision Process

Thus far, the MRI illustration has demonstrated that it is difficult to quantify a project's riskiness. It may be possible to reach the general conclusion that one project is more or less risky than another or to compare the riskiness of a project with the business as a whole, but it is difficult to develop a really good measure of project risk. This lack of precision in measuring project risk adds to the difficulties involved in incorporating differential risk into the capital budgeting decision.

There are two methods for incorporating project risk into the capital budgeting decision process: (1) the certainty equivalent method, in which a project's expected cash flows are adjusted to reflect project risk; and (2) the risk-adjusted discount rate method, in which differential risk is dealt with by changing the cost of capital. Although the risk-adjusted discount rate method is used by most businesses, the certainty equivalent method does have some theoretical advantages. Furthermore, it raises some interesting issues related to the risk-adjustment process.

The Certainty Equivalent Method

The *certainty equivalent (CE) method* follows directly from the economic concept of *utility*.[5]

Under the CE approach, managers must first evaluate a cash flow's risk, and then specify how much money, with certainty, would be required for an individual to be indifferent between the riskless (certain) sum and the risky cash flow's expected value. To illustrate the concept, suppose that a rich eccentric offered someone the following choices:

- **Flip a coin.** If it's a head, the individual receives $1 million; if it's a tail, the individual gets nothing. The expected value of the gamble is $(0.5 \times \$1,000,000) + (0.5 \times \$0) = \$500,000$, but the actual outcome will be either zero or $1 million, so the gamble is quite risky.
- **Do not flip the coin.** Simply pocket $400,000 in cash.

If the individual is indifferent to the two alternatives, $400,000 is defined to be his or her *certainty equivalent* amount for this particular risky expected $500,000 cash flow. The riskless $400,000 provides that individual with the same satisfaction (utility) as the risky $500,000 expected return.

In general, investors are risk averse; so the certainty equivalent amount for this gamble will be something less than the $500,000 expected value. But, each individual would have his or her own certainty equivalent value— the greater the individual's degree of risk aversion, the lower the certainty equivalent amount.

The CE concept can be applied to capital budgeting decisions, at least in theory, in this way:

- Convert each net cash flow of a project to its certainty equivalent value. Here, the riskiness of **each cash flow** is assessed, and a certainty equivalent cash flow is chosen on the basis of that risk. The greater the risk, the greater the difference between the expected value and its lower certainty equivalent value. (If a cash outflow is being adjusted, the certainty equivalent value is higher than the expected value. The unique risk adjustments required on cash outflows will be discussed in a later section.)
- Once each cash flow is expressed as a certainty equivalent, discount the project's certainty equivalent cash flow stream by the **risk-free rate** to obtain the project's *differential risk-adjusted NPV.*[6] Here, the term "differential risk-adjusted" implies that the unique riskiness of the project, as compared to the overall riskiness of the business, has been incorporated into the decision process. The risk-free rate is used as the discount rate because certainty equivalent cash flows are analogous to risk-free cash flows.
- A positive differential risk-adjusted NPV indicates that the project is profitable even after adjusting for differential risk.

The CE method is simple and neat. Furthermore, it can easily handle differential risk among the **individual** cash flows. For example, the final year's certainty equivalent cash flow might be adjusted downward an additional amount to account for salvage value risk if that risk is considered to be greater than the risk inherent in the operating cash flows.

Unfortunately, there is no practical way to estimate a risky cash flow's certainty equivalent value. There are no benchmarks available to help make the estimate, so each individual would have his or her own estimate, and these could vary significantly. Also, the risk assessment techniques—for example, scenario analysis—focus on profitability, and hence measure the stand-alone risk of a project in its entirety. This process provides no information about the riskiness of individual cash flows, so there is no basis for adjusting each cash flow for its own unique risk.

The Risk-Adjusted Discount Rate Method

In the *risk-adjusted discount rate (RADR) method*, expected cash flows are used in the valuation process, and the risk adjustment is made to the discount rate (the opportunity cost of capital). All average-risk projects are discounted at the business's corporate cost of capital, which represents the opportunity cost of capital for average-risk projects; high-risk projects are assigned a higher cost of capital; and low-risk projects are discounted at a lower cost of capital.

One advantage of the RADR method is that the process has a starting benchmark: the business's corporate cost of capital. This discount rate reflects the riskiness of the business in the aggregate, or the riskiness of the firm's average project. Another advantage is that project risk assessment techniques identify a project's aggregate risk—the combined risk of all of the cash flows—and the RADR applies a single adjustment to the cost of capital rather than attempts to adjust individual cash flows. However, the disadvantage is that typically there is no theoretical basis for setting the size of the RADR adjustment, so the amount of adjustment remains a matter of judgment.

The RADR method has one additional disadvantage. RADR combines the factors that account for time value (the risk-free rate) and the adjustment for risk (the risk premium): Project cost of capital = Differential risk-adjusted discount rate = Risk-free rate + Risk premium. The CE approach, on the other hand, keeps risk adjustment and time value separate—time value in the discount rate and risk adjustment in the cash flows. By lumping together risk and time value, the RADR method compounds the risk premium over time—just as interest compounds over time, so does the risk premium. This compounding of the risk premium means that the RADR method automatically assigns more risk to cash flows that occur in the distant future, and the farther into the future, the greater the implied risk. Because the CE method assigns risk to each cash flow individually, it does not impose any assumptions regarding the relationship between risk and time.

Consciously or unconsciously, the RADR method as it is normally used, with a constant discount rate applied to all cash flows of a project, implies that risk increases with time. This implication imposes a greater burden on long-term projects, so short-term projects will tend to look better financially than long-term projects. For most projects, the assumption of increasing risk over time is probably reasonable because cash flows are more difficult to forecast the farther one moves into the future. However, managers should be aware that the RADR approach automatically penalizes distant cash flows, and an additional explicit penalty based solely on cash flow timing is not warranted unless some specific additional risk can be identified.

Applying the RADR Method to the MRI Project

In most project risk analyses, it is impossible to assess quantitatively the project's corporate or market risk, and, similar to Ridgeland Memorial Hospital's MRI project, managers are left with only an assessment of the project's stand-alone risk. However, like the MRI project, most projects being evaluated are in the same line of business as the firm's other projects, and the profitability of most firms is highly correlated with the overall economy. Thus, stand-alone, corporate, and market risk are usually highly correlated, which suggests that managers can get a feel for the relative risk of most projects on the basis of the scenario and/or simulation analyses conducted to assess the project's stand-alone risk. In Ridgeland's case, its managers concluded that the MRI project has above-average corporate risk, which is the risk most relevant to not-for-profit firms, and hence the project was categorized as a high-risk project.

The business's corporate cost of capital provides the basis for estimating a project's differential risk-adjusted discount rate—average-risk projects are discounted at the corporate cost of capital, high-risk projects are discounted at a higher cost of capital, and low-risk projects are discounted at a rate below the corporate cost of capital. Unfortunately, there is no good way of specifying exactly how much higher or lower these discounts rates should be; given the present state of the art, risk adjustments are necessarily judgmental and somewhat arbitrary.

Ridgeland's standard procedure is to add 4 percentage points to its 10 percent corporate cost of capital when evaluating high-risk projects, and to subtract 2 percentage points when evaluating low-risk projects. Thus, to estimate the high-risk MRI project's differential risk-adjusted NPV, the project's expected (base case) cash flows shown in Table 13.1 are discounted at 10% + 4% = 14%. This rate is called the *project cost of capital*, as opposed to the corporate cost of capital, because it reflects the risk characteristics of a specific project rather than the aggregate risk characteristics of the business. The resultant NPV is −$200,017, so the project becomes unprofitable when the analysis is adjusted to reflect its high risk. Ridgeland's managers may still decide to go ahead with the MRI project, but at least they know that its expected profitability is not sufficient to make up for its riskiness.

<table>
<tr><td>

1. What are the differences between the certainty equivalent (CE) and risk-adjusted discount rate (RADR) methods for risk incorporation?
2. What assumptions about time and risk are inherent in the RADR method?
3. How do most businesses incorporate differential risk in the capital budgeting decision process?

</td><td>

Self-Test Questions

</td></tr>
</table>

Incorporating Debt Capacity into the Decision Process

Just as different businesses have different optimal capital structures, so do individual projects. Within any business, the overall optimal capital structure, which is reflected by the weights used in the corporate cost of capital estimate, represents an aggregation of the optimal capital structures of the business's individual projects. However, some projects probably support only a little debt, while other projects support a high level of debt. The proportion of debt in a project's, or a business's, optimal capital structure is called the project's, or business's, *debt capacity*.

One mistake that is often made when considering a project's debt capacity is to look at how the project is actually financed. For example, even though Ridgeland Community Hospital may be able to obtain a secured loan for the entire cost of the MRI equipment, the MRI project does not have a debt capacity of 100 percent. The willingness of lenders to furnish 100 percent debt capital for the MRI project is based more on Ridgeland's overall creditworthiness than it is on the financial merits of the MRI project because all of the hospital's operating cash flow, less interest payments on embedded debt, is available to pay the lender. Think of it this way: Would lenders provide 100 percent financing if Ridgeland were a start-up firm with the MRI project as its sole source of income?

The logical question that arises here is whether or not debt capacity differences should be taken into consideration in the capital budgeting process. In theory, if there are meaningful debt capacity differences between a project and the business, capital structure differentials, as well as risk differentials, should be taken into account in the capital budgeting process. For example, an academic health center might be evaluating two projects: (1) one involves research and development (R&D) of a new surgical procedure and (2) the other involves building a primary care clinic in a local upscale residential area. The R&D project would have relatively low debt capacity because it is a high business risk project with no assets suitable as loan collateral. Conversely, the clinic project would have relatively high debt capacity because it has low business risk and involves real estate that is suitable as collateral.

Incorporating capital structure differentials is mechanically easy. Merely change the weights used to compute the corporate cost of capital to reflect project debt capacity, as opposed to using the standard weights that reflect the business's target capital structure. Projects with higher-than-average debt capacity would use a relatively high value for the weight of debt and a relatively low value for the weight of equity, and vice versa. However, a problem arises when attempting to make debt capacity adjustments. We know from Chapter 11 that increased debt usage raises capital costs, so both the cost of debt and the cost of equity must increase as more and more debt financing is used. This dependency of capital costs on capital structure means that as the weights are changed in the cost of capital calculation, so should the component costs. However, it is very difficult, if not impossible, to estimate individual project costs of debt and equity that correspond to the project's optimal capital structure. Thus, capital structure adjustments quickly become a somewhat futile guessing game, so most businesses do not make such adjustments unless there are specific benchmark values that can be used for both a project's unique debt capacity and the corresponding capital costs.[7]

Self-Test Question

1. Discuss the pros and cons of incorporating debt capacity differences in the capital budgeting decision process.

Adjusting Cash Outflows for Risk

Some projects are evaluated on the basis of minimizing the present value of future costs rather than on the basis of the projects' NPVs. This evaluation is done because it is often impossible to allocate revenues to a particular project, and it is easier to focus on comparative costs when two projects will produce the same revenue stream. For example, suppose that Ridgeland Community Hospital must choose one of two ways for disposing of its medical wastes. There is no question about the need for the project, and the hospital's revenue stream is unaffected by which method is chosen. In this case, the decision will be based on the present value of expected future costs; the method with the lower present value of costs will be chosen.

Table 13.5 contains the projected annual costs associated with each method. The in-house system would require a large expenditure at Year 0 to upgrade the hospital's current disposal system, but the yearly operating costs are relatively low. Conversely, if Ridgeland contracts for disposal services with an outside contractor, it will only have to pay $25,000 up front to initiate the contract. However, the annual contract fee would be $200,000 a year. Note that inflation effects are ignored in this illustration to simplify the discussion.

If both methods were judged to have average risk, then Ridgeland's corporate cost of capital, 10 percent, would be applied to the cash flows to obtain the present value (PV) of costs for each method. Because the PVs of costs for the two waste disposal systems—$784,309 for the in-house system and $783,157 for the contract method—are roughly equal, Ridgeland's managers would be indifferent as to which method should be chosen on the basis of financial considerations only.

However, Ridgeland's managers believe that the contract method is much riskier than the in-house method. The cost of modifying the current system is known to the dollar, and operating costs can be predicted fairly well. Furthermore, with the in-house system, operating costs are under the control of Ridgeland's management. Conversely, if the hospital relies on the contractor for waste disposal, it is more or less stuck with continuing the contract because

	Cash Flows	
Year	In-House System	Outside Contract
0	($500,000)	($ 25,000)
1	(75,000)	(200,000)
2	(75,000)	(200,000)
3	(75,000)	(200,000)
4	(75,000)	(200,000)
5	(75,000)	(200,000)
Present Value of Costs at a Discount Rate of:		
10%	($784,309)	($ 783,157)
14%	—	($ 711,616)
6%	—	($867,473)

TABLE 13.5
Ridgeland Community Hospital: Waste Disposal Analysis

it will not have the in-house capability. Because the contractor was only willing to guarantee the price for the first year, perhaps the bid was low-balled, and large price increases will occur in future years. The two methods have about the same PV of costs when both are considered to have average risk, so which method should be chosen if the contract method is judged to have high risk? Clearly, if the costs are the same under a common discount rate, the lower-risk in-house project should be chosen.

Now, try to incorporate this intuitive differential risk conclusion into the quantitative analysis. Conventional wisdom is to increase the corporate cost of capital for high-risk projects, so the contract cash flows would be discounted using a project cost of capital of 14 percent, which is the rate that Ridgeland applies to high-risk projects. But, at a 14 percent discount rate, the contract method has a PV of costs of only $711,616, which is about $70,000 lower than that for the in-house method. If the discount rate were increased to 20 percent on the contract method, it would appear to be $161,000 cheaper than the in-house method. Thus, the riskier the contract method is judged to be, the better it looks.

Something is obviously wrong here. To penalize a cash outflow for higher-than-average risk, that outflow must have a **higher** present value, not a **lower** one. Therefore, a cash outflow that has higher-than-average risk must be evaluated with a lower-than-average cost of capital. Recognizing this, Ridgeland's managers actually applied a 10% − 4% = 6% discount rate to the high-risk contract method's cash flows. This produces a PV of costs for the contract method of $867,473, which is about $83,000 more than the PV of costs for the average-risk in-house method.

The appropriate risk adjustment for cash outflows is also applicable in other situations. For example, the City of Detroit offered Ann Arbor Health Systems the opportunity to use a city-owned building in one of the city's blighted areas for a walk-in clinic. The city offered to pay to refurbish the building, and all profits made by the clinic would accrue to Ann Arbor. However, after ten years, Ann Arbor would have to buy the building from the city at the then-current market value. The market value estimate that Ann Arbor used in its analysis was $2 million, but the realized cost could be much greater, or much less, depending on the economic condition of the neighborhood at that time. The project's other cash flows were of average risk, but this single outflow had high risk, so Ann Arbor lowered the discount rate that it applied to this one cash flow. This action created a higher present value on a cost (outflow), and hence lowered the project's NPV.

Self-Test Questions

1. Is there any difference between the risk adjustments applied to cash inflows and cash outflows? Explain your answer.
2. Can differential risk adjustments be made to single cash flows, or must the same adjustment be made to all of a project's cash flows?

Real Options

According to traditional capital budgeting analysis techniques, a project's NPV is the present value of its expected future cash flows when discounted at a rate that reflects the riskiness of those flows. However, as we discussed in Chapter 12 in the section on strategic value, such valuations generally do not incorporate the value inherent in additional actions that can be taken by the business only if the project is accepted. In other words, traditional capital budgeting can be likened to playing roulette, where a bet is made (the project is accepted) and the wheel is spun, but there is nothing that can be done to influence the outcome of the game. In reality, capital projects are more like playing draw poker. Here, although chance does play a role, the players can influence the final result by discarding the right cards and by assessing the actions of the other players.

The opportunities that managers have to change a project in response to changing conditions or to build upon a project are called *real*, or *managerial*, *options*. These terms denote that fact that such options arise from investments in real, rather than financial, assets and that the options are available to managers of businesses, as opposed to individual investors. To illustrate the concept of real options, we must first introduce decision tree analysis.

Decision Tree Analysis

Although risk analysis is an integral part of capital budgeting, managers are at least as concerned, or maybe more concerned, about managing risk than they are about measuring it. One way of managing risk is to structure large projects as a series of decision points that provide the opportunity to reevaluate decisions as additional information becomes available, and possibly to *cancel*, or once production begins, to *abandon*, the project if events take a turn for the worse.

Projects that are structured as a series of decision points over time are evaluated using *decision trees*. For example, suppose Medical Equipment International (MEI) is considering the production of a totally new and innovative intensive care monitoring system. The net investment for this project is broken down into three stages, as set forth in Figure 13.3. If the go ahead is given for Stage 1 (Year 0), the firm will conduct a $500,000 study of the market potential for the new monitoring system that will take about one year. If the results of the study are unfavorable, the project will be canceled; but if the results are favorable, MEI will (at Year 1) spend $1 million to design and fabricate several prototype systems. These systems would then be tested at two hospitals and the reactions of the hospital medical staffs would determine whether MEI will proceed with the project.

If reaction at the test hospitals is positive, MEI would establish a production line for the monitoring systems at one of its plants at a net cost of $10 million. If this stage were reached, then MEI's managers estimate that the project would generate net cash flows over the following four years,

FIGURE 13.3

Decision Tree Analysis (thousands of dollars)

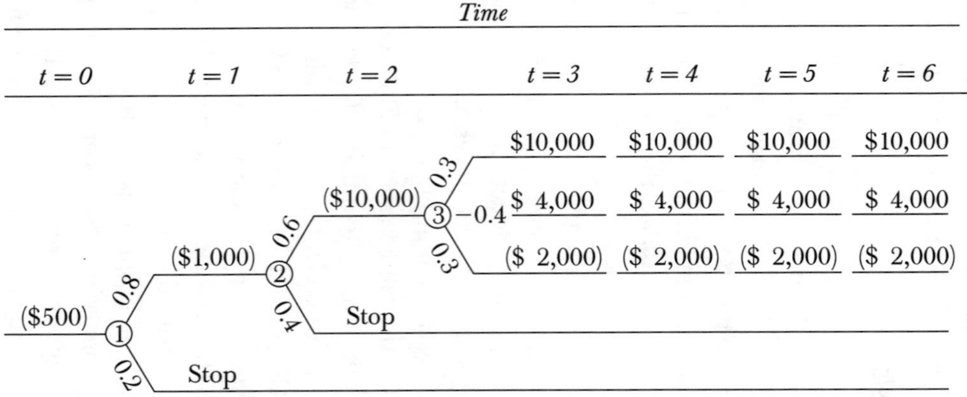

Time							Joint Probability	NPV	Product: Prob. NPV
$t = 0$	$t = 1$	$t = 2$	$t = 3$	$t = 4$	$t = 5$	$t = 6$			
			$10,000	$10,000	$10,000	$10,000	0.144	$15,250	$2,196
			$4,000	$4,000	$4,000	$4,000	0.192	436	84
			($2,000)	($2,000)	($2,000)	($2,000)	0.144	(14,379)	(2,071)
							0.320	(1,397)	(447)
($500)	($1,000)	($10,000)					0.200	(500)	(100)
							1.000	Expected NPV =	($ 338)
								$\sigma_{NPV} =$	$7,991

Nodes: ① 0.8 / 0.2 (Stop); ② 0.6 / 0.4 (Stop); ③ 0.3 / 0.4 / 0.3

which depend on the vitality of the hospital industry at that time and overall acceptance of the system.

A decision tree, such as the one in Figure 13.3, often is used to analyze such multistage, or sequential, decisions. Here, for simplicity, we assume that one year goes by between decisions. Each circle represents a decision point or stage. The dollar value to the left of each decision point represents the net investment required to go forward at that decision point, and the cash flows under the $t = 3$ to $t = 6$ headings represent the cash inflows if the project is carried to completion. Each diagonal line, which represents the beginning of a branch of the decision tree, has an estimated probability for moving along that branch based on information available to MEI's managers **today**. For example, management estimates that there is a probability of 0.8 that the initial study will produce favorable results, which leads to the expenditure of $1 million at Stage 2, and a 0.2 probability that the initial study will produce negative results, which leads to cancellation after Stage 1.

The joint probabilities shown in Figure 13.3 give the probability of occurrence of each final outcome—that is, the probability of moving completely along each branch. Each joint probability is obtained by multiplying together all the probabilities along a particular branch. For example, the probability that MEI will, if Stage 1 is undertaken, move through Stages 2 and 3 and that a strong demand will produce $10 million in net cash flows in each of the next four years is $0.8 \times 0.6 \times 0.3 = 0.144 = 14.4\%$.

The NPV of each final outcome is also given in Figure 13.3. MEI has a corporate cost of capital of 11.5 percent, and its management assumes initially that all projects have average risk. The NPV of the top (most favorable) outcome is about $15,250 (in thousands of dollars):

$$
\begin{aligned}
\text{NPV} = -\$500 &- \frac{\$1,000}{(1.115)^1} - \frac{\$10,000}{(1.115)^2} + \frac{\$10,000}{(1.115)^3} + \frac{\$10,000}{(1.115)^4} \\
&+ \frac{\$10,000}{(1.115)^5} + \frac{\$10,000}{(1.115)^6} \\
&= \$15,250.
\end{aligned}
$$

Other NPVs were calculated similarly.

The last column in Figure 13.3 gives the product of the NPV for each branch times the joint probability of that branch occurring, and the sum of the NPV products is the expected NPV of the project. Based on the expectations set forth in Figure 13.3, and assuming a cost of capital of 11.5 percent, the monitoring equipment project's expected NPV is −$338,000.

Because the expected NPV is negative, it would appear that this project is unprofitable, and hence should be rejected by MEI unless other considerations prevail. However, this initial judgment may not be correct. MEI must now consider whether this project is more, less, or about as risky as the firm's average project. The expected NPV is a negative $338,000, and the standard deviation of NPV is $7,991,000, so the coefficient of variation of NPV is quite large. This suggests that the project is highly risky in terms of stand-alone risk. Note also that there is a $0.144 + 0.320 + 0.200 = 0.664 = 66.4\%$ probability of incurring a loss. Based on all these findings, the project appears to be unacceptable financially unless it has some embedded real options that will increase its value and/or reduce its risk.

The Real Option of Abandonment

Abandonment, which we discussed in Chapter 12 in connection with estimating a project's economic life, is one type of real option that many projects possess. To illustrate the impact of this real option, suppose that MEI is not contractually bound to continue the project once production has begun. Thus, if sales are poor during Year 3 (t = 3) and MEI experiences a cash flow loss of $2 million, and similar results are expected for the remaining three years, MEI can abandon the project at the end of Year 3 rather than continue to suffer losses. In this situation, low first-year sales signify that the monitoring equipment is not selling well, so future sales will also be poor, and MEI has the opportunity to act on this new information once it becomes available.

The ability to abandon the project changes the branch of the decision tree in Figure 13.3 that contains the series of $2 million losses. It now looks like this (in thousands of dollars):

	Joint Probability	NPV	Product: Prob. × NPV
③ 0.3 ($2,000) ④ Stop	0.144	(10,883)	(1,567)

Changing this branch to reflect the results of choosing abandonment eliminates the $2 million cash losses in Years 4, 5, and 6, and thus causes the NPV for the branch to be higher, although still negative. This change increases the project's expected NPV from −$338,000 to about $166,000, and also lowers the project's standard deviation from $7,991,000 to $7,157,000. Thus, the abandonment real option changes the project's expected NPV from negative to positive, and also lowers its stand-alone risk as measured by either the standard deviation or coefficient of variation of NPV.

We can use the data just developed to estimate the value of the abandonment option. The NPV with the abandonment option is $166,000, while the NPV without this option is −$338,000, so the value of the real option is $166,000 − (−$338,000) = $504,000. However, this value understates the true value of the option because it also lowers the riskiness of the project. With lower risk, the difference between the two NPVs is greater than that calculated, although the added value of risk reduction would be relatively small in this illustration as well as difficult to quantify with any confidence. Because of this and similar complications, DCF techniques, when they can be used to value real options, generally will not give an accurate estimate of the option's value.

Here are some additional points to note concerning decision tree analysis and abandonment:

- Managers can reduce project risk if they can structure the decision process to include several decision points rather than just one. If MEI were to make a total commitment to the monitoring equipment project at $t = 0$, and sign contracts that would in effect require completion of the project, it might save some money and accelerate the project, but doing so would substantially increase the project's riskiness.
- Once production, or service, begins, the ability of the business to abandon a project can dramatically reduce the project's risk.
- The cost of abandonment generally is reduced if the firm has alternative uses for the project's assets. If MEI can convert the abandoned monitoring equipment production line to a different, more productive use, the cost of abandonment would be reduced, so the attractiveness of the monitoring equipment project would be enhanced.

Finally, note that capital budgeting is a dynamic process. Virtually all inputs to a capital budgeting decision change over time, and firms must periodically review both their expenditure plans and their ongoing projects. In the MEI example, conditions might change between Decision Points 1 and 2; if so, this new information should be used to develop revised probability and cash flow estimates. If a capital budgeting decision can be structured with multiple decision points, including abandonment, and if the firm's managers have the fortitude to admit it when a project is not working out as initially planned, then risks can be reduced and expected profitability can be increased.

Other Real Options

The MEI monitoring system project demonstrates that the real option of abandonment can add value to a project. In addition to abandonment, there are many other types of real options.

Flexibility Options

The *flexibility option* allows managers to switch inputs between alternative production or service processes. For example, by training clinical personnel to perform multiple tasks, individuals hired for a new service could potentially be used productively in other parts of the business. Thus, labor costs associated with the new service can be easily reduced if demand estimates are not met. This flexibility option reduces costs under poor utilization scenarios, and hence increases the value of the project.

Capacity Options

The *capacity option* allows businesses to manage their productive capacity in response to changing market conditions. If a project can be structured so that its level of operations can be reduced, or even suspended, if warranted rather than completely shut down, the value of the project is enhanced. Additionally, the option to expand new services from a relatively small scale to a large scale has value.

New Service Options It is easy to envision a situation in which a negative NPV project is accepted because embedded in it is the option to add complementary services or successive "generations of services." For example, the first move by a managed care organization into a new geographic area or the introduction of transplant services at a hospital. In such situations, the first project may not be profitable, but it could lead to additional opportunities that are.

Timing Options In our examples thus far, new projects brought with them embedded real options that could be exercised in the future, and hence added value to the project. *Timing options* can be somewhat different in that in some circumstances they involve the extinguishing of existing real options. Timing options were first analyzed in situations involving natural resources, in which decisions had to be made, such as when to harvest a forested area or how much oil to pump out of a field. Producing now gives immediate cash flows, but it eliminates the opportunity to obtain future cash flows from the same resource.

Of most interest to healthcare businesses is the *option to delay*, which is another type of timing option. If a project can be postponed, it might be more valuable in the future because, say, the service is worth more because of diminishing managed care power, or because technology has advanced, or because more information becomes available that decreases the project's risk. Of course, the option to delay is valuable only if it is worth more than the costs of delaying, which include time value of money costs, costs associated with competitor actions, and patient satisfaction costs. Thus, in general, the option to delay is most valuable to businesses that have proprietary technology or some other barrier to entry that lessens the costs associated with postponement.

Valuation of Projects That Have Real Options

In general, the true value of a project with real options can be thought of as the discounted cash flow (DCF) NPV plus the value of the real options:

$$\text{True NPV} = \text{DCF NPV} + \text{Value of real options.}$$

In most healthcare situations, it is not possible to place a dollar value on any real options associated with a project. However, managers should still think about the value of many projects in terms of the above equation. Here are some points to consider:

• Real options can add considerable value to many projects, so failure to consider such options leads to downward-biased NPVs, and thus to systematic underinvestment.

- In general, the longer a real option lasts before it must be "exercised," the more valuable it is. For example, suppose the real option is to expand into related services, such as expanding rehabilitative services into sports medicine services. The longer the expansion can be delayed and still retain its value, the more valuable the option.
- The more volatile the value of the underlying source of the real option, the more valuable the option. Thus, the more return volatility there is in the return on sports medicine services, the greater the value of a real option to expand into such services.
- The higher the cost of capital (the higher the general level of interest rates), the more valuable the real option. This point is not very intuitive, but we explain the rationale in Chapter 20 in our discussion of stock options.

1. How can the possibility of abandonment affect a project's profitability and stand-alone risk?
2. What are the costs and benefits of structuring large capital budgeting decisions in stages rather than as a single decision?
3. Why might DCF valuation underestimate the true value of a project?
4. What are some different types of real options?
5. How does the presence of real options influence the capital budgeting decision?

An Overview of the Capital Budgeting Decision Process

The discussion of capital budgeting thus far has focused on how managers evaluate individual projects. For capital planning purposes, healthcare managers also need to forecast the total number of projects that will be undertaken and the dollar amount of capital needed to fund these projects. The list of projects to be undertaken is called the *capital budget*, and the optimal selection of new projects is called the *optimal capital budget*.

While every healthcare provider estimates its optimal capital budget in its own unique way, some procedures are common to all businesses. The procedures followed by CALFIRST Health System are used to illustrate the process:

- The chief financial officer (CFO) estimates the system's corporate cost of capital. As discussed in Chapter 10, this estimate depends on market conditions, the business risk of CALFIRST's assets in the aggregate, and the system-wide optimal capital structure.
- The CFO then scales the corporate cost of capital up or down to reflect the unique risk and capital structure features of each division. To illustrate the concept, assume that CALFIRST has three divisions. For simplicity, the divisions are identified as LRD, ARD, and HRD, which stand for low-risk, average-risk, and high-risk divisions.
- Managers within each of the divisions evaluate the riskiness of the proposed projects within their divisions by categorizing each project as

having low risk (LRP), average risk (ARP), or high risk (HRP). These project risk classifications are based on the riskiness of each project relative to the **other projects in the division**, not to the system in the aggregate.

- Each project is then assigned a project cost of capital that is based on the **divisional cost of capital** and the project's relative riskiness. As discussed previously, this *project cost of capital* is then used to discount the project's expected net cash flows. From a financial standpoint, all projects with positive NPVs are acceptable, while those with negative NPVs should be rejected. Subjective factors are also considered, and these factors may result in a decision that differs from the one established solely on the basis of financial considerations.

Figure 13.4 summarizes CALFIRST's overall capital budgeting process. Here, the corporate cost of capital, 10 percent, is adjusted upward to 14 percent in the high-risk division and downward to 8 percent in the low-risk division. The same adjustment—4 percentage points upward for high-risk projects and 2 percentage points downward for low-risk projects—is applied to differential risk projects within each division. The end result is a range of project costs of capital within CALFIRST that runs from 18 percent for high-risk projects in the high-risk division to 6 percent for low-risk projects in the low-risk division.

FIGURE 13.4
CALFIRST:
Divisional and
Project Costs of
Capital

		High-risk project	18%
	HRD cost of capital = 14%	Average-risk project	14%
		Low-risk project	12%
Corporate cost of capital = 10%	ARD cost of capital = 10%	High-risk project	14%
		Average-risk project	10%
		Low-risk project	8%
	LRD cost of capital = 8%	High-risk project	12%
		Average-risk project	8%
		Low-risk project	6%

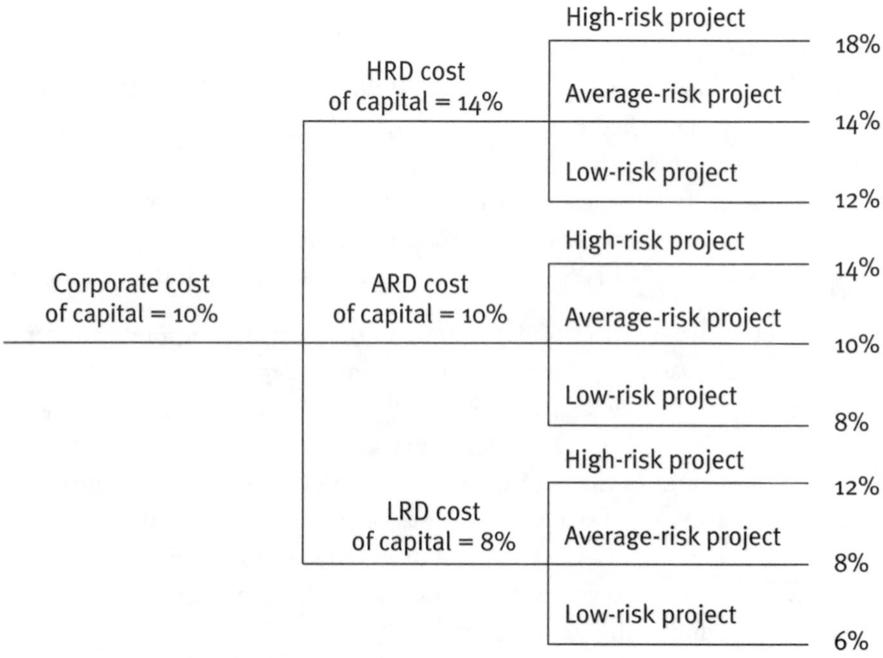

The final result is a financial analysis process that incorporates each project's debt capacity, at least at the divisional level, and riskiness. However, managers also must consider other possible risk factors that may not have been included in the quantitative analysis. For example, could the project being evaluated significantly increase the business's liability exposure? Conversely, does the project have any real option value or social value or other attributes that could impact its profitability or riskiness? Such additional factors must be considered, at least subjectively, before a final decision can be made. (A framework for considering multiple decision factors, the project scoring approach, is discussed in Chapter 12.) Typically, if the project involves new products or services and is large (in capital requirements) relative to the size of the business's average project, then the additional subjective factors will be very important to the final decision; one large mistake can bankrupt a firm, so "bet-the-firm" decisions are not made lightly. On the other hand, the decision on a small replacement project would be made mostly on the basis of numerical analysis.

Ultimately, capital budgeting decisions require an analysis of a mix of objective and subjective factors such as risk, debt capacity, profitability, medical staff needs, real option value, and social value. The process is not precise, and often there is a temptation to ignore one or more important factors because they are so nebulous and difficult to measure. Despite the imprecision and subjectivity, a project's risk, as well as its other attributes, should be assessed and incorporated into the capital budgeting decision process.

1. Describe a typical capital budgeting decision process.
2. Are decisions made solely on the basis of quantitative factors? Explain your answer.

Self-Test Questions

Capital Rationing

Standard capital budgeting procedures assume that businesses can raise virtually unlimited amounts of capital to meet capital budgeting needs. Presumably, as long as a business is investing the funds in profitable (i.e., positive NPV) projects, it should be able to raise the debt and equity needed to fund all projects that come along. Additionally, standard capital budgeting procedures assume that a business raises the capital needed to finance its optimal capital budget roughly in accordance with its target capital structure.

This picture of a business's capital financing/capital investment process is probably appropriate for most investor-owned firms. However, not-for-profit firms and small investor-owned businesses typically do not have unlimited access to capital. Their ability to raise equity capital often is limited, and their debt capital is constrained to the amount supported by the equity capital base. Thus, it is likely that such businesses will face periods in which the capital needed for investment in new projects will exceed the amount of capital available. This situation is called *capital rationing*.

If capital rationing exists, and hence a business has more acceptable projects than capital, then, from a financial perspective, the business should accept that set of capital projects that maximizes aggregate NPV and still meets the capital constraint. This approach could be called "getting the most bang from the buck" because it picks projects that have the most positive impact on the business's financial condition. In healthcare businesses, priority may be assigned to some low or even negative NPV projects, which is fine as long as these projects are offset by the selection of profitable projects, which would prevent the low-profitability, priority projects from eroding the business's financial condition.

Self-Test Questions

1. What is capital rationing?
2. From a financial perspective, how are projects chosen when capital rationing exists?

Key Concepts

This chapter discussed project risk definition, assessment, and incorporation. Here are its key concepts:

- Three separate and distinct *types of project risk* can be defined: (1) stand-alone risk, (2) corporate risk, and (3) market risk.
- A project's *stand-alone risk* is the risk the project would have if it were the sole project of a not-for-profit firm. It is measured by the variability of profitability, generally by the *standard deviation* or *coefficient of variation* of NPV. Stand-alone risk often is used as a proxy for both corporate and market risk because (1) corporate and market risk are often impossible to measure and (2) the three types of risk are usually highly correlated.
- *Corporate risk* reflects the contribution of a project to the overall riskiness of the business. It is measured conceptually by the project's *corporate beta*. Corporate risk ignores stockholder diversification, and it is the relevant risk for not-for-profit firms.
- *Market risk* reflects the contribution of a project to the overall riskiness of the owners' well-diversified investment portfolios. It is measured conceptually by the project's *market beta*. In theory, market risk is the relevant risk for investor-owned firms; but many people argue that corporate risk is also relevant to owners, especially the owner/managers of small businesses, and it is certainly relevant to a business's other stakeholders.
- Three techniques are commonly used to *assess a project's stand-alone risk*: (1) sensitivity analysis, (2) scenario analysis, and (3) Monte Carlo simulation.

- *Sensitivity analysis* shows how much a project's profitability—say, as measured by NPV—changes in response to a given change in an input variable such as volume, other things held constant.
- *Scenario analysis* defines a project's best, most likely, and worst cases and then uses these data to measure its stand-alone risk.
- Whereas scenario analysis focuses on only a few possible outcomes, *Monte Carlo simulation* uses continuous distributions to reflect the uncertainty inherent in a project's component cash flows. The result is a probability distribution of NPV, or IRR, that provides a great deal of information about the project's riskiness.
- Projects that require capital outlays in stages over time often are evaluated using *decision trees*. Here, the branches of the tree represent different outcomes, and, when subjective probabilities are assigned, the tree provides the profitability distribution for the project.
- In addition to the DCF-calculated NPV, some projects have additional value in the form of embedded *real options*.
- One type of real option is the ability to *abandon* a project once operations have begun. Such options can both increase a project's dollar return and decrease its riskiness, which has a twofold positive effect on value.
- There are two methods for incorporating project risk into the capital budgeting decision process: (1) the *certainty equivalent method*, in which a project's expected cash flows are adjusted to reflect project risk; and (2) the *risk-adjusted discount rate method*, in which differential risk is dealt with by changing the cost of capital.
- Projects are generally classified as *high risk*, *average risk*, or *low risk* on the basis of their stand-alone risk assessment. High-risk projects are evaluated at a discount rate greater than the firm's corporate cost of capital, average-risk projects are evaluated at the corporate cost of capital, and low-risk projects are evaluated at a rate less than the corporate cost of capital.
- When evaluating *risky cash outflows*, the risk adjustment process is reversed; that is, lower rates are used to discount more risky cash flows.
- Ultimately, capital budgeting decisions require an analysis of a mix of objective and subjective factors such as risk, debt capacity, profitability, medical staff needs, real option value, and social value. The process is not precise, but good managers do their best to ensure that none of the relevant factors are ignored.

This concludes our discussion of capital budgeting. In the next two chapters, we discuss financial and operating analyses and financial forecasting.

Selected References

Allen, Robert J. 1989. "Proper Planning Reduces Risk in New Technology Acquisitions." *Healthcare Financial Management* (December): 48–56.

Capettini, Robert, Chee W. Chow, and James E. Williamson. 1990. "Breakdown Approach Helps Managers Select Projects." *Healthcare Financial Management* (November): 48–56.

"Capital Management." 1992. J. Bruce Ryan and Matthews E. Ward, editors. *Topics in Health Care Financing* (Fall).

Gapenski, Louis C. 1992. "Accuracy of Investment Risk Models Varies" *Healthcare Financial Management* (April): 40–52.

———. 1992. "Project Risk Definition and Measurement in a Not-for-Profit Setting." *Health Services Management Research* (November): 216–224.

———. 1990. "Using Monte Carlo Simulation to Help Make Better Capital Investment Decisions." *Hospital & Health Services Administration* (Summer): 207–219.

Gup, Benton E., and S. W. Norwood III. 1981. "Divisional Cost of Capital: A Practical Approach." *Financial Management* (Spring): 20–24.

Hastie, K. Larry. 1974. "One Businessman's View of Capital Budgeting." *Financial Management* (Winter): 36–43.

Hertz, David B. 1964. "Risk Analysis in Capital Investments." *Harvard Business Review* (January–February): 96–106.

Holmes, Richard L., Rick E. Schroeder, and Laurie Frederick Harrington. 1999. "Using Microcomputers to Improve Capital Decision Making." *Journal of Health Care Financing* (Spring): 52–59.

Lewellen, Wilbur G., and Michael S. Long 1972. "Simulation versus Single-Value Estimates in Capital Expenditure Analysis." *Decision Sciences* (October): 9–33.

Ryan, J. Bruce and Joseph L. Gocke. 1988. "Incorporating Risk Into the Investment Decision." *Topics in Health Care Financing* (Fall): 49–65.

Weaver, Samuel C., Peter J. Clemmens III, Jack A. Gunn, and Bruce D. Danneburg. 1989. "Divisional Hurdle Rates and the Cost of Capital." *Financial Management* (Spring): 18–25.

Selected Web Sites

There are a multitude of web sites that pertain to this chapter.

Ohio State University maintains a web site with video clips by various finance professionals briefly discussing topics of relevance to this course. Unfortunately, the clips do not include healthcare executives. To access the clips, go to *www.cob.ohio-state.edu/fin/clips.htm*. Then, click on the clip of interest. For this chapter, try the clip by Steve Walsh titled "How We Do Capital Budgeting." Note that video clips are large files that are best accessed using a fast Internet link. Furthermore, player software is required to see the clips.

There are several spreadsheet add-in software packages available that perform Monte Carlo simulation. A demonstration version of one, called @RISK, can be downloaded from *www.palisade.com*. Then, click on the Trial Software tab near the top of the page.

Selected Cases

After covering both Chapters 12 and 13, the discussion of capital budgeting is complete. Thus, there are several cases in *Cases in Healthcare Finance* that can be used at this point:

Case 17: Grosse Pointe Hospital, which focuses on a "bread and butter" capital budgeting analysis of a proposed ambulatory surgery center.

Case 18: HEALTHWEST, which requires a staged entry (decision tree) analysis.

Case 19: Big Easy Health System, which involves a "make or buy" analysis regarding a health system's printing services.

Notes

1. The three types of risk relevant to capital budgeting decisions were first discussed in Chapter 5. A review of the applicable sections may be beneficial to some readers.

2. For an algebraic presentation of the relationships between the three types of risk, see Louis C. Gapenski, "Project Risk Definition and Measurement in a Not-For-Profit Setting," *Health Services Management*, November 1992, 216–224.

3. Spreadsheet programs have Data Table functions that automatically perform sensitivity analyses. After the table is roughed in, the spreadsheet automatically calculates and records a project's NPV, or some other value, in the appropriate cells in the table. This feature is explained in the Chapter 13 model on the Student Learning Diskette.

4. *Skewness* measures the degree of symmetry of a distribution. A skewness of zero indicates a symmetric distribution; positive skewness indicates a distribution that is skewed to the right, with a right tail longer than its left; and negative skewness indicates a distribution with a left tail that is longer than its right. The absolute value of the number indicates the degree of skewness—the larger the number, the more skewed the distribution.

5. Utility theory is used by economists to explain how individuals make choices among risky alternatives.

6. The risk-free rate does **not** incorporate the tax advantages of debt financing, so such benefits to taxable firms should be incorporated directly into the cash flows when the certainty equivalent method is used. Alternatively, the risk-free rate could be adjusted by using that rate instead of the costs of debt and equity in the corporate cost of capital equation.

7. One example where debt capacity adjustments are often made involves *project financing*. In project financing, lenders provide debt capital solely on the basis of the earnings power of the project because they have limited, or no, recourse against the business's other cash flows. In this situation, there is a readily identifiable cost of debt and debt capacity for the project.

Financial Analysis and Forecasting

Financial and Operating Analyses

Learning Objectives

After studying this chapter, readers should be able to:

- Explain the purposes of financial statement and operating analyses.
- Describe the primary techniques used in financial statement and operating analyses.
- Conduct basic financial statement and operating analyses to assess the financial condition of a business.
- Describe the problems associated with financial statement and operating analyses.

Introduction

Financial and operating analyses are of vital concern to healthcare managers, security analysts, investors, and lenders who use such analyses to make judgments about the financial soundness of businesses. The purposes of such analyses are to assess the financial condition of a business and, perhaps more importantly, to identify the operating factors that led to that condition. *Financial analysis* focuses on the data contained in a firm's financial statements such as revenues, operating costs, accounts receivable, and retained earnings. *Operating analysis*, on the other hand, focuses on operating factors such as occupancy (census), patient mix, length of stay, and labor productivity.

In this chapter, we discuss several techniques that extract information from a firm's financial statements and elsewhere and combine it in a form that facilitates making judgments about a business's financial condition and operations. Often, the end result of such analyses is a list of corporate strengths and weaknesses. In addition, some related topics, such as the problems inherent in such analyses, are discussed. For the most part, financial and operating analyses are applied to historical data, and hence the judgments made reflect the results of past managerial decisions. However, the more interesting question is what the business will do in the future. Therefore, managers invariably use the types of analysis discussed in this chapter as a springboard to predicting and planning for the future, which is the subject of the next chapter.

Financial Reporting in the Health Services Industry

Financial reporting in all industries follows standards set forth by the accounting profession called *generally accepted accounting principles (GAAP)*. The purpose of such standards is to ensure, to the extent possible, that financial information reported to outsiders is consistent across businesses and presented in a manner that facilitates interpretation and judgments. Because the health services industry has many unique features, including a high proportion of not-for-profit businesses, there are many organizations involved in setting reporting standards. Although the detail of establishing accounting standards is beyond the scope of this text, it should be noted that such standards are constantly being reviewed and modified as necessary to reflect changing economic conditions.[1]

Financial Statements

Accounting standards require businesses to prepare several *financial statements*, including three basic financial statements: (1) the *income statement*, (2) the *balance sheet*, and (3) the *statement of cash flows*. Taken together, these statements give an accounting picture of the firm's operations and its financial position. Detailed data are provided for the two or three most recent periods, plus brief historical summaries of key operating statistics for longer periods often are included.

Depending on size and ownership, a business's financial statements usually are made available to outside interested parties. Most large businesses prepare an *annual report*, which provides both the financial statements and a verbal description of the business's operating results during the past year along with a discussion of developments that will affect its future operations. In addition, large investor-owned firms must file even more detailed reports on an annual (called a 10-K) and quarterly (called a 10-Q) basis with the Securities and Exchange Commission (SEC). Finally, many larger firms also publish *statistical supplements,* which give financial statement data and key ratios going back about ten years. These reports, and similar reports that may be filed with state regulatory agencies, are often available from online sources including the business itself.

Income Statement

Table 14.1 contains simplified forms of the 1999 and 2000 income statements (also called statements of operations or statements of revenues and expenses) for Bayside Memorial Hospital, a 450-bed, not-for-profit, acute care hospital. Although a hospital is being used to illustrate financial and operating analysis techniques, they can be applied to any health services setting. Bayside had an excess of revenues over expenses, or net income, of $8,572,000 in 2000. Of course, being not-for-profit, the hospital paid no dividends, so it retained all of its net income. When looking at an income statement, it is also possible to get a rough idea of the organization's cash flow, which is approximately equal to its net income plus any noncash expenses. In 2000, Bayside's cash flow was $8,572,000 net income plus $4,130,000 depreciation expense, for a total estimated net cash flow of $12,702,000. Depreciation does not really *provide* funds; it is simply a noncash charge that is added back to net income to obtain an estimate of the business's net cash flow. Later in this section, we will discuss the statement of cash flows, which provides a better insight into Bayside's cash flows.

Note that the income statement reports on transactions *over a period of time*—for example, during Fiscal Year 2000. (Note that Bayside's fiscal year coincides with the calendar year.) The balance sheet, which we discuss next, may be thought of as a snapshot of the firm's asset, liability, and equity position *at a single point in time*—for example, on December 31, 2000.

Balance Sheet

Table 14.2 contains Bayside's 1999 and 2000 balance sheets. Although the assets are all stated in terms of dollars, only cash represents actual money. We see that Bayside could, if it liquidated its short-term investment securities, write checks at the end of 2000 for a total of $6,263,000 (versus total current liabilities of $13,332,000 due during 2001). The noncash current assets will presumably be converted to cash within a year, but they do not represent cash on hand.

The claims against assets are of two types: (1) liabilities, or money the firm owes, and (2) equity, also called net assets or fund capital.[2] Equity is a residual, so for 2000:

Assets	—	Liabilities	=	Equity
$151,278,000	—	($13,332,000 + $30,582,000)	=	$107,364,000.

	2000	1999
Net patient service revenue	$108,600	$ 97,393
Premium revenue	5,232	4,622
Other revenue	3,644	6,014
Total revenues	$117,476	$108,029
Expenses:		
Nursing services	$ 58,285	$ 56,752
Dietary services	5,424	4,718
General services	13,198	11,655
Administrative services	11,427	11,585
Employee health and welfare	10,250	10,705
Provision for uncollectibles	3,328	3,469
Provision for malpractice	1,320	1,204
Depreciation	4,130	4,025
Interest expense	1,542	1,521
Total expenses	$108,904	$105,634
Net income	$ 8,572	$ 2,395

TABLE 14.1
Bayside Memorial Hospital Statements of Operations (Income Statements) Years Ended December 31, 2000 and 1999 (in thousands)

TABLE 14.2

Bayside
Memorial
Hospital
Balance Sheets
December 31,
2000 and 1999
(in thousands)

	2000	1999
Cash	$ 4,263	$ 5,095
Short-term investments	2,000	0
Accounts receivable	21,840	20,738
Inventories	3,177	2,982
Total current assets	$ 31,280	$ 28,815
Gross plant and equipment	$ 145,158	$ 140,865
Accumulated depreciation	25,160	21,030
Net plant and equipment	$ 119,998	$ 119,835
Total assets	$ 151,278	$ 148,650
Accounts payable	$ 4,707	$ 5,145
Accrued expenses	5,650	5,421
Notes payable	825	4,237
Current portion of long-term debt	2,150	2,000
Total current liabilities	$ 13,332	$ 16,803
Long-term debt	$ 28,750	$ 30,900
Capital lease obligations	1,832	2,155
Total long-term liabilities	$ 30,582	$ 33,055
Net assets (equity)	$ 107,364	$ 98,792
Total liabilities and net assets	$ 151,278	$ 148,650

Liabilities consist of $13,332,000 of current liabilities plus $30,582,000 of long-term liabilities. If assets decline in value—suppose some of Bayside's fixed assets were sold at less than book value—liabilities remain constant, so the value of the equity capital declines.

A business's equity account is built up over time by retentions (retained earnings). In 2000, Bayside's income statement reported a net income of $8,572,000. As a not-for-profit organization, none of the net income can be paid out in dividends, so the entire amount must be retained in the business. Barring any asset sales or revaluations, Bayside's equity account should increase from year to year by the amount of net income. Thus,

$$
\begin{array}{lcll}
\text{2000 Equity balance} & = & \text{1999 Equity balance} & + & \text{2000 Net income} \\
\$107{,}364{,}000 & = & \$98{,}792{,}000 & + & \$8{,}572{,}000.
\end{array}
$$

Note that accumulated depreciation reported on the balance sheet is a *contra asset* account; that is, it is subtracted from gross fixed assets, so the larger a firm's accumulated depreciation, all else the same, the smaller its total assets. However, as noted earlier, the larger the amount of depreciation in any year, the greater the firm's cash flow because depreciation is a noncash expense. Accumulated depreciation on the balance sheet increases each year by the amount of depreciation expense reported on the income statement. For example,

$$\begin{array}{ccccc} \text{2000 Accumulated} & = & \text{1999 Accumulated} & + & \text{2000 Depreciation} \\ \text{depreciation} & & \text{depreciation} & & \text{expense} \\ \$25,160,000 & = & \$21,030,000 & + & \$4,130,000. \end{array}$$

Statement of Cash Flows

Some years ago, annual reports contained a statement called the "sources and uses of funds statement." The purpose of the statement was to report where the business had obtained funds during the past year and how it had used them. For example, had the business obtained most of its funds from such sources as bank loans and bond issues, or as retained earnings? Had it used those funds to retire debt, to build new facilities, to build up inventories, or to pay dividends? One could look at the statement and see the total sources and total uses, which were equal, and how funds were obtained and used; but there was no summary figure that could be used to judge whether the firm ended the year in a stronger or weaker financial position.

After several format revisions, organizations now report fund flows in the *statement of cash flows,* which typically is organized into three sections: (1) cash flow from operations, (2) cash flow from investing activities, and (3) cash flow from financing activities. Accountants adopted the new format because it provides information in the way most useful for financial analysis.

Table 14.3 contains Bayside's statement of cash flows, which focuses on the sources and uses of overall cash flow, for 2000. In the statement, cash coming into the hospital (inflows) are shown as positive numbers, while cash being spent (outflows) are shown as negative numbers (shown in parentheses). The top part lists cash generated by and used in operations. For Bayside, operations provided $11,196,000 in net cash flow. The income statement reported a rough cash flow estimate of Net income + Depreciation = $8,572,000 + $4,130,000 = $12,702,000, but as part of its operations, Bayside invested $1,297,000 in current assets (receivables and inventories) and lost $209,000 in spontaneous liabilities (payables and accruals). The end result, *net cash flow from operations,* was $12,702,000 − $1,297,000 − $209,000 = $11,196,000.

The next section of the statement of cash flows focuses on investments in fixed assets (plant and equipment), as opposed to investments in financial assets (securities). As noted in the statement, Bayside spent $4,293,000 on capital expenditures in 2000. Bayside's financing activities, as shown in the third section, highlight the fact that the hospital used cash to pay off previously incurred debt and to invest in marketable securities. The net effect of the hospital's financing activities was a *net cash outflow from financing* of $7,735,000.

When the three major sections are totaled, Bayside had a $11,196,000 − $4,293,000 − $7,735,000 = $832,000 *net decrease in cash* (i.e., net cash

TABLE 14.3

Bayside
Memorial
Hospital
Statement of
Cash Flows
Year Ended
December 31,
2000
(in thousands)

Cash Flows from Operating Activities:	
Net income	$ 8,572
Adjustments:	
Depreciation	4,130
Increase in accounts receivable	(1,102)
Increase in inventories	(195)
Decrease in accounts payable	(438)
Increase in accrued expenses	229
Net cash flow from operations	$ 11,196
Cash Flows from Investing Activities:	
Investment in plant and equipment	($ 4,293)
Cash Flows from Financing Activities:	
Investment in short-term securities	($ 2,000)
Repayment of long-term debt	(2,150)
Repayment of notes payable	(3,412)
Capital lease principal repayment	(323)
Change in current portion of LT debt	150
Net cash flow from financing	($ 7,735)
Net increase (decrease) in cash	($ 832)
Beginning cash	$ 5,095
Ending cash	$ 4,263

outflow) during 2000. The very bottom of Table 14.3 reconciles the 2000 net cash flow with the 2000 ending cash and equivalents balance shown on the balance sheet. Bayside began 2000 with $5,095,000 in cash, experienced a net cash outflow of $832,000 during the year, and ended the year with $5,095,000 − $832,000 = $4,263,000 in its cash account, as verified by the value reported on Table 14.2.

Bayside's statement of cash flows shows nothing unusual or alarming. It does show that the hospital's operations are inherently profitable (generated a positive cash flow), at least in 2000. Had the statement showed an operating cash drain, Bayside's managers would have had something to worry about; if it continued, such a drain could bleed the hospital to death. The statement of cash flows also provided easily interpreted information about Bayside's financing and fixed asset-investing activities for the year. For example, Bayside's cash flow from operations was used primarily to purchase new fixed assets, to invest in short-term securities, and to pay off notes payable and long-term debt. Such uses of operating cash flow do not raise any red flags regarding the hospital's financial actions. In fact, Bayside's ability to both increase securities investments and pay off debt indicates that 2000 was a very good year financially.

Managers and investors must pay close attention to the statement of cash flows. Financial condition is driven by cash flows, and the statement gives a good picture of the annual cash flows generated by the business.[3] An examination of Table 14.3, or, better yet, a series of such tables going back the last five years and projected five years into the future, would give Bayside's managers and creditors an idea of whether or not the hospital's operations are self-sustaining—that is, does the business generate the cash flows necessary to pay the expenses, including those associated with raising capital? Although the statement of cash flows is filled with valuable information, the bottom line tells little about the business's financial condition because operating losses can be covered by financing transactions such as borrowing or selling new common stock (if investor owned), at least in the short run.

Notes to the Financial Statements

The notes to the financial statements often contain information that can significantly affect a business's financial condition. For healthcare providers, these notes contain information on the firm's pension plan, its malpractice insurance, its noncapitalized lease agreements, the amount of charity care it provides, its accounting policies, and so forth. For example, the more important notes to Bayside's 2000 financial statements contained the following information:

- Inventories are valued at the lower of cost or market, with costs determined by the last-in, first-out (LIFO) method.
- Accounts receivable were reduced by $3,986,000 in 2000 and by $3,458.000 in 1999 to allow for doubtful accounts.
- Noncancelable operating lease commitments are estimated to be $858,000 in 2001, $842,000 in 2002, and $671,000 in 2003.
- The hospital's pension costs were $1,325,000 in 2000 and $1,214,000 in 1999. As of December 31, 2000, the hospital had a $20,985,000 actuarial present value of vested pension benefits and plan assets with a market value of $22,568,000, resulting in a pension plan excess of $1,580,000. (For simplicity, we excluded this amount from the balance sheet. Typically, any pension fund excess would be reported on the balance sheet as other assets. Annual pension expense is reported on the income statement in the employee health and welfare category.)
- Patient service revenue is reported net of provisions for charity care of $3,256,000 in 2000 and $2,985,000 in 1999. The amount of charity care provided is measured at the hospital's established rates.
- The hospital has agreements with third-party payers that provide for payments to the hospital at amounts less than its established rates. Net patient service revenue reported reflects the actual amounts agreed to by payers as opposed to charges.
- Premium revenue is that revenue collected from payers that is based on number of members as opposed to the amount of services provided.

- The hospital is self-insured for the purpose of protecting itself against professional and patient care claims. Professional insurance consultants have been retained to determine funding requirements. The amounts funded have been placed in a self-insurance trust account that is administered by a trustee. (The insurance trust account would normally be listed on the balance sheet as assets whose use is limited. Again, for simplicity, we have omitted that account from Bayside's illustrative balance sheet.)
- The hospital is an income beneficiary of the Robert A. Mitchell Charitable Trust. Because the assets of the trust are not controlled by the hospital, they are not included on the hospital's balance sheet. On December 31, 2000, the market value of the trust assets allocated to the hospital totaled $2,086,000. Income distributed to the hospital amounted to $168,000 in 2000 and $155,000 in 1999.

Clearly, the information contained in the notes to the financial statements has a bearing on Bayside's financial position, and it should be considered, either directly or indirectly, in any financial analysis. Indeed, professional analysts occasionally use the footnote information to recast financial statements before they even begin an analysis, and to such analysts the notes are especially vital.

Self-Test Questions

1. What governs financial reporting requirements in the health services industry?
2. Briefly, describe these three basic financial statements: (1) income statement, (2) balance sheet, and (3) statement of cash flows.
3. What type of information is provided by each type of statement?
4. What is the difference between net income and cash flow, and which is more meaningful to a firm's financial condition?
5. What types of information are contained in the notes to a business's financial statements?

Financial Statement Analysis

Financial statement analysis involves a number of techniques that extract information contained in a business's financial statements and combine it in a form that facilitates making judgments about the firm's financial condition. In the next sections, we discuss some common analytical techniques along with some problems inherent in such analyses.

Self-Test Question

1. What is financial statement analysis?

Ratio Analysis

Although a business's income statement and balance sheet contain a wealth of financial information, it is often difficult to make meaningful judgments about financial performance by merely examining the raw data. To illustrate the concept, consider that one managed care plan may have $5,248,760 in long-term debt and interest charges of $419,900, while another may have $52,647,980 in debt and interest charges of $3,948,600. The true burden of these debts, and each managed care plan's ability to pay the interest and principal due on them, cannot be easily assessed without additional comparisons, such as those provided by *ratio analysis*. In essence, ratio analysis combines data from the balance sheet and the income statement to create single numbers that have easily interpreted financial significance (i.e., numbers that measure various aspects of financial performance). In the case of debt and interest payments, ratios could be constructed that relate each plan's debt to its assets and the interest it pays to the income it has available for payment.

Unfortunately, an almost unlimited number of financial ratios can be constructed, and the choice of ratios depends in large part on the nature of the business being analyzed, the purpose of the analysis, and the availability of comparative data. Generally, ratios are grouped into categories to make them easier to interpret. In the paragraphs that follow, the data presented in Tables 14.1 and 14.2 are used to calculate an illustrative sampling of financial ratios for 2000 for Bayside Memorial Hospital, which are then compared with hospital industry average ratios.[4] Note that in a real analysis, many more ratios would be calculated and analyzed. Also, although a hospital is used to illustrate ratio analysis, the specific ratios used in any analysis depend on the type of healthcare provider. Some ratios are more meaningful for hospitals, some for managed care organizations, some for group practices, and so on.

Profitability Ratios

Profitability is the net result of a large number of managerial policies and decisions, so *profitability ratios* provide one measure of the aggregate financial performance of a business.

The *total margin*, often called the *total profit margin* or just *profit margin*, is **Total Margin** defined as net income divided by total revenues:

$$\text{Total margin} = \frac{\text{Net income}}{\text{Total revenues}} = \frac{\$8,572}{\$117,476} = 0.073 = 7.3\%.$$

Industry average $= 5.0\%$.

Bayside's total margin of 7.3 percent shows that the hospital makes 7.3 cents on every dollar of total revenues. The total margin measures the ability of the organization to control expenses. With all else the same, the higher the total margin, the lower the expenses relative to revenues. Bayside's total margin is above the industry average of 5.0 percent, which indicates relatively good expense control. How good? The industry data source also reports quartiles; for total margin, the upper quartile was 8.4 percent, which means that 25 percent of hospitals had total margins higher than 8.4 percent. Thus, although

Bayside's total margin was better than average, it was not as good as the top hospitals.

Bayside's relatively high total margin could mean that the hospital's gross charges are relatively high, its allowances are relatively low, its costs are relatively low, it has relatively high other (nonoperating) income, or some combination of these factors. A thorough operating analysis would help pinpoint the cause, or causes, of Bayside's high total margin.

When data are available, another useful margin ratio is the *operating margin*, which is defined as operating income divided by operating revenues. (Operating revenues are equal to patient service revenue plus premium revenue.) The advantage of this margin measure is that it focuses on core business operations, and hence removes the influence of nonoperating gains and losses, which often are transitory and unrelated to core operations. However, the current format of healthcare financial statements makes this ratio difficult to determine without additional information.

With only the data given in the financial statements, Bayside's operating margin can be estimated as follows. First, Bayside's operating revenue for 2000 was $108,600,000 + $5,232,000 = $113,832,000. If the assumption is that all expenses were operating expenses, Bayside's 2000 operating margin would be ($113,832 − $108,904) / $113,832 = $4,928 / $113,832 = 0.043 = 4.3%. Removing nonoperating revenue from the calculation lowers the profit margin.

Return on Assets (ROA)   The ratio of net income to total assets measures the *return on total assets*, usually just called *return on assets (ROA)*:

$$\text{Return on assets} = \frac{\text{Net income}}{\text{Total assets}} = \frac{\$8,572}{\$151,278} = 0.057 = 5.7\%.$$

Industry average = 4.8%.

Bayside's 5.7 percent ROA, meaning that each dollar of total assets generated 5.7 cents in profit, is well above the 4.8 percent average for the hospital industry. ROA tells managers how productively, in a financial sense, a business is using its assets. The higher the ROA, the greater the net income for each dollar invested in assets, and hence the more productive the assets. ROA measures both a firm's ability to control expenses, as expressed by the total margin, and its ability to use its assets to generate revenue.

Return on Equity (ROE)   The ratio of net income to total equity (net assets) measures the *return on equity (ROE)*:

$$\text{Return on equity} = \frac{\text{Net income}}{\text{Total equity}} = \frac{\$8,572}{\$107,364} = 0.080 = 8.0\%.$$

Industry average = 8.4%.

Bayside's 8.0 percent ROE is slightly below the 8.4 percent industry average.

The hospital was able to generate 8.0 cents of income for each dollar of equity investment, while the average hospital produced 8.4 cents. ROE is especially meaningful for investor-owned businesses. Owners are concerned with how well the business's managers are utilizing owner-supplied capital, and ROE gives one answer to this question. For not-for-profit businesses such as Bayside, ROE tells its board of trustees and managers how well, in financial terms, its community-supplied capital is being utilized.

Bayside's 2000 total margin and return on assets were above the industry averages, yet the hospital's ROE is below the average. As will be shown when Du Pont analysis is discussed, this seeming inconsistency is due to Bayside's relatively low use of debt financing.

Liquidity Ratios

One of the first concerns of most managers, and the major concern of a firm's creditors, is the business's *liquidity*. Will the business be able to meet its cash obligations in a timely manner as they become due? Bayside has debts totaling over $13 million (i.e., its current liabilities) that must be paid off within the coming year. Will the hospital be able to make these payments? A full liquidity analysis requires the use of a cash budget, which we will discuss in Chapter 15. However, by relating the amount of cash and other current assets to current obligations, ratio analysis provides a quick, easy-to-use, rough measure of liquidity.

The *current ratio* is computed by dividing current assets by current liabilities: **Current Ratio**

$$\text{Current ratio} = \frac{\text{Current assets}}{\text{Current liabilities}} = \frac{\$31,280}{\$13,332} = 2.3.$$

Industry average $= 2.0$.

The current ratio tells managers that the liquidation of Bayside's current assets at book value would provide 2.3 dollars of cash for every one dollar of current liabilities. If a business is getting into financial difficulty, it will begin paying its accounts payable more slowly, building up short-term bank loans (i.e., notes payable), and so on. If these current liabilities rise faster than current assets, the current ratio will fall, and this could spell trouble. Because the current ratio is an indicator of the extent to which short-term claims are covered by assets that are expected to be converted to cash in the near term, it is one commonly used measure of liquidity.

Bayside's current ratio is slightly above the average for the hospital industry. Because current assets should be converted to cash in the near future, it is highly probable that these assets could be liquidated at close to their stated values. With a current ratio of 2.3, the hospital could liquidate current assets at only 43 percent of book value and still pay off current creditors in full.[5]

Although industry average figures are discussed in detail later, it should be stated here that the industry average is not a magic number that all businesses should strive to achieve. In fact, some very well managed businesses will be above the average, while other good firms will be below it. However, if a firm's ratios are far removed from the average for the industry, its managers should be concerned about why this difference occurs.

Days Cash on Hand
The current ratio measures liquidity on the basis of balance sheet accounts as opposed to income statement items. However, the true measure of a business's liquidity is whether or not it can meet its payments as they become due, and so liquidity is more related to cash flows than it is to assets and liabilities. The *days-cash-on-hand ratio* moves closer to those factors that truly determine liquidity:

$$\text{Days cash on hand} = \frac{\text{Cash} + \text{Short-term investments (Marketable securities)}}{(\text{Expenses} - \text{Depreciation} - \text{Provision for uncollectibles})/365}$$

$$= \frac{\$4{,}263 + \$2{,}000}{(\$108{,}904 - \$4{,}130 - \$3{,}328)/365} = \frac{\$6{,}263}{\$277.93} = 22.5 \text{ days.}$$

Industry average $= 30.6$ days.

The denominator of the equation **estimates** average daily cash expenses by stripping out noncash expenses from reported total expenses. The numerator is the cash and securities that are available to make those cash payments. Because Bayside's days cash on hand is lower than the industry average, its liquidity position as measured by days cash on hand is worse than that of the average hospital.

For Bayside, the two measures of liquidity—(1) current ratio and (2) days cash on hand—give conflicting results. Perhaps the average hospital has a greater proportion of cash and marketable securities in its current assets than does Bayside. More analysis would be required to make a supportable judgment concerning Bayside's liquidity position. Remember, though, that the cash budget is the primary tool used by managers to ensure liquidity.

Debt Management (Capital Structure) Ratios

The extent to which a firm uses debt financing, or *financial leverage,* is an important measure of financial performance for several reasons. First, by raising funds through debt, owners of for-profit businesses can maintain control of the firm with a limited investment. For not-for-profit firms, debt financing allows the organization to provide more services than it could if it were solely financed with contributed and earned capital. Next, creditors look to owner-supplied funds to provide a margin of safety; if the owners have provided only a small proportion of total financing, the risks of the enterprise are borne mainly by its creditors. Finally, if the firm earns more on investments financed with borrowed funds than it pays in interest, the return on equity capital is magnified, or leveraged up.

Two types of ratios are used to assess debt management:

1. Balance sheet data are used to determine the extent to which borrowed funds have been used to finance assets. Such ratios are called *capitalization ratios*.
2. Income statement data are used to determine the extent to which fixed financial charges are covered by reported profits. Such ratios are called *coverage ratios*.

The two sets of ratios are complementary, so most financial statement analyses examine both types.

The ratio of total debt to total assets, generally called the *debt ratio*, measures the percentage of total funds provided by creditors:

Capitalization Ratio 1: Total Debt to Total Assets (Debt Ratio)

$$\text{Debt ratio} = \frac{\text{Total debt}}{\text{Total assets}} = \frac{\$43,914}{\$151,278} = 0.290, \text{ or } 29.0\%.$$

Industry average $= 42.3\%$.

In this definition, debt is defined as **all debt** and includes current liabilities, long-term debt, and capital lease obligations—everything but equity. However, this ratio has many variations, all of which use different definitions of what constitutes debt. Creditors prefer low debt ratios because the lower the ratio, the greater the cushion against creditors' losses in the event of bankruptcy and liquidation. Conversely, owners of for-profit firms may seek high leverage either to leverage up returns or because selling new stock would mean giving up some degree of control. In not-for-profit firms, managers may seek high leverage to offer more services.

Bayside's debt ratio is 29.0 percent. This means that its creditors have supplied somewhat less than one-third of the firm's total financing. Put another way, each dollar of assets was financed with 29 cents of debt, and consequently, 71 cents of equity. (The *equity ratio* is 1 − Debt ratio, so Bayside's equity ratio is 71 percent.) Because the average debt ratio for the hospital industry is over 40 percent, Bayside uses significantly less debt than the average hospital. The low debt ratio indicates that the hospital would find it relatively easy to borrow additional funds, presumably at favorable rates.

Another commonly used capitalization ratio is the *debt to equity ratio*. The debt ratio and debt to equity ratios are transformations of each other, and hence provide the same information, but with a slightly different twist:

Capitalization Ratio 2: Debt to Equity Ratio

$$\text{Debt to equity ratio} = \frac{\text{Total debt}}{\text{Total equity}} = \frac{\$43,914}{\$107,364} = 0.409, \text{ or } 40.9\%.$$

Industry average $= 73.3\%$.

This ratio tells analysts that Bayside's creditors have contributed 40.9 cents for each dollar of equity capital, while the industry average is 73.3 cents per dollar.

Both the debt ratio and debt to equity ratio increase as a business uses a greater proportion of debt financing, but the debt ratio rises linearly and approaches a limit of 100 percent, while the debt to equity ratio rises exponentially and approaches infinity.

Lenders, in particular, prefer the debt to equity ratio to the debt ratio. Their preference is based on the fact that it tells them how much capital creditors have provided to the business **per dollar of equity capital**. The higher this ratio, the riskier the creditors' position.

Coverage Ratio 1: Times- Interest- Earned Ratio

The *times-interest-earned (TIE) ratio* is determined by dividing earnings before interest and taxes (EBIT) by the interest charges. EBIT is used in the numerator because it represents the amount of income that is available to pay interest expense. For a not-for-profit business, which does not pay taxes, EBIT = Net income + Interest expense. For Bayside:

$$\text{TIE ratio} = \frac{\text{EBIT}}{\text{Interest expense}} = \frac{\$8,572 + \$1,542}{\$1,542} = \frac{\$10,114}{\$1,542} = 6.6.$$

Industry average = 4.0.

The TIE ratio measures the number of dollars of income available to pay each dollar of interest expense. In essence, it is an indicator of the extent to which income can decline before the business's earnings are less than its annual interest costs. Failure to pay interest can bring legal action by the firm's creditors, which could possibly result in bankruptcy.

Bayside's interest is covered 6.6 times, so it has 6.6 dollars of accounting income to pay each dollar of interest expense. Because the industry average TIE ratio is four times, the hospital is covering its interest charges by a relatively high margin of safety. Thus, the TIE ratio reinforces the previous conclusion based on the debt ratio—namely, that the hospital could easily expand its use of debt financing.

Coverage ratios are often better measures of a firm's debt utilization than capitalization ratios because coverage ratios discriminate between low-interest rate debt and high-interest rate debt. For example, a group practice might have $10 million of 4 percent debt on its balance sheet, while another might have $10 million of 8 percent debt. If both practices have the same income and assets, both would have the same debt ratio. However, the group paying 4 percent interest would have the lower interest charges, and hence would be in a better financial position than the group paying 8 percent. The better financial position that results from a lower interest rate is captured by the TIE ratio.

Coverage Ratio 2: Cash Flow Coverage Ratio

Although the TIE ratio is easy to calculate, it has two major deficiencies. First, leasing has become widespread in recent years. Also, many debt contracts require that principal payments be made over the life of the loan, rather than only at maturity. Thus, most businesses must meet fixed financial charges other than interest payments. Second, the TIE ratio ignores the fact that accounting income, whether measured by EBIT or net income, does not indicate the actual cash flow available to meet fixed charge payments. These deficiencies are corrected in the *cash flow coverage (CFC) ratio,* which shows the margin by which cash flow covers fixed financial requirements:

$$\text{CFC ratio} = \frac{\text{EBIT} + \text{Lease payments} + \text{Depreciation expense}}{\text{Interest expense} + \text{Lease payments} + \text{Debt principal}/(1 - T)}$$

$$= \frac{\$10{,}114 + \$1{,}368 + \$4{,}130}{1{,}542 + \$1{,}368 + \$2{,}000/(1 - 0)} = \frac{\$15{,}612}{\$4{,}910} = 3.2.$$

Industry average = 2.3.

Although not shown directly on Bayside's financial statements, the hospital had $1,368,000 of lease payments and $2 million of debt principal repayments in 2000.

What is the purpose of the $(1 - T)$ term applied to the debt principal? For investor-owned firms, the debt principal repayments, because they are paid with after-tax dollars, must be *grossed up* by dividing by $1 - T$. This gives the amount of pre-tax dollars, which are contained in the numerator, that are required to cover the principal repayments.

Like its TIE ratio, Bayside's CFC ratio exceeds industry standard, which indicates that Bayside is better at covering its total fixed payments with cash flow than is the average hospital. This fact should be reassuring both to creditors and management, and reinforces the view that Bayside has untapped debt capacity.

Asset Management (Activity) Ratios

The next group of ratios, the *asset management,* or *activity, ratios,* is designed to measure how effectively the business's assets are being managed. These ratios help to answer whether or not the total amounts of each type of asset as reported on the balance sheet seem reasonable, too high, or too low in view of current and projected operating levels. Bayside and other hospitals must borrow or raise equity capital to acquire assets. If they have too many assets, then their capital costs will be too high and their profits will be depressed. Conversely, if assets are too low, then profitable patient volume may be lost or vital services not offered.

The *fixed asset turnover ratio,* also called the *fixed asset utilization ratio,* **Fixed Asset** measures the utilization of plant and equipment, and it is the ratio of total **Turnover Ratio** revenues to net fixed assets:

$$\text{Fixed asset turnover} = \frac{\text{Total revenues}}{\text{Net fixed assets}} = \frac{\$117{,}476}{\$119{,}998} = 0.98.$$

Industry average = 2.2.

Bayside's ratio of 0.98 indicates that each dollar of fixed assets generated 98 cents in revenue. This value compares poorly with the industry average of 2.2 times, which indicates that Bayside is not using its fixed assets as productively as the average hospital. (The lower quartile value for the industry is 1.8; thus, Bayside falls in the bottom 25 percent of all hospitals in its fixed asset utilization.)

Before condemning Bayside's management for poor performance, it should be pointed out that a major problem exists with the use of the fixed asset turnover ratio for comparative purposes. Recall that all assets except cash and accounts receivable reflect historical costs rather than current value. Inflation and depreciation have caused the values of many assets that were purchased in the past to be seriously understated. Therefore, if an old hospital that had acquired much of its plant and equipment years ago is compared to a new hospital with the same physical assets, the old hospital, because of a much lower book value, would report a much-higher turnover ratio. This difference in fixed asset turnover is more reflective of the inability of financial statements to deal with inflation than of any inefficiency on the part of the new hospital's managers.

Total Asset Turnover Ratio

The *total asset turnover ratio* measures the turnover, or utilization, of all of the firm's assets. It is calculated by dividing total revenues by total assets:

$$\text{Total asset turnover} = \frac{\text{Total revenues}}{\text{Total assets}} = \frac{\$117,476}{\$151,278} = 0.78.$$

Industry average = 0.97.

Thus, each dollar of total assets generated 78 cents in total revenue. Bayside's total asset turnover ratio is below the industry average, but not as far below as its fixed asset turnover ratio. Thus, the hospital is utilizing its current assets better than its fixed assets, relative to the industry. Such judgments could be confirmed by examining Bayside's current asset turnover.[6]

Days in Patient Accounts Receivable

Days in patient accounts receivable is used to measure effectiveness in managing receivables. This measure of financial performance, which is sometimes classified as a liquidity ratio rather than an asset management ratio, has many names including *days in receivables, average collection period (ACP),* and *days' sales outstanding (DSO).* It is computed by dividing net patient accounts receivable by average daily patient revenue to find the number of days that it takes an organization, on average, to collect its receivables:

$$\text{Days in patient accounts receivable} = \frac{\text{Net patient accounts receivable}}{\text{Net patient service revenue} / 365}$$

$$= \frac{\$21,840}{\$108,600 / 365}$$

$$= 73.4 \text{ days.}$$

Industry average $= 64.0$ days.

In the calculation for Bayside, premium revenue has not been included because such revenue is collected before services are provided, and hence does not affect receivables.[7]

Bayside is not doing as well as the average hospital in collecting its receivables. The lower quartile value is 78.7 days, so a relatively large number of hospitals are doing worse. Still, as we will emphasize in Chapter 16, it is important that businesses collect their receivables as soon as possible. Clearly, Bayside's managers should strive to increase the hospital's performance in this key area.

Other Ratios

The final group of ratios examines other facets of a business's financial condition. For investor-owned firms, at least those with publicly traded stock, some ratios can be developed that relate the firm's stock price to its earnings and book value per share. Such *market value ratios* give managers an indication of what investors think of the firm's past performance and future prospects. If the firm's liquidity, asset management, debt management, and profitability ratios are all good, its stock price, and hence market value ratios, will be high.

The *average age of plant* gives a rough measure of the average age in years of a business's fixed assets: **Average Age of Plant**

$$\text{Average age of plant} = \frac{\text{Accumulated depreciation}}{\text{Depreciation expense}} = \frac{\$25,160}{\$4,130} = 6.1 \text{ years.}$$

Industry average $= 9.1$ years.

Bayside's physical assets are newer than those of the average hospital. Thus, the hospital offers more up-to-date facilities than average, and hence will probably have lower capital expenditures in the near future. On the other hand, Bayside's net fixed asset valuation will be relatively high, which biases the hospital's fixed asset and total asset turnover ratios downward. This fact raises serious questions about the validity of the turnover ratios calculated previously.

For investor-owned firms, the *price/earnings (P/E) ratio* shows how much **Price/Earnings** investors are willing to pay per dollar of reported profits. Suppose that the **Ratio** stock of General Home Care, an investor-owned home health care business, sells for $28.50, while the firm had 2000 earnings per share (EPS) of $2.20. Then, its P/E ratio would be 13.0:

$$\text{P/E ratio} = \frac{\text{Price per share}}{\text{Earnings per share}} = \frac{\$28.50}{\$2.20} = 13.0.$$

Industry average $= 15.2$.

P/E ratios are higher for firms with high growth prospects, other things held constant, but they are lower for riskier firms. General's P/E ratio is slightly below the average of other investor-owned home health care businesses, which suggests that the business is regarded as being somewhat riskier than most, as having poorer growth prospects, or both.

Market/Book Ratio The ratio of a stock's market price to its book value gives another indication of how investors regard the firm. Firms with relatively high rates of return on equity generally sell at higher multiples of book value than those with low returns. General reported $80 million in total equity on its 2000 balance sheet, and the firm had five million shares outstanding, so its book value per share is $80 / 5 = $16.00. Dividing the price per share by the book value per share gives a *market/book (M/B) ratio* of 1.8:

$$\text{M/B ratio} = \frac{\text{Price per share}}{\text{Book value per share}} = \frac{\$28.50}{\$16.00} = 1.8.$$

Industry average $= 2.1$.

Investors are willing to pay slightly less for each dollar of General's book value than for that of an average home health care business.

Comparative and Trend Analysis

When conducting ratio analysis, the value of a particular ratio, in the absence of other information, tells almost nothing. For example, if it is known that a nursing home business had a current ratio of 2.5, it is virtually impossible to say whether this is good or bad. Additional data are needed to help interpret the results of this ratio analysis. In the discussion of Bayside's ratios, the focus was on *comparative analysis;* that is, the hospital's ratios were compared with the average ratios for the industry. Another useful ratio analysis tool is *trend analysis*, in which the trend of a single ratio is analyzed over time. Trend analysis gives clues about whether a business's financial situation is improving, holding constant, or deteriorating.

It is easy to combine comparative and trend analyses in a single graph such as the one shown in Figure 14.1. Here, Bayside's ROE (the solid line) and industry average ROE data (the dashed lines) are plotted for the past five years. The graph shows that the hospital's ROE has been declining faster than the industry average from 1996 through 1999, but that it rose above the industry in 2000. Other ratios can be analyzed in a similar manner.

Self-Test Questions
1. What is the purpose of ratio analysis?
2. What are two ratios that measure profitability?
3. What are two ratios that measure liquidity?
4. What are two ratios that measure debt management?
5. What are two ratios that measure asset management?
6. What are two ratios that measure market value?

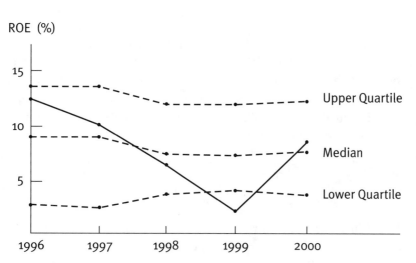

FIGURE 14.1

Bayside Memorial Hospital: ROE Analysis, 1996–2000

Return on Equity (ROE)

Year	Bayside	Industry		
		Lower Quartile	*Median*	*Upper Quartile*
1996	12.5%	2.6%	8.6%	13.3%
1997	10.0	2.5	8.6	13.3
1998	6.7	2.8	7.2	12.1
1999	2.4	4.1	7.2	12.1
2000	8.0	3.8	7.4	12.3

7. How can comparative and trend analyses be used to help interpret ratio results?

Tying the Ratios Together: Du Pont Analysis

A complete ratio analysis provides a detailed picture of a business's financial condition; but it does not provide an overview of a firm's condition nor does it tie any of the ratios together. *Du Pont analysis* provides an overview of a business's financial condition and helps managers and investors understand the relationships among several ratios. Essentially, Du Pont analysis, so named because managers at the Du Pont Company developed it, combines basic financial ratios in a way that provides valuable insights into a firm's financial condition. The analysis decomposes return on equity (ROE), which is one of the most important measures of a business's profitability, into the product of three other ratios, each of which has an important economic interpretation. The result is the *Du Pont equation*:

$$
\begin{aligned}
\text{ROE} &= \text{Total margin} \times \text{Total asset turnover} &\times& \quad \text{Equity multiplier} \\
&= \text{Return on assets} &\times& \quad \text{Equity multiplier.}
\end{aligned}
$$

Note that the Du Pont equation actually has two forms. One form has three factors on the right side of the equation, while the other recognizes that the product of the total margin and total asset turnover is return on assets. By combing these ratios, the second form has only two factors on the right side.

The mathematical validity of the Du Pont equation can easily be seen by expressing it in ratio form:

$$
\begin{aligned}
\frac{\text{Net income}}{\text{Total equity}} &= \frac{\text{Net income}}{\text{Total revenues}} \times \frac{\text{Total revenues}}{\text{Total assets}} \times \frac{\text{Total assets}}{\text{Total equity}} \\
&= \frac{\text{Net income}}{\text{Total assets}} \times \frac{\text{Total assets}}{\text{Total equity}}.
\end{aligned}
$$

By canceling like terms in the numerator and denominator, we see that the left side of the equation is equal to the right side.

Bayside's 2000 data are used to illustrate the Du Pont equation:

$$
\begin{aligned}
\frac{\$8,572}{\$107,364} &= \frac{\$8,572}{\$117,476} \times \frac{\$117,476}{\$151,278} \times \frac{\$151,278}{\$107,364} \\
7.98\% &= 7.30\% \times 0.78 \times 1.41 \\
&= 5.69\% \times 1.41.
\end{aligned}
$$

Bayside's 2000 total margin was 7.3 percent, so the hospital made 7.3 cents profit on each dollar of total revenue. Furthermore, assets were turned over, or created revenues, 0.78 times during the year, so the hospital earned a return of $7.30\% \times 0.78 = 5.69\%$ on its assets. This value for ROA, when rounded, is the same as was calculated previously in the ratio analysis section.

If the hospital used only equity financing, its 5.69 percent ROA would equal its ROE. However, creditors supplied 29 percent of Bayside's capital, while the equityholders (i.e., the community) supplied the rest. Because the 5.69 percent ROA belongs exclusively to the suppliers of equity capital, which comprises only 29 percent of total capital, Bayside's ROE is higher than 5.69 percent. Specifically, ROA must be multiplied by the *equity multiplier*, which shows the total assets working for each dollar of equity capital, to obtain the ROE of 7.98 percent. This 7.98 percent ROE could be calculated directly: ROE = Net income/Total equity = $\$8,572/\$107,364$ = 7.98%. However, the Du Pont equation shows how total margin, which measures expense control; total asset turnover, which measures asset utilization; and financial leverage, which measures debt utilization, interact to determine ROE.

Bayside's managers use the Du Pont equation to analyze ways of improving the hospital's financial performance. To influence the profit margin (i.e., expense control), the hospital's marketing staff can study the effects of raising charges, or lowering them to increase volume, moving into new services or markets with higher margins, entering into new contracts with managed care plans, and so on. Furthermore, management accountants can study the expense items and, while working with department heads and clinical staff, can seek ways to reduce costs.

Regarding total asset turnover (i.e., asset utilization), Bayside's analysts, while working with both clinical and marketing staffs, can investigate ways of reducing investments in various types of assets. Finally, the hospital's financial staff can analyze the effects of alternative financing strategies on the equity multiplier (i.e., debt utilization), seeking to hold down interest expenses and the risks of debt while still using debt to leverage up ROE.

The Du Pont equation provides a useful comparison between a business's performance as measured by ROE and the performance of an average hospital. For example, here is the comparative analysis for 2000:

Bayside:	ROE	=	7.3% × 0.78	×	1.41
		=	5.69%	×	1.41 ≈ 8.0%.
Industry average: ROE		=	5.0% × 0.97	×	1.73
		=	4.85%	×	1.73 ≈ 8.4%.

The Du Pont analysis tells managers and creditors that Bayside has a significantly higher profit margin, and thus better control over expenses, than does the average hospital. However, the average hospital has a better total asset turnover, and thus Bayside is getting below-average utilization from its assets. In spite of the average hospital's advantage in asset utilization, Bayside's superior expense control outweighs its utilization disadvantage because its ROA of 5.69 percent is higher than the industry average ROA of 4.85 percent. Finally, the average hospital has offset Bayside's advantage in ROA by using more financial leverage, although Bayside's lower use of debt financing decreases its risk. The end result is that Bayside gets somewhat less return on its equity capital than does the average hospital.

One potential problem with Du Pont and ratio analyses applied to not-for-profit organizations, especially hospitals, is that a large portion of their net income may come from other (nonoperating) sources rather than from operations. If the nonoperating income is highly variable and unpredictable, return on equity and the ratios, as previously defined, may be a poor measure of the hospital's inherent profitability. All applicable ratios, as well as the Du Pont analysis, could be recast to focus on operations by using net operating revenue in lieu of total revenues.

Self-Test Questions

1. Explain how the Du Pont equation combines several ratios to obtain an overview of a business's financial condition.
2. Why may a focus on operating revenue be preferable to a focus on total revenues?

Common Size Analysis

In *common size analysis*, all income statement items are divided by total revenues, and all balance sheet items are divided by total assets. Thus, a common size income statement shows each item as a percentage of revenues, and a common size balance sheet shows each account as a percentage of total assets. The significant advantage of common size statements is that they facilitate comparisons of income statements and balance sheets over time and across firms because they compensate for scale (size) differentials.

Table 14.4 contains Bayside's common size income statement for 2000, along with the common size statement for the hospital industry. A lower percentage of Bayside's revenue comes from capitated contracts and a higher percentage from nonoperating sources than is true of the average hospital. In addition, Bayside overall is doing a better job of controlling expenses, which results in a higher profit margin.

Table 14.5 contains Bayside's common size balance sheet for 2000, along with industry average data. Three striking differences are revealed: (1) Bayside's current assets are significantly lower than the industry average, (2) its net plant and equipment are significantly higher, and (3) Bayside uses far less debt financing than the average hospital.

Self-Test Questions
1. How are common size statements created?
2. What advantage do common size statements have over regular statements when conducting a financial statement analysis?

TABLE 14.4
Bayside Memorial Hospital: Common Size Income Statement for 2000

	Bayside	Industry Average
Net patient service revenue	92.4%	90.4%
Premium revenue	4.5	7.2
Other revenue	3.1	2.4
Total revenues	100.0%	100.0%
Expenses:		
Nursing services	49.6%	50.7%
Dietary services	4.6	4.7
General services	11.2	11.5
Administrative services	9.7	10.2
Employee health and welfare	8.7	9.2
Provision for uncollectibles	2.8	2.8
Provision for malpractice	1.1	1.0
Depreciation	3.5	3.0
Interest expense	1.3	1.9
Total expenses	92.7%	95.0%
Net income	7.3%	5.0%

Note: This table contains inconsistencies because values are rounded to the nearest tenth percent.

TABLE 14.5

Bayside Memorial Hospital: Common Size Balance Sheet for 2000

	Bayside	Industry Average
Cash and equivalents	2.8%	3.7%
Short-term investments	1.3	2.0
Accounts receivable	14.4	17.2
Inventories	2.1	2.5
Total current assets	20.7%	25.4%
Gross plant and equipment	96.0%	90.1%
Accumulated depreciation	16.6	15.5
Net plant and equipment	79.3%	74.6%
Total assets	100.0%	100.0%
Accounts payable	3.1%	3.9%
Accrued expenses	3.7	4.1
Notes payable	0.5	3.2
Current portion of long-term debt	1.4	2.1
Total current liabilities	8.8%	13.3%
Long-term debt	19.0%	36.5%
Capital lease obligations	1.2	0.9
Total long-term liabilities	20.2%	37.4%
Net assets (equity)	71.0%	49.3%
Total liabilities and net assets	100.0%	100.0%

Note: This table contains inconsistencies because values are rounded to the nearest tenth percent.

Percentage Change Analysis

Another frequently used technique when analyzing financial statements is percentage change analysis. Here, the percentage changes in the individual accounts on the balance sheet and items on the income statement over some time period are calculated and compared. In this format, it is easy to see which items are growing faster or slower than others, and hence to see which of them are under control and which are out of control. For example, Bayside's net patient service revenue plus premium revenue, which is the hospital's net operating revenue, grew at an 11.6 percent rate from 1999 to 2000. At the same time, nursing services expenses grew by only 2.7 percent. This information tells Bayside's managers that revenues associated with patients grew faster than nursing expenses, which is a positive trend for the hospital. Other items and accounts would be analyzed in a similar manner.

The conclusions reached in a percentage change analysis, as well as in a common size analysis, generally parallel those derived from ratio analysis. However, occasionally a serious deficiency is highlighted only by one of the three analytical techniques, while the other two techniques fail to bring the deficiency to light. Thus, a thorough financial statement analysis will include a Du Pont analysis to provide an overview, and will then include ratio, common size, and percentage change analyses.

1. What is percentage change analysis?
2. Why is it useful?
3. Which analytical techniques should be used in a complete financial statement analysis?

Market Value Added and Economic Value Added

Two financial performance measures that are being used by managers with increasing frequency focus directly on management's success or failure in creating value; they are: (1)Market Value Added (MVA) and (2) Economic Value Added (EVA). These measures are especially useful in investor-owned businesses because of their direct link with shareholder wealth maximization. However, as you will see, EVA also can be used within not-for-profit firms.

Market Value Added (MVA)

A primary financial goal of any investor-owned business is shareholder wealth maximization. This goal obviously benefits owners, and it also ensures that scarce resources are allocated as efficiently as possible. However, managerial zeal to enhance owners wealth does not mean that other stakeholders, including creditors, employees, patients, and so on, should be treated unfairly because such actions are both unethical and will ultimately be detrimental to owners.

Although the fundamental goal of shareholder wealth maximization is widely accepted, managers sometimes confuse shareholder wealth maximization with maximizing the total market value of the firm's stock. A firm's total market value—its stock price multiplied by the number of shares outstanding—can be increased by raising and investing as much equity capital as possible, which increases the size and aggregate value of the firm. Although size-increasing actions often result in higher managerial salaries and benefits, such a strategy rarely benefits shareholders because it ignores the fact that what is most relevant to shareholders is not the size of the firm, but rather the return that it earns on shareholder supplied capital.

Individual shareholder's wealth is actually maximized when a firm's managers maximize the **difference** between the market value of the firm's stock and the amount of capital that equity investors have supplied to the firm. This difference is called *Market Value Added (MVA)*:

$$\text{MVA} = \text{Market value of equity} - \text{Book value of equity}.$$

To illustrate the MVA concept, consider HCA. In May of 2000, its total market value of equity was 564 million shares outstanding $\times \$28.50$ stock price = $16.1 billion, while the amount of shareholder capital used (the book value of equity) was about $5.6 billion. Thus, HCA's MVA at that point in time was $16.1 − $5.6 = $10.5 billion. This amount represents the difference between the funds, including retained earnings, which HCA's equity investors have put into the corporation since its founding and the value of the cash they could get by selling the business. In other words, HCA's managers have created $10.5 billion of wealth for the firm's shareholders. (HCA's MVA had been significantly higher prior to the summer of 1997 when the firm became the target of a federal probe into Medicare fraud.)

In spite of some recent problems, the managers of HCA have done a good job overall of creating shareholder wealth. In contrast, consider the situation at Beverly Enterprises, a long-term care business. In May of 2000, Beverly Enterprises' total market value of equity was 102.5 million shares outstanding ×$3.38 stock price = $346 million, while its shareholders had supplied about $642 million in equity capital. Thus, Beverly Enterprises' MVA was $346 − $642 = −$296 million. In other words, Beverly Enterprises destroyed shareholder wealth while HCA created wealth. In per dollar of equity terms, HCA's managers created $16.1/$5.6 = $2.88 of wealth for every dollar supplied by its stockholders, while Beverly Enterprises' managers destroyed $296/$642 = $0.46 of wealth for every dollar of equity supplied.[8]

Clearly, the MVA concept is applicable only to investor-owned businesses because it focuses on how well managers have done in creating value for shareholders, and hence equity market value is needed for its calculation. However EVA, which is discussed in the next section, applies to both investor-owned and not-for-profit businesses.

Economic Value Added (EVA)

Whereas MVA measures the combined effect of managerial actions to create shareholder wealth since the inception of the business, *Economic Value Added (EVA)* focuses on managerial effectiveness in a given year.[9] The basic formula for EVA is:

EVA = After-tax operating profit − (Total capital × Corporate cost of capital).

In the EVA equation, operating profit can be thought of as revenues minus all operating costs including taxes, if applicable, but excluding interest expense. Total capital supplied is the sum of the book values of debt and equity, and hence total assets. Also, in the EVA context, after-tax operating profit is often called *net operating profit after taxes (NOPAT)*, and it is actually calculated as EBIT × (1 − T). Because the calculation of EVA does not require market value data, it can be applied to both for-profit and not-for-profit businesses.[10]

To illustrate the EVA concept, consider Birmingham Health Providers, a medical group practice. The group had $1 million in NOPAT in 2000 generated from $5 million of investor-supplied debt and equity capital. The firm's corporate cost of capital was 10 percent. With these assumptions, Birmingham Health Providers' 2000 EVA was $500,000:

$$EVA = \$1 - (\$5 \times 0.10) = \$1 - \$0.5 = \$0.5 \text{ million.}$$

EVA is an estimate of a business's true economic profit for the year, and it differs substantially from accounting profitability measures such as net income. EVA represents the residual income that remains after **all costs**, including the opportunity cost of the employed equity capital, have been recognized. Conversely, accounting profit is formulated without imposing a charge for equity capital. EVA depends on both operating efficiency and balance sheet management: without operating efficiency, profits will be low, and without efficient balance sheet management, there will be too many assets, and hence too much capital, which results in higher-than-necessary dollar capital costs.

For not-for-profit firms, equity capital is a scarce resource that must be managed well to ensure the financial viability of the organization, and hence its ability to continue to perform its stated mission. EVA lets managers know how well they are doing in managing this scarce resource because the higher the EVA in any year, the better job that managers are doing in using the organization's contributions and earnings to create value for the community. Of course, EVA measures only economic value; any social value created by the equity capital is ignored and, therefore, must be subjectively considered.

EVA, not MVA, can be applied to divisions as well as to entire businesses, and the charge for capital should reflect the riskiness and capital structure of the business unit, whether it is the aggregate business or an operating division. The specific calculation of EVA for a firm or division is much more complex than presented here because many accounting issues, such as inventory valuation, depreciation, amortization of research and development costs, and the like, must be addressed properly when estimating a firm's after-tax operating profit. Nevertheless, the brief discussion here illustrates that EVA tells managers that a business's true economic profitability depends on both income statement profitability and effective use of balance sheet assets.

Self-Test Questions
1. What is Market Value Added (MVA) and how is it measured?
2. What is Economic Value Added (EVA) and how is it measured?
3. Can MVA and EVA be applied to not-for-profit firms?
4. Why is EVA a better measure of financial performance than are accounting measures such as earnings per share and return on equity?

Benchmarking

Ratio analysis, as well as other financial performance evaluation techniques, requires comparisons to make meaningful judgments. In the previous examination of selected ratios, Bayside's ratios were compared to industry average ratios. However, similar to most businesses, Bayside's managers go one step further—they compare their ratios not only with industry averages, but also with the industry leaders, as well as their primary competitors. The technique of comparing ratios against selected standards is called *benchmarking*, while the comparative ratios are called *benchmarks*. Bayside's managers benchmark against industry averages; against National/GFB Healthcare and Pennant Healthcare, which are two leading for-profit hospital businesses; and against Woodbridge Memorial Hospital and St. Anthony's, which are its primary local competitors.

To illustrate the concept, consider how Bayside's analysts present total margin data to the firm's board of trustees:

	2000		*1999*
National/GFB	9.8%	National/GFB	9.6%
Industry top quartile	*8.4*	*Industry top quartile*	*8.0*
St. Anthony's	8.0	St. Anthony's	7.9
Bayside	**7.3**	Pennant Healthcare	5.0
Industry median	*5.0*	*Industry median*	*4.7*
Pennant Healthcare	4.8	**Bayside**	**2.2**
Industry lower quartile	*1.8*	*Industry lower quartile*	*2.1*
Woodbridge Memorial	0.5	Woodbridge Memorial	(1.3)

Benchmarking permits Bayside's managers to easily see exactly where the firm stands relative to its competition both in any given year and over time. As the data show, Bayside was roughly in the middle of the pack in 2000 with respect to its primary competitors and two large investor-owned hospital chains, although its showing was better than the average hospital. Its 1999 performance was significantly worse, so it improved substantially from 1999 to 2000. Although benchmarking is illustrated with one ratio, other ratios could be analyzed similarly. Also, for presentation purposes, comparative data can be color-coded for ease of recognition and interpretation.

All comparative analyses require comparative data. Such data are available from a number of sources including commercial suppliers, federal and state governmental agencies, and various industry trade groups. Each of these data suppliers uses a somewhat different set of ratios designed to meet its own needs. Thus, the comparative data source selected in a very real sense dictates the ratios that will be used in the analysis. Also, there are minor and sometimes major differences in ratio definitions between data sources; for example, one source may use a 365-day year while another uses a 360-day year. There are also numerous differences on using operating values versus total values when constructing ratios. It is **very important** to know the specific definitions used in the comparative data, for definitional differences between the ratios being calculated and the comparative ratios can lead to erroneous interpretations and conclusions. Thus, the first task in a ratio analysis is to make sure that the definitions used to develop the comparative data are understood.

1. What is benchmarking?

2. Why is it important to be familiar with the comparative data set?

Operating Analysis

Operating analysis goes one step beyond financial statement analysis in that operating analysis examines operating variables with the goal of **explaining** a business's financial performance. Like ratios, operating analysis *indicators* are typically grouped into major categories to make interpretation easier. For hospitals, the most commonly used categories are:

- Profit indicators;
- Price indicators;
- Volume (utilization) indicators;
- Length of stay indicators;
- Service intensity indicators;
- Efficiency indicators; and
- Unit cost indicators.

Because of the large number of indicators used in a typical operating analysis, it cannot be discussed in detail here. However, to give you an appreciation for this type of analysis, we will discuss seven commonly used hospital operating analysis indicators, one from each category. Note that much of the data needed to calculate operating analysis indicators are not contained in a business's financial statements. Thus, more complete data are required for this type of analysis, and hence the analysis is used more by managers than by outside analysts.

Profit per Discharge

Profit per discharge, a profit indicator, provides a measure of the amount of profit, as measured by net income, earned per discharge. Note that this a "raw" measure in the sense that it is not adjusted for case mix, which we discuss later, or local wage conditions. Often, operating indicators are calculated in both raw and adjusted forms. In 2000, Bayside's managerial accounting system reported $93,740,000 in inpatient service revenue, $84,865,000 in inpatient costs, and 18,281 patient discharges. Thus, Bayside's profit per discharge was $485:

$$\text{Profit per discharge} = \frac{\text{Inpatient profit}}{\text{Total discharges}} = \frac{\$93,740,000 - \$84,865,000}{18,281}$$

$$= \frac{\$8,875,000}{18,281} = \$485.$$

Industry average = $73.

Compared to the industry average, Bayside's inpatient services are highly profitable. It is not uncommon in today's tight reimbursement environment for hospitals to lose money (as measured by accounting profit) on inpatient services. In fact, with such a low median profit ($73), many hospitals are losing money on inpatient services. Most, however, make up the losses with profits either from other services or from nonoperating income.

Net price per discharge, which is one of many price indicators, measures the **Net Price per** average revenue collected on each inpatient discharge. Based on the data **Discharge** presented in the discussion of the previous indicator, Bayside's net price per discharge for 2000 was $5,128:

$$\text{Net price per discharge} = \frac{\text{Net inpatient revenue}}{\text{Total discharges}} = \frac{\$93,740,000}{18,281} = \$5,128.$$

Industry average = $5,556.

Bayside collects less per discharge than the average hospital, ignoring bad debt losses. However, we have already seen that Bayside makes a profit on each discharge, so its inpatient services cost structure must be proportionally even lower than the industry average. This could be caused by a lower-than-average case mix, which measures the average intensity of services provided, or to a very aggressive cost management program.

Occupancy rate, one of many volume indicators, measures the extent of uti- **Occupancy** lization of a hospital's **licensed** beds, and hence fixed assets. Because overhead **Percentage** costs are incurred on all assets, whether used or not, higher occupancy spreads **(Rate)** fixed costs over more patients, and hence increases per patient profitability. Based on 95,061 inpatient days in 2000, Bayside's occupancy rate was 57.9 percent:

$$\text{Occupancy rate} = \frac{\text{Inpatient days}}{\text{Number of licensed beds} \times 365} = \frac{95,061}{450 \times 365} = 57.9\%.$$

Industry average = 45.4%.

Bayside has a higher occupancy rate, and hence is using its fixed assets more productively than the average hospital. It is interesting to note that this conclusion is contrary to the financial analysis interpretation of the hospital's 2000 fixed asset turnover ratio. While that ratio is affected by inflation and accounting convention, the occupancy percentage is not. Hence, it is a superior measure of pure asset utilization, at least regarding inpatient utilization. On this basis, it appears that Bayside's managers are doing a good job, relative to the industry, of utilizing the hospital's inpatient fixed assets. Note that this measure can also be applied to **staffed** beds. In Bayside's case, the two measures of capacity are the same, but many hospitals have fewer staffed beds than licensed beds.

Length of Stay (LOS) or Average Length of Stay (ALOS)

Average length of stay (ALOS), or just *length of stay (LOS)*, is the number of days that an average inpatient is hospitalized with each admission. ALOS and an alternative version that is adjusted for case mix are the sole length-of-stay indicators. Bayside's 2000 LOS was 5.2 days:

$$\text{LOS} = \frac{\text{Inpatient days}}{\text{Total discharges}} = \frac{95,061}{18,281} = 5.2 \text{ days}.$$

Industry average = 4.7 days.

On average, Bayside keeps its patients in the hospital slightly longer than the average hospital does. In general, that longer stay is considered to have a negative impact on inpatient profitability because most hospitals have a reimbursement mix heavily weighted toward prospective (episodic) payment. With payment being fixed per discharge, lower LOS typically leads to lower costs and, hence, higher profitability.

All Patient Case Mix Index

The *all patient case mix index* is one of several intensity of service indicators. The concept of measuring case mix was first applied to Medicare patients, and hence many hospitals calculate both a Medicare case mix index and an all patient case mix index. Case mix is based on diagnosis, with those diagnoses requiring more complex treatments assigned a higher value. The idea here is to be able to differentiate (on average) between hospitals that provide relatively simple, and hence low cost, services from those that provide highly complex and costly services. Case mix values assigned to diagnoses are periodically recalibrated, with the intent of forcing the average hospital to have a case mix index of 1.0. In general, case mix is related to size because large hospitals typically offer a more complex set of services than do small hospitals. Furthermore, case mix values tend to be very high at teaching hospitals (about 1.4) because the most complex cases often are transferred to such hospitals.

Bayside's all patient case mix index was 1.12 for 2000, which is slightly below the industry average of 1.15. Thus, the patients that Bayside admits to the hospital require about the same intensity of services as do patients at the average hospital, which tells us that inpatient revenues and costs are not influenced by having a patient mix that is either relatively simple to treat or relatively complex.

Inpatient FTEs per Occupied Bed

The number of *inpatient full-time equivalent employees (FTEs) per occupied bed* is a measure of workforce productivity, and hence is an efficiency indicator. The lower the number, the more productive the workforce. When the focus is on inpatient productivity, inpatient FTEs are used. The measure can also be adapted to outpatient productivity. Needless to say, there are many situations within a hospital setting in which it is difficult to allocate FTEs to the type of service provided. With an inpatient workforce of 2,005 FTEs, Bayside's inpatient FTEs per occupied bed was 4.8 in 2000:

$$\text{Inpatient FTEs per occupied bed} = \frac{\text{Inpatient FTEs}}{\text{Average daily census}}$$

$$= \frac{2{,}005}{0.579 \times 450} = \frac{1{,}251}{260.55} = 4.8.$$

Industry average $= 5.6.$

Note that the average daily census (the number of patients hospitalized on an average day) was calculated by multiplying Bayside's occupancy rate (57.9 percent $= 0.579$) by the number of licensed beds (450). With higher-than-average labor productivity, it is no surprise that Bayside's inpatient services are profitable.

Salary per FTE, one of the unit cost indicators, provides a simple measure of the **Salary per FTE** relative cost of the largest resource item used in the hospital industry—labor. With total salaries of $83,038,613 in 2000 and 2,681 total FTEs, Bayside's salary per FTE in 2000 was $30,973:

$$\text{Salary per FTE} = \frac{\text{Total salaries}}{\text{Total FTEs}} = \frac{\$83{,}038{,}613}{2{,}681} = \$30{,}973.$$

Industry average $= \$32{,}987.$

Now, we can see that Bayside's profitability likely is a result of both worker productivity and control over wages and benefits.

For a full analysis, it would be useful to examine many more ratios and indicators. Still, as is apparent from the seven operating indicators presented, operating analysis goes beyond financial analysis in an attempt to identify the operating strengths and weaknesses that underlie a business's financial performance. Although operating analysis has been illustrated using the hospital industry, the concepts can be applied to any healthcare business, although the ratios selected would differ. Also, operating indicators are interpreted in the same way as financial ratios (i.e., by using comparative and trend analysis).

1. What is the difference between financial and operating analyses?   **Self-Test**
2. Why is operating analysis important?   **Questions**
3. Describe four indicators that are commonly used in operating analysis.

Limitations of Financial and Operating Analyses

While financial and operating analyses can provide a great deal of useful information concerning a business's operations and financial condition, such analyses have limitations that necessitate care and judgment. In this section, some of the problem areas are highlighted:

- Many large healthcare businesses operate a number of different divisions in quite different lines of business, and in such cases, it is difficult to develop meaningful comparative data. This problem tends to make financial statement and operating analyses somewhat more useful for firms with single product or service lines than for large, multiservice firms.

- Most businesses want to be better than average, although half will be above and half will be below average. Merely attaining average performance is not necessarily good. However, as was demonstrated earlier, compilers of industry data often report ratios in quartiles or other percentiles. Also, it is useful for managers to compare their firms not only with the industry average, but also with the top firms in the industry as well as their leading competitors. In the end, it is extremely important that senior managers establish their own standards of performance and ensure that all other managers are aware of these goals and are taking actions on a daily basis to achieve them; that is the purpose of the financial planning and control process.

- Generalizing about whether or not a particular ratio or indicator is good or bad is often difficult. For example, a high current ratio may show a strong liquidity position, which is good, or an excessive amount of receivables, which is bad. Similarly, a high asset turnover ratio may denote either a business that uses its assets efficiently or one that is undercapitalized and simply cannot afford to buy enough assets.

- Businesses often have some ratios and indicators that look good and others that look bad, which make the firm's financial position—strong or weak—difficult to determine. For this reason, significant judgment is required when analyzing financial and operating performance. Several methodologies have been proposed to reduce the information contained in a financial statement analysis to a single value, and hence make interpretation much easier. One method applied is *multiple discriminant analysis*, which attempts to divide firms into two groups on the basis of their probabilities of going bankrupt. Another method merely combines ratios selected judgmentally into a composite index, which is then compared to the industry average index. In spite of such attempts, the distillation of the wide variety of information contained in a ratio analysis into a single measure of financial condition has not proved very effective.[11]

- Different accounting practices can distort financial statement ratio comparisons. For example, firms can use different accounting conventions to value cost of goods sold and ending inventories. During inflationary periods these differences can lead to ratio distortions. Other accounting practices, such as those related to leases, can also create distortions.

- Inflation effects can distort both firms' balance sheets and income statements. Numerous reporting methods have been proposed to adjust accounting statements for inflation; but no consensus has been reached either on how to do this or even on the practical usefulness of the resulting data. Nevertheless, accounting standards encourage, but do not require, businesses to disclose supplementary data to reflect the effects of general inflation. Inflation effects tend to make ratio comparisons over time for a given firm, and across firms at any point in time, less reliable than would be the case in the absence of inflation.

1. Briefly, describe some of the problems encountered when performing financial statement and operating analyses.
2. Explain how inflation effects created problems in the Bayside illustration.

Key Concepts

The primary purpose of this chapter is to present the techniques used by managers and investors to assess a business's financial performance. The main focus is on financial performance as reflected in a business's financial statements, although operating data was also introduced to try to explain financial performance. Here are its key concepts:

- *Financial statement analysis*, which is used to assess a business's financial condition, focuses on the data contained in a business's financial statements. *Operating analysis* provides insights into why a firm is in a strong or weak financial condition.
- *Ratio analysis* is designed to reveal the relative strengths and weaknesses of a firm as compared to other firms in the same industry, and to show whether the firm's position has been improving or deteriorating over time.
- The *Du Pont equation* indicates how the total margin, the total asset turnover ratio, and the use of debt interact to determine the rate of return on equity. It provides a good overview of a business's financial performance.
- *Liquidity ratios* indicate the business's ability to meet its short-term obligations.
- *Asset management ratios* measure how effectively managers are utilizing the business's assets.
- *Debt management ratios* reveal the extent to which the firm is financed with debt; and the extent to which operating cash flows cover debt service and other fixed charge requirements.
- *Profitability ratios* show the combined effects of liquidity, asset management, and debt management on operating results.
- Ratios are analyzed using *comparative analysis*, in which a firm's ratios are compared with industry averages, or those of another firm, and *trend analysis*, in which a firm's ratios are examined over time.
- In a *common size analysis*, a business's income statement and balance sheet are expressed in percentages. This facilitates comparisons between firms of different sizes and for a single firm over time.
- In *percentage change analysis*, the differences in income statement items and balance sheet accounts over time are expressed in percentages. In this

way, it is easy to identify those items and accounts that are growing appreciably faster or slower than average.

- *Market Value Added (MVA)* and *Economic Value Added (EVA)* are two financial performance measures that focus directly on management's ability to enhance shareholder wealth. Although MVA is not applicable to not-for-profit businesses, EVA can be used to assess the performance of any business, regardless of ownership.
- *Benchmarking* is the process of comparing the performance of a particular firm with a group of benchmark firms, often industry leaders and primary competitors.
- Financial performance analysis is hampered by some serious problems including *development of comparative data, interpretation of results*, and *inflation effects*.

Although financial and operating analyses clearly have limitations, when used with care these analyses can provide a sound picture of a healthcare business's financial condition as well as identify those operating factors that contribute to that condition.

Selected References

Bazzoli, Gloria J., and William O. Cleverley. 1994. "Hospital Bankruptcies: An Exploration of Potential Causes and Consequences." *Health Care Management Review* (Summer): 41–51.

Beaver, William H., and Joan E. Horngren. 1991. "Ten Commandments of Financial Statement Analysis." *Financial Analysts Journal* (January–February): 9.

Bitter, Michael E., and Judith Cassidy 1992. "Perceptions of New AICPA Audit Guide." *Healthcare Financial Management* (November): 38–48.

Boles, Keith E. 1992. "Insolvency in Managed Care Organizations: Financial Indicators." *Topics in Health Care Financing* (Winter): 40–57.

Cleverley, William O., and Roger K. Harvey. 1992. "Is There a Link Between Hospital Profit and Quality?" *Healthcare Financial Management* (September): 40–45.

———. 1990. "Profitability: Comparing Hospital Results with Other Industries." *Healthcare Financial Management* (March): 42–52.

Cleverley, William O. 1995. "Understanding Your Hospital's True Financial Position and Changing It." *Health Care Management Review* (Spring): 62–73.

———. 1994. "Trends in the Hospital Financial Picture." *Healthcare Financial Management* (February): 56–63.

———. 1990. "ROI: Its Role in Voluntary Hospital Planning." *Hospital & Health Services Administration* (Spring): 71–82.

Coyne, Joseph S. 1990. "Analyzing the Financial Performance of Hospital-based Managed Care Programs: The Case of Humana." *Journal of Health Administration Education* (Fall): 571–642.

Donnelly, Joseph T. 1993. "RBRVS as a Financial Assessment Tool." *Healthcare Financial Management* (February): 45–51.

Duis, Terry E. 1993. "The Need for Consistency in Healthcare Reporting." *Healthcare Financial Management* (July): 40–44.

————. 1994. "Unraveling the Confusion Caused by GASB, FASB Accounting Rules." *Healthcare Financial Management* (November): 66–69.

Eastaugh, Steven R. 1992. "Hospital Strategy and Financial Performance." *Health Care Management Review* (Summer): 19–32.

Gapenski, Louis C., W. Bruce Vogel, and Barbara Langland-Orban. 1993. "The Determinants of Hospital Profitability." *Hospital & Health Services Administration* (Spring): 63–80.

Gardiner, Lorraine, Sharon L. Oswald, and John S. Jahera, Jr. 1996. "Prediction of Hospital Failure: A Post-PPS Analysis." *Hospital & Health Services Administration* (Winter): 441–460.

Harkey, John and Robert Vraciu 1992. "Quality of Health Care and Financial Performance: Is There a Link?" *Health Care Management Review* (Fall): 55–61.

Luecke, Randall W., and David T. Meeting. 1996. "SFAS 124, Accounting for Investments: The Rules Have Changed." *Healthcare Financial Management* (December): 58–63.

Lynn, Monty L., and Paul Wertheim.1993. "Key Financial Ratios Can Foretell Hospital Closures." *Healthcare Financial Management* (November): 66–70.

McCue, Michael J. 1991. "The Use of Cash Flow to Analyze Financial Distress in California Hospitals." *Hospital & Health Services Administration* (Summer): 223–241.

Pelfrey, Sandra. 1990. "How Proposed FASB Standards Would Affect Hospitals." *Healthcare Financial Management* (February): 54–67.

Prince, Thomas R. 1991. "Assessing Financial Outcomes of Not-for-Profit Community Hospitals." *Hospital & Healthcare Administration* (Fall): 331–349.

Robbins, Walter A., and Rick Turpin 1993. "Accounting Practice Diversity in the Healthcare Industry." *Healthcare Financial Management* (May): 111–114.

Sherman, Barnet.1990. "How Investors Evaluate the Creditworthiness of Hospitals." *Healthcare Financial Management* (March): 25–31.

Sylvestre, Jeanne and Frank R. Urbancic. 1994. "Effective Methods for Cash Flow Analysis." *Healthcare Financial Management* (July): 62–72.

Titera, William R. 1993. "FASB Proposes Changes in Not-for-Profit Reporting." *Healthcare Financial Management* (April): 39–49.

Titera, William R. 1995. "AICPA Seeks Comments on Proposed Accounting Changes." *Healthcare Financial Management* (August): 72–81.

Vogel, W. Bruce, Barbara Langland-Orban, and Louis C. Gapenski. 1993. "Factors Influencing High and Low Profitability Among Hospitals." *Health Care Management Review* (Spring): 15–26.

Zeller, Thomas L., Brian B. Stanko, and William O. Cleverly 1997. "A New Perspective on Hospital Financial Ratio Analysis." *Healthcare Financial Management* (November): 62–67.

Selected Web Sites

There are a multitude of web sites that pertain to this chapter.

One of the best ways to access corporate SEC filings is by using the 10K Wizard page found at *www.tenkwizard.com*. Then, enter the firm's ticker symbol or name to access the filings.

The Stern Stewart and Company web site contains information on EVA and MVA. Of particular interest is the video clip of corporate executives extolling the virtues of EVA; see *www.sternstewart.com*.

The American Hospital Directory has summary information, including financial data, on a large number of individual hospitals; see *www.ahd.com*. Then, click on Free Services.

The Center for Healthcare Industry Performance Studies (CHIPS) web site contains a great deal of information on the financial data products that it sells; see *www.chipsonline.com*.

InterStudy publications is the largest compiler and seller of HMO data. For more information on their range of publications, see *www.hmodata.com*.

Selected Cases

There are two cases in *Cases in Healthcare Finance* that are applicable to this chapter:

Case 1: Gateway Community Hospital (A), which focuses on conducting financial and operating analyses in a hospital setting.

Case 2: Gator Health Plans, which has the same focus, but applied to an HMO.

If time permits, both cases should be assigned because they illustrate how industry specific factors affect financial and operating analyses. In addition, Case 1 has a model that generates the ratios, and hence it focuses on interpretation. Case 2 also requires interpretation, but, in addition, students are required to calculate the ratios.

Notes

1. For more information on the various organizations involved in setting accounting principles for the healthcare industry, see Woodrin Grossman and William Warshauer, Jr., "An Overview of the Standard Setting Process," *Topics in Health Care Financing*, Summer 1990, 1–8.

2. One could divide liabilities into (1) interest-bearing debt owed to specific firms or individuals and (2) noninterest-bearing debt owed to suppliers, employees, and in the case of taxable firms, governments. We do not make this distinction, so the terms *debt* and *liabilities* are used synonymously. Also, note that an investor-owned firm would show common equity rather than net assets on its balance sheet.

3. Takeover specialists at investment banking firms always focus on an organization's cash flows. To them, cash flows are the primary determinant of a business's value. We will have more to say about this issue in Chapter 18.

4. Industry average ratios are available from many sources. For example, the Center for Healthcare Industry Performance Studies (CHIPS) publishes an annual almanac that provides hospital industry data on 33 financial ratios and 43 operating ratios. The ratios are reported in several groupings, such as by hospital size and geographic location. See William O. Cleverley, *Almanac of Hospital Financial & Operating Indicators* (Columbus, OH: CHIPS, published annually). The industry average ratios presented in this chapter are for illustrative

use only, and hence should not be used for making real-world comparisons. Also, note that in accordance with standard practice, we are calling the comparative data *averages*, but in reality they are *median* values. Median values are better for comparisons because they are not biased by extremely high or low values in the industry data set.

5. To determine the minimum proportion of current assets that must be converted to cash to meet current obligations, divide the number 1 by the current ratio. For Bayside, $1 / 2.3 = 0.43$, or 43 percent. This proportion is confirmed by noting that $0.43 \times \$31,280,000 = \$13,332,000$, the amount of current liabilities.

6. Bayside's 2000 current asset turnover ratio (Total revenues / Total current assets) is 3.8, compared to the industry average of 3.6, so the hospital is slightly above average in its utilization of current assets.

7. Because information on credit sales generally is not available from a business's financial statements, the assumption that all sales are on credit is typically used. Although almost all hospital services are provided on credit because of the third-party-payer system, other healthcare businesses might have a much lower proportion of credit sales than do hospitals. As the proportion of cash sales increases, the days in accounts receivable measure loses its usefulness. Also, note that it would be better to use **average** receivables in the calculation, either measured as an average of monthly receivables or by adding beginning and end of year receivables and then dividing by two.

8. Note that MVA does not account for time value, so comparisons between firms have little value unless the firms are about the same age.

9. The EVA concept was developed in detail and popularized by the consulting firm of Stern Stewart and Company. For a much more complete discussion of the concept, see G. Bennett Stewart, III, *The Quest for Value* (New York: HarperBusiness, 1991).

10. For an excellent discussion of the application of EVA in setting managerial compensation within not-for-profit businesses, see William O. Cleverley and Roger K. Harvey, "Economic Value Added—A Framework for Health Care Executive Compensation," *Hospital & Health Services Administration*, Summer 1993, 215–228.

11. For a general discussion of multiple discriminant analysis, see Eugene F. Brigham, Louis C. Gapenski, and Phillip R. Daves, *Intermediate Financial Management* (Fort Worth, TX: Dryden Press, 2000), Chapter 20. See William O. Cleverley, "Predicting Hospital Failure with the Financial Flexibility Index," *Healthcare Financial Management*, May 1985, 29–37, for a discussion of the financial flexibility index.

FINANCIAL FORECASTING

Learning Objectives

After studying this chapter, readers should be able to:

- Describe in general terms the overall planning process for businesses.
- Explain how the constant growth method can be used to forecast a business's financial statements.
- Describe the various methods used in practice to forecast income statement items and balance sheet accounts.
- Construct a cash budget for a business and explain its usefulness.

Introduction

In the last chapter, we saw how managers can analyze financial statements to identify a business's strengths and weaknesses. Now, we consider the actions managers can take to exploit a business's strengths and to overcome its weaknesses. As we shall see, managers are vitally concerned with *projected*, or *pro forma, financial statements*, and with the effects of alternative policies on these statements. An analysis of such effects is the key ingredient of financial planning. However, a good financial plan cannot, by itself, ensure that a business's goals will be met; the plan must be backed up by a financial control system for monitoring the situation, both to make sure that the plan is carried out properly and to facilitate rapid adjustments if economic and operating conditions change from those built into the plan.

Strategic Planning

Financial plans, which have financial forecasts as their foundation, are developed within the framework of the business's overall strategic planning process. Thus, we begin our discussion with an overview of this process.

Mission Statement

The strategic plan of any business should begin with a statement, called the *mission statement*, which defines the overall purpose of the organization. The mission can be defined either specifically or in general terms. For example, an investor-owned medical equipment manufacturer might state that its corporate mission is "to increase the intrinsic value of the firm's common stock." Another might say that its mission is "to maximize the growth rate in earnings and dividends per share while avoiding excessive risk." Yet another might state that its principal goal is "to provide our customers with state-of-the-art diagnostic systems at the lowest attainable cost, which in our opinion will also maximize benefits to our employees and stockholders."

Mission statements for not-for-profit businesses normally are stated in different terms; but the reality of competition in the health services industry forces all businesses, regardless of ownership, to operate in a manner consistent with financial viability. To illustrate a not-for-profit mission statement, consider the following statement of Bayside Memorial Hospital, a not-for-profit, acute care hospital:

> "Bayside Memorial Hospital, along with its medical staff, is a recognized, innovative healthcare leader dedicated to meeting the needs of the community. We strive to be the best comprehensive healthcare provider in our service area through our commitment to excellence."

This mission statement provides Bayside's managers with an overall framework for establishing the hospital's goals and objectives.

Corporate Goals

The mission statement contains the general philosophy and approach of the business, but it does not provide managers with specific operational goals. *Corporate goals* set forth specific goals that management strives to attain. Corporate goals generally are qualitative in nature, such as "keeping the firm's research and development efforts at the cutting edge of the industry." Multiple goals are established, and they should be changed over time as conditions change. Furthermore, a firm's corporate goals should be challenging, yet realistically attainable.

Bayside Memorial Hospital divides its corporate goals into five major areas as shown below:

1. *Quality and Customer Satisfaction*
   * To make quality performance the goal of each employee
   * To be recognized by our patients as the provider of choice in our market area
   * To identify and resolve as rapidly as possible areas of patient dissatisfaction
2. *Medical Staff Relations*
   * To identify and develop timely channels of communication among all members of the medical staff, management, and board of directors
   * To respond in a timely manner to all medical staff concerns brought to the attention of management
   * To make Bayside Memorial Hospital a more desirable location to practice medicine

- To develop strategies to enhance the mutual commitment of the medical staff, administration, and board of directors for the benefit of the hospital's stakeholders
- To provide the highest quality, most cost-effective medical care through a collaborative effort of the medical staff, administration, and board of directors

3. *Human Resources Management*
   - To be recognized as the customer service leader in our market area
   - To develop and manage human resources to make Bayside Memorial Hospital the most attractive location to work in our market area
4. *Financial Performance*
   - To maintain a financial condition that permits us to be highly competitive in our market area
   - To develop the systems necessary to identify inpatient and outpatient costs by unit of service
5. *Health Systems Management*
   - To be a leader in applied technology based on patient needs
   - To establish new services and programs in response to patient needs

Of course, these goals occasionally conflict, and when they do Bayside's senior managers have to make judgments regarding which one takes precedence.

Corporate Objectives

Once a business has defined its mission and goals, it must develop objectives designed to help it achieve its stated goals. *Corporate objectives* are generally quantitative in nature, such as specifying a target market share, a target ROE, a target earnings per share growth rate, or a target EVA (economic value added). Furthermore, the extent to which corporate objectives are met is commonly used as a basis for managers' compensation. To illustrate corporate objectives, consider Bayside's financial performance goal of maintaining a financial condition that permits the hospital to be highly competitive in its market area. These objectives are tied to that goal:

- To maintain or exceed the hospital's current 7.3 percent total margin
- Over time, to increase the hospital's debt ratio to the range of 35 to 40 percent. However, this objective will not be attained by accepting new projects that will lower the hospital's profit margin.
- To maintain the hospital's liquidity as measured by the current ratio in the range of 2.0 to 2.5
- Over time, to increase fixed asset utilization as measured by the fixed asset turnover ratio to 1.5

Corporate objectives give managers precise targets to shoot for. But the objectives must support the business's mission and goals, and must be chosen carefully so that they are challenging yet attainable.

1. Briefly, describe the nature and use of the following corporate planning tools:
   a. Mission
   b. Goals
   c. Objectives
2. Why do financial planners need to be familiar with the business's strategic plan?

Operating Plans

Operating plans can be developed for any time horizon, but most firms use a five-year horizon, and thus the term *five-year plan* has become common. In a five-year plan, the plans are most detailed for the first year, with each succeeding year's plan becoming less specific. The operating plan is intended to provide detailed implementation guidance to meet corporate objectives. The five-year plan explains in considerable detail who is responsible for what particular function and when specific tasks are to be accomplished.

Table 15.1 contains Bayside Memorial Hospital's annual planning schedule. This schedule illustrates the fact that for most organizations, the planning process is essentially continuous. Next, Table 15.2 outlines the key elements of the hospital's five-year plan, with an expanded section for finance. A full outline would require several pages, but Table 15.2 does at least provide insights into the format and content of a five-year plan. It should be noted that for Bayside, much of the planning function takes place at the department level, with technical assistance from the marketing, planning, and financial staffs. Larger businesses, with divisions, would begin the planning process at the divisional level. Thus, each division has its own mission and goals, as well as objectives designed to support its goals, and these plans are then consolidated to form the corporate plan.

1. What is the purpose of a business's operating plan?
2. What is the most common time horizon for operating plans?
3. Briefly, describe the contents of a typical operating plan.

The Financial Plan

The financial planning process can be broken down into five steps:

1. Set up a system of projected financial statements that can be used to analyze the effects of planned operations on the firm's financial condition. This system can also be used to monitor operations after the plan has been finalized and put into effect. Rapid awareness of deviations from plans is essential to a good control system, and such a system in turn is essential to corporate success in a changing world.

Months	Action	
April–May	Marketing department analyzes national and local economic factors likely to influence Bayside's patient volume and reimbursement rates. At this time, a preliminary volume forecast is prepared for each service line.	**TABLE 15.1** Bayside Memorial Hospital: Annual Planning Schedule
June–July	Operating departments prepare new project (capital budgeting) requirements, as well as operating-cost estimates based on the preliminary volume forecast.	
August–September	Financial analysts evaluate proposed capital expenditures and department operating plans. Preliminary forecasted financial statements and cash budgets are prepared with emphasis on Bayside's sources and uses of funds and forecasted financial condition.	
October–November	All previous input is reviewed and the hospital's five-year plan is drafted by the planning, financial, and departmental staffs. Any new information developed during the planning process "feeds back" into earlier actions.	
December	The five-year plan is approved by the hospital's executive committee, and then submitted to the board of directors for final approval.	

2. Determine the specific financial requirements needed to support the firm's five-year plan. This financial requirement includes funds for plant and equipment as well as for inventory and receivables buildups, for research and educational programs, and for major marketing campaigns.
3. Forecast the financing sources to be used over the next five years. This forecast involves estimating the funds that will be generated internally (primarily retentions), as well as those that must be obtained from external sources. Any constraints on planned operations imposed by financial limitations should be incorporated into the plan; examples include restrictions in debt covenants that limit the debt ratio, the current ratio, and coverage ratios.
4. Establish and maintain a system of controls governing the allocation and use of funds within the firm. Essentially, this step involves making sure that the basic plan is carried out properly.
5. Develop procedures for adjusting the basic plan if the forecasted economic conditions on which the plan was based do not materialize. For example, if Bayside's forecast on Medicare and Medicaid reimbursement used to develop the five-year plan proves to be too high or too low, the correct amounts must be recognized and reflected in operational and financial plans as rapidly as possible. Thus, Step 5 is really a "feedback loop" that triggers modifications to the plan.

TABLE 15.2
Bayside
Memorial
Hospital:
Five-Year Plan
Outline

Chapter 1	Corporate mission and goals
Chapter 2	Corporate objectives
Chapter 3	Projected business environment
Chapter 4	Corporate strategies
Chapter 5	Summary of projected business results
Chapter 6	Service line plans

A. Marketing
B. Operations
C. Finance
    1. Working capital
       a. Overall working capital policy
       b. Cash and marketable securities management
       c. Inventory management
       d. Credit policy and receivables management
    2. Financial forecast
       a. Current condition and forecast assumptions
       b. Capital budget
       c. Cash budget
       d. Pro forma financial statements
       e. External financing requirements
       f. Financial condition analysis
    3. Accounting budgets
    4. Control plan
D. Administration and human resources
E. New service lines

The principal components of the *financial forecast* are: (1) an analysis of the business's current financial condition; (2) a revenue (volume and reimbursement) forecast; (3) the capital budget; (4) the cash budget; (5) a set of pro forma, or projected, financial statements; (6) the external financing plan; and (7) an analysis of the firm's projected financial condition. In previous chapters, we discussed the capital budget and financial statement analysis. In the remainder of this chapter, we focus on some of the plan's other elements—the revenue forecast, pro forma financial statements, the external financing plan, and cash budgeting.

Self-Test Questions

1. What are the five steps of the financial planning process?
2. What are the principal components of the financial forecast?

Revenue Forecasts

The starting point, and most critical element, in the financial forecast is the *revenue forecast*. The reason why revenue forecasts are so important to the development of the financial plan is that all elements of the plan are derived from the volume forecast portion of the revenue forecast. If the volume projection is way off base, the rest of the financial plan will be almost worthless.

Revenue forecasts can be done in two ways: (1) from the top or (2) from the bottom. When forecasted from the top, historical trends in aggregate (organizational) revenues are examined and used as the basis for forecasting future revenues. When forecasting from the bottom, revenues are forecasted for individual services and then aggregated to create the organization forecast. Most large organizations use both methods, and then the last step in the process is to resolve inconsistencies. In this way, the best possible forecasts are made.

Forecasting from the Top

When forecasting from the top, the revenue forecast generally starts with a review of organizational revenues over the past five to ten years, which is expressed in a graph such as that in Figure 15.1. The first part of the graph shows actual total operating revenues for Bayside Memorial Hospital from 1996 through 2000. Over these five years (four growth periods), total operating revenue (net patient service revenue plus premium revenue) grew from $86,477,000 to $113,832,000, or at a compound annual growth rate of 7.1 percent. Alternatively, a time-series regression can be applied to total operating revenue. We used a spreadsheet to perform a log-linear regression on all five years of operating revenue data, with a resulting annual growth rate of 6.9 percent.[1] However, Bayside's revenue growth rate accelerated in the second half of the historical period, primarily as a result of new capacity that came online in 1998. Furthermore, a new, aggressive marketing program was instituted in late 1999 that resulted in a growth rate in operating revenues in 2000 of more than 11 percent.

On the basis of the recent trends in operating revenues, on anticipated service introductions, and on forecasts of local competition and third-party-payer trends, Bayside's planning group projects a growth rate of 11 percent for 2001, which produces a total operating revenue forecast of $126,354,000. It is very important to recognize that the operating revenue forecast is driven by two elements: (1) changes in volume (utilization) and (2) changes in reimbursement rates. Whereas volume changes tend to have a large impact on plant and staffing requirements, and hence costs, reimbursement rate changes, unless substantial, do not have as much of an effect on operating variables. Thus, it is important for managers to recognize whether operating revenue changes are a result of changes in volume, which indicates that the business is experiencing real changes in output, or a result of reimbursement effects, which may have no impact on volume.

If Bayside's volume forecast is off, the consequences can be serious. First, if the market for any particular service expands more than Bayside has expected and planned for, then the hospital will not be able to meet its patients'

FIGURE 15.1

Bayside
Memorial
Hospital:
Historical and
Projected
Revenues
(thousands of
dollars)

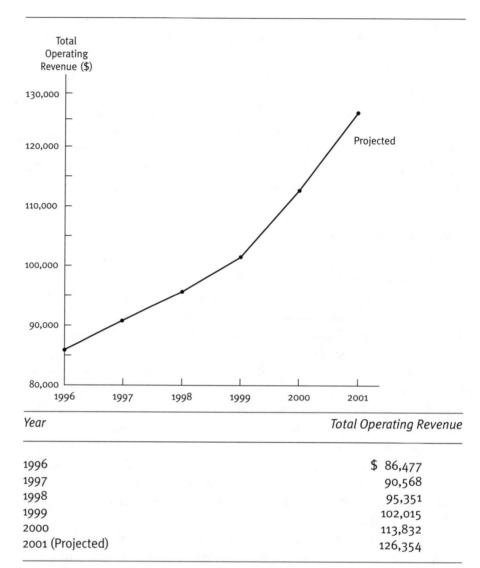

Year	Total Operating Revenue
1996	$ 86,477
1997	90,568
1998	95,351
1999	102,015
2000	113,832
2001 (Projected)	126,354

needs. Potential customers will end up going elsewhere, and Bayside will lose market share and perhaps miss a major opportunity. On the other hand, if its projections are overly optimistic, Bayside could end up with too much capacity, which means excess equipment, inventory, and staff. This excess would mean low turnover ratios, high costs for labor and depreciation, and possibly layoffs. All of these factors would result in low profitability, which could degrade the hospital's ability to compete in the future. If Bayside had financed the unneeded expansion primarily with debt, its problems would, of course, be compounded. Thus, an accurate volume forecast is critical to the well-being of any healthcare provider.

Finally, note that the operating revenue forecast, like virtually any forecast, is actually the expected value of a probability distribution of possible revenues. Because any forecast is subject to a greater or lesser degree of uncertainty, for financial planning purposes we are often just as interested in the degree of uncertainty inherent in the forecast (its standard deviation) as we are in the expected value.

Forecasting from the Bottom

To begin the process of forecasting operating revenue from the bottom, Bayside divides its services into four major groups: (1) inpatient, (2) outpatient, (3) ancillary, and (4) other. Each of these categories is broken down into individual services; for example, one of the services that is part of the overall inpatient services revenue forecast is neurosurgery.

Next, the level of population growth and disease trends is forecasted; for example, analysts predict the population growth in the hospital's service area, and any trend in disease patterns or technology that will affect the number of neurosurgeries performed. To illustrate the concept, consider the data obtained from a state health agency, which show that 523 neurosurgeries were performed in Bayside's service area in 2000. With a service area population of 756,508 in 2000, the neurosurgery rate in the service area was 69.1 per 100,000 population. With a population forecast of 788,700 for 2001, Bayside's managers predict that (788,700 / 100,000) × 69.1 = 545 neurosurgeries will be performed in 2001 in its service area.

Bayside's managers then look at the competitive environment. Consideration is given to such factors as the hospital's inpatient and outpatient capacities, its competitors' capacities, and new services or service improvements that either Bayside or its competitors might institute. For example, Bayside performed 127 neurosurgeries in 2000, so it had 24.3 percent of the neurosurgery market in that year. With an additional neurosurgeon now on the staff, increased marketing, and new managed care contracts, the hospital expects to increase its market share to 30 percent in 2001. Thus, the forecast for neurosurgeries in 2001 is 163.

Bayside's managers must then consider its pricing strategy and trends in reimbursement. Of course, some of the pricing strategy may have an impact on demand for services. It is important to know if the hospital has plans to raise outpatient charges to boost profit margins or to lower charges to gain market share and utilize excess capacity. If such actions are expected to affect volume forecasts, then these forecasts must be revised. Regarding neurosurgeries, Bayside has reimbursement data, as well as utilization data, by payer, so it can easily convert the estimate of the number of procedures into a revenue estimate. The end result is a utilization and revenue forecast for neurosurgeries.

Bayside creates a volume and revenue forecast for each individual service, and then aggregates these forecasts by service group. Independently, the hospital forecasts operating revenues by service group using the procedures discussed in the previous section. The aggregate forecast based on individual service forecasts are then compared with the service group forecasts. Differences are reconciled, and the resultant revenue forecast for the hospital is then compared to the organizational forecast. Further refinement is often necessary; but the end result is a total operating revenue forecast for the hospital, with breakdowns by major groups and by individual services.

Self-Test Questions

1. What are two approaches to the total operating revenue forecast?
2. Discuss some factors that must be considered when developing an operating revenue forecast.
3. Why is it necessary for planners to distinguish between volume changes and reimbursement changes?

Creating Pro Forma Financial Statements

The revenue forecast provides the starting point for creating a business's projected financial statements, which typically are called *pro forma financial statements*, or just *pro formas*. There are many techniques used to create the pro formas, most of which are either too complex or too detailed to discuss here. Thus, we will focus our attention more on concepts than on providing a cookbook approach to financial statement forecasting. We begin by discussing a conceptual framework for financial statement forecasting. Then, we consider some issues inherent in the forecasting process.

Self-Test Question

1. What are pro forma financial statements?

Constant Growth Forecasting

The *constant growth method*, also called the *percentage of revenues method* or, more commonly, *percentage of sales* method, is a simple technique for creating pro forma financial statements. Although this method has little value in practice, it provides an excellent introduction to the forecasting process and lays the groundwork for understanding the more complex methods that are used in practice.

Assumptions

The constant growth method is based on two assumptions: (1) Most income statement items and balance sheet accounts are tied directly to revenues, and (2) the current levels of most income statement items and balance sheet accounts are optimal for the current volume of services provided. The basic premise is that as revenues either increase or decrease, so will most income statement items and balance sheet accounts. Furthermore, the changes in items and accounts will be proportional to the change in revenues. These assumptions create a situation wherein all income statement items and balance sheet accounts are assumed to grow at the same rate—the rate of revenue growth.

Of course, revenue changes can be a result of either volume changes or reimbursement rate changes, which typically are driven by inflation. In most situations, revenue changes are a result of both factors. For example, Bayside's 11 percent increase in revenues might be a result of a projected 6 percent increase in the volume of services provided and a 5 percent inflationary increase in reimbursement rates. Because many of the income statement items and balance sheet accounts are affected by both volume and inflation changes, many financial statement variables would be expected to also increase by 11 percent. Those variables that are tied only to volume or to inflation would be expected to increase at a lower rate. However, the constant growth method as illustrated here assumes that all financial statement variables related to revenues are influenced by both volume and inflationary changes.

Illustration

We will illustrate the constant growth method with Bayside Memorial Hospital, whose 2000 financial statements are given in Column 1 of Tables 15.3 and 15.4. We will explain the other columns of these tables as we discuss the forecast for 2001.

To begin the process, we will assume (contrary to fact) that Bayside operated its fixed assets at full capacity to support the $113,832,000 in total operating revenue in 2000; that is, the hospital had no excess beds or outpatient facilities.[2] Because we are assuming no excess capacity, if volume is to increase in 2001, Bayside will need to increase its fixed assets along with its current assets.

If, as projected, Bayside's total operating revenue increases to $126,354,000, what will its pro forma 2001 income statement and balance sheet look like, and how much external financing will the hospital require during to support operations in 2001? The first step in using the constant growth method to forecast the business's financial statements is to identify those income statement items and balance sheet accounts that vary directly with revenues. For illustrative purposes, the increased operating revenue forecast for 2001 is expected to bring corresponding increases in all of the income statement items except interest expense; that is, operating costs and administrative expenses are assumed to be tied directly to total operating revenue, but interest expense is a function of financing decisions. Furthermore, other (nonoperating) revenue is also assumed to grow at the same rate.

Under such a naïve assumption, the first-pass forecasted, or pro forma, 2001 income statement is constructed as follows:

- Place the forecasted constant growth rate, 11.0 percent, in Column 2 in Table 15.3 for all items expected to increase with revenues. Those items calculated within the forecasted income statement, such as total operating costs, as well as those items not expected to increase proportionally with revenues, such as interest expense, have a NA (not applicable) in Column 2.
- Forecast the first-pass 2001 pro forma amounts by multiplying each applicable 2000 value by the growth rate. To illustrate the technique, note

TABLE 15.3
Bayside Memorial Hospital: Historical and Projected Income Statements (thousands of dollars)

	2000 (1)	Growth Rate (2)	2001 Projections		
			First Pass (3)	Second Pass (4)	Third Pass (5)
Total operating revenue	$ 113,832	11.0%	$ 126,354	$ 126,354	$ 126,354
Other revenue	3,644	11.0	4,045	4,045	4,045
Total revenues	$ 117,476	NA	$ 130,398	$ 130,398	$ 130,398
Expenses:					
Nursing services	$ 58,285	11.0%	$ 64,696	$ 64,696	$ 64,696
Dietary services	5,424	11.0	6,021	6,021	6,021
General services	13,198	11.0	14,650	14,650	14,650
Administrative services	11,427	11.0	12,684	12,684	12,684
Employee health and welfare	10,250	11.0	11,378	11,378	11,378
Provision for uncollectibles	3,328	11.0	3,694	3,694	3,694
Provision for malpractice	1,320	11.0	1,465	1,465	1,465
Depreciation	4,130	11.0	4,584	4,584	4,584
Interest expense	1,542	NA	1,542	1,820	1,842
Total expenses	$ 108,904	NA	$ 120,714	$ 120,992	$ 121,014
Net income	$ 8,572	NA	$ 9,685	$ 9,407	$ 9,385

TABLE 15.4

Bayside Memorial Hospital: Historical and Projected Balance Sheets (thousands of dollars)

	2000 (1)	Growth Rate (2)	2001 Projections First Pass (3)	2001 Projections Second Pass (4)	2001 Projections Third Pass (5)
Cash	$ 4,263	11.0%	$ 4,732	$ 4,732	$ 4,732
Short-term investments	2,000	11.0	2,220	2,220	2,220
Accounts receivable	21,840	11.0	24,242	24,242	24,242
Inventories	3,177	11.0	3,526	3,526	3,526
Total current assets	$ 31,280	NA	$ 34,721	$ 34,721	$ 34,721
Gross plant and equipment	$ 145,158	11.0%	$ 161,125	$ 161,125	$ 161,125
Accumulated depreciation	25,160	NA	29,744	29,744	29,744
Net plant and equipment	$ 119,998	NA	$ 131,381	$ 131,381	$ 131,381
Total assets	$ 151,278	NA	$ 166,102	$ 166,102	$ 166,102
Accounts payable	$ 4,707	11.0%	$ 5,225	$ 5,225	$ 5,225
Accrued expenses	5,650	11.0	6,272	6,272	6,272
Notes payable	825	11.0	916	916	916
Current portion of long-term debt	2,150	11.0	2,387	2,387	2,387
Total current liabilities	$ 13,332	NA	$ 14,799	$ 14,799	$ 14,799
Long-term debt	$ 28,750	NA	$ 28,750	$ 32,221	$ 32,499
Capital lease obligations	1,832	11.0	2,034	2,034	2,034
Total long-term liabilities	$ 30,582	NA	$ 30,784	$ 34,255	$ 34,555
Net assets (equity)	$107,364	NA	$ 117,049	$ 116,771	$ 116,749
Total liabilities and net assets	$ 151,278	NA	$ 162,631	$165,824	$166,080

that the 2001 forecast for nursing services expenses is $58,285,000 × 1.11 = $64,696,000.[3]

- Some items marked NA, such as interest expense, are carried over into 2001 at their 2000 values. We know that the interest expense in 2001 will be larger than in 2000 if Bayside will have to borrow additional funds, but we cannot predict the amount of interest increase until the first-pass financial statements have been completed. The remaining income statement items marked NA, such as total expenses, are calculated by merely adding or subtracting other forecasted items.
- When the first-pass income statement is completed (Column 3 in Table 15.3), we see that the projected net income is $9,685,000. Note that an 11 percent increase in net income would be $8,572,000 × 1.11 = $9,515,000. The forecasted amount is somewhat greater than an 11 percent increase because interest expense was held at its 2000 level.

Turning to the balance sheet, because we assumed that Bayside was operating at full capacity in 2000, fixed assets as well as current assets must increase if revenues are to increase. More cash will be needed for transactions, receivables will be higher, additional inventory must be stocked, new plant must be added, and so on.[4]

To construct the first-pass pro forma balance sheet contained in Column 3 in Table 15.4, we proceed as follows:

- All balance sheet accounts that are expected to increase with revenues are forecast in the same way as on the income statement. To illustrate the concept, consider the cash account. The 2001 forecast is created by multiplying the 2000 value by the growth rate, so $4,263,000 × 1.11 = $4,732,000, which is shown in Column 3 of Table 15.4.
- The forecasted 2001 depreciation expense from the income statement is added to the 2000 accumulated depreciation account on the balance sheet to obtain the 2001 accumulated depreciation forecast: $4,584,000 + $25,160,000 = $29,744,000.
- The long-term debt value is **initially** held at its 2000 value, $28,750,000. However, any external financing required in 2001 will be obtained by issuing more long-term debt. Alternatively, any excess funds generated would be used to retire long-term debt. In effect, long-term debt is the "plug" variable. It will be adjusted in the second and third passes to make the balance sheet balance.
- To forecast the 2001 equity amount, add the net income projected for 2001, which must all be retained within the business, to the 2000 balance sheet equity amount to obtain the projected amount for 2001: $9,685,000 + $107,364,000 = $117,049,000.
- Finally, fill in the missing values in Column 3 by merely adding or subtracting as necessary.

The projected 2001 asset accounts sum to $166,102,000. This sum is less than an 11 percent increase because accumulated depreciation, which is a contra (negative) asset account, increased by about 18 percent. Thus, to support a revenue increase of 11 percent, Bayside must increase its assets from $151,278,000 to $166,102,000. The projected liability and equity accounts sum to $162,631,000. Again, this sum is less than an 11 percent increase because (1) long-term debt was held at its 2000 level and (2) the equity account increased by less than 11 percent.

At this point, the balance sheet **does not balance**: Assets total $166,102,000, while only $162,631,000 of liabilities and equity is projected. Thus, we have a shortfall, or *external financing requirement (EFR)*, of $3,471,000, which will have to be raised by bank borrowings and/or by selling securities or by changing operating variables—such as charges—to generate more revenue and, hence, more retained earnings.

The External Financing Plan

Assuming no change in operating variables, Bayside could use short-term notes payable, long-term debt, increased solicitations, or a combination of these sources to make up the $3,471,000 shortfall. Ordinarily, Bayside would base this choice on its target capital structure, the relative costs of different types of securities, maturity matching considerations, its ability to increase contributions above the forecasted level, and so on. The decision as to how this shortfall will be financed is called the *external financing plan*.

However, our simplistic forecast assumes that Bayside will raise the required external funds by issuing additional long-term debt. However, the use of additional debt capital will change the first approximation income statement for 2001 as set forth in Column 3 of Table 15.3 because more debt will lead to higher interest expense. Bayside's managers are forecasting that new long-term debt will carry an interest rate of 8 percent. Thus, $3,471,000 of new long-term debt will increase the interest expense projected for 2001 by 0.08 × $3,471,000 = $278,000.

The projected 2001 income statement and balance sheet, including financing feedback effects, are shown in Column 4 (Second Pass) of Tables 15.3 and 15.4. We see that although $3,471,000 was added to Bayside's liabilities, the hospital is still $166,102,000 − $165,824,000 = $278,000 short in meeting its financing requirements. This new, but much smaller, shortfall is a result of the added interest expense; $278,000 of new interest decreases net income buy a like amount, and hence the equity balance falls to $117,049,000 − $278,000 = $116,771,000.

The process could be repeated yet again by adding an additional $227,000 of external (long-term debt) financing to create a third-pass income statement and balance sheet. As shown in Column 5 of Tables 15.3 and 15.4, the projected equity balance would be further reduced by additional interest requirements, but the balance sheet would be closer to being in balance because more long-term debt is added to the liabilities side. Successive iterations would continue to reduce the discrepancy. If the budget process were computerized, as would be true for most firms, an exact solution could be reached very rapidly. Even if the process is stopped after just a few iterations, the projected statements would generally be very close to being in balance, and they would certainly be close enough for practical purposes, given the uncertainty inherent in the projections themselves.

The base case pro forma financial statements, along with the corresponding financial and operating analyses that we discussed in Chapter 14, are then reviewed by Bayside's executive committee for consistency with the hospital's financial objectives. Generally, they will make changes in the initial assumptions that will result in a new set of pro forma financial statements, which are then analyzed and reviewed, and so on, until the forecast is finalized.

The forecasting process undertaken by Ann Arbor Health Systems, a for-profit hospital, is very similar to that used by Bayside. The only real difference is that a for-profit business has to deal with the fact that it uses stock rather than fund financing. This fact presents three complications. First, the firm may pay dividends, so net income must be reduced by the forecasted dividend payment to find the amount of capital that is retained within the firm, and hence which flows to the balance sheet. Second, the firm has the option of issuing common stock to meet its external financing needs. Third, the financing feedback effect must be expanded to include dividend payments, if the business is paying dividends, on any new common stock that is issued.

Finally, note that forecasted financial statements must be checked for internal consistency; that is, accumulated depreciation on the balance sheet must be consistent with the depreciation expense shown on the income statement, and the equity reported on the balance sheet must be consistent with the retentions shown on the income statement. It is imperative that pro forma statements recognize the dependencies between the income statement items and balance sheet accounts.

Self-Test Questions

1. Briefly, describe the mechanics of the constant growth forecasting method.
2. Why is the external financing requirement so important to the planning process?
3. Do you think that most healthcare businesses use the constant growth method to develop pro forma financial statements, or do they use some other methodology?

Factors That Influence the External Financing Requirement

The external funding requirement is one of the key pieces of information that stems from the pro forma financial statements. If the business is unable to fund this requirement, then its plans for the future must be altered. The five factors that have the greatest influence on the external financing requirement are: (1) projected revenue growth; (2) initial fixed asset utilization rate, or excess capacity situation; (3) capital intensity; (4) profit margin; and (5) for investor-owned businesses, dividend policy. In this section, we discuss each of these factors in some detail.

Revenue Growth Rate

The faster Bayside's revenues are forecasted to grow, the greater its need for external financing will be. At growth rates less than 8.7 percent, Bayside will need no external financing; indeed, all required funds can be obtained by spontaneous increases in current liability accounts plus retained earnings, and the hospital will even generate surplus capital. However, if Bayside's projected revenue growth rate is 8.7 percent or higher, then it must seek outside financing, and the greater the projected growth rate, the greater will be its external financing requirement. The reasoning here is as follows:

- Increases in revenues normally require increases in assets. If revenues are not projected to grow, no new assets will be needed.
- Any projected asset increases require financing of some type. Some of the required financing will come from spontaneously generated liabilities. Also, assuming a positive profit margin (and for investor-owned firms, a payout ratio of less than 100 percent), the firm will generate some retained earnings.
- If the revenue growth rate is low enough, spontaneously generated funds plus retained earnings will be sufficient to support the asset growth. However, if the growth rate exceeds a certain level, then external financing will be needed. If management foresees difficulties in raising this capital—perhaps because it has no more debt capacity—then the feasibility of the firm's expansion plans may have to be reconsidered.

Capacity Utilization

In determining Bayside's external financing requirement for 2001, we assumed that the hospital's fixed assets were being fully utilized. Thus, any significant increase in revenues would require an increase in fixed assets. What would be the effect if Bayside had been operating its fixed assets at less than full capacity? Assume that Bayside's managers consider 90 percent occupancy to be full capacity. Because the hospital had 57.9 percent occupancy in 2000, it was actually operating at 57.9 / 90 = 64% of capacity. Under this condition, fixed assets could remain constant until revenues reach that level at which fixed assets were being fully utilized, defined as *capacity sales*, which is calculated as follows:

$$\text{Utilization rate (\% of capacity)} = \frac{\text{Actual revenue}}{\text{Capacity sales}},$$

so

$$\text{Capacity sales} = \frac{\text{Actual revenue}}{\text{Utilization rate}}.$$

Because Bayside had been operating in 2000 at 64 percent of capacity, its capacity sales *without any new fixed assets* would be $113,832,000 / 0.64 = $177,862,000. In reality, Bayside could easily increase its revenue to $126,354,000 with no increase in fixed assets. Thus, its external financing requirement would decrease by $161,125,000 − $145,158,000 = $15,967,000 (the projected increase in gross plant and equipment), and hence Bayside's forecast would actually show surplus capital in 2001.

Capital Intensity

The amount of assets required per dollar of sales (total assets/sales) is often called the *capital intensity ratio*, which is the reciprocal of the total asset turnover ratio. Capital intensity has a major effect on capital requirements to support any level of sales growth. If the capital intensity ratio is low, such as for home health care businesses, then revenues can grow rapidly without much outside capital. However, if the firm is capital-intensive, such as a hospital, then even a small growth in output will require a great deal of outside capital if the firm is operating at full capacity.

Profitability

Profitability is also an important determinant of external financing requirements—the higher the profit margin, the lower the external financing requirement, other factors held constant. Bayside's profit (total) margin in 2000 was 7.3 percent. Now, suppose its profit margin increased to 10 percent through higher reimbursements and better expense control. This would increase net income, and hence retained earnings, which in turn would decrease the requirement for external financing.

Dividend Policy

For investor-owned firms, dividend policy also affects external capital requirements. When Ann Arbor Health Systems projects its 2001 financial statements, if it foresees difficulties in raising capital, it might want to consider a reduction in its dividend payout ratio. However, before making this decision, management should consider the possible effects of a dividend cut on stock price.[5]

Self-Test Question

1. How do the following factors affect the external financing requirement?
   a. Revenue growth rate
   b. Capacity utilization
   c. Capital intensity
   d. Profitability
   e. For investor-owned firms, dividend policy

Sustainable Growth

We have mentioned previously that investor-owned firms, other than start-up firms, generally try to avoid issuing new common stock. There are two reasons for this aversion: (1) High issuance costs must be incurred to sell common stock, but no such costs are incurred on retained earnings; and (2) information asymmetries lead investors to view stock issues as bad news, and hence stock prices typically decline when a new stock issue is announced. These two factors combine to make equity raised by selling stock much more costly than equity obtained by retaining earnings. In addition, not-for-profit businesses are unable to issue new common stock, so they must rely mainly on retained earnings as their source of equity. Therefore, regardless of ownership, managers are often confronted with this question: How fast can the business grow (or how many new services can be offered) using only earnings retentions and debt financing? In other words, what is the business's *sustainable growth rate*, or the growth rate that can be achieved without any new equity financing? If we make some assumptions, a relatively simple model can be used to answer that question.[6]

We begin by defining these key terms:

- PM = projected profit (total) margin, or net income divided by total revenues.
- b = target retention rate = 1 − Target payout ratio.
- D / E = target debt-to-equity ratio.
- A / S = ratio of total assets to sales (revenues), which is the reciprocal of the total asset turnover ratio.

If a business is operating at full capacity, and if it is currently at its target capital structure, then its sustainable growth rate (sustainable g) can be found using this equation:

$$\text{Sustainable g} = \frac{PM \times b \times (1 + D/E)}{A/S - [PM \times b \times (1 + D/E)]}.$$

To illustrate the use of the sustainable growth rate equation, consider the situation facing Bayside Memorial Hospital. From the data in Tables 15.3 and 15.4 presented earlier in the chapter, Bayside's 2000 profit (total) margin = 7.3%; because Bayside is a not-for-profit hospital, its retention rate = 1.00; its book value debt-to-equity ratio = Total debt / Total equity = ($151,278,000 − $107,364,000) / $107,364,000 = 0.41; and its assets-to-sales ratio = Total assets / Total revenues = $151,278,000 / $117,476,000 = 1.29. If we assume (1) that these values will hold for 2001; (2) that Bayside's current book value structure is also its target market value target; (3) that depreciation cash flows are being used to replace worn-out assets; and (4) that financing feedback effects are small, and hence can be ignored, then the firm's sustainable growth rate is 8.6 percent:

$$\text{Sustainable g} = \frac{\text{PM} \times \text{b} \times (1 + \text{D/E})}{\text{A/S} - [\text{PM} \times \text{b} \times (1 + \text{D/E})]}$$

$$= \frac{7.3\% \times 1.00 \times (1 + 0.41)}{1.29 - [0.073 \times 1.00 \times (1 + 0.41)]}$$

$$= \frac{10.29\%}{1.29 - 0.10} = \frac{10.29\%}{1.19} = 8.6\%.$$

Thus, according to the sustainable growth model, Bayside's revenues can grow as much as 8.6 percent in 2001 without requiring the hospital to increase its use of financial leverage. Note that this is essentially the same rate as we obtained using a spreadsheet model along with the constant growth method.

An actual revenue growth rate that differs from the sustainable rate has important implications for a business, and managers must actively develop growth targets and financial objectives that are mutually consistent. If the revenue growth rate is less than the sustainable rate, then the business will generate more than enough capital to meet its capital investment needs and its financial plans must call for an increase in cash and marketable securities; a reduction in the amount of debt outstanding; a merger program; stock repurchases or a dividend increase (for investor-owned firms); or some combination of these actions. Conversely, if the revenue growth rate is greater then the sustainable rate, then financial leverage must be increased, or for investor-owned firms, new equity must be sold or the payout ratio reduced. If these are not viable options, then the growth rate itself must be scaled back.

In Bayside's actual case, with its excess capacity and a forecasted revenue growth rate of only 11 percent, it did not require any external financing for 2001. However, Bayside's managers are well aware of its sustainable growth rate, and the implications of expanding beyond that rate.

Self-Test Question

1. Why is it important for managers to know their firms' sustainable growth rate?

Problems with the Constant Growth Approach

For the constant growth rate method to produce accurate forecasts, each item and account that is assumed to grow with revenues must increase at the same rate as revenues. Unfortunately, such a situation rarely exists. Here are some of the problems encountered in "real-world" forecasting.

Revenue Growth Is Due to Pricing Rather Than Volume Changes

Earlier we emphasized that revenue growth can be due to changes in either unit volume or pricing (reimbursement). If revenue growth is a result solely of reimbursement rate changes that are not caused by inflation, then there will be no impact on some income statement items, such as labor expenses, or on some balance sheet items, such as inventories, payables, and fixed asset requirements.

Because the constant growth method ties most items and accounts directly to dollar revenues, it can give very misleading forecasts when reimbursement rate changes, which are not the result of inflation, rather of volume changes, are driving the revenue forecast.

Economies of Scale

There are economies of scale in the use of many kinds of assets, and when they occur, the asset growth rates are less than volume growth rates. For example, healthcare businesses typically need to maintain base stocks of different inventory items, even when volume levels are quite low. Then, as volume expands, inventories tend to grow less rapidly than volume, so the use of a constant growth rate would overstate the amount of inventories required.

Lumpy Assets

In many industries, technological considerations dictate that if a business is to be competitive, it must add fixed assets in large, discrete units. For example, in the hospital industry, it is usually not economically feasible to add, say, five beds, so when hospitals expand capacity, they typically do so in relatively large increments. In such a situation, when capacity volume is reached, even a small increase in volume would require a hospital to significantly increase its fixed assets, so a small projected volume increase could bring with it a very large increase in fixed asset requirements.

Suboptimal Relationships

All of the asset projections in a forecast should be based on target, or optimal, relationships between revenues and assets, and not the relationships that actually exist. For example, in 2000 Bayside had $3,177,000 in inventories. Our constant growth forecast projected inventories to be $3,526,000 in 2001. The projection assumed that the 2000 inventory level was optimal for the actual revenues realized. However, if the 2000 inventory level was suboptimal, say, too large, it might be possible to grow revenues by 11 percent with no increase in inventories at all. Conversely, if the inventory level were too small in 2000, then the actual level of inventories required in 2001 would be greater than the forecast.

 If any of the problems noted here are encountered in practice, and generally many of them are, then the simple constant growth method should not be used. Rather, other techniques must be used to forecast asset and liability levels and the resulting external financing requirement. Some of these methods are discussed in the following section.

1. Describe several conditions under which the constant growth method can give questionable results.
2. Do these conditions happen often in "real-world" forecasting?

Self-Test Questions

Real-World Forecasting

We have emphasized that the constant growth method is not used in actual forecasting situations. The overall approach of first forecasting the firm's income statement, then its balance sheet, then its external financing requirement, and so on, is used, but techniques other than constant growth are used to forecast the specific income statement items and balance sheet accounts. In this section, we discuss the four forecasting techniques that are used in practice: (1) simple linear regression, (2) curvilinear regression, (3) multiple regression, and (4) specific item forecasting.

Simple Linear Regression

Simple linear regression often is used to estimate asset requirements. To illustrate the concept, consider Bayside's inventories and total operating revenue over the last five years, which are given in the lower section of Figure 15.2, and the regression plot, which is shown in the upper section. The estimated regression equation, as found using a spreadsheet, is as follows (in thousands of dollars):

$$\text{Inventories} = \$1,459 + (0.0150 \times \text{Net operating revenue}).$$

The plotted points are quite close to the regression line. In fact, the correlation coefficient between inventories and sales is +0.99, which indicates that there is a very strong linear relationship between these two variables. Why might this be the case for Bayside? According to the EOQ model, which we will discuss in Chapter 16, inventories should increase with the square root of revenues, which would cause the regression to be nonlinear—the true regression line would rise at a decreasing rate. However, Bayside has greatly expanded its number of service lines over the last decade, and the base stocks associated with these new services have caused inventories to rise. Also, inflation has had a similar impact on both revenues and inventory levels. These three influences—(1) economies of scale in existing services, (2) base stocks for new services, and (3) inflationary effects—are offsetting, resulting in the observed linear relationship between inventories and sales.

We can use the estimated relationship between inventories and revenues to forecast the 2001 inventory level. Because 2001 net operating revenue is projected at $126,354,000, 2001 inventories should be $3,354,000:

$$\text{Inventories} = \$1,459 + (0.0150 \times \$126,354)$$

$$= \$1,459 + \$1,895 = \$3,354.$$

This is $3,526,000 − $3,354,000 = $172,000 less than our earlier forecast based on the constant growth method. The difference occurs because the constant growth method assumes that the ratio of inventories to revenues remains constant, or, in other words, the regression line passes through the

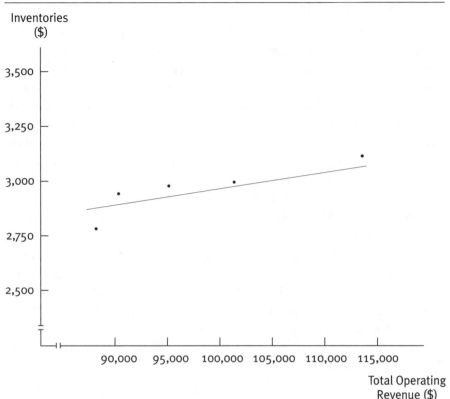

FIGURE 15.2
Bayside Memorial Hospital: Linear Regression on Inventories (thousands of dollars)

Year	Total Operating Revenue	Inventories
1996	$ 86,477	$2,752
1997	90,568	2,838
1998	95,351	2,896
1999	102,015	2,981
2000	113,832	3,177

Inventories = $1,459 + (0.0150 × Total operating revenue)

origin. But, as seen in Figure 15.2, the ratio actually declines because the inventory regression line does not pass through the origin.

We could run linear regressions on all the items on the income statement and all the accounts on the balance sheet that need to be forecasted to determine those that might be forecasted using this technique. Those items and accounts that produce a high correlation (those for which there is a strong linear relationship) may then be forecasted in this way. Then, we could use these relationships in Tables 15.3 and 15.4, in place of the constant growth rates, to create new pro forma financial statements based on linear regressions.

Curvilinear Regression

Simple linear regression is based on the assumption that a straight-line re-lationship exists between a particular variable and revenues, or some other variable. Although linear relationships between financial statement variables and revenue frequently do exist, these relationships often assume other forms. For example, if the EOQ relationship had dominated the inventory-revenue relationship, the correct plot of inventory versus revenue would be a concave curve rather than the straight line shown in Figure 15.2. If we forecasted the inventory level needed to support revenue growth using a linear relationship, our forecast would be too high.

Businesses have in their databases historical data on their own firms by divisions, by product lines, and by individual services. They also have or can easily obtain certain types of data for other firms in their industry. These data can be analyzed using computer programs based on advanced statistical techniques (1) to help determine whether a relationship is curvilinear or linear and (2) to estimate the curvilinear relationship should one exist. Once the best-fit relationship has been estimated, it can be used to project future levels of items such as inventories, given the revenue forecast.[7]

Multiple Regression

If the relationship between a variable, such as inventories, and revenues is such that the individual points are widely scattered about the regression line (and hence the correlation coefficient is low), but a curvilinear relationship does not appear to exist, then there is a good chance that other factors in addition to revenue affect the level of that variable. For example, inventory levels might be a function of both revenue level and the number of different services offered (or products sold). In this case, we would obtain the best forecast for inventory level by using multiple regression techniques, where inventories would be regressed against both revenue and the number of services offered. Then the projected inventories would be based on forecasts of number of services in addition to total revenue. Most computer installations now have complete regression software packages, which makes it easy to apply multiple and curvilinear regression techniques. One can even do multiple regression analysis with many spreadsheet programs.

Specific Item Forecasting

A final technique, and the one that is often most useful in practice, is to develop a specific model for each income statement item and balance sheet account that must be forecasted. For example, salaries could be projected using payroll records and expected salary increases; receivables could be forecasted by using the payments pattern approach; gross fixed assets could be forecasted on the basis of the firm's capital budget; and depreciation could be forecast on the basis of the firm's aggregate depreciation schedule.[8] Of course, projected volume typically remains an important element behind each of these specific item forecasts.

Specific item forecasting is especially useful when input costs and output prices are affected by different forces, and hence are expected to grow at different rates. In today's healthcare environment, this is probably the rule rather than the exception.

Comparison of Forecasting Methods

The constant growth method assumes that different financial statement variables are directly related to revenue. It is the easiest method, but often its forecasts are of questionable value. Simple linear regression differs from the constant growth method in that regression does not assume a constant relationship to revenue. This technique can improve the forecasts for many financial statement variables. Note, too, that curvilinear and multiple regression techniques can provide especially accurate forecasts when relationships either (1) are not linear or (2) depend on other variables in addition to sales. Finally, specific item forecasting that utilizes various decision models can be used.

As we move down the list of forecasting methods, accuracy may or may not increase, but costs are sure to increase. The need to employ more complicated, and consequently more costly, methods varies from situation to situation. As in all situations, the costs of using more refined techniques must be balanced against the benefits obtained. Unfortunately, there is no assurance that the use of more sophisticated forecasting methods will lead to better forecasts. Furthermore, the use of more complicated forecasting methods often hides the assumptions inherent in the forecast.

Self-Test Questions

1. Identify several techniques that can be used instead of constant growth forecasting.
2. Which techniques do you think would be the most accurate? The most costly?

Computerized Financial Planning Models

Although the types of financial forecasting described thus far in the chapter can be done with a hand calculator, even the smallest healthcare businesses now have at least a personal computer and can employ some type of computerized financial planning model. Such models can be programmed to show the effects of different volume and reimbursement rates, different relationships between volume and operating assets, and even different assumptions about reimbursement rates and input costs (labor, materials, and so forth). Plans are then made regarding how any projected external financing requirements are to be met—through short-term bank loans; selling long-term bonds; or, in the case of investor-owned firms, selling new common stock. Pro forma balance sheets, income statements, and statements of cash flows are generated under the different financing plans, and key risk and return ratios, such as the current ratio, debt/assets ratio, times-interest-earned ratio, return on assets, and return on equity, are calculated.

Depending on how these projections look, management may need to modify the base case, or initial, forecast. For example, management might conclude that the projected volume growth rate must be cut because external financing requirements exceed the firm's ability to raise money. Or management could decide to raise more funds internally, if possible. Alternatively, the firm might investigate service processes that require fewer fixed assets, or it might consider the possibility of contracting out some services rather than offering them in house.

Scenario Analysis

The most important benefit of a computerized forecasting model is that it permits managers to see the effects of changing both basic assumptions and specific financial policies. The pro forma financial statements could be rerun over and over, each time creating a new scenario that changes one or more of the basic operating assumptions inherent in the model. For example, what if there is a significant reduction in Medicare payments? What if we lose a large managed care contract to a competitor? What if we experience a nurses' strike during the coming year? What if a competitor opens a new outpatient surgery center? Changes in basic assumptions about Medicare reimbursement, labor costs, or competitors' actions have a significant effect on volume, reimbursement rates, cost relationships, profit margins, and so on. A computerized forecasting model permits managers to quickly develop forecasts to match numerous different assumptional scenarios, although the forecasts are only as good as the managers' ability to predict the impact of each scenario on key forecasting parameters.

Forecasting models also permit managers to assess the impact of changes in financial variables, such as changing the source of external financing or interest rate forecasts. It is important, however, to note (1) that managers still must interpret the results of all the forecasts and (2) that the analysis could encompass virtually hundreds of combinations of operating assumptions and financial policies, and thus hundreds of different sets of pro forma financial statements could easily be created.

One way to reduce the number of possible scenarios is to perform a sensitivity analysis to determine the effect of each assumption; assumptions that have little effect on the key financial integrity and profitability ratios need not be changed from their base case levels. Another approach to reducing the number of scenarios is to perform a Monte Carlo simulation analysis. For example, instead of specifying volume, reimbursement levels, labor costs, and so on at discrete levels, probability distributions could be specified. Then, the key results would be presented as distributions rather than as point estimates.[9]

1. Why are computerized planning models playing an increasingly important role in corporate management?

Self-Test Question

Financial Controls

Financial forecasting and planning is vital to corporate success, but planning is for naught unless the firm has a control system that both (1) ensures implementation of the planned policies and (2) provides an information feedback loop that permits rapid adjustments if the assumed market conditions change. In a financial control system, the key question is not "How is the firm doing in 2001 as compared with 2000?" Rather, it is "How is the firm doing in 2001 as compared with the forecasts, and if actual results differ from those expected, what can we do to get back on track?"

The basic tools of financial control are *budgets* and *pro forma financial statements*. These documents set forth expected performance, and hence they express management's target. These targets are then compared with actual corporate performance—on a daily, weekly, or monthly basis—to determine the *variances*, which are defined here as the difference between realized values and target values. Thus, the control system identifies those areas where performance is not meeting target levels. If a business's actuals are better than its targets, this could signify that its managers are doing a great job, but it could also mean that the targets were set too low and, thus, should be raised in the future. Conversely, failure to meet the financial targets could mean that market conditions are changing, that some managers are not performing up to par, or that the targets were set initially at unrealistic, unattainable levels. In any event, some action should be taken, and perhaps quickly if the situation is deteriorating rapidly. By focusing on variances, managers can "manage by exception," concentrating on those operations most in need of improvement and leaving alone those operations that are running smoothly.

Of course, entire textbooks have been written on financial controls, and much of the subject of financial control overlaps with managerial accounting. Here, we want only to emphasize that financial controls are as critical to financial performance as are financial planning and forecasting. We must also add that financial control systems are not costless. Thus, the control system must balance its costs against the savings it is intended to produce.

1. What are the purposes of a financial control system?
2. What are the basic financial control tools and how do they work?

Self-Test Questions

The Cash Budget

Thus far, our discussion of financial planning and forecasting has focused on projecting a business's financial statements. However, financial statements are prepared in accordance with accounting convention, and hence may not provide much information about a business's cash position. Even when a pro forma statement of cash flows is created, the information provided focuses on the end-of-year position, whereas managers need to have a feel for the business's cash position throughout the year. This situation is corrected by the *cash budget*.

To create a cash budget, managers forecast both fixed asset and inventory requirements, along with the times when such payments must be made. This information is combined with projections about the delay in collecting accounts receivable, wage payment dates, interest payment dates, and so on. All this information is then combined to show the organization's projected cash inflows and outflows over some specified period. Generally, businesses use a monthly cash budget forecasted over the next year, plus a more detailed daily or weekly cash budget for the coming month. The monthly cash budget is used for liquidity planning purposes and the daily or weekly budget for actual cash control.

Creating a cash budget does not require the application of a complex set of accounting rules. Rather, all the entries in a cash budget represent the actual movement of cash into or out of the organization. Table 15.5 contains a monthly cash budget that covers six months of 2001 for Madison Homecare, a small, for-profit home health care business. Madison's cash budget, which is broken down into four sections, is typical, although there is a great deal of variation in formats used by different organizations.

The first section of the cash budget contains the *collections worksheet*, which translates the billing for services provided into cash revenues. Because of its location in a summer resort area, Madison's patient volume, and hence billings, peak in July. However, like most health services organizations, Madison rarely collects when services are provided. What is relevant from a cash budget perspective is not when services are provided or when billings occur, but rather when cash is collected. Based on previous experience, Madison's managers know that most collections occur 30 to 60 days after billing. In fact, Madison's managers have a collections table that allows them to forecast, with some precision, the timing of collections. This table was used to convert the billings shown on Line 1 of Table 15.5 into the collection amounts shown on Lines 2 and 3.

The next section of Madison's cash budget is the *supplies worksheet*, which accounts for timing differences between when supplies are ordered and when they are paid for. Madison's patient volume forecasts, which are used to predict the billing amounts shown on Line 1, are also used to forecast the supplies (primarily medical) needed to support patient services. These supplies are ordered and received one month prior to expected usage, as shown on Line 4. However, Madison's suppliers do not demand immediate payment. Rather, Madison has, on average, 30 days to pay for supplies after they are received. Thus, the actual payment occurs one month after purchase, as shown on Line 5.

TABLE 15.5
Madison Homecare: May Through October Cash Budget

	Mar	Apr	May	Jun	Jul	Aug	Sep	Oct
Collections Worksheet:								
1. Billed charges	$50,000	$50,000	$100,000	$150,000	$200,000	$100,000	$100,000	$50,000
2. Collections:								
a. Within 30 days			19,600	29,400	39,200	19,600	19,600	9,800
b. 30–60 days			35,000	70,000	105,000	140,000	70,000	70,000
c. 60–90 days			5,000	5,000	10,000	15,000	20,000	10,000
3. Total collections			$ 59,600	$104,400	$154,200	$174,600	$109,600	$ 89,800
Supplies Worksheet:								
4. Amount of supplies ordered			$ 10,000	$ 15,000	$ 20,000	$ 10,000	$ 10,000	$ 5,000
5. Payments made for supplies			$ 10,000	$ 15,000	$ 20,000	$ 10,000	$ 10,000	$ 5,000
Net Cash Gain (Loss):								
6. Total collections (from Line 3)			$ 59,600	$104,400	$154,200	$174,600	$109,600	$ 89,800
7. Total purchases (from Line 5)			$ 10,000	$ 15,000	$ 20,000	$ 10,000	$ 10,000	$ 5,000
8. Wages and salaries			60,000	70,000	80,000	60,000	60,000	60,000
9. Rent			2,500	2,500	2,500	2,500	2,500	2,500
10. Other expenses			1,000	1,500	2,000	1,000	1,000	500
11. Taxes					20,000		20,000	
12. Payment for capital assets						50,000		
13. Total payments			$ 73,500	$109,000	$104,500	$123,500	$ 93,500	$ 68,000
14. Net cash gain (loss)			($ 13,900)	($ 4,600)	$ 49,700	$ 51,100	$ 16,100	$ 21,800
Borrowing/Surplus Summary:								
15. Cash at beginning with no borrowing			$ 15,000	$ 1,100	($ 3,500)	$ 46,200	$ 97,300	$113,400
16. Cash at end with no borrowing			$ 1,100	($ 3,500)	$ 46,200	$ 97,300	$113,400	$135,200
17. Target cash balance			10,000	10,000	10,000	10,000	10,000	10,000
18. Cumulative surplus cash (loan balance)			($ 8,900)	($ 13,500)	$ 36,200	$ 87,300	$103,400	$125,200

The next section combines data from the collections and supplies worksheets with other projected cash outflows to show the *net cash gain (loss)* for each month. Cash from collections is shown on Line 6. Lines 7 through 12 list cash payments that are expected to be made during each month, including payments for supplies. Then, all payments are summed, with the total shown on Line 13. The difference between expected cash receipts and cash payments, Line 6 minus Line 13, is the net cash gain or loss during the month, which is shown on Line 14. For May, there is a forecasted net cash outflow of $13,900, where the parentheses indicate a negative cash flow (or loss).

Although Line 14 contains the meat of the cash budget, Lines 15 through 18 (the *Borrowing/Surplus Summary*) extend the basic budget data to show Madison's forecasted cash position for each month. Line 15 shows the forecasted cash on hand at the beginning of each month, assuming that no borrowing takes place. Madison is expected to enter the budget period—the beginning of May—with $15,000 of cash on hand. For each succeeding month, Line 15 is merely the value shown on Line 16 for the previous month. The values on Line 16, which are obtained by adding Lines 14 and 15, show the cash on hand at the end of each month, assuming no borrowing takes place. For May, Madison expects a cash loss of $13,900 on top of a starting balance of $15,000, for an ending cash balance of $1,100, in the absence of any borrowing. This amount is the cash at beginning with no borrowing amount for June shown on Line 15.

To continue, note that Madison's target cash balance (i.e., the amount that it wants on hand at the beginning of each month) is $10,000, which is shown on Line 17. The target cash balance is subtracted from the forecasted ending cash with no borrowing amount to determine the firm's borrowing requirements (shown in parentheses), or surplus cash (shown without parentheses). Because Madison expects to have ending cash, as shown on Line 16, of only $1,100 in May, it will have to borrow $10,000 − $1,100 = $8,900 to bring the cash account up to the target balance of $10,000. Assuming that this amount is indeed borrowed, the total loan outstanding will be $8,900 at the end of May. (The assumption is that Madison will not have any loans outstanding on May 1 because the beginning cash balance exceeds the firm's target balance.)

The cumulative cash surplus or required loan balance is shown on Line 18; a positive value indicates a cash surplus, while a negative value indicates a loan requirement. The surplus cash or loan requirement shown on Line 18 is a **cumulative amount**. Thus, Madison is projected to borrow $8,900 in May; it has a cash shortfall during June of $4,600, as reported on Line 14, so its total loan requirement projected for the end of June is $8,900 + $4,600 = $13,500, as shown on Line 18.

The same procedures are followed in subsequent months. Patient volume and billings are projected to peak in July, accompanied by increased payments for supplies, wages, and other items. However, collections are projected to increase by a greater amount than costs, and Madison expects a $49,700 net cash inflow during July. This amount is sufficient to pay off the cumulative loan of $13,500 and have a $36,200 cash surplus on hand at the end of the month.

Patient volume, and the resulting operating costs, is expected to fall sharply in August, but collections will be the highest of any month because they will reflect the high June and July billings. As a result, Madison would normally be forecasting a healthy $101,100 net cash gain during the month. However, the firm expects to make a cash payment of $50,000 to purchase a new computer system during August, so the forecasted net cash gain is reduced to $51,100. This net gain adds to the surplus, so August is projected to end with $87,300 in surplus cash. If all goes according to the forecast, later cash surpluses will enable Madison to end this budget period with a surplus of $125,200.

The cash budget is used by Madison's managers for liquidity planning purposes. For example, the Table 15.5 cash budget indicates that Madison will need to obtain $13,500 in total to get through May and June. Thus, if the firm does not have any marketable securities to convert to cash, it will have to arrange for some type of financing to cover this period. Furthermore, the budget indicates a $125,200 cash surplus at the end of October. Madison's managers will have to consider how these funds can best be utilized. Perhaps the money should be paid out to owners as dividends or bonuses, or be used for fixed asset acquisitions, or be temporarily invested in marketable securities for later use within the business. This decision will be made on the basis of Madison's overall financial plan.

This brief illustration shows the mechanics and managerial value of the cash budget. However, before concluding this discussion of the cash budget, several additional points need to be made. First, if cash inflows and outflows are not uniform during the month, a monthly cash budget could seriously understate a business's peak financing requirements. The data in Table 15.5 show the situation expected on the last day of each month, but on any given day during the month it could be quite different. If all payments had to be made on the fifth of each month, but collections came in uniformly throughout the month, Madison would need to borrow cash to cover within-month shortages. For example, August's $123,500 of cash payments may occur before the full amount of the $174,600 in collections have been made. In this situation, some amount of cash would have to be obtained to cover shortfalls in August, even though the end-of-month cash flow after all collections have been made is positive. In this case, Madison would have to prepare a weekly or daily cash budget to indicate such borrowing needs.

Also, because the cash budget represents a forecast, all the values in the table are **expected** values. If actual patient volume, collection times, supplies purchases, wage rates, and so on, differ from forecasted levels, the projected cash deficits and surpluses will be incorrect. Thus, there is a reasonable chance that Madison may end up needing to obtain a larger amount of funds than is indicated on Line 18. Because of the uncertainty of the forecasts, spreadsheet programs are particularly well suited for constructing and analyzing cash budgets. For example, Madison's managers could change any assumption, say, projected monthly volume or the time third-party payers take to pay, and the cash budget would automatically and instantly be recalculated. This assumption would show Madison's managers exactly how the firm's cash position would change under alternative operating assumptions. Typically, such an analysis is used to determine how large a credit line to establish to cover temporary cash shortages.[10] In Madison's case, such an analysis indicated that a $20,000 line is sufficient.

Self-Test Questions

1. Considering all the information in projected financial statements, why do organizations need a cash budget?
2. Does the cash budget require an extensive knowledge of accounting principles?
3. In your view, what is the most important line of the cash budget?

Key Concepts

This chapter described in broad outline how firms forecast their financial statements, estimate their future financing requirements, and plan their cash needs. Here are its key concepts:

- The primary planning documents are *strategic plans, operating plans,* and *financial plans.*
- *Financial forecasting* generally begins with a forecast of the firm's revenues, in terms of both volume and reimbursement rates, for some future time period.
- *Pro forma,* or *projected, financial statements* are developed to estimate the firm's future financial condition and external financing requirements.
- The *constant growth method* of forecasting financial statements is based on the assumptions (1) that most income statement items and balance sheet accounts vary directly with revenues and (2) that the business's current levels of income statement items and balance sheet accounts are optimal for its current level of revenues.
- A business can determine the amount of the *external financing requirement* by estimating the amount of assets necessary to support the forecasted level of revenues and then subtracting from that amount the forecasted total claims. The business can then plan to raise the necessary funds through bank borrowing, by issuing securities, or both.
- Additional external capital means additional interest and/or dividends, which lowers the amount of forecasted retained earnings. Thus, raising external funds creates a *financing feedback* effect that must be incorporated in the forecasting process.

- Four factors have the greatest impact on the external financing requirement. (1) The higher a firm's *revenue growth rate*, the greater will be its need for external financing. (2) The greater the *capital intensity*, the greater the need for external capital. (3) The higher the *profit margin*, the lower the need. (4) Finally, the larger a for-profit business's *dividend payout*, the greater its need for external funds.
- A formula can be used to estimate a firm's *sustainable growth rate*, which is the growth rate that can be sustained without issuing new common stock.
- The constant growth method typically is inadequate to deal with real-world situations such as *nonoptimal relationships, economies of scale, excess capacity,* or *lumpy assets.*
- *Linear regression, curvilinear regression, multiple regression,* and *specific item forecasting techniques* can be used to forecast asset requirements when the constant growth method is not appropriate.
- Even the smallest businesses now use *computerized financial planning models* to forecast both their financial statements and their external financing needs.
- *Financial controls* should be an integral part of a firm's planning system.
- A *cash budget* is a forecast that shows projected cash inflows and outflows over some period. It is used to forecast cash shortages and surpluses, and hence is the primary tool for cash management purposes.

The type of forecasting described in this chapter is important for several reasons. First, if the projected operating results are unsatisfactory, management can "go back to the drawing board," reformulate its plans, and develop more reasonable targets for the coming year. Second, it is possible that the funds required to meet the forecast simply cannot be obtained; if so, it is obviously better to know this in advance and to scale back the projected level of operations than suddenly to run out of cash and have operations grind to a halt. Third, even if the required funds can be raised, it is desirable to plan for their acquisition well in advance.

Selected References

Anderson, Dave. 1985. "Impact of Strategic Financial Planning in the Health Care Industry." *Topics in Health Care Financing* (Summer): 1–6.

Armstrong, J. Scott. 1985. *Long Range Forecasting.* New York: Wiley.

Cook, Donald. 1990. "Strategic Plan Creates a Blueprint for Budgeting." *Healthcare Financial Management* (May): 21–27.

Dixon, Leslie H., and Susan K. Bossert. 1993. "The Commercial Bank as Investment Advisor for Hospital Investable Assets." *Topics in Health Care Financing* (Summer): 58–68.

Fallon, Robert P. 1991. "Not-For-Profit ≠ No Profit: Profitability Planning in Not-For-Profit Organizations." *Health Care Management Review* (Summer): 47–61.

Folger, James, C. 1989. "Integration of Strategic, Financial Plans Vital to Success." *Healthcare Financial Management* (January): 22–32.

Glenesk, Alan E. 1990. "Six Myths That Can Cloud Strategic Vision." *Healthcare Financial Management* (May): 38–43.

Green, Larry A. 1993. "Cash Management: Acceleration and Information Strategies." *Topics in Health Care Financing* (Summer): 44–57.

Kelly, Vincent K. 1993. "Banks As a Source of Capital." *Topics in Health Care Financing* (Summer): 21–34.

Makridakis, Spyros and Steven C. Wheelwright. 1983. *Forecasting Methods for Management.* New York: Wiley.

Nyp, Randall G., and Ingo Angermeier. 1990. "Financial Plan Charts a Hospital's Course for Success." *Healthcare Financial Management* (May): 30–36.

Scarborough, Sydney P. 1993. "Establishing Banking Relationships." *Topics in Health Care Financing* (Summer): 69–79.

Schmitz, Vincent, Guy M. Masters, and Walter Dilts. 1989. "Better Forecasting Ensures Profitability, Quality of Care." *Healthcare Financial Management* (January): 60–66.

Thomas, L. Murray and Richard R. Johnson. 1988. "Financial Modeling: Creating a Plan for the Future." *Healthcare Financial Management* (February): 70–78.

Selected Web Sites

There are two web sites maintained by professional organizations dedicated to forecasting. For the Institute of Business Forecasting (IBF), see *www.ibforecast.com*; and for the International Institute of Forecasters (IIF), see *forecasting.cwru.edu*.

The site listed below provides a great deal of information on forecasting, see *hops.wharton.upenn.edu/forecast*.

Selected Cases

There are two cases in *Cases in Healthcare Finance* that are applicable to this chapter:

Case 8: Park City Clinic, which examines the preparation and use of a cash budget.

Case 25: Gateway Community Hospital (B), which focuses on the creation of pro forma financial statements in a hospital setting. Note that this case is best used as a follow-on to Case 1.

Notes

1. In a log-linear regression, the operating revenue amounts are converted to natural logarithms and regressed against time. The slope coefficient of the regression line, which is $0.0669 = 6.69\%$ in this case, is the *continuous* growth rate over the five-year period. The continuous growth rate is converted to a *compound annual* growth rate as follows:

$$e^{0.0669} - 1 \approx 6.9\%.$$

2. This assumption does not imply that Bayside's 2000 occupancy rate was 100 percent. A hospital is operating at full capacity when its average occupancy is somewhere around 80 to 90 percent. A few times during the year, a hospital may operate at 100 percent capacity, but most hospital managers prefer to maintain a reserve capacity to meet emergency situations.

3. We generated the forecast with a spreadsheet model, so some of the amounts shown on the financial statements may be different from those obtained by a calculator.

4. Some assets, such as short-term investments, clearly are not tied directly to operations, and hence would not vary directly with revenues. In fact, Bayside could reduce its short-term investments to zero, thereby reducing any external funding requirements. However, the naïve methodology applied here assumes that almost all balance sheet accounts would automatically increase with revenues.

5. Most managers believe that dividend cuts have a severe negative impact on stock price, and this belief is generally supported by empirical testing. For a complete discussion of dividend policy, see Chapter 17.

6. For a more complete discussion of sustainable growth, see Robert C. Higgins, "How Much Growth Can a Firm Afford?" *Financial Management*, Fall 1977, 7–16.

7. Often, a plot of the data will suggest a nonlinear relationship. The data—inventories in this case—can then be converted to logarithms if it appears that the regression points slope down, or raised to a power if the slope of the points seems to be increasing. The graphics capabilities of spreadsheets can be used to identify nonlinear relationships.

8. We will discuss the payments pattern approach to receivables management in Chapter 16.

9. This is a good time to mention the basic axiom of computer modeling: GIGO, which means "garbage in, garbage out." Stated another way, the output of a financial model is no better than the assumptions and other inputs used to construct it. So when you build models, proceed with caution. Note, though, that one advantage of computer modeling is that it does bring the key assumptions out into the open, where their realism can be examined. One strong advocate of models made this statement: "Critics of our models generally attack our assumptions, but they forget that in their own forecasts, they simply assume the answer."

10. A *credit line* is an agreement between a borrower and a financial institution that obligates the institution to furnish credit over a time period, typically a year, up to the agreed-upon amount. The borrower may use some, all, or none of the credit line. Usually, credit lines require borrowers to pay an upfront fee for the credit guarantee called a *commitment fee*.

Other Topics

WORKING CAPITAL MANAGEMENT

Learning Objectives

After studying this chapter, readers should be able to:

• Discuss in general terms how businesses manage cash and marketable securities.
• Discuss the key elements of receivables and inventory management.
• Explain the role of accruals in a business's financing mix.
• Measure the cost-of-trade credit and determine when costly trade credit is preferable to other short-term debt sources.

Introduction

In the discussion of healthcare financial management leading up to this chapter, the general focus has been on long-term, strategic decisions. Another important element of healthcare finance involves the management of short-term (current) assets, which is commonly called *working capital management.* The term "working capital" originated in the early years in the United States when Yankee peddlers were the main source of goods for many farmers in remote areas of the Northeast. These merchants would load up their wagons with goods and then set off on a regular route to peddle their wares. Following the economic definitions of capital (assets) versus labor, the peddler's horse and wagon constituted the business's fixed capital, while the merchandise was called "working capital" because it was what was sold, or turned over, to produce a profit.

How important is working capital management? The average hospital has almost 10 percent of its assets in cash and short-term investments (marketable securities) plus almost 15 percent in accounts receivable. In addition, not-for-profit hospitals have another 20 percent of assets invested in *funded depreciation,* which is depreciation cash flow that is being accumulated on the balance sheet to purchase fixed assets when current plant needs to be replaced. Thus, hospitals, on average, have close to half of their assets invested in accounts that require management techniques discussed in this chapter. In addition to the management of short-term assets, this chapter also covers accruals and trade credit. Although these are sources of short-term debt financing as opposed to assets, accruals and trade credit typically are considered to be part of working capital management.

In general, the goal of working capital management is to support the operations of the business at the lowest possible cost. However, the implementation of working capital management principles is very dependent on the size and nature of the healthcare business. For example, working capital management within a large hospital differs significantly from that within a small home health agency. Thus, this chapter focuses on basic concepts only—the implementation details for different healthcare businesses must be learned in a more specialized setting.

Cash Management

All businesses need *cash*, which includes both actual cash and funds held in commercial checking accounts, to pay for labor, materials, and supplies; to buy fixed assets; to pay taxes; to service debt; and so on. However, cash earns no return, and hence is classified as a *nonearning asset*. In spite of the fact that cash itself earns no return, every dollar on the asset side of the balance sheet, including dollars of cash, must be financed; that is, there must be a corresponding dollar on the liabilities and equity side of the balance sheet. Because each dollar of financing has either a direct or an indirect (opportunity) cost, the goal of cash management is to minimize the amount of cash the business must hold to conduct its normal activities, but at the same time, have sufficient cash on hand to support operations.

Cash Management Techniques

A key element in a business's cash management process is the cash budget, which is discussed in Chapter 15. In essence, the cash budget tells managers how effective they are in applying the cash management techniques discussed in the following sections.[1]

Cash Flow Synchronization If an individual received income once a year, he or she would probably put it in the bank, draw down the account during the year as cash is needed, and have an average balance over the year equal to about half the annual income. If the individual received income monthly instead of once a year, he or she would operate similarly, but the average balance would be much smaller. If the individual could arrange to receive income daily and to pay for rent, food, and other charges on a daily basis, and further was quite confident of the forecasted inflows and outflows, he or she could, at least in theory, hold a zero cash balance.

Exactly the same situation applies to businesses. By improving cash flow forecasts and by taking steps to match cash receipts with required cash outflows, businesses can reduce their cash balances to a minimum. Recognizing this point, some firms bill customers on a regular billing cycle throughout the month that matches their own outflows. This improves the *synchronization of cash flows,* which in turn enables a business to reduce its cash balances, decrease its bank loans, lower interest expenses, and boost profits.

Float is defined as the difference between the balance shown on a business's or individual's checkbook and the balance shown on the bank's records. Suppose that a business writes, on the average, checks in the amount of $5,000 each day, and it takes six days for these checks to clear and to be deducted from the business's bank account. This will cause the business's own checkbook to show a balance that is $6 \times \$5,000 = \$30,000$ smaller than the balance on the bank's records. This difference is called *disbursement float*.

Managing Float

Suppose that the business also receives checks in the amount of $5,000 daily, but it loses four days while they are being deposited and cleared. This difference will result in $4 \times \$5,000 = \$20,000$ of *collections float*. In total, the business's *net float*—the difference between the $30,000 disbursement float and the $20,000 collections float—will be $10,000.

If the business's own collection and clearing process is more efficient than that of the recipients of its checks, which is generally true of more-efficient businesses, the business could actually show a negative balance on its own books, but have a positive balance on the records of its bank. Some businesses that are good at managing float indicate that they *never* have positive book cash balances. In fact, one medical equipment manufacturer stated that its bank's records show an average cash balance of about $200,000, while its own *book* balance is *minus* $200,000—it has $400,000 of net float. Obviously the firm must be able to forecast its disbursements and collections accurately to make such heavy use of float.

Basically, a firm's net float is a function of its ability to speed up collections on checks received and to slow down collections on checks written. Efficient businesses go to great lengths to speed up the processing of incoming checks, thus putting the funds to work faster, and they try to stretch their own payments out as long as possible, without engaging in unethical or illegal practices.

Managers have searched for ways to collect receivables faster since the day that credit transactions began. Although cash collection is the responsibility of a firm's managers, the speed with which checks are cleared is dependent on the banking system. Several techniques are now used both to speed collections and to get funds where they are needed, but the three most popular are lockbox services, concentration banking, and electronic claims processing. Here are some points to note about lockbox services and concentration banking. The discussion of electronic claims processing occurs later in this chapter.

Acceleration of Receipts

Lockboxes are one of the oldest cash management tools, and virtually all banks that offer cash management services also offer lockbox services. In a lockbox system, incoming checks are sent to post office boxes rather than to corporate headquarters. For example, Health SouthWest, a regional HMO headquartered in Oklahoma City, has its Texas members send their payments to a box in Dallas, its New Mexico members send their checks to Albuquerque, and so on, rather than have all checks sent to Oklahoma City. Several times a day, a local bank collects the contents of each lockbox and deposits the checks into the firm's local account. The bank then provides the HMO with daily records of the receipts collected, usually by electronic data transmission, in a format that permits online updating of the firm's receivables accounts.

A lockbox system reduces the time required for a business to receive incoming checks, to deposit them, and to get them cleared through the banking system so that the funds are available for use more quickly. This time reduction occurs because mail time and check collection time are both reduced if the lockbox is located in the geographic area where the customer (check writer) is located. Lockbox services can often increase the availability of funds by one to four days over the regular system for businesses with customers over a large geographical area.

Lockbox systems, although efficient in speeding up collections, result in the business's cash being spread around among many banks. The primary purpose of *concentration banking* is to mobilize funds from decentralized receiving locations, whether they are lockboxes or decentralized firm locations, into one or more central cash pools. In a typical concentration system, the firm's collection banks record deposits received each day. Based on disbursement needs, the funds are then transferred from these collection points to a concentration bank. Concentration accounts allow businesses to take maximum advantage of economies of scale in cash management and investment. Health SouthWest uses an Oklahoma City bank as its concentration bank. The HMO cash manager then uses this pool for short-term investing or reallocation among its other banks.

One of the keys to concentration banking is the ability to quickly transfer funds from collecting banks to concentration banks, and electronic systems make such transfers easy. *Automated clearinghouses* are communications networks that provide a means of sending data from one financial institution to another. Instead of using paper checks, computer files are created, and all entries for a particular bank are placed on a single file that is sent to that bank. Some banks send and receive their data on tapes, while others have direct computer links to the clearinghouse. In addition to automated clearinghouses, the *Federal Reserve wire system* can be used for cash concentration or for other cash transfers. This system is used to move large sums that occur on a sporadic basis, such as would occur if Health SouthWest borrowed $10 million in the commercial paper market.

Disbursement Control

Accelerated collections represent one side of using float, and controlling funds outflows is the flip side of the coin. Efficient cash management can only result if both inflows and outflows are effectively managed.

No single action controls disbursements more effectively than *payables centralization*. This permits the firm's managers to evaluate the payments coming due for the entire firm and to schedule cash transfers to meet these needs on an organization-wide basis. Centralized disbursement also permits more efficient monitoring of payables and float balances. However, centralized disbursement can have a downside—centralized offices may not be able to make prompt payment for services rendered, which can create ill will with suppliers.

Zero-balance accounts (ZBAs) are special disbursement accounts that have a zero-dollar balance on which checks are written. Typically, a firm establishes several ZBAs in the concentration bank and funds them from a *master account.* As checks are presented to a ZBA for payment, funds are automatically transferred from the master account. If the master account goes negative, it is replenished by borrowing from the bank against a line of credit or by selling some securities from the firm's marketable securities portfolio. Zero-balance accounts simplify the control of disbursements and cash balances, and hence reduce the amount of idle (i.e., noninterest-bearing) cash.

Whereas zero-balance accounts are typically established at concentration banks, *controlled disbursement accounts* can be set up at any bank. In fact, controlled disbursement accounts were initially used only in relatively remote banks, so this technique was originally called *remote disbursement.* The basic technique is simple: Controlled disbursement accounts are not funded until the day's checks are presented against the account. The key to controlled disbursement is the ability of the bank that has the account to report the total amount of checks received for clearance each day by 11 a.m., Eastern Standard Time. This early notification gives a firm's managers sufficient time to wire funds to the controlled disbursement account to cover the checks presented for payment, and to invest excess cash at midday, when money market trading is at a peak.

Matching the Costs and Benefits of Cash Management

Although a number of techniques have been discussed to reduce cash balance requirements, implementing these procedures is not a costless operation. How far should a business go in making its cash operations more efficient? As a general rule, a business should incur these expenses only so long as the marginal returns exceed the marginal costs.

The value of careful cash management depends on the opportunity costs of funds invested in cash, which in turn depends on the current rate of interest. For example, in the early 1980s, with interest rates at relatively high levels, businesses were devoting a great deal of care to cash management. Today, with interest rates much lower, the value of cash management is reduced. Clearly, larger businesses, with larger cash balances, can better afford to hire the personnel necessary to maintain tight control over their cash positions. Cash management is one element of business operations in which economies of scale are present. Banks also have placed considerable emphasis on developing and marketing cash management services. Because of scale economies in cash management operations, smaller businesses generally find bank-supplied services to be less costly than operating in-house cash management systems.

1. What is float?
2. How do businesses use float to increase cash management efficiency?
3. What are some methods that businesses can use to accelerate receipts?
4. What are some methods that businesses can use to control disbursements?
5. How should cash management actions be evaluated?

Marketable Securities Management

Many businesses hold large portfolios of temporary financial investments historically called *marketable securities.* On the balance sheet, such securities often are labeled *short-term investments.* Typically, such investments are held as a substitute for cash balances. Thus, although discussed in separate sections, cash and marketable securities management cannot be separated in practice because management of one implies management of the other. In addition to marketable securities, which are held to meet short-term needs, many providers also hold portfolios of securities that will be used for long-term as opposed to short-term purposes. These portfolios will be discussed in the next major section.

Specific Rationales for Holding Marketable Securities

Most businesses hold portfolios of marketable securities in lieu of larger cash balances. Then, part of the portfolio is liquidated periodically to increase the cash account when cash outflows exceed inflows. In addition, most businesses also rely on bank credit lines to meet unforeseen needs, but they may still hold some marketable securities to guard against a possible shortage of bank credit. Of course, the motivation to hold marketable securities instead of cash is the ability to convert a nonearning asset into an earning asset. Even if the yield on marketable securities is low, it is clearly more than the yield on cash.

In addition to holding marketable securities as a substitute for cash, they are also used to accumulate funds to meet large payments that are anticipated to occur in the near term. Thus, funds might be accumulated in marketable securities to pay for an expected liability settlement or to make a tax payment that is coming due. The key here is that marketable securities are carried to either account for uncertainty in cash flows or to fund a known short-term need.

Criteria for Selecting Marketable Securities

In general, the key characteristics sought in marketable securities investments are safety and liquidity. Thus, most healthcare managers are willing to give up some return to ensure that funds are available, in the amounts expected, when needed.

Large businesses, with large amounts of surplus cash, often directly own Treasury bills, commercial paper, negotiable certificates of deposit, and even Euromarket securities (i.e., dollar denominated loans held outside the United

States). Such securities, which are highly liquid and free of interest rate and default risk are known as *cash equivalents*. In addition, large taxable firms often hold floating rate preferred stock because of its 70 percent dividend exclusion from federal income taxes. Conversely, smaller businesses are more likely to invest with a bank or with a money market or preferred stock mutual fund because a small business's volume of investment simply does not warrant hiring specialists to manage its marketable securities portfolio. Small businesses often use a mutual fund and then literally write checks on the fund to bolster the cash account as the need arises.[2] Interest rates on mutual funds are somewhat lower than rates on direct investments of equivalent risk because of management fees. However, for smaller firms, net returns may well be higher on mutual funds because no in-house management expense is required.

To illustrate a typical investment mix of marketable securities, note that the average hospital marketable securities portfolio consists of 3 percent domestic stocks, 9 percent bonds, and 88 percent cash equivalents. Clearly, hospital managers are willing to sacrifice return for safety when securities are chosen for short-term purposes.

1. Why do businesses hold marketable securities portfolios?
2. What are some securities that are commonly held as marketable securities?
3. Why are these the securities of choice?

Self-Test Questions

Long-Term Securities Management

Not-for-profit providers, and hospitals in particular, often have large portfolios of long-term security holdings, which is something that is not common in other industries. These holdings are listed on the balance sheet as *long-term investments*. The reasons that not-for-profit hospitals typically carry large amounts of long-term securities are:

- Not-for-profit hospitals often set aside funds for future fixed asset replacement rather than acquire the funds at time of replacement. Because the funds for this purpose generally stem from depreciation-generated cash flow, as opposed to net income, such a portfolio is called the *funded depreciation* portfolio.
- Many hospitals self-insure at least part of their professional liability exposure, and hence establish an investment pool to meet actuarial needs.
- Many hospitals have defined benefit pension plans, which require a firm-sponsored pension fund.
- Not-for-profit hospitals receive endowment gifts that must be managed over time.

The selection of securities for long-term investment portfolios obviously is quite different from those selected for marketable securities portfolios. With time now on their side, managers are more willing to take risks to gain a return edge. For example, the typical hospital's funded depreciation account (portfolio) consists of 29 percent domestic stocks, 46 percent bonds, 23 percent cash equivalents, and 2 percent international stocks. Furthermore, the typical endowment fund consists of 46 percent domestic stock, 38 percent bonds, 13 percent cash equivalents, and 3 percent international stocks. It is clear that hospital managers, and especially managers at large hospitals and hospital systems with large amounts of money to invest, are willing to create riskier portfolios in the search for higher returns. The 1990s were good to those businesses that held higher risk portfolios, but there is no assurance that every decade will be as kind. Still, with time on the side of long-term investment portfolios, a series of years with below-average results can still be salvaged by a few years with above-average performance.

Self-Test Questions

1. Why do businesses, mostly not-for-profit hospitals, hold long-term investment portfolios?
2. Why do the securities held differ from those held in marketable securities portfolios?

Receivables Management

Generally, businesses would rather sell for cash than on credit, but competitive pressures force most firms to offer credit. The problem is most acute in the health services industry where the third-party-payment system forces providers to extend credit to most patients. In a credit sale, goods are shipped or services are provided, revenues are booked, and an account receivable is created. Eventually, the customer or third-party payer will pay the account, at which time the business will receive cash and its receivables will decline.

The Accumulation of Receivables

The total amount of accounts receivable outstanding at any given time is determined by two factors: (1) the volume of credit sales and (2) the average length of time between sales and collections. For example, suppose Home Infusion, Inc., a home health care business, begins operations on January 1, and on the first day starts to provide services to patients billed at $1,000 each day. For simplicity, assume that all patients have the same insurance, that it takes Home Infusion two days to submit patients' bills, and it takes the insurer another 18 days to make the payments. Thus, it takes 20 days from delivery of service to receipt of payment.

At the end of the first day, Home Infusion's accounts receivable will be $1,000; they will rise to $2,000 by the end of the second day; and by January 20, they will have risen to $20,000. On January 21, another $1,000 will be added to receivables, but, assuming that the insurer pays the full amount for services provided 20 days earlier, payments for services provided on January 1 will reduce receivables by $1,000, so total accounts receivable will remain constant at $20,000. If either the volume of credit sales or the collection period changes, such changes will be reflected in the amount of receivables.

What is the cost implication of carrying $20,000 in receivables? The $20,000 on the left side of the balance sheet must be financed by a like amount on the right side. Home Infusion uses a bank loan to finance its receivables, which has an interest rate of 12 percent. Thus, over a year, the firm must pay the bank $0.12 \times \$20,000 = \$2,400$ in interest to carry its receivables balance. The cost associated with carrying other current assets can be thought of in a similar way.[3]

Monitoring the Receivables Position

If a sale is made for cash, the profit is definitely earned, but if the sale is on credit, the profit is not actually earned until the account is collected. If the account is never collected, the profit is never earned. Thus, healthcare managers must monitor receivables to ensure that they are being collected in a timely manner and to uncover any deterioration in the "quality" of receivables. Early detection can help managers take corrective action before the situation has a significant negative impact on the organization's financial condition.

Suppose Adolph Weiss & Sons, a manufacturer of surgical instruments, manufactures and sells 200,000 instruments a year at an average sales price of $198 each. Furthermore, assume that all sales are on credit, with terms of 2/10, net 30, which means that customers must pay within 30 days, but they receive a 2 percent discount if they pay within 10 days. Finally, assume that 70 percent of the firm's customers take discounts and pay on Day 10, while the other 30 percent pay on Day 30.

Average Collection Period (ACP)

Weiss's *average collection period (ACP)*, often called *days sales outstanding (DSO)* or *days in receivables*, is 16 days:

$$\text{ACP} = (0.7 \times 10 \text{ days}) + (0.3 \times 30 \text{ days}) = 16 \text{ days}.$$

Weiss's *average daily sales (ADS)*, assuming a 360-day year, is $110,000:

$$\text{ADS} = \frac{\text{Annual sales}}{360} = \frac{\text{Units sold} \times \text{Sales price}}{360} = \frac{200,000 \times \$198}{360}$$

$$= \frac{\$39,600,000}{360} = \$110,000.$$

If the firm had made cash as well as credit sales, the analysis would focus on credit sales only, and the calculated amount would have been average daily *credit* sales.

Weiss's accounts receivable, assuming a constant, uniform rate of sales during the year, will at any point in time be $1,760,000.[4]

$$\text{Receivables balance} = \text{ADS} \times \text{ACP}$$

$$= \$110,000 \times 16 = \$1,760,000.$$

The ACP is a measure of the average length of time it takes Weiss's customers to pay off their credit purchases, and the ACP is often compared to the industry average ACP. For example, if all surgical instrument manufacturers sell on the same credit terms, and if the industry average ACP is 25 days versus Weiss's 16-day ACP, then Weiss either has a higher percentage of discount customers or else its credit department is exceptionally good at ensuring prompt payment.

The ACP can also be compared with the firm's own credit terms. For example, suppose Weiss's ACP had been running at a level of 35 days versus its 2/10, net 30 credit terms. With a 35-day ACP, some customers would obviously be taking more than 30 days to pay their bills. In fact, if some customers were paying within ten days to take advantage of the discount, the others would, on average, have to be taking much longer than 35 days. One way to check this possibility is to use an aging schedule.

Aging Schedules An *aging schedule* breaks down a firm's receivables by age of account. Table 16.1 contains the December 31, 2000, aging schedules of two surgical instrument manufacturers—Weiss and Cutright. Both firms offer the same credit terms, 2/10, net 30, and both show the same total receivables balance. However, Weiss's aging schedule indicates that all of its customers pay on time: 70 percent pay on Day 10, while 30 percent pay on Day 30. Cutright's schedule, which is more typical, shows that many of its customers are not abiding by its credit terms: 27 percent of its receivables are more than 30 days past due, even though Cutright's credit terms call for full payment by Day 30.

Aging schedules cannot be constructed from the type of summary data that are reported in a business's financial statements, they must be

TABLE 16.1
Aging Schedules for Two Firms

Age of Account (Days)	Weiss		Cutright	
	Value of Account	Percentage of Total Value	Value of Account	Percentage of Total Value
0–10	$1,232,000	70%	$ 825,000	47%
11–30	528,000	30	460,000	26
31–45	0	0	265,000	15
46–60	0	0	179,000	10
Over 60	0	0	31,000	2
Total	$1,760,000	100%	$1,760,000	100%

developed from the accounts receivable ledger. However, well-run businesses have computerized accounts receivable records. Thus, it is easy to determine the age of each invoice, sort electronically by age categories, and thus generate an aging schedule.

The primary point in analyzing the aggregate accounts receivable situation **The Payments** is to see if payers are slowing down their payments. If so, the firm will have **Pattern** to increase its receivables financing, which will increase its cost of carrying **Approach** receivables. Furthermore, the payment slowdown may signal an increase in bad debt losses down the road. The ACP and aging schedule are useful in monitoring credit operations, but both are affected by increases and decreases in a firm's level of sales. Thus, changes in sales levels, including normal seasonal or cyclical changes, can change a firm's ACP and aging schedule even though its customers' payment behavior has not changed at all. For this reason, a procedure called the *payments pattern approach* has been developed to measure any changes that might be occurring in customers' payment behavior.

To illustrate the payments pattern approach, consider the credit sales of Hanover Pharmaceutical Company, a small drug manufacturer that commenced operations in January 2000. Table 16.2 contains Hanover's credit sales and receivables data for 2000. Column 2 shows that Hanover's credit sales are seasonal, with the lowest sales in the fall and winter months and the highest sales during the summer.

Now, assume that 10 percent of Hanover's customers pay in the same month that the sale is made, that 30 percent pay in the first month following the sale, that 40 percent pay in the second month, and that the remaining 20 percent pay in the third month. Furthermore, assume that Hanover's customers have the same payment behavior throughout the year—that is, they always take the same length of time to pay. On the basis of this payment pattern, Column 3 of Table 16.2 contains Hanover's receivables balance at the end of each month. For example, during January, Hanover has $60,000 in sales. Ten percent of the customers paid during the month of sale, so the receivables balance at the end of January was $60,000 - (0.1 \times \$60,000) = (1.0 - 0.1) \times \$60,000 = 0.9 \times \$60,000 = \$54,000$. By the end of February, 10% + 30% = 40% of the customers had paid for January's sales, and 10 percent had paid for February's sales. Thus, the receivables balance at the end of February was $(0.6 \times \$60,000) + (0.9 \times \$60,000) = \$90,000$. By the end of March, 80 percent of January's sales had been paid, 40 percent of February's had been paid, and 10 percent of March's had been paid, so the receivables balance was $(0.2 \times \$60,000) + (0.6 \times \$60,000) + (0.9 \times \$60,000) = \$102,000$; and so on.

Columns 4 and 5 give Hanover's average daily sales (ADS) and average collection period (ACP) respectively, as these measures would be calculated from quarterly statements. For example, in the April–June quarter, ADS = ($60,000 + $90,000 + $120,000) / 90 = $3,000, and the end-of-quarter

TABLE 16.2

Hanover Pharmaceutical Company: Receivables Data (thousands of dollars)

Month (1)	Credit Sales (2)	Receivables (3)	Quarterly ADS (4)	Quarterly ACP (5)	Year to Date ADS (6)	Year to Date ACP (7)
January	$ 60	$ 54				
February	60	90				
March	60	102	$2.00	51	$2.00	51
April	60	102				
May	90	129				
June	120	174	3.00	58	2.50	70
July	120	198				
August	90	177				
September	60	132	3.00	44	2.67	49
October	60	108				
November	60	102				
December	60	102	2.00	51	2.50	41

Notes: (a) ADS = Average daily sales.
(b) ACP = Average collection period (in days).

(June 30) ACP = $174,000 / $3,000 = 58 days. Columns 6 and 7 also show ADS and ACP, but, here, they are calculated on the basis of accumulated sales throughout the year. For example, at the end of June, ADS = $450,000 / 180 = $2,500 and ACP = $174,000 / $2,500 = 70 days. (For the entire year, sales are $900,000, ADS = $2,500, and ACP at year-end = 41 days. These last two figures are shown in the lower right corner of the table.)

The data in Table 16.2 illustrate two major points. First, when the level of sales changes, the ACP changes, which suggests that customers are paying faster or slower, even though we know that customers' payment patterns are actually not changing at all. The rising monthly sales trend causes the calculated ACP to rise, whereas falling sales (as in the third quarter) cause the calculated ACP to fall, even though customers' payment patterns are actually not changing. Second, we see that the ACP depends on an averaging procedure, but regardless of whether quarterly, semiannual, or annual data are used, the ACP is still unstable even though payment patterns are not changing. Therefore, it is difficult to use the ACP as a monitoring device if the firm's sales exhibit seasonal or cyclical patterns.

Seasonal or cyclical variations also make it difficult to interpret aging schedules. Table 16.3 contains Hanover's aging schedules at the end of each quarter of 2000. At the end of June, Table 16.2 shows that Hanover's receivables balance was $174,000. Eighty percent of April's $60,000 of sales had been collected, 40 percent of May's $90,000 of sales had been collected,

TABLE 16.3

Hanover Pharmaceutical Company: Aging Schedules (thousands of dollars)

Age of Account (Days)	Value and Percentage of Value at the End of Each Quarter							
	March 31		June 30		September 30		December 31	
0–30	$ 54	53%	$108	47%	$ 54	41%	$ 54	53%
31–60	36	35	54	31	54	41	36	35
61–90	12	12	12	7	24	18	12	12
Total	$102	100%	$174	100%	$132	100%	$102	100%

and 10 percent of June's $120,000 of sales had been collected. Thus, the end-of-June receivables balance consisted of 0.2 × $60,000 = $12,000 of April sales, 0.6 × $90,000 = $54,000 of May sales, and 0.9 × $120,000 = $108,000 of June sales. Note again that Hanover's customers had not changed their payment patterns. However, rising sales during the second quarter created the impression of faster payments when judged by an aging schedule, and falling sales after July created the opposite appearance. Thus, neither the ACP nor the aging schedule provides managers with an accurate picture of customers' payment patterns if sales fluctuate during the year or if they are trending up or down.

With this background, we can now examine the *uncollected balances schedule*, which is shown in Table 16.4. At the end of each quarter, the dollar amount of receivables remaining from each of the three month's sales is divided by that month's sales to obtain three receivables-to-sales ratios. For example, at the end of the first quarter, $12,000 of the $60,000 January sales, or 20 percent, are still outstanding; 60 percent of February sales are still out; and 90 percent of March sales are uncollected. Exactly the same situation is revealed at the end of each of the next three quarters. Thus, Table 16.4 shows that the payments pattern of Hanover's customers has remained constant.

Recall that at the beginning of the example, we assumed the existence of a constant payments pattern. In a normal situation, the payments pattern would probably vary somewhat over time. Such variations would be shown in the last column of the uncollected balances schedule. For example, suppose customers began, in the second quarter, to pay their accounts slower. That payment might cause the second quarter uncollected balances schedule to look like this (in thousands of dollars):

Quarter and Month	Sales	Remaining Receivables	Receivables/Sales Ratio
Quarter 2			
April	$ 60	$ 16	27%
May	90	70	78
June	120	110	92
		$196	197%

TABLE 16.4
Hanover
Pharmaceutical
Company:
Uncollected
Balances
Schedule
(thousands of
dollars)

Quarter and Month	Sales	Remaining Receivables	Receivables/Sales Ratio
Quarter 1			
January	$ 60	$ 12	20%
February	60	36	60
March	60	54	90
		$102	170%
Quarter 2			
April	$ 60	$ 12	20%
May	90	54	60
June	120	108	90
		$174	170%
Quarter 3			
July	$120	$ 24	20%
August	90	54	60
September	60	54	90
		$132	170%
Quarter 4			
October	$ 60	$ 12	20%
November	60	36	60
December	60	54	90
		$102	170%

We see that the receivables-to-sales ratios are now higher than in the corresponding months of the first quarter. This increase causes the total uncollected balances percentage to rise from 170 to 197 percent, which in turn should alert Hanover's managers that customers are paying slower than they did earlier in the year.

The uncollected balances schedule permits a business to monitor its receivables better, and it can also be used to forecast future receivables balances. When Hanover's pro forma 2001 quarterly balance sheets are constructed, management can use the receivables-to-sales ratios, coupled with the 2001 sales estimates, to project each quarter's receivables balance using the historical payments pattern from 2000. For example, Hanover's projected end-of-June 2001 receivables balance might be forecasted as follows:[5]

Projected Quarter 2	Projected Sales	Receivables/Sales Ratio	Projected Receivables
April	$ 70,000	20%	$ 14,000
May	100,000	60	60,000
June	140,000	90	126,000
		Total projected receivables =	$200,000

The payments pattern approach permits managers to remove the effects of seasonal and/or cyclical sales variation and to construct an accurate measure of customers' payments patterns. Thus, it provides financial managers with better aggregate information than such crude measures as the average collection period or aging schedule.

Unique Problems Faced by Healthcare Providers

Although the general principles of receivables management discussed up to this point are applicable to all businesses, healthcare providers face some unique problems. The most obvious problem is the complexities in billing created by the third-party-payer system. For example, rather than having to deal with a single billing system that applies to all customers, providers have to deal with the rules and regulations of many different governmental and private insurers using different payment methodologies. Thus, providers have to maintain large staffs of specialists that operate under the firm's *patient accounts manager.*

To illustrate the problem, consider Table 16.5, which contains the receivables mix for the hospital industry. There are multiple payers within many of the categories listed in the table, so the actual number of different payers can easily run into the hundreds or thousands.

Table 16.6 provides information on how long it takes hospitals to collect receivables. Because of the large number of payers, and the complexities involved with billing and follow-up actions, which lead to high error rates, hospitals clearly have a great deal of difficulty in collecting bills in a timely manner. On average, collecting a receivable takes 62.8 days. However, this number has decreased in recent years as hospital managers have become increasingly aware of the costs associated with carrying receivables, and as automated systems have made the collections process more efficient. In spite of the positive trend, 24.9 percent of receivables still were over 90 days old. In addition, 5.2 percent of patient bills were never paid at all, with 3.4 percent being charged off as bad debt losses, and 1.8 percent going to charity care.

TABLE 16.5 Hospital Industry's Receivables Mix

Payer	Percentage of Total Accounts Receivable
Medicare	30.2%
Commercial insurers	19.5
Medicaid	14.0
Self-pay	13.4
HMO/PPO	9.7
Blue Cross	8.1
CHAMPUS	5.1
	100.0%

Source: Zimmerman Associates, *Hospital Accounts Receivable Analysis (HARA),* published quarterly.

TABLE 16.6
Hospital
Industry's
Collection
Performance

Aggregate Aging Schedule

Age of Account (Days)	Percentage of Total Accounts Receivable
0–30	42.5%
31–60	21.4
61–90	11.2
91–120	7.8
Over 120	17.1
	100.0%

Days in Patient Accounts Receivable

Percentile Values	Average Collection Period (Days)
10th	43.9 days
25th	52.7
Median	62.8
75th	73.6
90th	87.9

Sources: Zimmerman Associates, *Hospital Accounts Receivable Analysis (HARA)*, published quarterly.
Center for Healthcare Industry Performance Studies, *1998–99 Almanac of Hospital Financial and Operating Indicators.*

One development of note in provider collections is the movement toward electronic claims processing. In the early 1990s, new standards were promulgated for the *electronic data interchange (EDI)* of healthcare claims that facilitate widespread adoption of electronic claims processing and payment systems over time. In such a system, claims information is electronically transmitted over telephone lines in a standard format that can be processed by receiving firms without human intervention. Because the health services reimbursement system is paper intensive, mountains of paper claims are currently produced, which lead to high error rates and numerous delays. Although Medicare intermediaries, as well as other third-party payers, are currently passing information to providers on magnetic tape, these systems tend to be payer-unique and require providers to have relatively sophisticated computer systems.[6]

To help providers collect in a timely fashion from managed care plans, many states have enacted laws that mandate "prompt" payment. For example, New York State requires that all undisputed claims by providers be paid by plans within 45 days of receipt. If prompt payment is not made, fines are assessed. In its first year of enactment (1999), New York assessed $266,000 in fines to plans for late payment.

Self-Test Questions

1. Explain how a business's receivables balance is built up over time and why there are costs associated with carrying receivables.
2. Briefly, discuss three means by which a firm can monitor its receivables position.

3. What are some of the unique problems faced by healthcare providers in managing receivables?
4. What trends are occurring in billing and collections?

Credit Policy

The success or failure of a business depends primarily on the demand for its products or services—as a rule, the higher its sales, the larger its profits and the better its financial condition. Sales, in turn, depend on a number of factors, some of which are exogenous, but others are under the control of the firm. The major controllable variables that affect demand are sales prices, product or service quality, marketing, and the firm's *credit policy*. Credit policy, in turn, consists of four variables:

1. The *credit period*, which is the length of time buyers (payers) are given to pay for their purchases
2. The *credit standards*, which refer to the minimum financial strength of acceptable credit customers, and the amount of credit available to different customers
3. The firm's *collection policy*, which is measured by its toughness or laxity in following up on slow-paying accounts
4. Any *discounts* given either for bulk purchases such as contracts with managed care plans or for early payment, including the discount amount and period

In general, healthcare businesses have only limited control over credit policy because much of it is more-or-less dictated to them. For example, providers are prohibited from setting credit standards because they must treat all patients who need care (at least sufficiently to stabilize the condition). In addition, credit period is more dependent on the payment system and payer policies than it is on policies established by the provider. Still, healthcare businesses do have discretion regarding some aspects of credit policy. Collection policy is probably the most important credit policy variable for healthcare providers.

At large health services organizations, credit policy usually is administered by a person with the title of *patient accounts manager*. However, the credit policy itself normally is established by the organization's executive committee, which usually consists of the business's president and vice presidents in charge of finance, marketing, and operations.

Collection policy refers to the procedures that a business follows to collect past-due accounts. For example, a letter may be sent to a patient (or third-party payer) when a bill is ten days past due; a more severe letter, followed by a telephone call, may be used if payment is not received within 30 days; and the account may be turned over to a collection agency after 90 days. One of the keys to an effective collections policy is to collect as quickly as possible.

To illustrate the concept, consider Table 16.7, which lists the probability of collecting a self-pay account as time passes by. After two years, the probability of collecting is only about 12 percent, which confirms that timeliness is one of the most important factors in collections.

The collection process can be expensive in terms of both out-of-pocket expenditures and lost goodwill, but, at least, some firmness is needed to prevent an undue lengthening of the collection period and to minimize outright losses. As in similar situations, a balance must be struck between the costs and benefits of different collection policies.

The key to a good collections program is to first identify which patients can be collected from immediately, and how much. Then, the patients must be segregated into categories on the basis of probability of payment—say, (1) most likely to pay full amount, (2) likely to pay partial amount, and (3) unlikely to pay. This classification allows the patient accounts manager to best use the provider's collection resources. Most effort should be directed toward the "most likely to pay" patients, while the least effort should be applied to the "unlikely to pay" patients. A rationale approach to collection policy should result in the greatest amount of collections for the lowest cost.

Many providers are now accepting credit card payments from patients to collect copays and deductibles, and even full charges from self-pay patients. Although credit card payments are somewhat reduced by fees paid to sponsoring banks, credit card payments represent almost instant cash in hand. Additionally, money collected at the time services are provided reduces the need for later billing and collections, which is a very costly process.

The key factor in determining whether or not a receivable will be collected is *credit quality,* which is defined in terms of the probability of default. The probability estimate for a given patient is, for the most part, a subjective judgment, but credit evaluation is a well-established practice, and a good patient accounts manager can make reasonably accurate judgments regarding the probability of default by different classes of patients.

Although most credit decisions are subjective, many businesses use a

TABLE 16.7
Relationship Between Age and Collectibility

Probability of Collecting	Age of Receivable
96%	Less than 30 days
92	1 month
85	2 months
72	3 months
56	6 months
42	9 months
25	12 months
12	24 months

Source: The Health Care Collector, July 1995. Gaithersburg, MD: Aspen Publishers.

sophisticated statistical method called *multiple discriminant analysis (MDA)* to assess credit quality. MDA is similar to multiple regression analysis. The dependent variable is, in essence, the probability of default, and the independent variables are factors associated with financial strength and the ability to pay off the debt if credit is granted. For example, if a firm such as Walgreen Drug Stores evaluated consumers' credit quality, then the independent variables in the credit-scoring system might be: (1) Does the credit applicant own his or her own home? (2) How long has the applicant worked on his or her current job? (3) What is the applicant's outstanding debt in relation to his or her annual income? (4) Does the potential customer have a history of paying his or her debts on time?

One major advantage of an MDA credit-scoring system is that a customer's credit quality is expressed in a single numerical value, rather than as a subjective assessment of various factors. This automated procedure is a tremendous advantage for a large firm, which must evaluate many customers in many different locations using many different credit analysts, because without it, the firm would have a hard time applying equal standards to all credit applicants. To illustrate credit scoring, suppose Hanover Pharmaceuticals has historical information on 500 of its customers, all of whom are retail drug stores. Of these 500, assume that 400 have always paid on time, but the other 100 either paid late or, in some cases, went bankrupt and did not pay at all. Furthermore, the firm has historical data on each customer's quick ratio, times-interest-earned ratio, debt ratio, years in existence, and so on. Multiple discriminant analysis relates the experienced record, or historical probability, of late payment or nonpayment with various measures of a firm's financial condition, and MDA assigns weights for the critical factors. In effect, MDA produces an equation that looks much like a regression equation, and when data on a customer are plugged into the equation, then a credit score for that customer is produced.

1. What are the four credit policy variables?
2. Which one is most important to healthcare providers? Explain your answer.
3. What is a credit-scoring system?

Self-Test Questions

Inventory Management

Inventories are an essential part of virtually all business operations. As is the case with accounts receivable, inventory levels depend heavily on patient volume, and hence revenues. However, whereas receivables build up after services have been provided, inventories must be acquired before hand. This is a critical difference, and the necessity of forecasting volume before establishing target inventory levels makes inventory management a difficult task. Also, because errors in the establishment of inventory levels quickly lead either to lost revenues or to excessive carrying costs, inventory management is as important as it is difficult. In the health services industry, inventory management is even more critical than in other industries because an inventory shortage could lead to catastrophic consequences for patients.

Proper inventory management requires close coordination among the marketing, purchasing, patient services, and finance departments. The patient services departments are generally the first to spot changes in volume. These changes must be worked into the business's purchasing and operating schedules, and the financial manager must arrange any financing that will be needed to support the inventory buildup. Improper communication among departments, poor volume forecasts, or both, can lead to disaster.

Larger businesses employ *computerized inventory control systems*. The computer starts with an inventory count in memory. As withdrawals are made, they are recorded in the computer, and the inventory balance is revised. When the order point is reached, the computer automatically places an order, and when the order is received, the recorded balance is increased.

A good inventory control system must be dynamic. A large provider may stock thousands of different items. The usage of these various items can rise or fall quite separately from rising or falling aggregate utilization. As the usage rate for an individual item begins to rise or fall, the inventory manager must adjust its balance to avoid running short or ending up with obsolete items. If the change in the usage rate appears to be permanent, then the *base inventory* level should be recomputed, the *safety stock* should be reconsidered, and the computer model used in the control process should be reprogrammed.

A relatively new approach to inventory control called *just-in-time (JIT)* is gaining popularity in all industries, including health services. To illustrate the use of just-in-time systems among providers, consider the following example. One large hospital used to maintain a 25,000 square foot warehouse to hold its medical supplies. However, as cost pressures mounted, the hospital closed its warehouse and sold the inventory to a major hospital supplier. Now, the supplier is a full-time partner of the hospital in the ordering and delivering of supplies of both the supplier itself and of some 400 other firms.

The inventory streamlining process began with daily deliveries to the hospital's loading dock, but soon expanded to a JIT system called *stockless inventory*. Now, the supplier fills orders in exact, sometimes small, quantities and delivers them directly to the hospital's departments, including the operating rooms and nursing floors. The hospital's managers estimate that the stockless system has saved about $1.5 million a year since it was instituted, including $350,000 from staff reductions and $650,000 from inventory reductions. Additionally, the hospital has converted space that was previously used as storerooms to patient care and other cash-generating uses. The suppliers that offer stockless inventory systems typically add 3 to 5 percent service fees, but many hospitals still can realize savings on total inventory costs.

The stockless inventory concept has its own set of problems. The major concern is that a *stock-out,* which occurs when an inventory item is not in stock, will cause a serious problem. "We walk very carefully and slowly because we can't afford a glitch," said a spokesperson for the supplier. "The first morning that an operating room doesn't open, we've got a problem." Some hospital managers are concerned that such systems create too much dependence on a single supplier, and eventually the cost savings will disappear as prices are increased.

As stockless inventory systems become more prevalent in hospitals, more and more hospitals are decreasing their in-house inventory management, or *materials management,* as it is often called, in favor of outside contractors who assume both inventory management and supplier roles. In effect, hospitals are beginning to outsource inventory management. For example, some hospitals are experimenting with an inventory management program known as *point-of-service distribution,* which is one generation ahead of stockless systems. Under point-of-service programs, the supplier delivers supplies, intravenous solutions, medical forms, and so on, to the supply rooms. The supplier owns the products in the supply rooms until used by the hospital, at which time the hospital pays for the items.

In addition to reducing inventories, outside inventory managers often are better at ferreting out waste than are their in-house counterparts. For example, an inventory management firm recently found that one hospital was spending $600 for products used in a single open-heart surgery, while another was spending only $420. Because there was no meaningful difference in the procedure or outcomes, the higher-cost hospital was able to change the type of medical supplies used in the surgery and to pocket the difference.

In an even more advanced form of inventory management, some hospitals are just beginning to negotiate with suppliers to furnish materials on the basis of how much medical care is delivered, rather than the type and number of products used. In such agreements, providers pay suppliers a set fee for each unit of patient service provided—for example, $125 for each case-mix-adjusted patient day. Under this type of system, a hospital ties its supplies expenditures to its revenues, which, at least for now, are for the most part tied to the number of units of patient service. The end of the evolution of inventory management techniques for healthcare providers is expected to be some form of capitated payment, whereby providers will pay suppliers a previously agreed-upon fee regardless of actual future patient volume, and hence regardless of the amount of materials actually consumed.

1. Why is good inventory management important to a business's success?
2. Describe some recent trends in inventory management by healthcare providers.

Self-Test Questions

The Economic Ordering Quantity (EOQ) Model

Inventories are obviously necessary, but it is equally obvious that a business's profitability will suffer if it has too much or too little inventory. How can we determine the optimal inventory level? In general, inventory levels are set on the basis of experience, which, after all, is the best teacher. However, managers can gain a feel for those factors that affect inventory levels by examining the *economic ordering quantity (EOQ) model.* The EOQ model examines the costs associated with inventory, and then identifies the level that minimizes these costs. Inventory costs typically are broken down into three categories: (1) carrying costs, (2) ordering costs, and (3) stockout costs. *Stockout costs,* which are the costs associated with running out of an item of inventory, tend to be difficult to measure, and hence will not be included in our discussion of the EOQ model.

Carrying Costs

Carrying costs generally rise in direct proportion to the average amount of inventory carried. Inventories carried, in turn, depend on the frequency with which orders are placed. To illustrate the concept, consider the following example. If a hospital uses S units per year, and if it places equal-sized orders N times per year, then S / N units will be purchased with each order. If the inventory is used evenly over the year, and if no safety stocks are carried, then the average inventory, A, will be:

$$A = \frac{\text{Units per order}}{2} = \frac{S/N}{2}.$$

For example, if S = 120,000 units per year, and N = 4, then the hospital will order 30,000 units at a time, and its average inventory will be 15,000 units.

$$A = \frac{S/N}{2} = \frac{120,000/4}{2} = \frac{30,000}{2} = 15,000 \text{ units.}$$

Just after a shipment arrives, the inventory will be 30,000 units; just before the next shipment arrives, it will be zero; and on average, 15,000 units will be carried.

Now, assume the hospital purchases its inventory at a price P = $2 per unit. The average inventory value is, thus, P × A = $2 × 15,000 = $30,000. If the hospital uses short-term debt with a cost of 10 percent to finance its inventory, it will incur $3,000 in interest expense to carry the inventory for one year. Furthermore, assume that each year the hospital incurs $2,000 of storage costs (space, utilities, security, taxes, and so forth), that its inventory insurance costs are $500, and that it must mark down inventories by $1,000 because of depreciation and obsolescence. Then, the hospital's total costs of carrying the $30,000 average inventory is $3,000 + $2,000 + $500 + $1,000 = $6,500, so the annual percentage cost of carrying the inventory is $6,500 / $30,000 = 0.217 = 21.7%.

Defining the annual percentage carrying cost as C, we can, in general, find the annual total carrying cost, TCC, as the percentage carrying cost, C, times the price per unit, P, times the average number of units, A:

$$TCC = \text{Total carrying cost} = C \times P \times A.$$

In our example,

$$TCC = 0.217 \times \$2 \times 15{,}000 = \$6{,}500.$$

Ordering Costs

Although we assume that carrying costs are entirely variable and rise in direct proportion to the average size of inventories, we assume that all *ordering costs* are fixed. For example, the costs of placing and receiving an order—interoffice memos, long-distance telephone calls, costs to the supplier of setting up a production run (if necessary), and taking delivery—are essentially fixed regardless of the size of an order, so this part of inventory costs is simply the fixed cost of placing and receiving orders times the number of orders placed per year.[7] If the fixed costs associated with ordering inventories are designated F, and if we place N orders per year, the total ordering cost is given by this equation:

$$\text{Total ordering cost} = TOC = F \times N.$$

Substituting $N = S / 2A$ into the equation produces this result:

$$TOC = F \times \left(\frac{S}{2A}\right).$$

To illustrate the use of the total ordering cost equation, assume that F = \$100, S = 120,000 units, and A = 15,000 units. With these data, the total annual ordering cost is \$400:

$$TOC = \$100 \times \left(\frac{120{,}000}{30{,}000}\right) = \$100 \times 4 = \$400.$$

Total Inventory Costs

The expressions for total carrying cost and total ordering cost can be combined to find total inventory costs, TIC, as follows:

$$TIC = TCC + TOC$$

$$= [C \times P \times A] + \left[F \times \left(\frac{S}{2A}\right)\right].$$

Recognizing that the average inventory carried is $A = Q / 2$, or one-half the size of each order quantity, Q, we can rewrite the total inventory costs equation as follows:

$$TIC = \left[C \times P \times \left(\frac{Q}{2} \right) \right] + \left[F \times \left(\frac{S}{Q} \right) \right].$$

Here, we see that total carrying cost equals average inventory in units, Q / 2, multiplied by unit price, P, times the percentage annual carrying cost, C. Total ordering cost equals the number of orders placed per year, S / Q, multiplied by the fixed cost of placing and receiving an order, F.

The EOQ Model

Figure 16.1 illustrates the basic premise on which the EOQ model is built; namely, that some costs rise with larger inventories while other costs decline, and there is an optimal order size (and associated average inventory) that minimizes the total costs associated with inventories. In essence, carrying costs rise with larger orders because larger order size leads to larger average inventories. On the other hand, ordering costs decline with larger orders because larger orders lead to fewer orders being placed.

The sum of the carrying and ordering cost curves in Figure 16.1 represents total inventory costs. The point where TIC is minimized defines the *economic ordering quantity (EOQ)*, which, in turn, determines the optimal average inventory level. The EOQ is found by differentiating the total inventory costs (TIC) equation with respect to ordering quantity, Q, and then

FIGURE 16.1

The EOQ
Concept

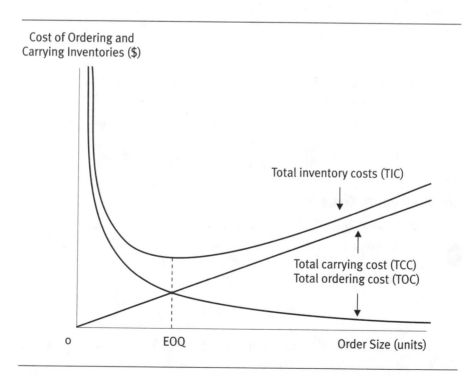

setting the derivative equal to zero. The end result is this equation, called the
EOQ model:

$$EOQ = \sqrt{\frac{2 \times F \times S}{C \times P}}.$$

Here,

EOQ = economic ordering quantity, or the optimum quantity to be ordered
each time an order is placed.

F = fixed costs of placing and receiving an order.

S = annual usage in units.

C = annual carrying costs expressed as percentage of average inventory
value.

P = purchase price the firm must pay per unit of inventory.

To illustrate the EOQ model, consider the following data, supplied by
Bayside Memorial Hospital. One of the items used by several of Bayside's
laboratories is a biological hazard bag used to dispose of biological wastes.
For this item:

F = fixed cost per order = $100.

S = annual usage = 11,250 bags per year.

C = percentage carrying cost = 25 percent of inventory value.

P = purchase price per bag = $1.00 per bag.

Substituting these data into model results in an EOQ of 3,000 bags:

$$EOQ = \sqrt{\frac{2 \times F \times S}{C \times P}} = \sqrt{\frac{2 \times \$100 \times 11{,}250}{0.25 \times \$1.00}} = \sqrt{9{,}000{,}000} = 3{,}000.$$

With an EOQ of 3,000 bags and annual usage of 11,250 bags, Bayside will place 11,250 / 3,000 = 3.75 orders per year. Notice that average
inventory holdings depend directly on the EOQ. Immediately after an order
is received, 3,000 bags are in stock. Because the weekly usage rate is 216 bags
(11,250 / 52 weeks), inventories are drawn down by this amount each week.
Thus, the actual number of units held in inventory will vary from 3,000 bags
just after an order is received to zero just before a new order arrives. With
a 3,000 beginning balance, a zero ending balance, and an assumed uniform
usage rate, inventories will average one-half the EOQ, or 1,500 bags, during
the year. At a cost of $1.00 per bag, the average investment in inventories will
be 1,500 × $1.00 = $1,500. If inventories are financed by bank loans, the
loan balance will vary from a high of $3,000 to a low of $0, but the average
amount outstanding over the course of a year will be $1,500.

Notice that the EOQ, and hence average inventory holdings, rises with
the square root of usage. Therefore, a given increase in volume, and hence

usage, will result in a less-than-proportional increase in inventories, so the revenues/sales ratio will tend to decline as a business grows. For example, Bayside's EOQ is 3,000 bags at an annual usage of 11,250, and the average inventory is 1,500 bags, or $1,500. However, if usage of biological hazard bags were to increase by 100 percent, to 22,500 bags per year, the EOQ would rise only to 4,243 units, or by about 41 percent, and the average inventory would rise by this same percentage. This suggests that there are economies of scale in holding inventories.[8]

Finally, what is Bayside's total inventory costs for the year, assuming that the EOQ is ordered each time. Using the equation developed earlier, total inventory costs are calculated to be $750:

$$\text{TIC} = \left[C \times P \times \left(\frac{Q}{2} \right) \right] + \left[F \times \left(\frac{S}{Q} \right) \right].$$

$$= [0.25 \times \$1.00 \times 3,000] + \left[\$100 \times \left(\frac{11,250}{3,000} \right) \right]$$

$$= \$375 + \$375 = \$750.$$

Note two points. First, the $750 total inventory cost represents the total of carrying costs and ordering costs, but this amount does not include the 11,250 × $1.00 = $11,250 annual purchasing price of the inventory itself. Second, as we see both in Figure 16.1 and in the numbers just preceding, at the EOQ, total carrying cost (TCC) equals total ordering cost (TOC). This property is not unique to the Bayside illustration; it always holds.

The EOQ model can be used to examine such issues as reorder points, safety stocks, and the impact of quantity discounts on inventory decisions. However, as stated at the beginning, the model is more useful for understanding inventory decisions than for making them. Thus, we will leave further discussion to other books.

Self-Test Questions

1. What are some of the costs associated with inventories?
2. Briefly, describe the EOQ model and its implications for inventory management.

Accruals

At this point in the chapter, we have concluded our discussion of current asset management. Now, we turn our attention to two current liability accounts: (1) accruals and (2) accounts payable. Although sources of short-term debt, the management of accruals and trade credit generally is considered to be part of working capital management, and hence they are discussed in this chapter rather than in Chapter 6.

Businesses generally pay employees on a weekly, biweekly, or monthly basis, even though wages actually are earned on a daily basis. Similarly, the business's estimated income taxes (if applicable), the social security and income taxes withheld from employee payrolls, and the sales taxes collected are generally paid on a weekly, monthly, or quarterly basis, even though the obligations are created on a daily basis. The wages and taxes that a business owes because of these timing differentials are listed on the balance sheet as *accruals.*

Accruals increase automatically, or *spontaneously*, as a business's operations expand. Furthermore, this type of short-term debt is free in the sense that no explicit interest is paid on accruals. For these two reasons, accruals are an important source of short-term financing for businesses, especially those that are growing rapidly. However, a business cannot ordinarily control its accruals because the timing of wage payments is set by economic forces and industry custom, while tax payment dates are established by law. Thus, businesses should use all the accruals they can because they represent free financing, but managers have little control over the levels of such accounts.

1. What is meant by the term "spontaneous financing?"
2. What are accruals, and what should a business's policy be regarding the use of accrual financing?

Self-Test Questions

Accounts Payable (Trade Credit)

Healthcare businesses often make purchases from other firms on credit. Such debt is recorded on the balance sheet as an *account payable*. Accounts payable, or *trade credit*, is the largest single category of short-term debt for many businesses. Because small businesses often do not qualify for financing from other sources, they rely especially heavily on trade credit.

The Cost of Trade Credit

Like accruals, trade credit is a spontaneous source of financing in the sense that it arises from ordinary business transactions. For example, suppose that a hospital purchases an average of $2,000 a day of supplies on terms of net 30, which means that it must pay for goods 30 days after the invoice date. On average, the hospital will owe 30 times $2,000, or $60,000, to its suppliers, assuming that the hospital's managers act rationally and do not pay before the credit is due. If the hospital's volume, and consequently its purchases, were to double, its accounts payable would also double to $120,000. Simply by growing, the hospital would have spontaneously generated an additional $60,000 of financing. Similarly, if the terms under which it bought supplies were extended from 30 to 40 days, the hospital's accounts payable would expand from $60,000 to $80,000. Thus, a supplier that lengthens the credit period, as well as expands volume, and hence purchases, generates additional financing for a business.

Firms that sell on credit have a *credit policy* that includes certain *terms of credit*. For example, Midwestern Medical Supply Company sells on terms of 2/10, net 30, which means that a 2 percent discount is given if payment is made within ten days of the invoice date, with the full invoice amount being due and payable within 30 days if the discount is not taken. Suppose that Chicago Health System, Inc., buys an average of $12 million of medical and surgical supplies from Midwestern each year, less a 2 percent discount, for net purchases of $11,760,000 / 360 = $32,666.67 per day. For the sake of simplicity, suppose that Midwestern is Chicago Health System's only supplier. If Chicago Health System takes the discount, paying at the end of the tenth day, its payables will average $10 \times \$32,666.67 = \$326,667$, so Chicago Health System will, on average, be receiving $326,667 of credit from its only supplier, Midwestern Medical Supply Company.

Suppose now that the health system's managers decide not to take the discount. What effect will this decision have on the system's financial condition? First, Chicago Health System will begin paying invoices in 30 days, so its accounts payable will increase to $30 \times \$32,666.67 = \$980,000$. Midwestern will now be supplying Chicago Health System with $980,000 − $326,667 = $653,333 of **additional** trade credit. The health system could use this additional credit to pay off bank loans, to expand inventories, to increase fixed assets, to build up its cash account, or even to increase its own accounts receivable.

Chicago Health System's additional credit from Midwestern has a cost—it is foregoing a 2 percent discount on its $12 million of purchases, so its costs will rise by $240,000 per year. Dividing this $240,000 dollar cost by the amount of additional credit provides the implicit approximate percentage cost of the added trade credit:

$$\text{Approximate percentage cost} = \frac{\$240,000}{\$653,333} = 36.7\%.$$

Assuming that Chicago Health System can borrow from its bank or from other sources at an interest rate less than 36.7 percent, it should not expand its payables by foregoing discounts.

The following equation can be used to calculate the approximate percentage cost, on an annual basis, of not taking discounts:

$$\text{Approximate \% cost} = \frac{\text{Discount percent}}{100 - \text{Discount percent}}$$
$$\times \frac{360}{\text{Days credit received} - \text{Discount period}}.$$

The numerator of the first term, Discount percent, is the cost per dollar of credit, while the denominator in this term, 100 − Discount percent, represents the funds made available by not taking the discount. Thus, the first term is the periodic cost rate of the trade credit. In this example, Chicago Health System must spend \$2 to gain \$98 of credit, for a cost rate of $2 / 98 = 0.0204 = 2.04\%$. The second term shows how many times each year this cost is incurred; in this example, $360/(30 - 10) = 360/20 = 18$ times. Putting the two terms together, the approximate cost of not taking the discount when the terms are 2/10, net 30, is computed as follows:

$$\text{Approximate \% cost} = \frac{2}{98} \times \frac{360}{20} = 0.0204 \times 18$$
$$= 0.367 = 36.7\%.$$

The cost of trade credit can be reduced by paying late—that is, by paying beyond the date that the credit terms allow. Such a strategy is called *stretching*. If Chicago Health System could get away with paying Midwestern in 60 days rather than in the specified 30, the effective credit period would become $60 - 10 = 50$ days, and the approximate cost would drop from 36.7 percent to $(2 / 98) \times (360 / 50) = 14.7\%$. In recessionary periods, businesses may be able to get away with late payments to suppliers, but they will also suffer a variety of problems associated with stretching accounts payable and being branded a slow payer.

On the basis of the preceding discussion, it is clear that trade credit consists of two distinct components:

1. *Free trade credit* involves credit received during the discount period.
2. *Costly trade credit* involves credit in excess of the free credit, and whose cost is an implicit one based on the foregone discount.

From a finance perspective, managers should view trade credit in this way. First, the actual price of supplies is the discounted price—that is, the price that would be paid on a cash purchase. Any credit that can be taken without an increase in price is free credit that should be taken. Second, if the discounted price is the actual price, then the added amount that must be paid if the discount is not taken is, in reality, a *finance charge* for granting additional credit. A business should take the additional credit only if the finance charge is less than the cost of alternative credit sources.

In the example, Chicago Health System should take the \$326,667 of free credit offered by Midwestern Medical Supply Company. Free credit is good credit. However, the cost rate of the additional \$653,333 of costly trade credit is approximately 37 percent. The health system has access to bank loans at a 9.5 percent rate, so it does not take the additional credit. Under the terms of trade found in most industries, the costly component will involve a relatively high percentage cost, so stronger firms will avoid using it.

Self-Test Questions

1. What is trade credit?
2. What is the difference between free and costly trade credit?
3. How should businesses make the decision as to how much trade credit to use?

Key Concepts

This chapter examined working capital management, including accruals and trade credit. Here are its key concepts:

- The essence of working capital management is to support the business's operations at the lowest possible cost.
- The *primary goal of cash management* is to reduce the amount of cash held to the minimum necessary to conduct business.
- *Cash management techniques* generally fall into four categories: (1) *synchronizing cash flows*, (2) *using float*, (3) *accelerating collections*, and (4) *controlling disbursements*.
- *Lockboxes* are used to accelerate collections. A *concentration banking system* consolidates the collections into a centralized pool that can be managed more efficiently than a large number of individual accounts.
- Three techniques for controlling disbursements are: (1) *payables centralization*, (2) *zero-balance accounts*, and (3) *controlled disbursement accounts*.
- The implementation of a sophisticated cash management system is costly, and all cash management actions must be evaluated to ensure that the benefits exceed the costs.
- Firms can reduce their cash balances by holding *marketable securities*, which serve both as a *substitute for cash* and as a *temporary investment* for funds that will be needed in the near future. Safety is the primary consideration when selecting marketable securities.
- When a firm sells goods to a customer on credit, an *account receivable* is created.
- Businesses can use *aging schedules* and the *average collection period (ACP)* measure to help keep track of their receivables position and to help avoid the buildup of possible bad debts.
- The four credit policy variables are: (1) *credit period*, (2) *credit standards*, (3) *collection policy*, and (4) *discounts*.
- Because of unique circumstances, the credit policy variable most controllable by healthcare providers is collection policy.
- Proper *inventory management* requires close coordination among the marketing, purchasing, patient services and finance departments. Because the cost of holding inventory can be high, inventory management is important.
- *Just-in-time (JIT)* systems are used to minimize inventory costs and, simultaneously, to improve operations.
- *Inventory costs* can be divided into two types for purposes of the EOQ model: (1) carrying costs and (2) ordering costs. In general, *carrying costs* increase as the level of inventory rises, but ordering costs decline with larger inventory holdings.
- The *economic ordering quantity (EOQ) model* is a formula for determining

the order quantity that will minimize total inventory costs. It provides many insights into inventory management, but its real-world use is limited.

- *Accruals* are a source of short-term financing that result from the build up of wages and taxes due. Because they are a costless source of financing, businesses should take all the accruals that they can get.
- *Accounts payable*, or *trade credit*, is a source of short-term financing that stems from buying supplies on credit.
- Businesses should take all of the *free trade credit* available, but should take *costly trade credit* only if the implied cost is less than that on other sources of short-term credit.

Our discussion of working capital management has been brief. However, the concepts covered enable readers to at least have some appreciation for the issues involved. For additional information, see any of the large number of references given next.

Selected References

"Accounts Receivable Management." 1993. Roland S. Funsten, editor. *Topics in Health Care Financing* (Fall).

Adams, William T., Gregory M. Snow, and Paul M. Helmick. 2000. "Automated Charge Processing Streamlines Data Entry." *Healthcare Financial Management* (May): 50–53.

Anderson, Alexander M. 1993. "Enhancing Hospital Cash Reserves Management." *Healthcare Financial Management* (July): 91–95.

Anderson, Howard J. 1989. "Patient Accounts Managers Share Views on Receivables." *Healthcare Financial Management* (December): 42–46.

Berling, Robert J., Jr., and John T. Geppi. "Hospitals Can Cut Materials Costs by Managing Supply Pipeline." *Healthcare Financial Management* (April): 9–26.

Bruch, Nancy M., and Lynn L. Lewis 1994. "Using Control Charts to Help Manage Accounts Receivable." *Healthcare Financial Management* (July): 44–48.

Cantone, Lisa and Ann Bullock. 2000. "Getting Tough with Home Health Receivables." *Healthcare Financial Management* (April): 44–49.

Dias, Kathie and Dale Stockamp. 1992. "Nursing Process Approach Improves Receivables Management." *Healthcare Financial Management* (September): 55–64.

Dixon, Leslie H., and Susan K. Bossert. "The Commercial Bank as Investment Advisor for Hospital Investable Assets." *Topics in Health Care Financing* (Summer): 58–68.

Edwards, Donald E., William C. Hamilton, and Rex Hauser. 1991. "Financial Reserve: Hospitals Leery of Credit Lines, Factoring Receivables." *Healthcare Financial Management* (October): 82–88.

Ferconio, Sandra and Michael R. Lane. 1991. "Financing Maneuvers: Two Opportunities to Boost a Hospital's Working Capital." *Healthcare Financial Management* (October): 74–80.

Folk, Mark D., and Peter R. Roest. 1995. "Converting Accounts Receivable into Cash." *Healthcare Financial Management* (September): 74–78.

Frohlich, Robert M., Jr. 1994. "Effective Reassignment of Accounts Can Decrease Bad Debt." *Healthcare Financial Management* (July): 37–42.

Green, Larry A. 1993. "Cash Management: Acceleration and Information Strategies." *Topics in Health Care Financing* (Summer): 44–57.

Groenevelt, Claudia J. 1990. "Applying Japanese Management Tips to Patient Accounts." *Healthcare Financial Management* (April): 46–55.

Haavik, Stan. 2000. "Building a Demand-Driven, Vendor-Managed Supply Chain." *Healthcare Financial Management* (February): 56–61.

Hauser, Rexford C., Donald E. Edwards, and Judy T. Edwards. 1991. "Cash Budgeting: An Underutilized Resource Management Tool in Not-for-Profit Health Care Entities." *Hospital & Health Services Administration* (Fall): 439–446.

Karpinski, Joseph P. 1997. "Designing a Successful Investment Program." *Healthcare Financial Management* (February): 58–63.

Kelly, Vincent K. 1993. "Banks As a Source of Capital." *Topics in Health Care Financing* (Summer): 21–34.

Kincaid, Timothy J. 1993. "Selling Accounts Receivable to Fund Working Capital." *Healthcare Financial Management* (May): 27–32.

Kowalski, Jamie C. 1991a. "Materials Management Crucial to Overall Efficiency." *Healthcare Financial Management* (January): 40–44.

———. 1991b. "Inventory to Go: Can Stockless Deliver Efficiency." *Healthcare Financial Management* (November): 21–34.

Ladewig, Tommy L., and Bill A. Hecht. 1993. "Achieving Excellence in the Management of Accounts Receivable." *Healthcare Financial Management* (September): 25–32.

Lane, Michael R. 1997. "Can Earning Prompt-Payment Discounts Really Save Money?" *Healthcare Financial Management* (September): 72–75.

"Managing Accounts Receivable." 1990. John F. Clarkin, editor. *Topics in Health Care Financing* (Fall).

Marshall, Steve. 1993. "Cost Justifying the Electronic Billing Decision." *Healthcare Financial Management* (June): 68–72.

Masonson, Leslie N. 1992. "Banks Aggressively Marketing Cash Management Services." *Healthcare Financial Management* (December): 59–60.

Moynihan, James J. 1993. "Improving the Claims Process with EDI." *Healthcare Financial Management* (January): 48–52.

Newton, Robert L. 1993. "Measuring Accounts Receivable Performance: A Comprehensive Method." *Healthcare Financial Management* (May): 33–36.

Prince, Thomas R., and Ramachandran Ramanan. 1992. "Collection Performance: An Empirical Analysis of Not-for-Profit Community Hospitals." *Hospital & Health Services Administration* (Summer): 181–196.

Reiss, John B., and Stephen J. Di Cioccio. 1991. "Where There's a Will: How to Finance Medicare Receivables—Legally." *Healthcare Financial Management* (October): 90–96.

Robinson, Edward F. 1989. "Automated Collection Systems Improve Cash Flow." *Healthcare Financial Management* (December): 31–40.

Seidner, Alan G. 1987. "Reviewing the Basics of Investment Management." *Healthcare Financial Management* (October): 68–72.

Sen, Sunasir and James P. Lawler. 1995. "Securitizing Receivables Offers Low-Cost

Financing Option." *Healthcare Financial Management* (May): 32–37.

Slater, Robin Michaels, Ronald Corti, and Joseph Privitera. 1991. "Giving Receivables an 'Outside' Chance." *Healthcare Financial Management* (October): 56–66.

Smith, DeFord and Lesley C. McPherson. 1988. "Improving Hospital Investments Using a Disciplined Approach." *Healthcare Financial Management* (July): 32–41.

Souders, Richard V. 1990. "Electronic Claims Can be a Remedy for Cash Flow Troubles." *Healthcare Financial Management* (June): 62–68.

Spiegel, Mel. 1989. "Selling Accounts Receivable Can Improve Cash Flow." *Healthcare Financial Management* (September): 40–46.

Swarzman, Gerald F. 1994. "Does Your Patient Accounting System Pass the Systems Test?" *Healthcare Financial Management* (July): 27–34.

Wallace, Robin. 1999. "Accounts Receivable Reports: Underutilized Mining Tools." *Medical Group Management Journal* (November/December): 28–31.

Zimmerman, David 1993. *Cash is King*. Franklin, WI: Eagle Press.

Selected Web Sites

To learn more about the cash management services offered by large banks, see First Union's cash management site at *www.firstunion.com/business/cashman*.

For some insights as to what the credit card industry is doing regarding patient payments, see *www.mastercard-visa.com*. Then, click on Visa Easy Pay.

Selected Cases

There are two cases in *Cases in Healthcare Finance* that are applicable to this chapter:

Case 23: Gulf Pharmaceuticals, which focuses on the basic concepts of receivables management.

Case 24: Grand Forks Medical Center, which covers inventory management, with emphasis on the EOQ model.

Notes

1. This discussion of cash management is necessarily brief. For a much more detailed discussion of cash management within the health services industry, see Alan G. Seidner and William O. Cleverley, *Cash and Investment Management for the Health Care Industry* (Gaithersburg, MD: Aspen, 1990).

2. Money market mutual funds cannot be used as a replacement for commercial checking accounts because the number of checks that can be written against such funds normally is limited to just a few per month.

3. To be precise, the full amount of the receivables account does **not** require financing. The cash costs associated with providing the services that produce the $20,000 in revenues do need to be financed, but the profit component does not. For example, assume that Home Infusion has cash costs of $800 associated with each day's revenues of $1,000. Then, 20 days of receivables would actually require only 20 × $800 = $16,000 in financing. The remaining $4,000 of

receivables, which represent profits, would be offset on the balance sheet by increasing the retained earnings (equity) account by a like amount.

4. If the accounts receivable balance and average daily credit sales (ADS) are known, the ACP can be calculated as follows:

$$ACP = \frac{\text{Receivables}}{\text{ADS}} = \frac{\$1,760,000}{\$110,000} = 16 \text{ days.}$$

5. This forecast for accounts receivable, one of Hanover's balance sheet accounts, is an example of the specific item forecasting method discussed in Chapter 15.

6. Medicare has spent over $100 million to develop an all-encompassing electronic payment system that was supposed to have been in operation in 2000. However, the project was plagued by unexpected problems and delays, so its implementation has been indefinitely postponed.

7. Note that in reality both carrying and ordering costs can have variable and fixed cost elements, at least over certain ranges of inventory. For example, security and utilities charges are probably fixed in the short run over a wide range of inventory levels. Similarly, labor costs in receiving inventory could be tied to the quantity received, and hence could be variable. To simplify matters, the EOQ model treats all carrying costs as variable and all ordering costs as fixed.

8. Note, however, that these scale economies relate to each particular item, and not to the entire business. For example, a large distributor of hospital supplies might have a higher inventory/sales ratio than a much smaller distributor if the small firm has only a few high-sales-volume items while the large firm distributes a great many low-volume items.

DISTRIBUTIONS TO OWNERS: BONUSES, DIVIDENDS, AND REPURCHASES

Learning Objectives

After studying this chapter, readers should be able to:

- Discuss the three theories of dividend policy.
- Describe the information content and clientele effect hypotheses.
- Explain the residual dividend model and how managers use it to help establish dividend policy.
- Explain stock dividends and stock splits and the rationale for their use.
- Discuss stock repurchase programs and the reasons for their current popularity.

Introduction

Successful businesses earn income. That income can then be reinvested in operating assets, used to acquire securities, used to retire debt, or, in the case of investor-owned businesses, distributed to owners. If the decision is made to distribute income to owners, three key issues arise: (1) What percentage should be distributed? (2) What form should the distribution take—bonuses, cash dividends, or stock repurchases? (3) How stable should the distribution be— that is, should the funds paid out from year to year be stable and dependable, which owners may prefer, or be allowed to vary with the business's cash flows and investment requirements, which might be better for the business? These three issues are the primary focus of this chapter, but we also consider two related issues: (1) stock dividends and (2) stock splits.

Distributions in Small Businesses

In general, the distribution to owners in small businesses differs from that in large businesses. In this section, we focus on small businesses. The remainder of the chapter is devoted to distributions in large publicly held corporations.

The reason for a separate treatment of small businesses is twofold. First, small businesses often are organized as proprietorships or partnerships. If they are organized as corporations, taxes typically are filed under Chapter S, which means that, like a proprietorship or partnership, the earnings of the business is prorated among the owners and taxed as ordinary income, regardless of whether or not the earnings are reinvested in the business. Second, as owners/managers of the business, small businesses can return earnings to owners in the form of increased compensation, either directly as wages or indirectly as perquisites. In large corporations, there is a "firewall" between the managers and the owners, and hence the only ways to distribute earnings to owners (the stockholders) is through dividends and stock repurchases.

These inherent differences between small and large businesses, as well as the limited resources available to devote to the finance and accounting function, create an incentive for small businesses to use the *cash basis* of accounting, as opposed to the *accrual basis* that is favored by large businesses. In the cash method, revenues and costs are reported on the income statement as they occur, rather than when the obligations occur. Furthermore, because the financial statements of small businesses are not presented to outside owners, the statements are used both for control purposes and for tax purposes. For the most part, small businesses report as little net income as possible, unless funds are specifically required to be retained in the business.

To illustrate the situation facing a typical small healthcare provider, consider Table 17.1, which shows the income statements for the Bismarck Clinic, a two-physician family practice. The left-side column shows the income statement as it typically would be constructed. However, this format gives the impression that there is no ownership value to the business because the net income is zero. To determine the value of ownership, any bonuses paid to the two owners/physicians must be explicitly shown on the income statement.

TABLE 17.1
Bismarck Clinic: Standard and Recast Income Statements

	Standard Format	Recast Format
Revenues:		
Professional fees	$ 950,000	$ 950,000
Other income	50,000	50,000
Total revenues	$1,000,000	$1,000,000
Expenses:		
Physician compensation	$ 320,000	$ 280,000
Staff compensation	300,000	300,000
Clinical supplies	85,000	85,000
Office supplies	50,000	50,000
Rent	50,000	50,000
Insurance	25,000	25,000
Telephone and utilities	25,000	25,000
Outside laboratory fees	25,000	25,000
Other expenses	120,000	120,000
Total expenses	$1,000,000	$ 960,000
Net income	$ 0	$ 40,000

Although not an easy task, some judgments must be made regarding what portion of the $320,000 in physician compensation ($160,000 for each owner/physician) is for actual professional services and what portion is, in reality, a return on owners capital. Assume that current studies indicate that the median compensation for salaried primary care physicians in the area is $140,000. Assuming that this amount is the "fair" compensation for the work being done by the two owners/physicians of Bismarck Clinic, their compensation of $160,000 implies that they are receiving a bonus of $20,000 each, for a total of $40,000 in bonuses. The right-side column of the income statement does not list the $40,000 in bonuses from physician compensation, and hence shows a net income for the practice of $40,000. Because the practice is a partnership, the $40,000 is taxed at each physician's personal tax rate regardless of whether it is received as salary (bonuses) or earnings (net income).

With no differential tax consequences, the two income statements create the same cash flows to the owners/physicians. The value of recasting is that the compensation is broken down into the portion that is a result of employment at the clinic and the portion that is a result of owning the clinic. Indeed, Bismarck Clinic has $100,000 of assets, so its implied return on assets (ROA) is $40,000 / $100,000 = 40%, as opposed to zero indicated initially. Furthermore, if the clinic has $20,000 in debt financing (with the interest expense shown in the other expenses category), the implied return on equity (ROE) to the owners/physicians is $40,000 / $80,000 = 50%.[1]

Although recasting the income statement as we have done in Table 17.1 seems like much ado about nothing, it is essential in some circumstances. For example, if the clinic is put up for sale, it will be necessary to convince potential buyers that it has economic value to a new owner. This can be done only if the business can generate a positive net income (cash flow) for its new owner. Showing a zero net income to prospective buyers will not generate much interest.

1. How can a small business's income statement be recast to show the value of employment versus the value of ownership?
2. Why is such a recasting necessary?

Self-Test Questions

Dividends Versus Capital Gains: Does It Matter To Investors?

In this section, and in the remainder of the chapter, we discuss the decisions involving distributions to owners of a large firm, where stockholders and managers are separated. When deciding how much cash to distribute to stockholders, managers must keep in mind that the firm's primary objective is to maximize shareholder value. Consequently, the *target payout ratio*—defined as the percentage of net income to be paid out as cash dividends—should be based in large part on investors' preferences for dividends versus capital gains: Do investors prefer (1) to have the firm distribute income as cash dividends or (2) to have it either repurchase stock or else plow the earnings back into the business, both of which should result in capital gains?

This preference can be considered in terms of the constant growth stock valuation model, which was first presented in Chapter 8:

$$E(P_0) = \frac{E(D_1)}{R(R_e) - E(g)}.$$

If the firm increases the payout ratio, it raises $E(D_1)$. This increase in the numerator, taken alone, would cause the stock price, $E(P_0)$ to rise. However, if $E(D_1)$ is raised, then less money will be available for reinvestment, which will cause the expected growth rate, $E(g)$, to decline, and hence would tend to lower the stock's price, which illustrates that any change in payout policy will have two opposing effects. Thus, the *optimal dividend policy* depends on the relationship between dividend policy and the required rate of return on (cost of) equity, $R(R_e)$. The policy that results in the lowest cost of equity will maximize stock price.

In this section, we examine three theories of investor preference: (1) the dividend irrelevance theory, (2) the "bird-in-the-hand" theory, and (3) the tax preference theory. In essence, these theories focus on whether or not dividend policy affects the cost of equity. If it does, then, like capital structure policy, the dividend policy that produces the lowest cost of equity will be optimal because it will produce the highest stock price.

Dividend Irrelevance Theory

The principal proponents of the *dividend irrelevance theory* are Merton Miller and Franco Modigliani (MM), who argued that dividend policy has no effect on a business's cost of equity, and hence on stock price.[2] If this is true, then dividend policy would be irrelevant. The essence of dividend irrelevance is that a business's value is determined solely by its earning power and its business risk. In other words, MM argued that the value of a business depends only on the income produced by its assets, and not on how this income is split between dividends and retained earnings.

To understand MM's argument that dividend policy is irrelevant, recognize that any shareholder can construct his or her own dividend policy. For example, if a firm does not pay dividends, a shareholder that wants a 5 percent dividend can "create" it by selling 5 percent of his or her stock. Conversely, if a firm pays a higher dividend than an investor desires, the investor can use the unwanted dividends to buy additional shares of the firm's stock. If investors could buy and sell shares and, thus, create their own dividend policy **without incurring costs**, then the firm's dividend policy would truly be irrelevant. However, investors who want additional dividends must incur brokerage costs to sell shares and perhaps pay capital gains taxes, and investors who do not want dividends must first pay taxes on the unwanted dividends and then incur brokerage costs to purchase shares with the after-tax dividends.

Because taxes and brokerage costs do exist, dividend policy may well be relevant. However, the merit of any theory is based on how well it describes reality, and not on the number or realism of its assumptions. Therefore, the validity of the dividend irrelevance theory must be judged by empirical testing, the results of which will be discussed in a later section.

Bird-in-the-Hand Theory

The principal conclusion of the dividend irrelevance theory—that dividend policy does not affect the cost of equity—has been hotly debated in academic circles. In particular, Myron Gordon and John Lintner argued that the cost of equity decreases as the dividend payout is increased because investors are more certain of receiving dividends than they are of capital gains, which are supposed to result from profit retentions.[3] Gordon and Lintner said, in effect, that investors value a dollar of expected dividends more highly than a dollar of expected capital gains because the dividend yield component, $E(D_1) / P_0$, is less risky than the capital gains component, $E(g)$, in the total expected return equation, $E(R) = E(D_1) / P_0 + E(g)$.

MM disagreed. They argued that the cost of equity is independent of dividend policy, which implies that investors are indifferent between dividends and capital gains. Furthermore, they called the Gordon-Lintner argument the *bird-in-the-hand* fallacy because, in their view, most investors plan to reinvest their dividends in the stock of the same or similar firms, and, in any event, the riskiness of a business's cash flows to investors in the long run is determined by the riskiness of operating cash flows rather than by dividend policy.

Tax Preference Theory

There are three tax-related reasons for thinking that investors might prefer a low dividend payout to a high payout. First, long-term capital gains are taxed at a maximum rate of 20 percent (10 percent if in the lowest bracket), whereas dividend income is taxed at effective rates that go up to 39.6 percent. Therefore, high-income investors (who own most of the stock and receive most of the dividends) might prefer to have firms retain and plow earnings back into the business. Earnings growth would presumably lead to higher stock prices, and thus lower-taxed capital gains would be substituted for higher-taxed dividends. Second, taxes are not paid on the gain until a stock is sold. Because of time value effects, a dollar of taxes paid in the future has a lower effective cost than a dollar paid today. Third, if a stock is held until the stockholder dies, no capital gains tax is due at all—the beneficiaries who receive the stock can use the stock's value on the day of death as their cost basis and, thus, completely escape the capital gains tax on the gain thus far.

Because of these tax advantages, investors may prefer to have firms retain most of their earnings, which in turn would lead to a lower cost of equity. If so, investors would be willing to pay more for low-payout firms than for otherwise similar high-payout firms.

The Empirical Evidence

These three theories offer contradictory advice to the managers of investor-owned corporations, so which, if any, should we believe? The most logical way to proceed is to test the theories empirically. Many such tests have been conducted, but their results have been mixed. There are two reasons for this: (1) For a valid statistical test, things other than dividend policy must be held constant; that is, the sample firms must differ only in their dividend policies; and (2) we must be able to measure with a high degree of accuracy each sample firm's cost of equity. Neither of these two conditions holds: (1) We cannot find a set of publicly owned firms that differ only in their dividend policies, and (2) we cannot obtain precise estimates of firms costs of equity.

Therefore, the studies have been unable to establish a clear relationship between dividend policy and the cost of equity. In other words, no study has shown that in the aggregate investors prefer either higher or lower dividends. Nevertheless, individual investors do have strong preferences. Some prefer high dividends, while others prefer all capital gains. These differences among individuals help explain why it is difficult to reach any definitive conclusions regarding the optimal dividend payout. Even so, both evidence and logic suggest that investors prefer firms that follow a *stable, predictable* dividend policy (regardless of the payout level). We will consider the issue of dividend stability later in the chapter.

Self-Test Questions

1. What variable must dividend policy affect to have an impact on stock price?
2. Briefly, explain the dividend irrelevance, bird-in-the-hand, and tax preference theories.
3. What did Modigliani and Miller assume about taxes and brokerage costs when they developed their dividend irrelevance theory?
4. How did the bird-in-the-hand theory get its name?
5. In what sense does MM's theory represent a middle-ground position between the other two theories?
6. What have been the results of empirical tests of the dividend theories?

Other Dividend Policy Issues

Before we discuss how dividend policy is set in practice, we must examine two other theoretical issues that could affect our views toward dividend policy: (1) the information content, or signaling, hypothesis; and (2) the clientele effect.

Information Content (Signaling) Hypothesis

When MM set forth their dividend irrelevance theory, they assumed that everyone—investors and managers alike—has identical information regarding the firm's future earnings and dividends. In reality, however, different investors have different views on both the level of future dividend payments and the uncertainty inherent in those payments. Furthermore, managers have better information about future prospects than do outside stockholders.

It has been observed that an increase in the dividend amount is often accompanied by an increase in the price of the stock, while a dividend cut generally leads to a stock price decline. This observation could mean that investors, in the aggregate, prefer dividends to capital gains. However, MM argued differently. They noted the well-established fact that corporations are reluctant to cut dividends, and hence will not raise dividends unless they anticipate good earnings in the future. Thus, MM argued that a higher-than-expected dividend increase is a "signal" to investors that the firm's management forecasts good future earnings. Conversely, a dividend reduction, or a smaller-than-expected increase, is a signal that management is forecasting poor earnings in the future. Thus, MM argued that investors' reactions to changes in dividend policy do not necessarily show that investors prefer dividends to retained earnings. Rather, they argued that price changes following dividend actions simply indicate that there is an important *information (signaling) content* in dividend announcements.

Interestingly, it also has been suggested that managers can use capital structure as well as dividends to give signals concerning firms' future prospects. For example, a firm with good earnings prospects can carry more debt than a similar firm with poor earnings prospects. This theory, called *incentive signaling*, rests on the premise that signals with cash-based variables (either debt interest or dividends) cannot be mimicked by unsuccessful firms because such firms do not have the future cash-generating power to maintain the announced interest or dividend payment. Thus, investors are more likely to believe a glowing verbal report when it is accompanied by a dividend increase or a debt-financed expansion program.[4]

Like most other aspects of dividend policy, empirical studies of the signaling hypothesis have had mixed results. There is clearly some information content in dividend announcements. However, it is difficult to tell whether the stock price changes that follow increases or decreases in dividends reflect only signaling effects or both signaling and dividend preferences. Still, signaling effects should be considered when a firm is contemplating a change in dividend policy.

Clientele Effect Hypothesis

As we indicated earlier, different groups, or *clienteles*, of stockholders prefer different dividend payout policies. For example, retired individuals and university endowment funds generally prefer cash income, so they may want the firm to pay out a high percentage of its earnings. Such investors, and pension funds, are often in low or even zero tax brackets, so taxes are of no concern. On the other hand, stockholders in their peak earning years might prefer reinvestment because they have less need for current investment income and would simply reinvest dividends received, after first paying income taxes on those dividends.

If a firm retains and reinvests income rather that paying dividends, those stockholders who need current income would be disadvantaged. The value of their stock might increase, but they would be forced to go to the trouble and expense of selling off some of their shares to obtain cash. Also, some institutional investors, or trustees for individuals, would be legally precluded from selling stock and then "spending capital." On the other hand, stockholders who are saving, rather than spending, dividends might favor a low dividend policy because the less the firm pays out in dividends, the less these stockholders will have to pay in current taxes and the less trouble and expense they will have to go through to reinvest their after-tax dividends. Therefore, investors who want current investment income should own shares in high-dividend-payout firms, while investors with no need for current investment income should own shares in low-dividend-payout firms. For example, investors who seek high cash income might invest in electric utilities, which have had a 60 percent payout in recent years, while those who favor growth could invest in the semiconductor industry, in which the payout is only 3 percent. (For comparison, the average payout ratio for the S&P 500 firms is 24 percent.)

To the extent that stockholders can switch firms, a firm can change from one dividend payout policy to another and then let stockholders who do not like the new policy sell to other investors who do. However, frequent switching would be inefficient because of (1) brokerage costs, (2) the likelihood that stockholders who are selling will have to pay capital gains taxes, and (3) a possible shortage of investors who like the firm's newly adopted dividend policy. Thus, management should be hesitant to change its dividend policy because a change might cause current shareholders to sell their stock, which would force the stock price down. Such a price decline might be temporary, but it might also be permanent—if few new investors are attracted by the new dividend policy, then the stock price would remain depressed. Of course, the new policy might attract an even larger clientele than the firm had before, in which case the stock price would rise.

Evidence from many studies suggests that there is in fact a *clientele effect*. MM and others have argued that one clientele is as good another, so the existence of a clientele effect does not necessarily imply that one dividend policy is better than any other. MM may be wrong, though, and neither they nor anyone else can prove that the aggregate makeup of investors permits firms to disregard clientele effects. This issue, like most others concerning dividend policy, is still up in the air.

Self-Test Question

1. Define (a) information content and (b) the clientele effect, and explain how they affect dividend policy.

Dividend Stability

The stability of dividends is as important as the level. Profits and cash flows vary over time, as do investment opportunities. Taken alone, this suggests that corporations should vary their dividends over time, increase them when cash flows are large and the need for internal funds is low, and lower them when cash is in short supply relative to investment opportunities. However, many stockholders rely on dividends to meet expenses, and they would be seriously inconvenienced if the dividend stream were unstable. Furthermore, reducing dividends to make funds available for capital investment could send incorrect signals to investors who might then push down the stock price because they interpreted the dividend cut to mean that the firm's future earnings prospects had been diminished. Thus, maximizing its stock price requires a firm to balance its internal needs for funds against the needs and desires of its stockholders.

How should this balance be struck—that is, how stable and dependable should a firm attempt to make its dividends? It is impossible to give a definitive answer to this question, but here are some points to consider. Virtually every publicly owned firm makes a five- to ten-year financial forecast of earnings and dividends. Such forecasts are never made public; they are used for internal planning purposes only. However, security analysts construct similar forecasts and do make them available to investors. Furthermore, almost all internal forecasts for a "normal" firm show a trend of higher earnings and dividends. Both managers and investors know that economic conditions may cause actual results to differ from forecasted results, but "normal" firms expect to grow over time.

Years ago, when inflation was not persistent, the term "stable dividend policy" meant a policy of paying the same dollar dividend year after year. For example, AT&T paid $9 per year ($2.25 per quarter) for 25 straight years. Today, though, most firms and stockholders expect earnings to grow over time as a result of retentions and inflation, both of which tend to increase future earnings. Thus, dividends are normally expected to grow more or less in line with earnings, and, today, a "stable dividend policy" generally means increasing the dividend at a reasonably steady rate. Indeed, some firms, in their annual reports, inform investors of dividend growth expectations. Firms with volatile earnings and cash flows would be reluctant to make a commitment to increase the dividend each year, so they would not make such announcements. Even so, most firms would like to be able to exhibit dividend stability, and they try to come as close to it as they can.

Dividend stability has two components: (1) How dependable is the growth rate, and (2) can stockholders count on at least receiving the current dividend in the future? The most stable policy, from an investor's standpoint, is that of a firm whose dividend growth rate is predictable—such a firm's total return (dividend yield plus capital gains yield) would be relatively stable over the long run, and its stock would be a good hedge against inflation. The second most stable policy is where stockholders can be reasonably sure that the current dividend will not be reduced—it may not grow at a steady rate, but management will probably be able to avoid cutting the dividend. The least stable situation is where earnings and cash flows are so volatile that investors cannot count on the firm to maintain the current dividend over a typical business cycle.

Most observers believe that dividend stability is desirable. Assuming this position is correct, investors prefer stocks that pay more predictable dividends to stocks that pay the same average amount of dividends but in a more erratic manner. This means that the cost of equity will be minimized, and the stock price maximized, if a firm stabilizes its dividends as much as possible.

Self-Test Questions
1. What does "stable dividend policy" mean?
2. What are the two components of dividend stability?

Establishing the Dividend Policy in Practice

In the preceding sections, we saw that investors may or may not prefer dividends to capital gains, but that they do prefer predictable to unpredictable dividends. In this section, we describe how firms actually set their dividend policies.

Setting the Target Payout Ratio: The Residual Dividend Model

Before we begin our discussion of the model, note that the term "payout ratio" can be interpreted in two ways: (1) the conventional way, where the payout ratio means the percentage of net income paid out as **cash dividends**, or (2) in a more global context, in which the ratio includes both cash dividends and share repurchases. In this section, we assume that no repurchases occur. Increasingly, though, firms are using the residual model to determine "distributions to shareholders" and then making a separate decision as to the form of that distribution. (Repurchases are discussed in a later section.)

When deciding how much cash to distribute to stockholders, two points should be kept in mind: (1) The overriding objective is to maximize shareholder value, and (2) the firm's cash flows really belong to its shareholders, so management should refrain from retaining income unless it can be reinvested to produce returns higher than shareholders could themselves earn by investing the cash in investments of similar risk. On the other hand, internal equity (retained earnings) is cheaper than external equity (new common stock). This encourages firms to retain earnings because they add to the equity base and, thus, reduce the likelihood that the firm will have to raise external equity at a later date to fund future real-asset investments.

When establishing a dividend policy, one size does not fit all. Some firms produce a lot of cash but have limited investment opportunities—this is true for firms in profitable, but mature, industries where few opportunities for growth exist. Such firms typically distribute a large percentage of their cash to shareholders, thereby attracting investment clienteles that prefer high dividends. Other firms generate little or no excess cash but have many good investment opportunities—this is often true of new firms in rapidly growing industries. These firms generally distribute little or no cash but enjoy rising earnings and stock prices, thereby attracting investors who prefer capital gains.

Dividend payouts and dividend yields for firms vary considerably, even within the healthcare sector. Generally, firms in stable, cash-producing industries pay relatively high dividends, whereas firms in unstable or rapidly growing industries pay lower dividends. In general, the healthcare sector has been buffeted by significant economic change in recent years. Other than the pharmaceutical industry, which has a 41 percent payout ratio, the other healthcare industries are below the 24 percent payout of the S&P 500.

For a given firm, the optimal payout ratio is a function of four factors: (1) stockholder's preferences for dividends versus capital gains, (2) the firm's investment opportunities, (3) its target capital structure, and (4) the availability and cost of external capital. The last three elements are combined in what we call the *residual dividend model*. Under this model, a firm follows these four steps when deciding its target payout ratio: (1) It determines the optimal capital budget; (2) it determines the amount of equity needed to finance that budget, given its target capital structure; (3) it uses retained earnings to meet equity requirements to the extent possible; and (4) it pays dividends only if more earnings are available than are needed to support the optimal level of new investment. The word "residual" implies leftover, and the residual policy implies that dividends are paid out of "leftover" earnings.

If a firm rigidly follows the residual dividend policy, then dividends paid in any given year can be expressed as follows:

Dividends = Net income − Retained earnings required for new investments

= Net income − (Target equity ratio × Total capital budget).

For example, if net income is $100, the target equity ratio is 60 percent (meaning a target debt ratio of 40 percent), and the firm plans to spend $50 on capital projects, then its dividends under the residual model would be $100 − (0.6 × $50) = $100 − $30 = $70. So, if the firm had $100 of earnings and a capital budget of $50, it could use $30 of the retained earnings plus $50 − $30 = $20 of new debt to finance the capital budget, and this would keep its capital structure on target. Note that the amount of equity needed to finance new investments might exceed the net income; in our example, this would happen if the capital budget were $200. In such instances, no dividends would be paid, and the firm would have to raise external equity if it wanted to maintain its target capital structure and undertake all desired projects.

Most firms have a target capital structure that calls for at least some debt, so new financing is done partly with debt and partly with equity. As long as the firm finances with the optimal mix of debt and equity, and provided it uses only internally generated equity (retained earnings), then the marginal cost of each new dollar of capital will be minimized. Internally generated equity is available for financing a certain amount of new investment, but beyond that amount, the firm must turn to more expensive new common stock. At the point where new stock must be sold, the cost of equity, and consequently the marginal cost of capital, rises.

Because investment opportunities and earnings will surely vary from year to year, strict adherence to the residual dividend policy would result in unstable dividends. One year the firm might pay zero dividends because it needed the money to finance good investment opportunities, but the next year it might pay a large dividend because investment opportunities were poor and it, therefore, did not need to retain many earnings. Similarly, fluctuating earnings could also lead to variable dividends, even if investment opportunities were stable. Therefore, following the residual dividend policy would almost certainly lead to fluctuating, unstable dividends. Thus, the residual policy would be optimal only if investors were not bothered by fluctuating dividends. However, because investors prefer stable, dependable dividends, the cost of equity would be higher, and the stock price lower, if the firm followed the residual model in a strict sense rather than attempted to stabilize its dividends over time. Therefore, many firms use this modified residual model:

- Estimate the earnings and investment opportunities, on average, over the next five or so years.
- Use this forecasted information to find the residual model average payout ratio during the planning period, which then becomes the firm's target long-run payout ratio.
- Although the target payout ratio is one input, many other factors are considered when setting each year's dollar dividend.

Firms with very stable operations can plan their dividends with a fairly high degree of confidence. Other firms, especially those in cyclical industries, have difficulty maintaining in bad times a dividend that is really too low in good times. Historically, such firms have set a very low "regular" dividend and then supplemented it with an "extra" dividend when times were good. In essence, such firms announced a low regular dividend that it was reasonably sure could be maintained, even in bad times, so stockholders could count on receiving this dividend under almost all conditions. Then when times were good and profits and cash flows were high, the firms paid a clearly designated extra dividend. Investors recognized that the extra dividend might not be maintained in the future, so they did not interpret them as a signal that the firms' earnings were going up permanently, nor did they take the elimination of an extra dividend as a negative signal. In recent years, however, many firms that were following this *low-regular-dividend-plus-extras policy* have replaced the "extras" with stock repurchases.

Earnings, Cash Flows, and Dividends

We normally think of earnings as being the primary determinant of dividends, but, in reality, cash flows are even more important. This point should be more or less intuitive because dividends clearly depend more on cash flows, which reflect the firm's ability to pay dividends, than on current earnings, which are heavily influenced by accounting practices and which do not necessarily reflect the ability to pay dividends. Because of this relationship, dividends (or better yet cash to investors) divided by cash flow is probably a better measure of payout than is dividends divided by net income. Still, historical precedent is to express the payout ratio on the basis of earnings.

Quarterly Versus Annual Dividends

Traditionally, U.S. investor-owned corporations have paid dividends quarterly. In fact, the term "quarterly dividend" is a permanent part of the financial lexicon—that is, up until recently. Over the last few years, firms have been throwing historical precedent out and changing to a single annual dividend. In 2000, Baxter International, a medical supplies firm, joined the ranks, which already included such blue-chip firms as Disney and McDonald's.

The reason for the move from quarterly to annual dividends is simple: It cuts costs. First, paying only one dividend instead of four saves the printing and distribution costs associated with three dividend payments. These savings can be considerable, especially for firms with large numbers of small shareholders, many of which send out over a million checks with each declared dividend. Second, there is a time value of money savings. To illustrate the concept, assume that about $370 billion was paid out as dividends in 2000. If this money were paid out annually, instead of quarterly, shareholders would lose the opportunity to invest the intra-year (quarterly) payments. At a 5 percent annual rate, the loss, which represents a savings to issuing firms, would total over $8 billion.

Although the incentive to switch to an annual dividend payment is strong, many firms are reluctant to switch because of shareholder resistance. When Baxter switched, there were many unhappy shareholders, but, according to a firm spokesman, "they were calmed by the $1.5 million in annual savings." Many corporate executives are predicting that a majority of publicly owned firms will pay annual dividends by the end of the decade.

Payment Procedures

In spite of the discussion in the previous section, dividends today typically are paid quarterly. For example, HCA (then Columbia/HCA) paid $0.02 per quarter in 2000, for an annual dividend rate of $0.08. The actual payment procedure is as follows:

- **Declaration date.** On the *declaration date*—say, on November 9—the directors meet and declare the regular dividend, issuing a statement similar to the following: "On November 9, 2000, the directors of HCA met and declared the regular quarterly dividend of 2 cents per share, payable to holders of record on December 11, payment to be made on January 4, 2001." For accounting purposes, the declared dividend becomes an actual liability on the declaration date. If a balance sheet were constructed, the total amount of the dividend would appear as a current liability, and retained earnings would be reduced by a like amount.
- **Holder-of-record date.** At the close of business on the *holder-of-record date*, December 11, the firm closes its stock transfer books and makes up a list of shareholders as of that date. If HCA is notified of the sale before 5 p.m. on December 11, then the new owner receives the dividend. However, if notification is received on or after December 12, the previous owner gets the dividend check.
- **Ex-dividend date.** Suppose Jean Buyer buys 100 shares of stock from John Seller on December 7. Will the firm be notified of the transfer in time to list Buyer as the new owner and, thus, pay the dividend to her? To avoid conflict, the securities industry has set up a convention under which the right to the dividend remains with the stock until four business days prior to the holder-of-record date; on the fourth day before that date, the right to the dividend no longer goes with the shares. The date when the right to the dividend leaves the stock is called the *ex-dividend date*. In our example, the ex-dividend date is four business days prior to December 11, or December 5 (December 9 and 10 are nonbusiness days). Therefore, if Buyer is to receive the dividend, she must buy the stock on or before December 4. If she buys it on December 5 or later, Seller will receive the dividend because he will be the official holder of record. Although the HCA dividend is only $0.02 per share, the ex-dividend date is still important. Barring fluctuations in the stock market, one would normally expect the price of the stock to drop by approximately the amount of the dividend on the ex-dividend date.[5]
- **Payment date.** The firm actually mails the checks to the holders of record on January 4, the *payment date*.

Changing Dividend Policies

From our previous discussion, it is obvious that firms should try to establish a rational dividend policy and then stick with it. Dividend policy can be changed, but this change can cause problems because such changes can inconvenience the firm's existing stockholders, send unintended signals, and convey the impression of dividend instability, all of which can have negative implications for stock prices. Still, economic circumstances do change, and, occasionally, such changes dictate that a firm should alter its dividend policy.

In general, when a change in dividend policy occurs, it is essential that the firm fully inform stockholders of the rationale for the change. Good communications between the firm and investors can mitigate the potential negative consequences of the change. This point is especially critical when dividends are being cut or omitted. Although there may be "good and just" reasons for the change, many stock investors still believe the old adage—"like diamonds, dividends are forever."

1. Explain the logic of the residual dividend model and why it is more likely to be used to establish a long-run payout target than to set the actual year-by-year dollar payment.
2. Which are more critical to the dividend decision, earnings or cash flow? Explain your answer.
3. Why are many firms changing from quarterly to annual dividend payments?
4. Explain the procedures used to actually pay the dividend.
5. Why do firms change their dividend policies and what is the best strategy in such situations?

Summary of the Factors Influencing Dividend Policy

In earlier sections, we described both the major theories of investor preference and some issues concerning the effects of dividend policy on the value of a firm. We also discussed the residual dividend model for setting a firm's long-run target payout ratio. In this section, we discuss several other factors that affect the dividend decision. These factors may be grouped into three broad categories: (1) constraints on dividend payments, (2) investment opportunities, and (3) availability and cost of alternative sources of capital. Each of these categories has several subparts, which we discuss in the following paragraphs.

Constraints

- **Bond indentures.** Debt contracts often contain restrictive covenants that limit dividend payments to earnings generated after the loan was granted. Also, debt contracts often stipulate that no dividends can be paid unless the current ratio, times-interest-earned ratio, or some other measure of financial soundness meet stated minimums.
- **Preferred stock restrictions.** Typically, common dividends cannot be paid if the firm has omitted a dividend on any preferred stock that had been issued. Any preferred arrearages must be satisfied before common dividends can be resumed.
- **Impairment of capital rule.** Dividend payments cannot exceed the amount shown in the retained earnings account on the balance sheet. This legal restriction, known as the *impairment of capital rule*, is designed to

protect creditors. Without the rule, a firm that is in trouble could sell off most of its assets and distribute the proceeds to stockholders, leaving the creditors holding an "empty bag." (*Liquidating dividends* can be paid out of capital, but they must be indicated as such, and they must not reduce capital below the limits stated in debt contracts.)

- **Availability of cash.** Cash dividends can be paid only with cash. Thus, a shortage of cash in the bank can restrict dividend payments. However, the ability to borrow can offset this factor.

- **Penalty tax on improperly accumulated earnings.** To prevent wealthy individuals from using corporations to avoid personal taxes, the tax code provides for a special surtax on improperly accumulated income. Thus, if the IRS can demonstrate that a firm's dividend payout ratio is being deliberately held down to help its stockholders avoid personal taxes, the firm is subject to heavy penalties. This factor is relevant only to privately owned firms—we have never heard of a publicly owned firm being accused of improperly accumulating earnings.

Investment Opportunities

- **Number of profitable investment opportunities.** If a firm typically has a large number of profitable investment opportunities, this will tend to produce a low target payout ratio, and vice versa if the firm's profitable investment opportunities are few in number.

- **Possibility of accelerating or delaying projects.** The ability to accelerate or to postpone projects will permit a firm to adhere more closely to a stable dividend policy.

Alternative Sources of Capital

- **Cost of selling new stock.** If a firm needs to finance a given level of investment, it can obtain equity by retaining earnings or by issuing new common stock. If flotation costs (which include both issuance costs and any negative signaling effects of a stock offering) are high, the cost of new equity will be well above the cost of retained earnings, making it better to set a low payout ratio and to finance through retention rather than through sale of new common stock. On the other hand, a high dividend payout ratio is more feasible for a firm whose flotation costs are low. Flotation costs differ among firms; for example, the flotation percentage is generally higher for small firms, so they tend to set low payout ratios.

- **Ability to substitute debt for equity.** A firm can finance a given level of investment with either debt or equity. As noted above, low stock flotation costs permit a more flexible dividend policy because equity can be raised either by retaining earnings or by selling new stock. A similar situation holds for debt policy: if the firm can adjust its debt ratio without raising costs sharply, it can pay the expected dividend, even if earnings fluctuate, by using a variable debt ratio.

• **Control.** If management is concerned about maintaining control, it may be reluctant to sell new stock, and hence the firm may retain more earnings than it otherwise would. However, if stockholders want higher dividends and a proxy fight looms, then the dividend will be increased.

It should be apparent from our discussion that dividend policy decisions are truly exercises in informed judgment, not decisions based on quantified rules. Even so, to make rational dividend decisions, financial managers must take into account all the points discussed in the preceding sections.

1. What constraints affect dividend policy?
2. How do investment opportunities affect dividend policy?
3. How do the availability and cost of outside capital affect dividend policy?

Self-Test Questions

The Dividend Policy Decision Process

In many ways, our discussion of dividend policy parallels our discussion of capital structure: We have presented the relevant theories and issues, and we have listed some additional factors that influence dividend policy, but we have not come up with any hard-and-fast guidelines that managers can follow. Dividend policy decisions are exercises in informed judgment, not decisions based on a precise mathematical model. In practice, dividend policy is not an independent decision—the dividend decision is made jointly with capital structure and capital budgeting decisions. The underlying reason for this joint decision process is asymmetric information, which influences managerial actions in two ways:

1. In general, managers do not want to issue new common stock. First, new common stock involves issuance costs—commissions, fees, and so on—and those costs can be avoided by using retained earnings to finance the firm's equity needs. Also, asymmetric information causes investors to view new common stock issues as negative signals and, thus, lowers expectations regarding the firm's future prospects. The end result is that the announcement of a new stock issue usually leads to a decrease in the stock price. Considering the total costs involved, including both issuance and asymmetric information costs, managers strongly prefer to use retained earnings as their primary source of new equity.
2. Dividend changes provide signals about managers' beliefs as to their firms' future prospects. Thus, dividend reductions, or worse yet, omissions, generally have a significant negative effect on a firm's stock price. Because managers recognize this, they try to set dollar dividends low enough so that there is only a remote chance that the dividend will have to be reduced in the future. Of course, unexpectedly large dividend increases can be used to provide positive signals.

The effects of asymmetric information suggest that, to the extent possible, managers should avoid both new common stock sales and dividend cuts because both actions tend to lower stock prices. Thus, in setting dividend policy, managers should begin by considering the firm's future investment opportunities relative to its projected internal sources of funds. The firm's target capital structure also plays a part, but because the optimal capital structure is a range, firms can vary their actual capital structures somewhat from year to year. Because it is best to avoid issuing new common stock, the target long-term payout ratio should be designed to permit the firm to meet all of its equity capital requirements with retained earnings. In effect, managers should use the residual dividend model to set dividends, but in a long-term framework. Finally, the current dollar dividend should be set so that there is an extremely low probability that the dividend, once set, will ever have to be lowered or omitted.

Of course, the dividend decision is made during the planning process, so there is uncertainty about future investment opportunities and operating cash flows. Thus, the actual payout ratio in any year will probably be above or below the firm's long-range target. However, the dollar dividend should be maintained, or increased as planned, unless the firm's financial condition deteriorates to the point where the planned policy simply cannot be maintained or the basic nature of the business changes. A steady or increasing stream of dividends over the long run signals that the firm's financial condition is under control. Furthermore, investor uncertainty is decreased by stable dividends, so a steady dividend stream reduces the negative effect of a new stock issue should one become absolutely necessary.

In general, firms with superior investment opportunities should set lower payouts, and hence retain more earnings, than firms with poor investment opportunities. The degree of uncertainty also influences the decision. If there is a great deal of uncertainty in the cash flow, then it is best to be conservative and to set a lower current dollar dividend. Also, firms with investment opportunities that can be delayed can afford to set a higher dollar dividend because, in times of stress, investments can be postponed for a year or two, which increases the cash available for dividends. Finally, firms whose cost of capital is largely unaffected by changes in the debt ratio can also afford to set a higher payout ratio because they can, in times of stress, more easily issue additional debt to maintain the capital budgeting program without having to cut dividends or issue stock.

Firms have only one opportunity to set the dividend payment from scratch. Therefore, today's dividend decisions are constrained by policies that were set in the past, hence setting a policy for the next five years necessarily begins with a review of the current situation.

Although we have outlined a rational process for managers to use when setting their firms' dividend policies, dividend policy still remains one of the most judgmental decisions that firms must make. For this reason, dividend policy is always set by the board of directors—the financial staff analyzes the situation and makes a recommendation, but the board makes the final decision.[6]

1. Describe the dividend policy decision process. Be sure to discuss all the factors that influence the decision.

Self-Test Question

Stock Dividends and Stock Splits

Stock dividends and stock splits are related to the firm's cash dividend policy. The rationale for stock dividends and splits can best be explained through an example. We will use Porter Surgical, a $700 million medical equipment manufacturer, for this purpose. Since its inception, Porter's markets have been expanding, and the firm has enjoyed strong sales and earnings growth. Some of its earnings have been paid out in cash dividends, but most have been retained, causing earnings per share and stock price to grow. Because the firm had only a few million shares outstanding, each of Porter's shares had a very high stock price, so many potential investors could not afford to buy a *round lot* of 100 shares. This high price limited the demand for the stock and, thus, kept the total market value of the firm below what it would have been if more shares, at a lower price, had been outstanding. To correct this situation, Porter "split its stock," as described in the next section.

Stock Splits

Although there is little empirical evidence to support the contention, there is nevertheless a widespread belief in financial circles that an *optimal price range* exists for stocks. "Optimal" means that if the price is within this range, the price/earnings ratio, hence the firm's value, will be maximized. Many observers, including Porter's management, believe that the best range for most stocks is from $20 to $80 per share. Accordingly, if the price of Porter's stock rose to $80, management would probably declare a two-for-one *stock split*, which would double the number of shares outstanding, halve the earnings and dividends per share, and thereby lower the stock price. Each stockholder would have more shares, but each share would be worth less. If the post-split price were $40, Porter's stockholders would be exactly as well off as they were before the split. However, if the stock price were to stabilize above $40, stockholders would be better off. Stock splits can be of any size; for example, the stock could be split two-for-one, three-for-one, one and a half-for-one, or in any other way.[7]

Stock Dividends

Stock dividends are similar to stock splits in that they "divide the pie into smaller slices" without affecting the fundamental position of the current stockholders. On a 5 percent stock dividend, the holder of 100 shares would receive an additional five shares (without cost); on a 20 percent stock dividend, the same holder would receive 20 new shares; and so on. Again, the total number of shares is increased, so earnings, dividends, and price per share all decline.

If a firm wants to reduce the price of its stock, should it use a stock split or a stock dividend? Stock splits are generally used after a sharp price run-up to produce a large price reduction. Stock dividends used on a regular annual basis will keep the stock price more or less constrained. For example, if a firm's earnings and dividends were growing at about 10 percent per year, its stock price would tend to go up at about that same rate, and it would soon be outside the desired trading range. A 10 percent annual stock dividend would maintain the stock price within the optimal trading range. Note, though, that small stock dividends create bookkeeping problems and unnecessary expenses, so firms today use stock splits far more often than stock dividends.

Price Effects

If a firm splits its stock or declares a stock dividend, will this increase the market value of its stock? Several empirical studies have sought to answer this question, and here is a summary of their findings.

- On average, the price of a firm's stock rises shortly after it announces a stock split or dividend.
- However, these price increases probably result from the fact that investors take stock splits/dividends as signals of higher future earnings and dividends. Because only firms whose managers are optimistic about the future tend to split their stocks, the announcement of a stock split is taken as a signal that earnings and cash dividends are likely to rise, which then causes the stock price to rise.
- However, if the firm does not announce an increase in earnings and dividends within a few months of the stock split or dividend, then its stock price will drop back to the earlier level.
- As we noted earlier, brokerage commissions are generally higher in percentage terms on lower-priced stocks. This means that it is more expensive to trade low-priced than high-priced stocks, and this, in turn, means that stock splits may reduce the liquidity of a firm's shares. This particular piece of evidence suggests that stock splits or dividends might actually be harmful, although a lower price does mean that more investors can afford to trade in round lots (100 shares), which carry lower commissions than do odd lots (less than 100 shares).

What do we conclude from all this? From a pure economic standpoint, stock dividends and splits are just additional pieces of paper that do not themselves create value. They can be likened to a story about Yogi Berra ordering pizza. When the counterman asked him whether he wanted the pizza cut into six or eight pieces, he reportedly said, "Make it eight, I'm feeling hungry tonight."

In spite of the lack of inherent value in stock splits and dividends, they do provide management with a relatively low-cost way of signaling that the firm's prospects look good. Furthermore, we should note that since few large, publicly owned stocks sell at prices above several hundred dollars, we simply do not know what the effect would be if highly successful firms had never split their stocks, and consequently had sold at prices in the thousands or even tens of thousands of dollars. All in all, it probably makes sense to employ stock splits when a firm's prospects are favorable, especially if the price of its stock has gone beyond the normal trading range.[8]

1. What are stock dividends and stock splits?
2. What impact do stock dividends and splits have on stock prices? Why?
3. In what situations should managers consider the use of stock dividends?
4. In what situations should managers consider the use of stock splits?

Self-Test
Questions

Stock Repurchases

Several years ago, a *Fortune* article entitled, "Beating the Market by Buying Back Stock" discussed the fact that during a one-year period, more than 600 major corporations repurchased significant amounts of their own stock. It also gave illustrations of some specific firms' repurchase programs and their effects on stock prices. The article's conclusion was that "buy-backs have made a mint for shareholders who stay with the firms carrying them out." Since then, research on *stock repurchases* has shown that the dramatic gains to stockholders trumpeted in the article are not universal. Still, it is clear that stock repurchases are now playing a much more important role in how firms distribute earnings to shareholders. Indeed, in the last few years 800 firms have announced stock repurchase programs, and $50 billion of repurchases were announced in the first two months of 2000 alone.

To illustrate the concept, consider HCA. We previously indicated that the firm is paying a quarterly dividend of 2 cents. If one considers only cash dividends, it appears that the payout is much too low for a firm whose "rightsizing" has resulted in the recent sale of over 100 hospitals. However, HCA announced in late 1999 that it would repurchase up to $1 billion of its common stock. With a total annual dividend of less than $50 million, it would take 20 years of cash dividends to return to stockholders the amount stated in the repurchase announcement.

In the remainder of this section, we explain what a stock repurchase is, how it is carried out, and how managers should analyze a possible repurchase program.

Types of Repurchases

There are two principal types of repurchases: (1) *non-capital-structure related*, where the firm has cash from operations available for distribution to its stockholders, and it distributes this cash by repurchasing shares rather than by paying cash dividends; and (2) *capital-structure related*, where the firm concludes that its capital structure is too heavily weighted with equity, and then it sells debt and uses the proceeds to buy back its stock. Stock that has been repurchased by a firm is called *treasury stock*. If some of the outstanding stock is repurchased, fewer shares will remain outstanding. Assuming that the repurchase does not adversely affect the firm's future earnings, the earnings per share on the remaining shares will increase, presumably resulting in a higher stock price. As a result, capital gains are substituted for dividends.

Repurchase Methods

Stock repurchases are generally made in one of three ways:

1. A publicly owned firm can simply buy its own stock through a broker on the open market.
2. The firm can make a tender offer, under which it permits stockholders to tender (send in) their shares to the firm in exchange for a specified price per share. In this case, it generally indicates that it will buy up to a specified number of shares within a particular time period (usually about two weeks); if more shares are tendered than the firm wishes to purchase, purchases may be made on a pro rata basis.
3. The firm can purchase a block of shares from one large holder on a negotiated basis. If a negotiated purchase is employed, care must be taken to ensure that this one stockholder does not receive preferential treatment over other stockholders or that any preference given can be justified by "sound business reasons." Historically, this method has been used to pay *greenmail*, which is the act of buying the stock owned by a potential "raider" who had expressed interest in taking over the firm. However, such deals, which often were at prices well above the current market price, were followed by a spate of lawsuits that have dampened managerial enthusiasm for the practice.

The Effects of Stock Repurchases

The effects of a repurchase can be illustrated with data on Atlanta Diabetes Counselors (ADC), Inc. The firm expects to earn $4.4 million in 2001, and 50 percent of this amount, or $2.2 million, has been allocated for distribution to common shareholders. There are 1.1 million shares outstanding, and the market price is $20 a share. ADC believes that it can either use the $2.2 million to repurchase 100,000 of its shares through a tender offer at $22 a share or pay a cash dividend of $2 a share.

The effect of a cash dividend is obvious—investors get $2 per share with no change in the number of shares outstanding. The effect of the repurchase can be analyzed in the following way:

$$\text{Current EPS} = \frac{\text{Total earnings}}{\text{Number of shares}} = \frac{\$4.4 \text{ million}}{1.1 \text{ million}} = \$4 \text{ per share.}$$

$$\text{P/E ratio} = \frac{\$20}{\$4} = 5.$$

EPS after repurchasing 100,000 shares

$$= \frac{\$4.4 \text{ million}}{1.0 \text{ million}} = \$4.40 \text{ per share.}$$

Expected market price after repurchase

$$= \text{P/E} \times \text{EPS} = 5 \times \$4.40 = \$22 \text{ per share.}$$

Note that this example proves that investors would receive the same before-tax benefits regardless of the distribution choice, either in the form of a $2 cash dividend or a $2 increase in the stock price. However, this result occurs because we assumed (1) that shares could be repurchased at exactly $22 a share and (2) that the P/E ratio would remain constant. If shares could be bought for less than $22, the repurchase would be even better for remaining stockholders, but the reverse would hold if ADC had to pay more than $22 a share. Furthermore, the P/E ratio might change as a result of the repurchase, rising if investors viewed it favorably and falling if they viewed it unfavorably. Some factors that might affect P/E ratios are considered next.

Although it may appear that ADC's stockholders would be indifferent between the two distribution methods, there are clear advantages and disadvantages to stock repurchases, which we examine in the next sections.

Advantages of Repurchases

- Repurchase announcements are viewed as positive signals by investors because the repurchase is often motivated by management's belief that the firm's shares are undervalued.
- The stockholders have a choice when the firm distributes cash by repurchasing stock—they can sell or not sell. With a cash dividend, on the other hand, stockholders must accept a dividend payment and pay the tax. Thus, those stockholders who need cash can sell back some of their shares, while those who do not want additional cash can simply retain their stock. From a tax standpoint, a repurchase permits both types of stockholders to get what they want.
- A repurchase can remove a large block of stock that is "overhanging" the market and keeping the price per share down.
- Dividends are "sticky" in the short run because managers are reluctant to

raise the dividend if the increase cannot be maintained in the future—managers dislike cutting cash dividends because of the negative signal a cut gives. Thus, if the excess cash flow is thought to be only temporary, management may prefer to make the distribution in the form of a share repurchase rather than to declare an increased cash dividend that cannot be maintained.

• Firms can use the residual model to set a *target cash distribution* level, then divide the distribution into a *dividend component* and a *repurchase component*. The dividend payout ratio will be relatively low, but the dividend itself will be relatively secure, and it will grow as a result of the declining number of shares outstanding. The firm has more flexibility in adjusting the total distribution than it would if the entire distribution were in the form of cash dividends because repurchases can be varied from year to year without sending negative signals.

• Repurchases can be used to produce large-scale changes in capital structures. For example, several years ago Consolidated Healthcare repurchased $400 million of its common stock to increase its debt ratio. The repurchase was necessary because even if the firm financed its capital budget only with debt, it would still take several years to get the debt ratio up to the target level. With a repurchase, a capital structure change can be almost instantaneous.

• Many firms grant large numbers of stock options to employees. If these firms have repurchased stock, these shares can be reissued when options are exercised. This practice avoids the dilution that would occur if new shares were sold to cover exercised options.

Disadvantages of Repurchases

• Stockholders may view large repurchases as a signal that the firm has limited investment opportunities, and hence a sign of slow growth ahead.

• Stockholders may not be indifferent between dividends and capital gains, and the price of the stock might benefit more from cash dividends than from repurchases. Cash dividends are generally dependable, but repurchases are not.

• The selling stockholders may not be fully aware of all the implications of a repurchase, or they may not have all pertinent information about the corporation's present and future activities. However, firms generally announce repurchase programs before embarking on them to avoid potential stockholder suits.

• The corporation may pay too high a price for the repurchased stock, to the disadvantage of remaining stockholders. If its shares are not actively traded, and if the firm seeks to acquire a relatively large amount of its stock, then the price may be bid above its equilibrium level and then fall after the firm ceases its repurchase operations.

Conclusions on Stock Repurchases

When all the pros and cons on stock repurchases have been totaled, where do we stand? Our conclusions may be summarized as follows:

- Because of the lower capital gains tax rate and the deferred tax on capital gains, repurchases have a significant tax advantage over dividends as a way to distribute income to stockholders. This advantage is reinforced by the fact that repurchases provide cash to stockholders who want cash, but allow those who do not need current cash to delay its receipt. On the other hand, dividends are more dependable and are, thus, better suited for those who need a steady source of income.
- Because of signaling effects, firms should not vary their dividends—this would lower investors' confidence in a firm and adversely affect its cost of equity and its stock price. However, cash flows vary over time, as do investment opportunities, so the "proper" dividend in the residual model sense varies. To get around this problem, a firm can set its dividend at a level low enough to keep dividend payments from constraining operations and then use repurchases as needed to distribute excess cash. Such a procedure would provide regular, dependable dividends plus additional cash flow to those stockholders who want it.
- Repurchases are also useful when a firm wants to make a large shift in its capital structure within a short period of time, or when it wants to distribute cash from a one-time event such as the sale of a subsidiary.

Increases in the size and frequency of stock repurchases in recent years suggest that managers believe that the advantages outweigh the disadvantages.

Self-Test Questions

1. Explain how repurchases can (1) help stockholders hold down taxes and (2) help firms change their capital structures.
2. What is treasury stock?
3. What are three ways a firm can repurchase its stock?
4. What are some advantages and disadvantages of stock repurchases?
5. How can stock repurchases help a firm operate in accordance with the residual dividend model?

Key Concepts

Managers must make decisions regarding whether earnings should be returned to owners or retained for reinvestment in the firm. Here are this chapter's key concepts:

- *Dividend policy* involves three issues: (1) What fraction of earnings should be distributed, on average, over time?; (2) should the distribution be in the form of cash dividends or stock repurchases?; and (3) should the firm maintain a steady, stable dividend growth rate?

- The *optimal dividend policy* strikes a balance between current dividends and future growth to maximize the firm's stock price.
- Miller and Modigliani (MM) developed the *dividend irrelevance theory*, which holds that a firm's dividend policy has no effect on either the value of its stock or its cost of capital.
- The *bird-in-the-hand theory* holds that a firm's value will be maximized by a high dividend payout ratio because cash dividends are less risky than potential capital gains.
- The *tax preference theory* states that because long-term capital gains are subject to lower taxes than dividends, investors prefer to have firms retain earnings rather than pay them out as dividends.
- *Empirical tests* of the three theories have been inconclusive. Therefore, theory cannot tell corporate managers how a given dividend policy will affect stock prices and capital costs.
- Dividend policy should take account of the *information content of dividends (signaling)* and the *clientele effect* hypotheses. The information content effect relates to the fact that investors regard an unexpected dividend change as a signal of management's forecast of future earnings. The clientele effect suggests that a firm will attract investors who like the firm's dividend payout policy. Both factors should be considered by firms that are considering a change in dividend policy.
- In practice, most firms try to follow a policy of paying a *steadily increasing dividend*. This policy provides investors with stable, dependable income, and departures from it give investors signals about management's expectations for future earnings.
- Most firms use the *residual dividend model* to set the long-run target payout ratio at a level that will permit the firm to satisfy its equity requirements with retained earnings.
- *Legal constraints, investment opportunities, availability and cost of funds from other sources,* and *taxes* are also considered when firms establish dividend policies.
- A *stock split* increases the number of shares outstanding. In theory, splits should reduce the price per share in proportion to the increase in shares because splits merely "divide the pie into smaller slices." However, firms generally split their stocks only if (1) the price is quite high and (2) management thinks the future is bright. Therefore, stock splits often are taken as positive signals and, thus, boost stock prices.
- A *stock dividend* is a dividend paid in additional shares of stock rather than in cash. Both stock dividends and splits are used to keep stock prices within an "optimal" trading range.
- Under a *stock repurchase plan*, a firm buys back some of its outstanding stock, thereby decreasing the number of shares, which should increase both EPS and the stock price. Repurchases are useful for making major

changes in capital structure, as well as for distributing temporary excess cash.

This concludes our discussion of distributions to shareholders. In the next chapter, we discuss business valuation, mergers, and acquisitions.

Selected References

Baker, H. Kent, Aaron L. Phillips, and Gary E. Powell. 1995. "The Stock Distribution Puzzle: A Synthesis of the Literature on Stock Splits and Stock Dividends." *Financial Practice and Education* (Spring/Summer): 24–37.

Baker, H. Kent, Gail E. Farrelly, and Richard B. Edelman. 1985. "A Survey of Management Views on Dividend Policy." *Financial Management* (Autumn): 78–84.

Brealy, Richard A. 1983. "Does Dividend Policy Matter?" *Midland Corporate Finance Journal* (Spring): 17–25.

Healy, Paul M., and Krishna G. Palepu. 1989. "How Investors Interpret Changes in Corporate Financial Policy." *Journal of Applied Corporate Finance* (Fall): 59–64.

Miller, Merton H. 1987. "Behavioral Rationality in Finance: The Case of Dividends." *Midland Corporate Finance Journal* (Winter): 6–15.

Woolridge, J. Randall and Chinmoy Ghosh. 1985. "Dividend Cuts: Do They Always Signal Bad News?" *Midland Corporate Finance Journal* (Summer): 20–32.

Selected Web Sites

For a web site that contains links to various stories and papers concerning dividend policy, see *www.morevalue.com/themes/dividend.html.*

Notes

1. Although the ROE is leveraged up by the use of debt financing, so is the riskiness to the physician/owners. Because they can shelter the income of the business by giving themselves bonuses, there is no true economic advantage to the use of debt financing—the increase in ROE is exactly offset by the increase in riskiness. See Chapter 11 for a more complete discussion.

2. See Merton H. Miller and Franco Modigliani, "Dividend Policy, Growth, and the Valuation of Shares," *Journal of Business*, October 1961, 411–433.

3. See Myron J. Gordon, "Optimal Investment and Financing Policy," *Journal of Finance*, May 1963, 264–272; and John Lintner, "Dividends, Earnings, Leverage, Stock Prices, and the Supply of Capital to Corporations," *Review of Economics and Statistics*, August 1962, 243–269.

4. See Stephen A. Ross, "The Determination of Financial Structure: The Incentive-Signaling Approach," *The Bell Journal of Economics*, Spring 1977, 23–40.

5. In reality, tax effects cause the price decline on average to be less than the full amount of the dividend.

6. Before we close our discussion of dividend policy, note that many businesses have *dividend reinvestment plans (DRIPs)*, which allow stockholders to buy more stock instead of receiving a cash dividend. DRIPs are discussed in Chapter 7.

7. *Reverse splits*, which reduce the number of shares outstanding, can even be used. For example, a firm whose stock sells for $5 might employ a one-for-five reverse split, exchanging one new share for five old ones and raising the value of the shares to about $25, which is within the optimal price range.

8. It is interesting to note that Berkshire Hathaway, which is controlled by billionaire Warren Buffett, one of the most successful financiers of the twentieth century, has never had a stock split. In mid-2000, it was selling on the NYSE for $55,000 per share, but it had reached a high of $80,000 in March of 1999. However, in response to investment trusts that were being formed to sell fractional units of the stock, Buffett created a new class of Berkshire Hathaway stock (Class B) worth about one-thirtieth of a Class A (regular) share.

BUSINESS VALUATION, MERGERS, AND ACQUISITIONS

Learning Objectives

After studying this chapter, readers should be able to:

- Discuss the history of merger activity in the United States.
- Describe the most popular motives for mergers and make judgments regarding their validity.
- Explain both the discounted cash flow and market multiple approaches to business valuation.
- Discuss the unique problems that arise when small businesses are being valued and when not-for-profit businesses are acquired by investor-owned businesses.

Introduction

Most of the growth in health services organizations occurs through internal expansion, which takes place when a business's existing operations grow through normal capital budgeting activities. However, the most dramatic examples of growth result from mergers and acquisitions. For some purposes, it is necessary to distinguish between mergers and acquisitions, but those distinctions do not affect the fundamental business and financial considerations involved. Thus, we generally will refer to all combinations in which a single business unit is formed from two or more existing units as a *merger*. We will begin our discussion of mergers with some general background information. Later, we will focus on mergers in the health services industry, including a discussion of the factors that must be considered when investor-owned and not-for-profit firms merge. In addition, we will discuss business valuation, which is a key element in any merger analysis.

Level of Merger Activity

To better understand mergers, it is useful to review the level of merger activity in the United States, including activity in the health services industry.

Merger Waves

Five major *merger waves* have occurred in the United States. The first was in the late 1800s, when consolidations took place within the oil, steel, tobacco, and other basic industries. The second occurred in the 1920s, when the buoyant stock market helped promoters consolidate businesses in a number of industries including utilities, communications, and automobiles. The third was in the 1960s, when conglomerate mergers (mergers among unrelated firms) were the rage.

The fourth wave of mergers was the "merger mania" of the 1980s. This wave was fueled by many factors including (1) the relatively depressed condition of the stock market at the beginning of the decade (in early 1982, the Dow Jones Industrial Index was below its 1968 level); (2) the unprecedented level of inflation that existed during the 1970s and early 1980s, which increased the replacement value of firms' assets; (3) a political climate that fostered a more tolerant attitude toward mergers; (4) the general belief among major natural resource firms that it was cheaper to "buy reserves on Wall Street" than to explore and find them in the field; (5) the development of an active junk bond market, which helped acquirers obtain the capital needed to do the deals; and (6) the decline of the dollar, which made U.S. firms relatively cheap for foreign businesses to acquire, combined with huge U.S. trade deficits, which gave these businesses large pools of funds to invest in the United States.

The final merger wave began in 1992, and it is still going strong in 2000. The current wave is significantly different from the wave of the 1980s. Most 1980s mergers were primarily financial transactions in which acquirers were seeking to buy firms that were selling at less than their true long-run values as a result of poor temporary economic trends or management. If a firm could be better managed, if redundant assets could be sold, or if administrative or operating costs could be cut, then cash flows and stock price would rise. In the current merger wave, however, most mergers are strategic in nature—firms are merging to enable the consolidated enterprise to better position itself to compete in the future. Indeed, many of the recent mergers have involved businesses in the banking, computer, health services, media, pharmaceutical, and telecommunications industries, all of which are undergoing structural changes and intense competition.

Another major difference between mergers in the 1990s and those in the 1980s is the way in which they are financed and the form of payment to the acquired firms' stockholders. In the 1980s wave, cash was the preferred method of payment because a cash offer that was large enough could convince even the most reluctant shareholders to approve the deal, and this put great pressure on the managers of target firms. Moreover, the cash for the deal was generally obtained by borrowing, often with junk bonds, which gave the combined enterprise a heavy debt burden that left it vulnerable to economic downturns. In the current wave, the preferred method of payment has been the stock swap because (1) there are fewer lenders willing to supply debt for mergers; and (2) in strategic mergers, it is easier to convince shareholders and managers of target firms that the merger should take place, so stock swaps are easier to sell. Also, in a stock swap, managers of target firms are much more motivated to work for the common good of the new enterprise if a merger does take place. Even the cash mergers have tended to be different: In the 1980s, firms typically borrowed the cash needed, but in the 1990s, corporate cash flows have often been high enough to fund acquisitions internally, especially smaller ones.

Merger Activity in the Health Services Industry

Prior to the current wave, mergers in the health services industry were neither as frequent nor as large as mergers in some other industries. First, the health services industry, at least in its current form, is relatively new—not having really developed until after World War II. Second, the motivations that fueled the wave of the 1980s only partially applied to health services, so the industry was not one of the major participants in that wave, although there were some spectacular mergers between for-profit hospital chains. However, the current wave of mergers in the health services industry has been very strong, with 1997 setting the record for the greatest number of deals. Table 18.1 provides some feel for the current level of merger activity. Although not shown in the table, merger activity in the health services industry declined 11 percent in 1998 from its 1997 peak. Furthermore, activity has fallen off an additional 38 percent from 1998 to 1999.

Several factors have been suggested to account for the decrease in merger activity in the health services industry since 1997. First, the Balanced Budget Act of 1997 (BBA), which placed significant restrictions on the growth of Medicare reimbursement rates, has lessened the values of many health-care providers—primarily nursing home, rehabilitation, and home health care businesses. Second, the results of merger activity that occurred earlier in the

	1998		1999	
Sub-Industry	Number of Deals	Dollar Volume	Number of Deals	Dollar Volume
Behavioral	53	$ 1.1	44	$ 0.3
Home health care	83	0.4	62	0.1
Hospital	140	16.2	110	7.4
Laboratories	94	0.8	51	3.1
Long-term care	149	8.8	79	1.9
Managed care	61	5.1	66	1.8
Medical practices	263	1.7	135	1.5
Rehabilitation	46	0.1	28	0.7
Other*	254	31.2	138	4.2
Total	1,143	$65.4	713	$21.0

TABLE 18.1

Merger Activity in the Health Services Industry: 1998 and 1999 (billions of dollars)

*This category includes dental practices, outpatient surgery centers, and hospices, among others.
Source: The Health Care M&A Year in Review, March 2000. New Canaan, CT: Irving Levin Associates.

decade are now in, and the verdict on many types of mergers is not good. Specifically, physician management firms have not delivered the cost savings and profits as promised. Additionally, the backlash against managed care has slowed the merger activity in that sub-industry. Finally, many mergers designed to create large, integrated delivery systems have not lived up to their promise of managerial and operational efficiencies, and some of these mergers are now being undone. Although only time will tell if merger activity returns to previous levels as never ending changes in the healthcare environment materialize, merger activity in the health services industry will always be a fact of life.

To illustrate some healthcare mergers, consider the following deals completed in 1999:

- IASIS Healthcare Corporation, a privately held firm, acquired 10 hospitals from Tenet Healthcare for $520 million in cash and 5 hospitals from Paracelsus Healthcare for $280 million in cash. IASIS was formed in 1998 by senior healthcare executives, many of whom were from HCA, expressly to acquire and operate hospitals. Tenet and Paracelsus were willing to sell the hospitals because they did not fit well into their strategic plans.
- Quest Diagnostics acquired the clinical laboratory operations of SmithKline Beecham for $1.0 billion in cash and 12.6 million shares of common stock valued at $300 million. The acquisition allowed Quest Diagnostics, whose primary business is diagnostic testing, to double its market share. At the same time, shedding its diagnostic testing business allowed SmithKline Beecham to focus on its primary business—pharmaceuticals. The transaction gave SmithKline Beecham 29.5 percent ownership of Quest Diagnostics, as well as two seats on the board of directors, and further guaranteed that Quest Diagnostics will be the supplier of all diagnostic testing required in SmithKline Beecham's pharmaceutical trials.
- Anthem, Inc., acquired Blue Cross and Blue Shield of Colorado for $200 million in cash. As part of the transaction, $155 million went to the Caring for Colorado Foundation, which was specially formed to continue the charitable mission of the acquired business. Anthem is an Indiana-based mutual insurance firm that provides healthcare management and insurance products and services. (*Mutual firms* are taxable entities that are owned by policyholders rather than shareholders.) Anthem also is the Blue Cross and Blue Shield licensee for Indiana, Kentucky, Ohio, Connecticut, New Hampshire, and Nevada.
- Team Health, the country's largest provider of physician services to hospitals, was purchased from MedPartners for $335 million in cash. Because the managers of Team Health, with the backing of several private equity firms, bought the enterprise, the deal is classified as a *management buyout (MBO)*. Team Health contracts with hospitals to provide physician

services in such areas as emergency medicine, radiology, and anesthesia. The transaction helped MedPartners to follow its strategy of reinventing itself from a physician management firm to a pharmaceutical services firm called Caremark.

Self-Test Questions

1. What are the five major merger waves that have occurred in the United States?
2. What are the differences between the waves of the 1980s and the 1990s?
3. Are mergers in the health services industry rising or falling? Explain your answer.
4. Describe one recent merger in the health services industry.

Motives for Mergers: The Good, The Bad, and The Ugly

In the previous section, we presented some factors that fueled merger waves in the past. In this section, we take a more detailed look at some of the motives behind business mergers, along with some views regarding the validity of these motives.

Synergy

From an economic perspective, the best motivation for mergers is to increase the value of the combined enterprise. If Firms A and B merge to form Firm C, and if C's value exceeds that of A and B taken separately, then *synergy* is said to exist. When synergy drives a merger, value is created, and hence society benefits. Furthermore, such a merger can be beneficial to both A's and B's stockholders if the firms are investor-owned.

Synergistic effects can arise from four sources:

1. **Operating economies.** Operating economies result from economies of scale in management, marketing, contracting, operations, or distribution, including mergers that better position a business strategically.
2. **Financial economies.** Financial economies can result in lower transactions costs, access to additional capital markets, and better coverage by security analysts.
3. **Differential efficiency.** When differential efficiency is involved, inefficient management is replaced by a better one, which results in the business's assets being used more productively.
4. **Increased market power.** Increased market power (reduced competition) can create synergistic effects by increasing the contracting clout of the enterprise.

Operating and financial economies are socially desirable, as are mergers that increase managerial efficiency. To some extent, increased market power can also be beneficial to society, such as the contracting savings that result when major purchasers buy healthcare services. However, too much market power can result in monopoly or monopsony power, which can be harmful to society, and hence is both undesirable and illegal.[1]

Availability of Excess Cash

Mergers are an easy, perhaps too easy, way for managers to get rid of excess cash. If a business has a shortage of internal investment opportunities compared with its cash flow, it could (1) increase its dividend or repurchase stock if investor-owned, (2) invest in marketable securities, or (3) purchase another business. Marketable securities often provide a good temporary parking place for money, but, generally, the rate of return on such securities is less than the return on real-asset investments.

Although there is nothing inherently wrong with using excess cash to buy other firms, the acquisition must create value to be economically worthwhile. Just making a firm larger may benefit managers, but it does not necessarily benefit stockholders or society at large. If the return on a potential acquisition is not as high as the opportunity cost of the capital used, then the capital should be used for other purposes. If the business is investor-owned, the capital should be returned to the firm's investors, while if the firm is not-for-profit, the capital should be used to retire debt or invested temporarily in securities until better uses can be found.

Purchase of Assets at Below Replacement Cost

Sometimes a business will be touted as a possible acquisition candidate because the cost of replacing its assets is considerably higher than its market value. For example, suppose that a small, rural hospital can be acquired for $5 million, while the cost to construct a similar hospital from the ground up is $10 million. There might be a strong temptation to say that the hospital is a "good buy" because it can be bought for less than its replacement value.

However, the true value of any business should be based on its earning power, which sets the economic value of its assets. The real question, then, is not whether the hospital can be acquired for less than its replacement cost, but rather whether it can be acquired for less than its *economic value*, which is a function of the cash flows that the hospital is expected to produce in the future. If the rural hospital's earning power gives it a value of $7 million, then it is a good buy at $5 million, but this conclusion is based on economic, not replacement, value.

Diversification

Managers often claim that diversification into other lines of business is a reason for mergers. They contend that diversification helps to stabilize the business's earnings stream, and thus benefits its owners. Stabilization of earnings is certainly beneficial to managers, employees, suppliers, customers, and other stakeholders, but its value is less certain from the standpoint of stockholders. If a stockholder is worried about the variability of a firm's earnings, he or she could diversify more easily than could the firm. Why should Firms A and B merge to stabilize earnings when a stockholder in Firm A could sell half of his or her stock in A and use the proceeds to purchase stock in Firm B? Stockholders can create diversification more easily than can the firm.

Also, if a stockholder is concerned about the relative performance of different industry segments, he or she can solve the problem more easily through portfolio diversification than can managers through mergers. For example, assume that a stockholder who holds primarily hospital stocks is concerned that the increased purchasing power of managed care plans will erode hospital profits, and hence value, over time. It is easier for the stockholder to purchase a managed care company's stock than it is for hospitals to diversify into managed care.

Of course, there are some situations where mergers for diversification do make sense from a stockholder's perspective. For example, if you were the owner/manager of a closely held business, it might be nearly impossible for you to sell part of your ownership interest to diversify because this would dilute your ownership and perhaps also generate a large capital gains tax liability. In this case, a diversification merger might well be the best way to achieve personal diversification. Also, as mentioned earlier, diversification mergers that better position businesses to deal with future events are worthwhile because such mergers can create operating synergies.

Even though diversification, without synergy, does not benefit shareholders directly, it clearly benefits a firm's other stakeholders. Thus, diversification-motivated mergers can be beneficial to not-for-profit businesses. Furthermore, stockholders can obtain indirect benefits from diversification because making the firm less risky to managers, creditors, suppliers, customers, and the like could have positive implications for the owners of the business.

Personal Incentives

Economists like to think that business decisions are based solely on economic considerations. However, there can be no question that some business decisions are based more on managers' personal motivations than on economic analyses. Many people, business leaders included, like power, and more power is attached to running a larger business than a smaller one. Obviously, no executive would ever admit that his or her ego was the primary reason behind a merger, but knowledgeable observers are convinced that egos do play a prominent role in many mergers. It has also been observed that executive salaries, prestige, and perquisites are highly correlated with the firm's size— the bigger the firm, the higher the executive benefits. This factor could also play a role in the aggressive acquisition programs of some corporations.

Managers' personal incentives as a basis for mergers constitute another example of the *agency problem*. Of course, there is nothing wrong with executives feeling good about increasing the size of their firms, or with their getting a better compensation package as a result of growth through mergers, provided that the mergers make economic sense.

Self-Test Questions
1. Define synergy. Is synergy a valid rationale for mergers?
2. Describe several situations that might produce synergistic gains within the health services industry.
3. Suppose your firm could purchase another firm for only half of its replacement value. Would this be sufficient justification for the acquisition?
4. Discuss the merits of diversification as a rationale for mergers.
5. Can managers' personal incentives motivate mergers? Explain your answer.

Types of Mergers

Economists have traditionally classified mergers into three primary categories:

1. **Horizontal.** A *horizontal merger* occurs when one firm combines with another in its line of business; for example, when one hospital acquires another or one home health care business merges with a second. The merger of Columbia/HCA Healthcare and Healthtrust was a horizontal merger because both firms were in the hospital industry.
2. **Vertical.** A *vertical merger* occurs when a firm merges with a supplier or when one type of provider acquires another. An example of a vertical merger is a drug manufacturer's acquisition of a pharmaceutical distribution firm, such as Eli Lilly's acquisition of PCS Health Systems. Another example is the acquisition of medical practices and home health care businesses by hospitals.
3. **Conglomerate.** A *conglomerate merger* occurs when unrelated enterprises combine. Because most health services organizations are in related business lines, mergers between such firms are rarely classified as conglomerate.

Operating economies, and anticompetitive effects, are, at least partially, dependent on the type of merger involved. Vertical and horizontal mergers generally provide the greatest synergistic operating benefits, but they are also the ones most likely to be attacked by federal or state authorities as anticompetitive. In any event, it is useful to think of these economic classifications when analyzing the feasibility of a prospective merger.

Self-Test Questions
1. What are the three primary economic classifications of mergers?
2. Briefly, describe the characteristics of each classification.

Hostile Versus Friendly Takeovers

In the vast majority of merger situations, a firm (the *acquirer*) simply decides to buy another firm (the *target*), negotiates a price with the target firm's management, and then acquires the firm. Occasionally, the acquired firm will initiate the action, but it is much more common for a firm to seek acquisitions than to seek to be acquired.

Once an acquiring firm has identified a possible target it must (1) establish a suitable price, or range of prices, and (2) tentatively set the terms of payment: Will it offer cash, its own common stock, bonds, or a mix of securities? Next, the acquiring firm's managers must decide how to approach the target firm's managers. If the acquirer has reason to believe that the target's management will support the merger, then it will simply propose a merger and try to work out suitable terms. If an agreement is reached, then the two management groups will issue statements indicating that they approve the merger and, if the firms are investor-owned, recommend that stockholders agree to the merger. Generally, the stockholders of acquiring firms must merely vote to approve the merger, but the stockholders of target firms are asked to *tender,* or send in, their shares to a designated financial institution, along with a signed power of attorney that transfers ownership of the shares to the acquiring firm. The target firm's stockholders then receive the specified payment, be it common stock of the acquiring firm (in which case, the target firm's stockholders become stockholders of the acquiring firm), cash, bonds, or some mix of cash and securities. This type of merger is called a *friendly merger*, or a *friendly tender offer*.

The acquisition of HCA (Hospital Corporation of America) by Columbia Healthcare typifies a friendly merger. First, the boards of directors of the two firms announced that HCA had agreed to be acquired by Columbia in a stock-swap transaction. (HCA stockholders received 1.05 shares of Columbia stock for each share held.) The merger was approved by shareholders of both firms and by the Justice Department, and then the acquisition was completed. Richard Scott, Columbia's CEO, said that the merger would provide Columbia with broader opportunities to achieve economies of scale and increased market share in selected markets, which would enable it to negotiate better contracts with managed care organizations. In addition, operating economies would be achieved in markets where Columbia and HCA hospitals provided duplicative services. Of course, in the end, the results of the Columbia/HCA deal fell far short of expectations. Size, government probes, and prosecutions for fraud all had negative impacts on the firm. Today, the renamed firm, HCA—The Healthcare Company, is much smaller and more focused than Columbia/HCA was at its zenith.

Often, however, the target firm's management resists the merger. Perhaps the managers feel that the price offered for the stock is too low, or perhaps they simply want to retain their autonomy. In either case, the acquiring firm's offer is said to be *hostile* rather than friendly, and the acquiring firm must make a direct appeal to the target firm's stockholders. In a *hostile merger*, the acquiring firm will again make a tender offer, and again it will ask the stockholders of the target firm to tender their shares in exchange for the offered price. This time, though, the target firm's managers will urge stockholders not to tender their shares, generally stating that the price offered (cash, bonds, or stocks in the acquiring firm) is too low.

Although many hostile takeover bids fail, most eventually succeed. It is very difficult to defend against a hostile takeover attempt if the bidder has a large amount of resources that it is willing to spend on the battle. In such situations, the acquiring firm can offer enough cash to shareholders to overcome even the most-adamant managerial resistance.

Self-Test Questions

1. What is the difference between a hostile and a friendly merger?
2. Describe the mechanics of a typical friendly takeover and of a typical hostile takeover.

Merger Regulation

Merger regulation falls into two broad categories: (1) regulation of the procedures that acquiring firms must follow in making hostile bids and (2) antitrust regulation to ensure that mergers do not lead to monopoly power.

Bid Procedure Regulation

Prior to the mid-1960s, friendly acquisitions generally took place through simple exchange-of-stock mergers, and the *proxy fight* was the primary weapon used in a hostile control battle. (In a proxy fight, a dissident group attempts to gain control of the board of directors by placing alternative candidates on the proxy statement, who, if elected, would bring in other managers.) However, in the mid-1960s, corporate raiders began to operate differently. First, they noted that it took a long time to mount a proxy fight—they had to first request a list of the target firm's stockholders, then be refused, and finally get a court order forcing management to turn over the list. During that time, management could think through and then implement a strategy to fend off the raider. As a result, the instigator lost most proxy fights.

That lengthy process led raiders to turn from proxy fights to tender offers, which have a much shorter response time. For example, the stockholders of a firm whose stock was selling for $20 might be offered $25 per share and be given two weeks to accept. The raider, meanwhile, would have accumulated a substantial block of the shares in open market purchases, and additional shares might have been purchased by institutional friends of the raider who promised to tender their shares in exchange for the tip that a raid was to occur, even though such actions are illegal.

Faced with a well-planned raid, managers generally were overwhelmed and unable to plan a timely counter action. Although the stock might still be undervalued at the offered price in the opinion of management of the target firm, they simply did not have time to get this message across to stockholders, or to find a friendly competing bidder (called a *white knight*), or to take any other action. This situation was thought to be unfair, and as a result, Congress passed the Williams Act in 1968. This law had two main objectives: (1) to regulate the way in which acquiring firms can structure takeover offers and (2) to force acquiring firms to disclose more information about their offers. Basically, Congress wanted to put target managers in a better position to defend against hostile offers. Additionally, Congress believed that shareholders needed easy access to information about tender offers, including information on any securities that might be offered in lieu of cash, to make a rational decision.

The Williams Act placed the following three major restrictions on the activities of acquiring firms:

1. Acquirers must disclose their current holdings and future intentions within ten days of amassing at least 5 percent of a firm's stock, and they must disclose the source of the funds to be used in the acquisition.
2. The target firm's shareholders must be allowed at least 20 days to tender their shares—that is, the offer must be "open" for at least 20 days.
3. If the acquiring firm increases the offer price during the 20-day open period, all shareholders who tendered prior to the improved offer must receive the higher price.

In total, these restrictions were intended to reduce the ability of the acquiring firm to surprise management and to stampede target shareholders into accepting the offer. Prior to the Williams Act, offers were generally made on a first-come, first-served basis, and they were often accompanied by an implicit threat to lower the bid price after 50 percent of the shares were in hand. The legislation also gave target managers more time to mount a defense, and it gave rival bidders and white knights a chance to enter the fray, and thus help a target's stockholders obtain a better price.

Many states have also passed laws designed to protect firms in their states from hostile takeovers. At first, these laws focused on disclosure requirements, but by the late 1970s, several states had enacted takeover statutes so restrictive that they virtually precluded hostile takeovers. The constitutionality of state laws regulating takeover bids was challenged, and, at first, the state laws were struck down. But, in 1987, the U.S. Supreme Court upheld an Indiana law that radically changed the rules of the takeover game. Specifically, the Indiana law first defined "control shares" as enough shares to give an investor 20 percent of the vote, and it went on to state that when an investor buys control shares, those shares can be voted only after approval by a majority of "disinterested shareholders," which are defined as those who are neither officers nor inside directors of the firm, nor associates of the raider. Thus, a hostile acquirer that owned 20 percent of a target firm's shares could not force a takeover by gaining only 31 percent more, but rather would have to get 51 percent of the remaining 80 percent, or 41 percent more. The law also gives the buyer of control shares the right to insist that a shareholders' meeting be called within 50 days to decide whether the shares may be voted. The Indiana law dealt a major blow to raiders mainly because it slowed down the action. Delaware (the state in which most large firms are incorporated) later passed a similar bill, and so did many other states.

The new state laws also have some features that protect target stockholders from their own managers. Included are limits on the use of *golden parachutes*, which are lucrative compensation plans given to managers who lose their jobs as a result of takeovers, and the elimination of some types of *poison pills*, which are actions that managers of beleaguered firms can take to "kill off their own companies" to make them less attractive as targets. Because these types of state laws do not regulate tender offers per se, but govern the practices of firms in the state, they have thus far withstood all legal challenges.

Antitrust Regulation

Antitrust laws are intended to ensure that no organization attains enough market power to act as a monopoly. Such laws are based on the assumption that vigorous competition is the most effective way to ensure that consumers receive the best possible goods and services at the lowest cost. Although both federal and state laws are involved, two primary federal laws govern antitrust litigation: (1) the Sherman Act and (2) the Clayton Act. The *Sherman Act*, which dates back to 1890, prohibits contracts, conspiracies, and combinations that restrain trade. The *Clayton Act*, which was passed in 1914, prohibits all mergers, acquisitions, and joint ventures that may substantially lessen competition or allow creation of a monopoly. Merger laws contain notification clauses, which require firms involved in mergers to file certain information with federal and state agencies. These agencies then have 30 days to request additional information, approve the deal, or file suit to prevent the merger.

The two agencies that are charged with enforcing antitrust laws are (1) the *Federal Trade Commission (FTC)* and (2) the *Justice Department (JD)*. The FTC and JD classify potential antitrust violations into two categories: per se or rule of reason. *Per se* violations are those so unlikely to produce redeeming consumer benefits that they are immediately presumed to be illegal. Examples would be two hospitals agreeing to fix prices for certain procedures or agreeing to allocate specific markets. Actions that are not considered per se violations are evaluated using *rule of reason* analysis. Under rule of reason analysis, the FTC or JD must first determine whether a merger, or other combination, will enable a business to exercise market power in an anticompetitive manner. If so, the agency must then analyze whether the activity produces economic efficiencies that outweigh the anticompetitive effects. If the benefits outweigh the anticompetitive consequences, then the merger is allowed to take place.

Mergers within the health services industry generally fall into the rule of reason category, so a great deal of leeway exists in implementing the antitrust laws.

Clearly, the manner in which antitrust laws are enforced have a significant impact on merger activity, and hence on the future structure of the healthcare system. Before the 1990s, when fee-for-service insurance prevailed, physicians competed with one another for patients and hospitals competed for inpatient business. Today, however, the health services industry is being transformed by the growth of managed care, selective contracting, and vertical integration, which can create single organizations that are capable of providing both insurance and medical services. This transformation means that the FTC and JD have a difficult task in deciding how and when to apply antitrust laws. For example, two hospitals may merge to increase their bargaining power with insurers. If insurers now have fewer hospitals with which to negotiate, they cannot drive nearly as hard a bargain as before, so the merger may be anticompetitive. But, by merging, the hospitals may be able to reduce duplicative services and achieve other operating efficiencies that could lead to lower prices, which would be good for the insurers, and ultimately for consumers. The question then becomes which merger policy—vigorous or lax enforcement—should the FTC and JD follow to ensure good health policy?

With encouragement from the Clinton administration, in late 1994, the FTC and JD issued a joint policy statement containing "safety zone" guidelines. The statement describes circumstances under which mergers between hospitals, physician/network joint ventures, and other healthcare combinations will not be challenged. For example, a hospital merger will not be challenged if one or both of the hospitals has fewer than 100 beds, less than 40 patients per day, and is more than five-years old. Also, a physician network will not be contested if the network has no more than 20 percent of the physicians in a specialty in a particular geographical market. Although the guidelines have no effect on court decisions, and hence are no guarantee of legality, most industry representatives agree that the guidelines are helpful in establishing ground rules for future merger activity.

The consolidation of the health services industry has produced different views on how aggressively antitrust laws should be enforced. Physicians and hospitals tend to support lenient enforcement, arguing that they can achieve efficiencies only through mergers, acquisitions, and joint ventures. In particular, there is concern over the fact that an insurer or managed care plan can sign up, say, 70 percent of the physicians in a community, while antitrust laws prohibit even 40 or 50 percent of the physicians in a market from joining together to form their own network. According to an American Medical Association spokesman, "It doesn't make any sense to prevent doctors from getting together. They won't fix prices; they will be subject to market discipline from buyers." Insurers and managed care firms, however, tend to argue for strict enforcement of antitrust laws on the grounds that competition will produce maximum efficiency and innovation in the healthcare system.

States are also involved in the antitrust field, as both supporters and challengers of proposed mergers. For example, four states requested information concerning the impact of the Columbia/HCA–Healthtrust merger on individual markets, and state actions have caused hospital chains involved in large mergers to agree to sell off hospitals in particular markets to avoid antitrust actions. However, for the most part, states have been supportive of mergers in the health services industry. Many states have passed certificate of public advantage (COPA) laws, which grant immunity from federal antitrust laws. However, COPA laws generally require merging hospitals to return to the community any savings that result from the merger. Furthermore, hospitals must file annual reports with the state that prove that the specific COPA requirements set down for the merger are being met. Finally, there is always the possibility that the FTC or JD might challenge activities permitted by state immunity doctrine legislation because of lax supervision.

Self-Test Questions

1. Is there a need to regulate mergers? Explain your answer.
2. Do the states play a role in merger regulation, or is it all done at the federal level?
3. What is the difference between bidding regulation and antitrust regulation?
4. What two federal agencies enforce antitrust laws?
5. Do you think that enforcement of antitrust laws should be aggressive or lenient for health services industry mergers? Support your position.

Business Valuation

Businesses are valued for many purposes including acquisitions, business split-ups, and the assessment of taxes. Our discussion here focuses on valuation for acquisition purposes, but the basic principles of valuation are applicable for all purposes. A very key point to remember throughout this discussion is that **business valuation is a very imprecise process**. The best that can be done, even by professional *appraisers* who conduct these valuations on a regular basis, is to attain a reasonable valuation, as opposed to a precise one.

Many different approaches can be used to value businesses, but we will confine our discussion to the two most commonly used in the health services industry: (1) discounted cash flow and (2) market multiple. However, regardless of the valuation approach, it is crucial to recognize two factors that affect acquisition valuations. First, the business being valued typically will not continue to operate as a separate entity, but rather will become part of the acquiring business's portfolio of assets. Thus, any changes in ownership form or operations that occur as a result of the proposed merger that would affect the value of the target business must be considered in the analysis. Second, the goal of merger valuation is to set the value of the target business's equity, or ownership position, because a business is acquired from its owners, not from its creditors. Thus, although we use the phrase "business valuation," the ultimate goal is to value the ownership stake in the business rather than its total value.

Discounted Cash Flow Approach

The *discounted cash flow (DCF)* approach to valuing a business involves the application of classical capital budgeting procedures to an entire business rather than to a single project. To apply this approach, two key items are needed: (1) a set of pro forma statements that develop the incremental cash flows expected to result from the merger; and (2) a discount rate, or cost of capital, to apply to these cash flows. There are two primary methods of DCF analysis: (1) the free operating cash flow method and (2) the free cash flow to equityholders method. The methods differ in how the cash flows and discount rates are formulated.

The development of accurate postmerger cash flow forecasts is, by far, the most important step in the DCF approach. In a pure *financial merger*, in which no synergies are expected, the incremental postmerger cash flows are simply the expected cash flows of the target firm if it were to continue to operate independently. However, even in this situation, the cash flows for a healthcare provider may be quite difficult to forecast because the nature of the industry is changing so rapidly. In an *operational merger*, in which the operations are to be integrated, the acquiring firm usually intends to change the target's operations to get better results, so forecasting future cash flows is even more complex.

Table 18.2 contains projected generic cash flow statements for Doctors' Hospital, an investor-owned hospital that is being evaluated as a possible acquisition by United Health Services Corporation (UHSC), a large integrated healthcare business. These statements are formatted like income statements, but they (1) focus on cash flows rather than on accounting income and (2) do not have to conform with generally accepted accounting principles (GAAP). The projected data are for the postmerger period, so all synergistic effects have been included in the estimates. Doctors' currently uses 50 percent debt, and if it were acquired, UHSC would maintain Doctors' debt ratio at 50 percent.[2] Doctors' has a 30 percent marginal tax rate, but UHSC faces a 40 percent marginal federal-plus-state tax rate.

Line 1 of Table 18.2 contains the forecast for Doctors' net revenues, including both patient services revenue and other revenue. Note that all contractual allowances and other adjustments to charges, including collection delays, have been considered, so Line 1 represents actual cash revenues. Note also that any change in Doctors' stand-alone forecasted revenues resulting from synergies have been incorporated into the Line 1 amounts. Lines 2 and 3 contain the cash expense forecasts, while Line 4 lists depreciation, a noncash expense. Again, the expense amounts pertain to Doctors' subsidiary, assuming that the merger takes place, so savings due to operational efficiencies

TABLE 18.2
Doctors'
Hospital:
Projected
Cash Flow
Statements and
Retention
Estimates
(millions of
dollars)

	2001	2002	2003	2004	2005
1. Net revenues	$105.0	$126.0	$151.0	$174.0	$191.0
2. Patient services expenses	80.0	94.0	111.0	127.0	137.0
3. Other expenses	9.0	12.0	13.0	16.0	16.0
4. Depreciation	8.0	8.0	9.0	9.0	10.0
5. Earnings before interest and taxes (EBIT)	$ 8.0	$ 12.0	$ 18.0	$ 22.0	$ 28.0
6. Interest	4.0	4.0	5.0	5.0	6.0
7. Earnings before taxes (EBT)	$ 4.0	$ 8.0	$ 13.0	$ 17.0	$ 22.0
8. Taxes (40 percent)	1.6	3.2	5.2	6.8	8.8
9. Net profit	$ 2.4	$ 4.8	$ 7.8	$ 10.2	$ 13.2
10. Estimated retentions	$ 4.0	$ 4.0	$ 7.0	$ 9.0	$ 12.0

are included. Line 5, which is merely Line 1 minus Lines 2, 3, and 4, contains the earnings before interest and taxes (EBIT) projection for each year.

In the cash flow forecasts, interest expense is shown on Line 6. Note that any required principal repayments must be included on Line 6. Also, the interest on any new debt expected to be issued to help fund future growth must be included here. Line 7 contains the earnings before taxes (EBT), and Line 8 lists the taxes based on a 40 percent marginal rate, which is the rate that would be applied to the combined enterprise. Line 9 lists each year's profit, or loss. Finally, because some of Doctors' assets are expected to wear out or become obsolete, and because UHSC plans to expand Doctors' subsidiary should the acquisition occur, some equity funds must be retained and reinvested in the subsidiary to pay for asset replacement and growth. These retentions, which are not available for transfer from the hospital subsidiary to the UHSC parent, are shown on Line 10.

Of course, the postmerger cash flows attributable to the target firm are extremely difficult to estimate. But, in a friendly merger, the acquiring firm would send a team consisting of literally dozens of accountants, financial analysts, engineers, and so forth, to the target firm to go over its books; to estimate required maintenance expenditures; to set values on assets such as real estate; and the like. This work would be done as part of a "due diligence" analysis, which we discuss in a later section.

Table 18.3 provides relevant cost of capital data for Doctors'. These data will be used to set the discount rates used in the DCF valuations.

Free Operating Cash Flow Method

As its name implies, the *free operating cash flow* method focuses on operating cash flows, and hence values the entire business. Because our aim is to value the ownership position in a business, the value of the debt financing must be stripped out from the overall valuation.

Free operating cash flow is defined as net operating profit after taxes (EBIT × [1 − T]) plus noncash expenses (depreciation) less operating cash

TABLE 18.3

Doctors' Hospital: Selected Cost of Capital Data and Calculations

Cost of equity	18.2%
Cost of debt	12.0%
Proportion of debt financing	0.50
Proportion of equity financing	0.50
Tax rate	40.0%

$$CCC = [w_d \times R(R_d) \times (1 - T)] + [w_e \times R(R_e)]$$
$$= [0.50 \times 12.0\% \times (1 - 0.40)] + [0.50 \times 18.2\%]$$
$$= 3.6\% + 9.1\% = 12.7\%.$$

Note: If necessary, see Chapter 10 for a discussion of the corporate cost of capital (CCC).

flow needed for reinvestment in the business. Table 18.4 uses the data contained in Table 18.2 to forecast the free operating cash flows for Doctors'. In merger valuations, the term "free" means cash flows that are available to the enterprise, or to shareholders, after all other expenses, including asset replacement and growth, have been taken into account.

Now, because these cash flows are operating cash flows, as are the cash flows in a conventional capital budgeting analysis, the appropriate discount rate is the corporate cost of capital. Should it be UHSC's corporate cost of capital? No; the cost of capital must reflect the riskiness of the cash flows being discounted, and hence the appropriate rate is that for Doctors', which was estimated in Table 18.3 to be 12.7 percent.[3] At this discount rate, the present value of the free operating cash flows shown in Table 18.4, discounted back to the end of 2000 (the beginning of 2001), is $41.9 million.

Finally, we have projected only five years of cash flows, but UHSC would likely operate Doctors' for many years, perhaps 20 or 30 or more. If the free operating cash flows given in Table 18.4 are assumed to grow at a constant rate after 2005, the constant growth model can be used to estimate Doctor's *terminal value.* Assuming a constant 5 percent growth rate in free operating cash flow forever, the terminal value is estimated to be $201.8 million:

$$\text{Terminal value} = \frac{2005 \text{ Cash flow} \times (1 + \text{Growth rate})}{\text{Required rate of return} - \text{Growth rate}}$$

$$= \frac{\$14.8 \times 1.05}{0.127 - 0.05} = \frac{\$15.54}{0.077}$$

$$= \$201.8 \text{ million.}$$

TABLE 18.4

Doctors' Hospital: Projected Free Operating Cash Flows (millions of dollars)

	2001	2002	2003	2004	2005
1. EBIT $\times$ (1 − T)	$4.8	$ 7.2	$10.8	$13.2	$16.8
2. Plus depreciation	8.0	8.0	9.0	9.0	10.0
3. Less retentions	4.0	4.0	7.0	9.0	12.0
4. Free operating cash flow	$8.8	$ 11.2	$12.8	$13.2	$14.8

The terminal value of Doctors', which represents the value at the end of 2005 of all cash flows beyond 2005, has a value of $111.0 million when discounted back to 2000 at 12.7 percent.[4]

The final estimate of the total value of Doctors' to UHSC is $41.9 + $111.0 = $152.9 million. However, Doctors' has debt outstanding that has a current market value of $86.6 million, so the ownership (equity) value of the hospital is $152.9 − $86.6 = $66.3 million.

Free Cash Flow to Equityholders Method

The *free cash flow to equityholders* method focuses solely on the cash flows that would be available to UHSC's stockholders, which are developed in Table 18.5. Because the cash flows shown on Line 4 belong to UHSC's stockholders, they should be discounted at the cost of equity rather than at the corporate cost of capital. Furthermore, the cost of equity used must reflect the riskiness of the free cash flows in the table, and hence the discount rate is more closely aligned with the cost of equity of Doctors' than with the cost of equity of either UHSC or the consolidated enterprise.

As before, the current value of Doctors' to UHSC is the present value of the free cash flows given in Table 18.5 plus the terminal value, all discounted at the 18.2 percent cost of equity. The present value of the Table 18.5 cash flows is $27.7 million. The terminal value, calculated in a similar manner as in the previous free operating cash flow method, is $89.1 million, and its present value is $38.6 million. Thus, the equity value of Doctors' is $27.7 + $38.6 = $66.3 million.

Of course, we "cooked the books" to ensure that the value came out to be the same under both of the DCF methods. Still, in real-world valuations, the two methods would be relatively consistent, so either one could be used. Obviously, UHSC would try to buy Doctors' at as low a price as possible, while Doctors' managers would hold out for the highest possible price. The final price is determined by negotiation, with the stronger negotiator capturing most of the incremental value. The larger the synergistic benefits, the more room for bargaining and the higher the probability that the merger will actually be consummated. We will have more to say about setting the bid price in a later section.

Although we will not illustrate it here, UHSC would perform a risk analysis on both the Table 18.4 and Table 18.5 cash flows just as it does on any set of capital budgeting flows. Generally, scenario analysis and Monte

TABLE 18.5

Doctors' Hospital: Projected Free Cash Flow to Equityholders (millions of dollars)

	2001	2002	2003	2004	2005
1. Net profit	$2.4	$4.8	$7.8	$10.2	$13.2
2. Plus depreciation	8.0	8.0	9.0	9.0	10.0
3. Less asset reinvestments	4.0	4.0	7.0	9.0	12.0
4. Free cash flow to equityholders	$6.4	$8.8	$9.8	$10.2	$11.2

Carlo simulation would be used to give UHSC's management some feel for the risks involved with the acquisition and resulting range of valuations. In the illustration, as with many healthcare mergers, the target firm is investor-owned but not publicly traded, so it is not possible to obtain a market beta on Doctors' stock. However, we can obtain market betas of the stocks of the major investor-owned hospital chains, and this value could be used to help estimate the capital costs given in Table 18.3.

Market Multiple Analysis

Another method of valuing a business is *market multiple analysis*, which applies a market-determined multiple to some proxy for value—typically some measure of revenues or earnings. Like the DCF valuation approach, the basic premise here is that the value of any business depends on the cash flows that the business produces. The DCF approach applies this premise in a precise manner, while market multiple analysis is more ad hoc.

To illustrate the concept, suppose that in recent hospital mergers, acquirers have been willing to pay four to five times the EBITDA of the target. EBITDA is one of the more common proxies for value used in market multiple analysis. It means *earnings before interest, taxes, depreciation, and amortization (EBITDA)*. Thus, we would say that the EBITDA market multiple is 4–5. To estimate the value of Doctors', using this method, note that Doctors' 2001 EBITDA estimate is $8 million in EBIT plus $8 million in deprecation, or $16 million. Multiplying EBITDA by the 4–5 market multiple gives a range for the value of Doctors' of $64 to $80 million. Because equity multiples are typically used in these analyses, the resulting value is the equity, or ownership, value of the business.

Clearly, the valuation of a business can only be considered a rough estimate. Although the DCF approach has strong theoretical support, one has to be very concerned over the validity of the estimated cash flows, growth rates, and discount rates applied to those flows. It doesn't take much variation in these estimates to create large differences in estimated value.

The market multiple method is more ad hoc, but its proponents argue that a proxy estimate for a single year, such as measured by EBITDA, is more likely to be accurate than a multiple-year cash flow forecast. Furthermore, the market multiple approach avoids the problem of having to estimate a terminal value. Of course, the market multiple approach has problems of its own. One concern is the comparability between the business being analyzed and the firm (or firms) that set the market multiple. Another concern is how well one year, or even an average of several years, of EBITDA captures the value of a business that will be operated for many years into the future, and whose EBITDA could soar as a result of merger-related synergies.

1. Briefly, describe two approaches commonly used to value acquisition candidates.

Self-Test Questions

2. What are some problems that occur when valuing target firms?
3. Which approach do you believe to be best? Explain your answer.

Unique Problems in Valuing Small Businesses

It should be obvious that the valuation of potential takeover candidates is a very difficult task, even when the target is a large, publicly traded firm. One of the primary difficulties in the process is estimating the right market *capitalization rate*, either the discount rate in the DCF approach or the market multiple in the market multiple approach. When the acquirer or target is a small, privately owned firm—say, a medical practice—several additional factors, such as the ones listed below, arise that might require modification of a rate based on the analysis of publicly traded firms.

- **Geographic and business line diversification.** Capitalization rates based on large business transactions typically involve businesses that have geographic and business line diversification. If the transaction behind the valuation does not have the same diversification benefits, then the capitalization rates may need to be adjusted. For example, the acquisition of one hospital by a large national chain places the target in a large diversified portfolio of hospitals. The same acquisition by a neighboring stand-alone hospital lacks such a diversification benefit. This fact makes the acquisition riskier for the neighbor than for the national chain, and hence argues for a higher discount rate, or lower market multiple. Of course, there may be more synergies inherent in merging with the neighbor, which would show up in the valuation as higher cash flow projections. Still, the added risk needs to be considered in the valuation process.
- **Owners' diversification.** When a large, publicly traded firm makes an acquisition, the target business is being added to the well-diversified personal investment portfolios of the acquiring firm's stockholders. Thus, the owners see only market risk in the transaction as opposed to corporate risk. When merger transactions take place between smaller businesses, or when the acquirer is a not-for-profit business, market risk is not relevant. Thus, the portfolio benefit associated with owners' personal diversification is not applicable, which may raise the riskiness inherent in the transaction.
- **Liquidity (marketability).** The ownership of a small business lacks liquidity (marketability), which lowers its value relative to the stock of a large firm that is publicly traded on a major exchange or in the over-the-counter market. In effect, a liquidity premium should be assessed when valuing small businesses, which will raise the discount rate used in the DCF approach and lower the multiple used in the market multiple approach. Of course, the effect of all three of these adjustments is to lower the value of the target firm. It is very difficult to judge how much lower the value should be because of lack of diversification or liquidity, but it has

been suggested that the value loss is quite large—as high as 50 percent or more.[5]

- **Control.** The final factor that often arises in valuing closely held businesses is that of control. The ability to control a business is very important and, as such, it has value. For example, assume that a business that is valued at $100,000 has three owners—one with 50.2 percent of the stock and two each with 24.9 percent. The value of the stock owned by the controlling stockholder is worth more than the proportionate amount—that is, worth more than $50,200, perhaps a great deal more. Similarly, the stock of each of the minority stockholders is worth less than $24,900, which is their proportionate share. The value of *control interests*, as opposed to *minority interests*, must be taken into account when assessing value, especially when the acquisition will not be for 100 percent of the stock of the target firm. Furthermore, control issues need to be considered when setting the terms of the acquisition offer.

- **Cash flows of medical practices.** As discussed in the previous chapter, small medical practices typically use a modified cash-basis accounting methodology. Furthermore, at the end of each year, any net income generated in excess of that required for retentions is paid out to the owner/physicians as bonuses. To determine the true cash flows that would accrue to an acquirer, the statements must be recast with the bonuses "backed out." The assumption, of course, is that physicians would be willing to work as hard in the future in the absence of bonuses as they do today. This assumption has spelled disaster for many medical practice acquisitions.

1. What unique considerations arise when valuing small, privately held businesses?

Self-Test Question

Setting the Bid Price

Assume that after a thorough valuation, UHSC concludes that Doctors' is worth $70 million. Furthermore, assume that Doctors' has 1 million shares of stock outstanding and that some shares sold recently in a private sale at $50 a share, so Doctors' total market value is assumed to be $50 million. With an estimated value of $70 million to UHSC, it could offer as much as $70 per share for Doctors' without diluting the value of its own stock.

Figure 18.1 illustrates the situation facing UHSC's managers as they set the bid price. The $70 per share maximum offer price is shown as a point on the horizontal axis, which plots bid price. If UHSC pays less—say, $65 a share—its stockholders will gain $5 per share, or $5 million in total, from the merger. On the other hand, if UHSC pays more than $70 per share, its stockholders will lose value. The line that shows the impact of the per share bid price on UHSC's stockholders is a 45-degree downward-sloping line that

FIGURE 18.1

Evaluating the
Takeover Bid

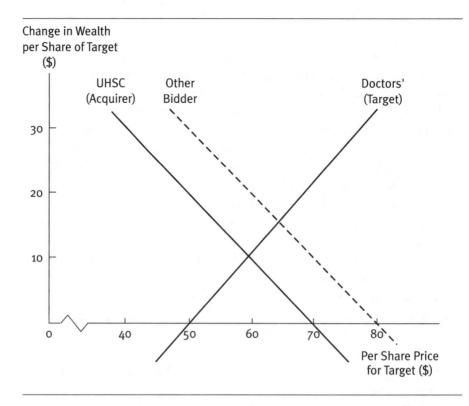

cuts the X-axis at $70. The distance between this diagonal line and the X-axis is the amount that UHSC's stockholders will gain, or lose, for each share of Doctors' acquired. The situation facing Doctors' shareholders is depicted by a 45-degree upward-sloping line that crosses the X-axis at $50. If the hospital is acquired for more than $50 per share, its shareholders will gain value, while they would lose value if the price were less than $50.

Note that there is a bid price range between $50 and $70 where the shareholders of both UHSC and Doctors' benefit from the merger. The range exists because the merger has synergistic benefits that can be divided between the two groups of stockholders. The greater the synergistic benefits, the greater the range of feasible bid prices and the greater the chance that the merger will be consummated.

The issue of how to divide the synergistic benefit is critically important in any merger analysis. Obviously, both parties will want to gain as much as possible. If Doctors' shareholders knew the maximum price that UHSC is willing to pay, $70, it would hold out for that price. UHSC, on the other hand, will try to acquire the hospital at a price as close to $50 a share as possible. Where within the $50 to $70 range should UHSC set its initial bid? The answer depends on a number of factors, including whether UHSC will pay with cash or securities, whether the managers of UHSC or Doctors' have the better negotiating skills, and whether another bidder is likely to enter the picture.

The likelihood of a bidding war for Doctors' plays an important role in setting the initial bid. Suppose first that no other bidder is likely. In this situation, UHSC might make a relatively low take-it-or-leave-it offer, and Doctors' shareholders might take it because some gain is better than no gain. On the other hand, assume that Doctors' has a unique situation that makes it attractive to several competing health systems. Now, when UHSC announces its bid, other bidders may enter the fray, and the final price will likely be close to $70 per share. Perhaps another potential acquirer could achieve even greater synergies with Doctors' Hospital than could UHSC, as shown in Figure 18.1 by the "Other Bidder" dashed line. If so, the bid price could rise above $70, in which case UHSC should drop out of the bidding.

UHSC would, of course, want to keep its maximum bid secret, and it would plan its bidding strategy carefully and consistent with the situation. If UHSC thought that other bidders would emerge, or that Doctors' management would resist a bid to protect their jobs, UHSC might decide to make a high *preemptive*, or *knockout*, *bid* in hopes of scaring off competing bids, eliminating management resistance, or both. On the other hand, if no other bidders were expected, UHSC might make a low-ball bid in hopes of "stealing" the hospital.

Another factor that influences the initial bid is the employment/control situation. First, consider the situation in which a small, owner-managed firm sells out to a larger concern. The owner/manager may be anxious to retain a high-status position, and he or she may also have developed a close relationship with the employees and, thus, be concerned about keeping operating control of the organization after the merger. These points are often stressed during the merger negotiations. When a publicly owned firm not controlled by its managers is merged into another firm, the acquired firm's management is also worried about its postmerger position. If the acquiring firm agrees to retain the old management, then management may be willing to support the merger and to recommend its acceptance to the stockholders. If the old management is to be removed, then it will probably resist the merger.

Self-Test Questions

1. What impact does the amount of synergistic benefit have on the likelihood of a merger being consummated?
2. What are some factors that influence the starting and final bid price?

Structuring the Takeover Bid

If the acquiring firm is investor-owned, its offer to the target shareholders can be in the form of cash, stock of the acquiring firm, debt of the acquiring firm, or a combination of the three. The structure of the bid is extremely important because it affects (1) the capital structure of the postmerger firm,

(2) the tax treatment of both the acquiring firm and the target's stockholders, (3) the ability of the target firm's stockholders to reap the rewards of future merger-related gains, and (4) the types of federal and state regulations to which the acquiring firm will be subjected. In this section, we focus on how taxes and regulation influence the way in which acquiring firms structure their offers.

The form of payment offered to the target shareholders determines the personal tax treatment of the target's stockholders. Target shareholders do not have to pay taxes on the transaction if they maintain a substantial equity position in the combined firm, defined by the IRS to mean that at least 50 percent of the payment to target shareholders must be in shares (either common or preferred) of the acquiring firm. In such nontaxable offers, target shareholders do not realize any capital gains or losses until the equity securities they receive in the takeover are sold. However, capital gains must be taken and treated as income in the transaction year if an offer consists of over 50 percent of either cash or debt securities, or some combination of the two.

All other things being equal, target stockholders prefer nontaxable offers, especially when they believe that the combined firm will perform well, because they can (1) benefit from the continuing good performance of the combined firm and (2) postpone the realization of capital gains and the payment of taxes. Most target shareholders are, thus, willing to sell their stock for a lower price in a nontaxable offer than in a taxable offer. As a result, one might expect nontaxable bids to dominate; however, other factors are at work. If a firm pays more than book value for a target firm's assets in a taxable merger, it can write up those assets; depreciate the marked-up value for tax purposes; and, thus, lower the postmerger firm's taxes vis-a-vis the taxes of the two firms operating separately. However, if the acquiring firm writes up the target firm's assets for tax purposes, then the target firm must pay capital gains taxes in the year the merger occurs. (These taxes can be avoided if the acquiring firm elects not to write up acquired assets and depreciates them on their old basis.)

Securities laws also have an effect on the construction of the offer. As we discussed in Chapter 7, the Securities and Exchange Commission (SEC) has oversight over the issuance of new securities, including stock or debt issued in connection with a merger. Therefore, whenever a corporation bids for control of another firm through the exchange of equity or debt, the entire process must take place under the scrutiny of the SEC. The time required for such reviews allows target management to implement defensive tactics and other firms to make competing offers, and, as a result, most hostile tender offers are for cash rather than securities.

Self-Test Questions

1. What are some alternative ways of structuring takeover bids?
2. How do taxes influence the payment structure?
3. How do securities laws affect the payment structure?

Due Diligence Analysis

One of the most important aspects of a merger is *due diligence analysis*.[6] The primary purposes of a due diligence analysis are (1) to uncover issues that would prevent the acquirer from pursuing the acquisition and (2) to provide the acquirer with insights into the day-to-day operations of the target firm so that an appropriate transaction can take place. Due diligence requires a uniform, disciplined approach to the merger analysis, which presumably will minimize the risk of overlooking issues that are key to the acquisition.[7]

Due diligence analysis normally takes place after a letter of intent has been signed between the acquiring and target firms, but before the terms of the transaction have been completed. It is normally carried out by a team that has been specially assembled for the task. Typically, the team will include one or two top executives, plus specialists from applicable staffs such as finance, legal, medical, nursing, personnel, risk management, and engineering. The team may consist entirely of personnel from the acquiring firm or it may contain consultants in addition to the in-house members.

The due diligence team will gather and analyze information about the acquisition. The end result is a report that summarizes the team's findings and makes recommendations as to whether or not to proceed with the acquisition and how the deal, if recommended, should be structured. The time required to conduct a due diligence analysis varies depending on the number of individuals on the team, the nature of the acquisition, and the accessibility of information. Generally, however, due diligence analyses take about 60 to 90 days, so acquirers must allow sufficient time for due diligence analysis when developing merger time tables.

Conducting a thorough due diligence analysis is a necessary component of the acquisition process. In addition to protecting the acquirer against a poor acquisition, it can establish a relationship between acquiring and target firms' management that not only facilitates successful negotiations but, more importantly, can help lead to a successful merger.

1. What is due diligence analysis?
2. Why is due diligence analysis so important to the merger process?

Self-Test Questions

The Role of Investment Bankers

The investment banking community is involved with mergers in a number of ways: (1) helping to arrange mergers; (2) helping target firms develop and implement defensive tactics; (3) helping in due diligence analysis, especially valuing target firms; (4) helping to finance mergers; and (5) speculating in the stocks of potential merger candidates.

Arranging Mergers

The major investment banking firms have merger and acquisition groups that operate within their corporate finance departments. (Corporate finance departments offer advice, as opposed to underwriting or brokerage services, to firms.) Members of these groups strive to identify businesses with excess cash that might want to buy other firms; firms that might be willing to be bought; and firms that might, for a number of reasons, be attractive to others. Similarly, dissident stockholders of firms with poor track records might work with investment bankers to oust management by helping to arrange a merger.

Developing Defensive Tactics

Target firms that do not want to be acquired generally enlist the help of an investment banking firm, along with a law firm that specializes in helping to block mergers. Defenses include such tactics as: (1) changing the bylaws so that only one-third of the directors are elected each year or that a 75 percent approval (a super majority) versus a simple majority is required to approve a merger, or both; (2) trying to convince the target firm's stockholders that the price being offered is too low; (3) raising antitrust issues in the hope that the FTC or the JD will intervene; (4) repurchasing stock in the open market in an effort to push the price above that being offered by the potential acquirer; (5) getting a white knight who is more acceptable to the target firm's management to compete with the potential acquirer; (6) getting a *white squire* who is friendly to current management to buy some of the target firm's shares, and (7) taking a poison pill, as described next.

    Poison pills, which occasionally really do amount to committing economic suicide to avoid a takeover, are such tactics as: (1) borrowing on terms that require immediate repayment of all loans if the firm is acquired, (2) selling off at bargain prices the assets that originally made the firm a desirable target, (3) granting such lucrative golden parachutes to target executives that the cash drain from these payments would render the merger infeasible, and (4) planning defensive mergers that would leave the firm with new assets that have questionable value and a huge debt load to service. Currently, the most popular poison pill is for a firm to give its stockholders *stock purchase rights* that allow them to buy at half price the stock of an acquiring firm should the firm be acquired. The blatant use of poison pills is constrained by directors' awareness that excessive use could trigger personal suits by stockholders against directors who voted for them, and, perhaps in the near future, by laws that would further limit management's use of such poison pills. Still, investment bankers and acquisition lawyers are busy thinking up new poison pill formulas, and others are just as actively trying to come up with antidotes.

Establishing a Fair Value

If a friendly merger is being worked out between two firms' managers, it is important to be able to document that the agreed-upon price is a fair one; otherwise, the stockholders of either firm may sue to block the merger. Therefore, in many large mergers, each side will hire an investment banking firm to evaluate the target firm and to help establish the fair price. Even if the merger is not friendly, investment bankers may still be asked to help establish a price. If a surprise tender offer is to be made, the acquiring firm will want to know the lowest price at which it might be able to acquire the stock, while the target firm may seek help in "proving" that the price being offered is too low.

Arranging Financing

Many mergers are financed with the acquiring firm's excess cash. At other times, however, the acquiring firm has no excess cash; hence, it requires a source of funds to pay for the target firm. Perhaps the single most important factor behind the 1980s merger wave was the widespread use of junk bonds, and the system that was developed to market these bonds. To be a successful investment banker in the mergers and acquisitions business, a banker must be able to offer a financing package to clients, whether they are acquirers that need capital for acquisitions or target firms that need capital to finance stock repurchase plans or other defenses against takeovers.

Risk Arbitrage

Arbitrage generally means simultaneously buying and selling the same commodity or security in two different markets at different prices, and pocketing a risk-free return. However, the major brokerage houses, as well as some wealthy private investors, are engaged in a different type of arbitrage called *risk arbitrage*. The *arbitrageurs*, or "arbs" as they are called, speculate in the stocks of firms that are likely takeover targets. Vast amounts of capital are required to speculate in a large number of securities and, thus, reduce risk, and also to make money on narrow spreads; however, many institutional investors have the wherewithal to play the game. To be successful, arbs need to be able to sniff out likely targets, assess the probability of offers reaching fruition, and move in and out of the market quickly and with low transaction costs.

1. What are some roles that investment bankers play in mergers?
2. What are some defensive tactics that firms can use to resist hostile takeover attempts?
3. What is the difference between pure arbitrage and risk arbitrage?

Self-Test Questions

Who Wins: The Empirical Evidence

The most recent merger waves have been notable for both the large number of businesses that have combined and the size of the mergers. With all of this activity and wealth transfer, the following questions have emerged: Do corporate acquisitions create value? If so, how is the value shared between the parties involved?

Financial researchers have classified corporate acquisitions as part of "the market for corporate control." Under this concept, management teams are viewed as facing constant competition from other management teams. If the team that currently controls a firm is not maximizing the value of the firm's assets, then an acquisition will likely occur and increase the value of the firm by replacing its poor managers with better ones. Furthermore, under this model, intense competition will cause managers to combine or divest assets whenever such steps would increase the value of the firm.

The validity of the competing views on who gains from corporate mergers can be tested by examining the stock price changes that occur around a merger announcement. Such changes in the stock prices of the acquiring and target firms represent market participants' beliefs about the value created by the merger, and about how this value will be divided between the target and acquiring firms' shareholders. As long as market participants are neither systematically wrong nor biased in their perceptions of the effects of mergers, examining a large sample of stock price movements will shed light on the issue of who gains from mergers.

One cannot simply examine stock prices around merger announcements dates because other factors influence stock prices. For example, if a merger were announced on a day when the entire market advanced, the fact that the stock price of a firm involved in a merger rose would not necessarily signify that the merger created value. Hence, studies examine the *abnormal returns* associated with merger announcements, where abnormal returns are defined as that part of a stock price change caused by factors other than changers in the general stock market.

Many studies have examined both acquiring and target firms' stock price responses to mergers and tender offers. Jointly, these studies have covered nearly every acquisition involving publicly traded firms from the early 1960s to the present, and they are remarkably consistent in their results: On average, the stock price of target firms increases by about 30 percent in hostile tender offers, while in friendly mergers the average increase is about 20 percent. However, for both hostile and friendly deals, the stock prices of acquiring firms, on average, remain constant. Thus, the evidence strongly indicates (1) that acquisitions do create value, but (2) that shareholders of target firms reap virtually all of the benefits.

In hindsight, these results are not too surprising. First, target firms' shareholders can always say no, so they are in the driver's seat. Second, takeovers are a competitive game, so if one potential acquirer does not offer full value for a target firm, then another potential acquirer will generally jump in with a higher bid. Finally, managers of acquiring firms might well be willing to give up all the value created by the merger because the merger would enhance the acquiring managers' personal positions with no explicit cost to their shareholders.

1. Explain how researchers can study the effects of mergers on shareholder wealth.
2. Do mergers create value? If so, where does this value go?
3. Do the research results discussed in this section seem logical? Explain your answer.
Self-Test Questions

Corporate Alliances

Mergers are one way for two firms to join forces, but many firms are striking cooperative deals, called *corporate alliances*, which fall short of merging. Whereas mergers combine all of the assets of the firms involved, as well as managerial and technical expertise, alliances allow firms to create combinations that focus on specific business lines that have the most potential for synergies. These alliances take many forms—from straightforward marketing agreements to joint ownership of world-scale operations.

A common form of corporate alliance is the *joint venture*, in which parts of firms are joined together to achieve specific, limited objectives. A joint venture is controlled by a management team consisting of representatives of the two, or more, parent firms. Joint ventures are becoming more prevalent in the health services industry as it strives to consolidate both insurance and provider functions. For example, both state officials and the Justice Department blocked the merger of two not-for-profit hospitals—Morton Plant and Mease—because the combined entity would dominate acute care delivery in an area near St. Petersburg, Florida. However, the hospitals were allowed to form a joint venture to consolidate billing and record keeping and to offer expensive high-tech services such as open-heart surgery, magnetic resonance imaging, and neonatal care. By forming a joint venture, the hospitals were able to gain at least some benefits of merging, yet satisfy antitrust laws.

A joint venture analysis is similar to a merger analysis, except that there are multiple classes of equity investors. Thus, in such analyses, the venture's cash flows must be broken down into distributions to each of the joint venture partners, and each partner must analyze its flows on the basis of their riskiness to determine if the venture is in its best interest.

1. What is the difference between a merger and a corporate alliance?
2. What is a joint venture? Give some reasons why joint ventures may be advantageous to the parties involved.
Self-Test Questions

Mergers Involving Not-for-Profit Businesses

One of the unique aspects of the health services industry is the large proportion of not-for-profit firms. Although the general principles discussed up to this point apply to all businesses, there are some problems that arise when not-for-profit firms are involved in mergers. In general, the merger of two not-for-profit firms does not require special consideration, but the acquisition of a not-for-profit firm by an investor-owned acquirer presents two significant problems.

The first problem involves the *charitable trust doctrine*. This doctrine, which was first developed in English common law and has been adopted by most states, holds that assets used for charitable purposes must be held in trust. This doctrine shaped the state incorporation laws for not-for-profit firms, which require that assets being used for charitable purposes must be used for such purposes in perpetuity (forever). The end result is that the proceeds from the sale of a not-for-profit corporation to an investor-owned business must be held in trust and continue to be used for charitable purposes. These laws place two requirements on the board of trustees of a not-for-profit firm about to be acquired by an investor-owned firm. First, the trustees must ensure that the acquisition price reflects the full fair market value of the assets being acquired. This assurance is normally obtained by getting the opinion of an investment banker or professional appraiser. Second, the trustees must establish a charitable entity to administer the proceeds from the sale for a charitable purpose. The usual vehicle for continuing the charitable purpose of the not-for-profit corporation is the tax-exempt *foundation*.

Many foundations have been spawned by the sales of not-for-profit businesses to investor-owned firms, primarily in the hospital industry and primarily as a result of acquisitions by Columbia/HCA Healthcare. Note, however, that foundations have also been created by sales of HMOs and other not-for-profit healthcare businesses. To illustrate the foundation concept, consider that Presbyterian Health Foundation was created in 1985 when Presbyterian Hospital in Oklahoma City was acquired by Hospital Corporation of America (HCA). The foundation began with $60 million in assets, but these have grown substantially over time. By law, at least 5 percent of assets of charitable foundations must be distributed each year, and Presbyterian Health Foundation has given a total of $30 million alone for rural outreach programs at the University of Oklahoma Health Science Center.

Although merger-related foundations are clearly doing a lot of good work with their vast amounts of assets, they have their critics. Most of the criticism stems from the close relationships that many foundations have with the for-profit providers that created them. Indeed, some foundations, instead of being funded entirely with cash, have ownership interests in the newly created for-profit entity, and it is easy for conflicts of interest to occur. One not-for-profit foundation even lost its tax-exempt status because it squandered millions of dollars on overpriced clinics, excessive compensation, and extravagant spending on personal items for managers and employees. At least not-for-profit hospitals are constrained somewhat by competitive forces, whereas the burden of oversight at charitable foundations falls completely on the board of trustees.

Many states have passed laws in recent years to ensure that hospital conversions are subject to full public scrutiny and oversight. In general, these laws, more than anything else, require full disclosure. For example, Georgia's law requires not-for-profit hospitals that are being sold or merged to file with the state attorney general's office, regardless of whether the merger is with a for-profit or not-for-profit business. Such filings, which become public information, must include the merger plan plus any financial gain that would accrue to board members, physicians, or managers. Furthermore, the state has the power to hold public hearings to determine whether or not the buyer is paying fair market value for the target hospital.

The second major problem in the acquisition of a not-for-profit provider by an investor-owned firm involves the tax-exempt, or municipal, debt that is often outstanding. Typically, such debt is issued for the sole purpose of funding plant and equipment owned by not-for-profit corporations. Furthermore, such debt usually has covenants that constrain the provider from merger activity that would lower the creditworthiness of the bonds or negatively affect the bonds' tax-exempt status.

To ease somewhat the conversion problems associated with municipal debt, many not-for-profit providers now include the so-called "Columbia clause" in their municipal bond indentures. In most indentures, the issuing hospital lists the circumstances under which the bonds may be redeemed prior to maturity. The Columbia clause allows bonds to be redeemed in the instance of a sale, lease, or joint venture with a for-profit firm involving a facility that had been financed with tax-exempt debt. Prior to placing such clauses in municipal bond indentures, hospitals selling to for-profit entities had to obtain private-letter rulings from the IRS to retire the bonds or make a tender offer to bondholders, and both of these mechanisms are relatively expensive compared to a call triggered by the clause.

Clearly, the restrictions on mergers involving not-for-profit firms and for-profit firms make such activities much more complicated than mergers involving only for-profits or only not-for-profits. Nevertheless, as evidenced by the amount of merger activity, these kinds of mergers do occur, and their volume is likely to increase, not decrease, in the future.

1. What are the unique problems inherent in the acquisition of a not-for-profit business by an investor-owned business?

Self-Test Question

Goodwill

We close this chapter by briefly discussing the concept of *goodwill*. Goodwill is primarily an accounting concept that is used to account for the fact that businesses usually are acquired for a price that exceeds the value of the assets purchased. The following is an overview of how goodwill works. When a business is acquired, its balance sheet (real) assets often are increased, or written up, to account for the fact that their true value is greater than their book value. Under *purchase accounting* rules, the dollar amount of the write-up is added to the book value of equity to obtain a new equity value, called the *net asset value*.[8] Then, if the purchase price exceeds the net asset value, this excess is placed on the balance sheet of the combined enterprise in an asset account called goodwill. The theory is that the business being acquired has some intangible asset, such as a trademark or consumer (patient) loyalty, that creates value above the value of the business's tangible assets.

To illustrate the concept, assume that Big Hospital is acquiring Small Hospital (SH) for $20 million. SH's pre-merger balance sheet has $10 million in liabilities and $10 million in equity. Furthermore, SH's total assets will be written up from $20 million to $25 million. The result is a net asset value for SH of $10 + $5 = $15 million. Now, with a purchase price of $20 million versus a net asset value of $15 million, the merger will create $5 million in goodwill that will appear on the asset side of the combined balance sheet.

What happens to goodwill? Under current accounting guidelines, it is written off over 40 years, so $5,000,000 / 40 = $125,000 in goodwill amortization expense will appear on the combined income statement for the next 40 years. Because it is not a cash expense, the amortization of goodwill does not affect a business's cash flow, but it does lower reported income and earnings per share. Thus, many managers believe that the current accounting treatment of goodwill dampens merger activity, and the shortening of the write-off period to 20 years would have an even greater negative effect. (See footnote 8.)

Note that goodwill represents a residual of the merger valuation rather than a component; that is, often you will hear someone ask "Where is the premium for goodwill?" Any amount paid for goodwill must stem from the valuation process described previously. If this process does not identify a value that exceeds the balance sheet net asset value, the business has no goodwill, or at least none that raises its value above that stated on the balance sheet.

Self-Test Question

1. Describe the concept of goodwill.

Key Concepts

This chapter examined mergers and acquisitions, including business valuation. Here are its key concepts:

- A *merger* occurs when two firms combine to form a single firm.
- In most mergers, one firm (the *acquirer*) initiates action to take over another (the *target*).
- There have been five prominent *merger waves* in the United States. The current wave includes a great deal of activity in the health services

industry, which, for the most part, involves mergers that aim to better position firms to respond to the changing healthcare marketplace.

- The primary *motives* for mergers are (1) synergy, (2) excess cash, (3) purchase of assets below replacement cost, (4) diversification, and (5) personal incentives.

- A *horizontal* merger occurs when two firms in the same line of business combine. A *vertical* merger is the combination of a firm with one of its customers or suppliers. A *conglomerate* merger occurs when firms in totally different industries combine.

- In a *friendly merger*, the managers of both firms approve the merger, whereas in a *hostile merger*, the target firm's management opposes the merger.

- Merger regulation falls into two broad categories: (1) *bid procedure regulation* and (2) *antitrust regulation.*

- *Merger analysis* consists of three tasks: (1) valuing the target firm, (2) setting the bid price, and (3) structuring the bid.

- Two approaches are most commonly used to *value businesses*: (1) the discounted cash flow approach and (2) the market multiple approach.

- The discounted cash flow approach has two variations: (1) the *free operating cash flow method* focuses on operating cash flows, which are available to both service debt and equity investors; and (2) the *free cash flow to equityholders method* focuses on cash flows available solely to equityholders.

- The *market multiple approach* uses some proxy for value, such as earnings before interest, taxes, depreciation, and amortization (EBITDA), and then multiplies it by a multiple derived from recent merger transactions.

- The discounted cash flow approach has the strongest theoretical basis, but its inputs, the projected cash flows and discount rate, are very difficult to estimate. The market multiple approach is somewhat ad hoc, but it requires a much simpler set of inputs.

- The valuation of *small businesses* is complicated by several factors including (1) lack of geographic and business line diversification, (2) lack of owners' diversification, (3) and lack of liquidity.

- Potential acquirers undertake *due diligence analysis* (1) to uncover issues that would prevent the acquirer from pursuing the acquisition and (2) to provide the acquirer with insights into the day-to-day operations of the target firm so that an appropriate transaction can take place.

- *Investment bankers* are involved in mergers in a number of ways: (1) they help arrange mergers, (2) they help target firms develop and implement defensive tactics, (3) they help value target firms, (4) they help finance mergers, and (5) they speculate in the stocks of potential merger candidates.

- Many studies have been conducted to determine who wins in mergers.

These studies indicate that mergers do create value, but that most of this value goes to the shareholders of target firms.

- Mergers are one way for two firms to join forces, but many firms are striking cooperative deals, called *corporate alliances*, which fall short of merging. A *joint venture* is a corporate alliance in which two or more firms combine some of their resources to achieve a specific, limited objective.
- Some unique problems arise when not-for-profit firms are involved in mergers with for-profit firms. The two largest are (1) a *charitable foundation* must be created from the merger proceeds, and (2) all *tax-exempt debt* must be refunded.
- *Goodwill*, a balance sheet asset account, is created when a business is acquired for more than its *net asset value*. Goodwill is amortized over time and deducted from revenues on the income statement.

This concludes our discussion of business valuation, mergers, and acquisitions. In the next chapter, we discuss capitation and risk sharing.

Selected References

Anthony, Michael F. 1997. "Tax-Exempt/Proprietary Partnerships: How the Deal Gets Done." *Healthcare Financial Management* (January): 45–49.

Baumann, Barbara H., and Marjorie R. Oxaal. 1993. "Estimating the Value of Group Medical Practices." *Healthcare Financial Management* (December): 58–65.

Becker, Scott and John Callahan. 1996. "Physician-Hospital Transactions: Developing a Process for Handling Valuation-Related Issues." *Journal of Health Care Finance* (Winter): 19–31.

Becker, Scott and Robert J. Pristave. 1995. "Physician-Based Transactions: The Sale of Medical Practices, Ambulatory Surgery Centers, and Dialysis Facilities." *Journal of Health Care Finance* (Winter):13–26.

Boo, Michael and Paul Louiselle. 1994. "Structuring Medical Practice Acquisitions." *Healthcare Financial Management* (December): 23–27.

Bryant, L. Edward, Jr. 1993. "Avoiding Antitrust Compliance Difficulties in Mergers and Acquisitions." *Healthcare Financial Management* (August): 48–58.

Clement, Jan P., and Michael J. McCue. 1996. "The Performance of Hospital Corporation of America and Healthtrust Hospitals After Leveraged Buyouts." *Medical Care* (July): 672–685.

Cleverley, William O. 1997. "Factors Affecting the Valuation of Physician Practices." *Healthcare Financial Management* (December): 71–73.

Cody, Marisue. 1996. "Vertical Integration Strategies: Revenue Effects in Hospital and Medicare Markets." *Hospital & Health Services Administration* (Fall): 343–357.

Collins, Hobart and Glenda Simpson. 1995. "Avoiding Pitfalls in Medical Practice Valuation." *Healthcare Financial Management* (March): 20–22.

Evans, Christopher J. 2000. "Measuring the Value of Healthcare Business Assets." *Healthcare Financial Management* (April): 58–64.

Federa, R. Danielle and Jonathan S. Ketcham. 1993. "The Valuation of Medical Practices." *Topics in Health Care Financing* (Spring): 67–75.

Hahn, William. 1994. "Determining a Healthcare Organization's Value." *Healthcare Financial Management* (August): 40–44.

———. 1998. "Payment Reform Will Shift Home Health Agency Valuation Parameters." *Healthcare Financial Management* (December): 31–34.

Harris, Jay and Atul Dhir. 1998. "A Successful PPMC Acquisition Strategy: Vision, Focus, and Discipline." *Healthcare Financial Management* (October): 54–60.

Hill, John E., and Jennifer Wild. 1995. "Survey Provides Data on Practice Acquisition Activity." *Healthcare Financial Management* (September): 54–72.

McCue, Michael J. 1996. "A Premerger Profile of Columbia and HCA Hospitals." *Health Care Management Review* (Spring): 38–45.

"Mergers and Acquisitions." 1989. Terence M. Meiling, editor. *Topics in Health Care Financing* (Summer).

Moore, Bettina E. 1999. "Nonprofit to For-Profit Hospital Transactions: All Roads Lead to the Attorney General's Office." *Journal of Health Care Financing* (Spring): 29–36.

Nanda, Sudhir and Andrew Miller. 1996. "Risk Analysis in the Valuation of Medical Practices." *Health Care Management Review* (Fall): 26–32.

Ortiz, John P. 1997. "Ensuring the Profitability of Acquired Physician Practices." *Healthcare Financial Management* (January): 71–72.

Peregrine, Michael W. 1997. "Creative Alliances Offer Alternatives to Corporate Mergers." *Healthcare Financial Management* (January): 52–55.

Peregrine, Michael W., and D. Louis Glaser. "Legal Issues in Medical Practice Acquisitions." *Healthcare Financial Management* (February): 70–76.

Principles and Practices Board. 1997. "Statement No. 20: Healthcare Mergers, Acquisitions, and Collaborations." *Healthcare Financial Management* (October): 104–111.

Reilly, Robert F. 1990. "The Valuation of a Medical Practice." *Health Care Management Review* (Summer): 25–34.

Reilly, Robert F., and James R. Rabe. 1997. "The Valuation of Health Care Intangible Assets." *Health Care Management Review* (Spring): 55–64.

Rimmer, Timothy B. 1995. "Physician Practice Acquisitions: Valuation Issues and Concerns." *Hospital & Health Services Administration* (Fall): 415–425.

Robinson, James C. 2000. "Capital Finance and Ownership Conversion in Health Care." *Health Affairs* (January/February): 56–71.

Schwartzben, Dov and Steven A. Finkler. 1998. "Combining Accounting Approaches to Practice Valuation." *Healthcare Financial Management* (June): 70–76.

Unland, James J. 1989. *Valuation of Hospitals and Medical Centers.* Chicago: Health Management Research Institute.

Ward, Matthews E., and Susanna E. Krentz. 1988. "Diversification: Myths versus Realities." *Topics in Health Care Financing* (Fall): 32–39.

Wilkins, Aaron S., and Peter D. Jacobson. 1998. "Fiduciary Responsibilities in Nonprofit Health Care Conversions." *Health Care Management Review* (Winter): 77–90.

Williams, Latham. 1995. "Structuring Managed Care Joint Ventures." *Healthcare Financial Management* (August): 32–36.

Selected Web Sites

To learn more about merger activity in the health services industry, see the Irving
Levin Associates site at *www.levinassociates.com*.

The web site of BVS (Business Valuation Services) offers some insights into the problems inherent in valuing small businesses; see *www.bvs-inc.com*. Of particular
interest are the articles and publications that can be accessed by clicking on the
Articles & Publications icon along the left side of the page.

Ohio State University maintains a web site with video clips by various finance professionals briefly discussing topics of relevance to this course. Unfortunately,
the clips do not include healthcare executives. To access the clips, go to
www.cob.ohio-state.edu/fin/clips.htm. Then, click on the clip of interest. For this
chapter, try the clip by T. Boone Pickens on white knights. Note that video
clips are large files that are best accessed using a fast Internet link. Furthermore,
player software is required to see the clips.

Selected Cases

There are three cases in *Cases in Healthcare Finance* that are applicable to this chapter:

Case 20: University Hospital, which focuses on the valuation and acquisition of one
hospital by another.

Case 21: Medical Partners, which examines the feasibility of a proposed joint venture.

Case 22: Community Physicians, Inc., which focuses on the valuation of a medical
practice.

Notes

1. *Monopsony* power arises when there is a single buyer, so managed care
   organizations could, in least in theory, become monopsonies.
2. For simplicity, we are holding the target's debt ratio at its current level. If the
   target has excess debt capacity, then the amount of new debt initially supported
   by the target increases the value of the target. Look at this in another way: Any
   new debt that can be issued up front on the basis of the target's assets reduces
   the amount of funds that the acquirer must put up to make the acquisition.
3. If the merger will affect the riskiness of the cash flows being discounted, then an
   adjustment must be made to the target's corporate cost of capital.
4. The use of the constant growth model to estimate a target's terminal value
   could create an upward bias in the valuation estimate because it assumes that
   the target will be operated forever. However, the contribution of cash flows
   after 40–50 years to the terminal value of the business is inconsequential, so the
   constant growth model does not really require constant growth into perpetuity.
   Still, if there is some doubt as to the life of the target, it might be best to either
   subjectively reduce the resulting constant growth terminal value estimate or to
   use some other methodology to estimate the terminal value.
5. See Ernest W. Walker and J. William Petty II, *Financial Management of the Small
   Firm* (Englewood Cliffs, NJ: Prentice-Hall, 1986), Chapter 13.

6. For more information on due diligence analysis, see Paul Louiselle, "Conducting Financial Due Diligence Analysis of Medical Practices," *Healthcare Financial Management*, December 1995, 29–33.

7. For an example of a due diligence checklist, see HFMA Principles and Practices Board, "Practice Acquisition: A Due Diligence Checklist" *Healthcare Financial Management*, December 1995, 36–39.

8. There are currently two methods of accounting for mergers: (1) *pooling of interests* and (2) *purchase accounting*. Under a pooling of interests, the balance sheet of the combined enterprise is merely the sum of the balance sheets of the two businesses. Under purchase accounting, goodwill is created as described in the text. The Financial Accounting Standards Board (FASB) is expected to issue a ruling in late 2000 that will require all mergers to use purchase accounting. Furthermore, the new ruling is expected to shorten the write-off period from 40 years to 20 years, which as we explain in the text, will increase the dollar amortization expense taken in each year.

CAPITATION, RATE SETTING, AND RISK SHARING

Learning Objectives

After studying this chapter, readers should be able to:

- Discuss, both in qualitative and quantitative terms, the incentives and risks inherent in capitation reimbursement.
- Describe how premium rates are developed.
- Explain the risk-sharing process, including its goals and implementation problems.

Introduction

Thus far, we have focused on making financial management decisions in what might be termed a *conventional reimbursement* environment. In such an environment, providers are reimbursed on the basis of each patient encounter. Thus, each hospital stay in an inpatient setting and each patient visit in an outpatient setting will generate additional revenue. The basis for payment may be charges, discounted charges, prospective payment, per diem, or some other methodology, but the key feature of conventional reimbursement is that higher patient volume leads to increased revenues. Also, in most conventional payment methodologies, the greater the intensity of service provided, and hence the higher the costs, the greater the reimbursement amount.

Under *capitation*, providers receive a fixed fee for each member (patient) enrolled, regardless of the amount or intensity of services provided. Clearly, capitation represents a reimbursement methodology that requires a different approach to financial management decision making than that used under conventional reimbursement. The basic cornerstones of finance, such as discounted cash flow analysis, risk and return, and opportunity costs, remain unchanged, but the manner in which these concepts are applied must recognize the unique features of capitation.

In this chapter, we first present some background information about capitation and discuss the mechanics of capitation and its implications for healthcare financial management. Then we present some techniques for setting rates on capitation contracts. Finally, we present some information on risk sharing among provider components within integrated delivery systems.

An Overview of Capitation

Formally defined, capitation is a flat periodic payment per enrollee to a health-care provider; it is the sole reimbursement for providing services to a defined population. The word "capitation" is derived from the term "per capita," which means per person. Generally, capitation payments are expressed as some dollar amount *per member per month (PMPM)*, where the word "member" typically means enrollee in some managed care plan, which is usually a health maintenance organization (HMO). For example, a primary care physician may receive a capitated payment of $15 PMPM for attending to the healthcare needs of 250 members of BetterCare, a regional HMO. Under this contract, the physician would receive $15 \times 250 \times 12 = $45,000 in total capitation payments over the year, and this amount must cover all of the primary care services offered to the patient population specified in the contract. Usually, capitated payments are adjusted for age and gender, but no other adjustments typically are made.

Figure 19.1 presents a comparison of the conventional and capitation payment systems. In the conventional system, as illustrated here by fee-for-service (FFS), the financial risk of providing healthcare services is shared between purchasers and insurers. Hospitals, physicians, and other providers bear negligible risk because they are paid on the basis of services provided. Insurers bear short-term risk in that in any year, payments to providers can exceed the amount of premiums collected. However, poor profitability by insurers in one year usually can be offset by price increases to purchasers the

FIGURE 19.1

Comparison of Conventional and Capitation Payment Systems

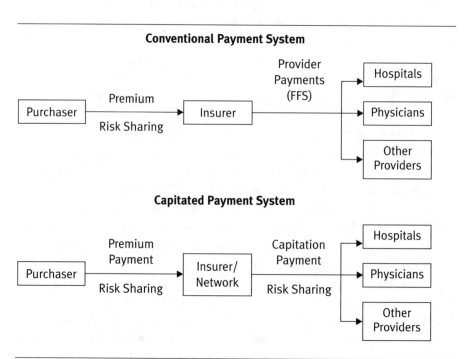

next year, so the long-term risk of financing the healthcare system is borne by purchasers.

Under capitation, fixed payments are made to providers regardless of the volume of services rendered, so risk sharing occurs among all three parties. Providers bear the short-term risk that the costs of providing service, including opportunity costs (profits), might exceed the capitation payment. Insurers/networks bear a longer-term risk, in that provider costs can increase when contracts are renewed, but purchasers still bear the ultimate risk of having to support the cost of the healthcare system.

1. What is capitation?
2. What are the primary differences between a conventional payment system and capitation?

Self-Test Questions

Provider Incentives Under Capitation

Capitation has a dramatic impact on provider incentives, and hence on provider behavior. Consider Figure 19.2, which depicts revenues and costs to a provider under both fee-for-service and capitation. Regardless of the payment system, total costs (TC), which are merely the sum of fixed costs (FC) and variable costs (VC), are tied directly to volume, so the greater the volume of services delivered, the greater the amount of total costs. The difference between the two graphs is the revenue line, and how profits and losses are realized. Under fee-for-service, the revenue line (Rev) is upward sloping, and it starts at the origin. At zero volume, the provider receives zero revenue, but at any positive volume, the greater the volume the higher the revenue. Under capitation, assuming a fixed number of enrollees, revenues are fixed independently of volume, and hence the revenue line is horizontal. On each graph, breakeven (BE) occurs when revenues equal total costs.

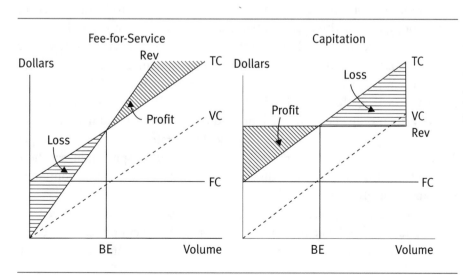

FIGURE 19.2
Revenue and Cost Structures Under Fee-for-Service and Capitation

Although the graphs are somewhat similar in general appearance, there is a profound difference in how profits and losses occur. First, consider fee-for-service. All volumes to the left of breakeven produce a loss for the provider, while all volumes to the right of breakeven produce a profit. Thus, the incentive for providers is to increase utilization because increased volume leads to increased profits. Now, look at the capitation graph. Here, all volumes to the left of breakeven produce a profit, whereas all volumes to the right of breakeven result in a loss. Under capitation, providers have the incentive to decrease utilization because decreased volume leads to increased profits. The only way to increase revenues is to increase the number of covered lives (enrollees).

Capitation completely reverses the actions that providers must take to assure financial success, and many providers find it difficult to adjust to the new, perverse (by conventional reimbursement standards) incentive system. Under fee-for-service, the keys to success are to work harder, increase volume, and hence increase profits; under capitation, the keys to profitability are to work smarter and decrease volume. Because the primary means to profitability with fee-for-service is increased volume, increased reimbursement rates, or both, the primary task of managers is to maximize utilization and reimbursement rates. Furthermore, any deficiencies in cost control often can be overcome by higher volume. Under capitation, the primary path to profitability is through cost control, so the key to success is lower volume and cost-effective treatment plans.

In general, capitation motivates providers to provide only needed services, and to provide those services in the lowest cost setting. Has capitation influenced provider behavior? It is difficult to fully assess the impact of capitation because few providers are fully capitated. Indeed, capitation is used most widely for primary care physicians, less so for specialists, and even less for hospitals. In fact, there is some recent evidence that managed care plans are cutting back somewhat on their use of capitation. Still, even relatively limited use of capitation, coupled with aggressive utilization management, can influence an entire market because it will set the standard for low-cost services. Evidence indicates that capitation accompanied by aggressive utilization management can reduce inpatient days from the national average of about 700 per 100,000 population to less than 250. If 85 percent occupancy is considered to be full capacity, then only about 0.8 beds are required per 1,000 population versus the current need, based on national average usage rates, of about 2.3 beds per 1,000 population. In spite of recent downsizing in the hospital industry, these data indicate that the industry still has too much capacity and that continued shrinkage is likely to occur.

Regarding physicians' behavior, the key feature is that managed care and capitation, with its emphasis on wellness and prevention as opposed to treatment, requires a different mix and fewer physicians than currently exists.

Although studies in this area are far from consistent, most indicate that the managed care system, as compared to a fee-for-service system, will require about the same number of primary care physicians, but 25–50 percent fewer specialists. Furthermore, managed care plans use more physician extenders, such as nurse practitioners and physician assistants, than are currently utilized. Of course, not all predictions come true, and the structure of the health services industry may not change as drastically as these data indicate. However, the handwriting on the wall suggests two powerful trends: (1) fewer hospital beds and (2) a physician mix that contains a greater proportion of primary care physicians. Most importantly, the data tell us that historical utilization rates based on conventional reimbursement methodologies are not good predictors of future utilization when the payment system is capitation or some other system that encourages aggressive utilization control.

Although much has been written about the negative aspects of capitation, particularly the incentive to withhold needed services, it must also be recognized that there are positive aspects to capitation. Here are some potential benefits associated with capitation:

- Providers receive a fixed payment regardless of whether services are actually rendered. Capitation revenues are predictable and timely, and thus are less risky than revenues from conventional payment methodologies that are tied to volume.
- Capitation payments are received before services are rendered, so, in effect, payers are extending credit to providers rather than vice versa, as under conventional reimbursement.
- Capitation supports national healthcare goals—primarily increased emphasis on cost control as well as wellness and prevention.
- Capitation may ease the reimbursement paperwork burden, and hence reduce expenditures on administrative costs.
- Capitation aligns the economic interests of physicians and hospitals because risk-sharing systems are typically established that allow all providers in a capitated system to benefit from reducing costs.
- Similarly, capitation encourages utilization of lower-cost treatments, such as outpatient surgery and home health care, as opposed to higher-cost inpatient alternatives. Thus, capitation creates incentives to use those services that are typically preferred by patients when such alternatives are clinically appropriate.

Self-Test Questions

1. What are the differences in provider incentives under conventional reimbursement and capitation?
2. What are the advantages of a capitated payment system?
3. What does current experience under managed care tell us about the look of the future healthcare delivery system?

Financial Risk Under Capitation

One of the key issues facing providers under capitation is its impact on financial risk. To examine this issue, we will first present a descriptive picture of financial risk, then examine the nature of financial risk, and finally present the results of an analysis that examines the financial risk inherent in capitation contracts.

Descriptive Risk

One way to assess the risk inherent in capitation versus other reimbursement contracts is to describe the nature of the risks incurred. Table 19.1 lists the most common provider-reimbursement methodologies and describes the financial risks inherent in each system.

    Fee-for-service is the least risky because the only risk facing providers is the risk that volume will be too low to cover fixed costs, assuming that the charge is set high enough to cover variable costs. Note that regardless of the reimbursement method, providers bear the cost of service risk in that costs can exceed revenues. However, a primary difference among the reimbursement types is the ability of the provider to influence the revenue/cost ratio. If providers set fees for each type of service provided, they can most easily ensure that revenues exceed costs. Furthermore, if providers have the power to set

TABLE 19.1
Descriptive Risk Under Various Reimbursement Methodologies

Contract Type	Provider Risks
Fee-for-service (charges)	Volume too low to cover fixed costs
Discounted fee-for-service (Discounted charges)	Volume too low to cover fixed costs
Prospective payment	Volume too low to cover fixed costs Case intensity Length of stay (for inpatients)
Per diem	Volume too low to cover fixed costs Case intensity Case mix Payer-limited length of stay
Global pricing	Volume too low to cover fixed costs Case intensity Pre- and post-operative care Physician services
Capitation	Utilization Case intensity Case mix Actuarial accuracy

rates above those that would exist in a truly competitive market, fee-for-service becomes even less risky. Finally, providers can increase usage by *churning*—creating more visits, ordering more tests, extending inpatient stays, and so on—which, in turn, increases revenues and reduces risks. *Discounted fee-for-service* may lower the profit potential of providers, but it does not alter the risks borne by providers.

Prospective payment, in which a fixed payment is made on the basis of each patient's diagnosis or procedure, adds a second dimension of risk to reimbursement contracts because the bundle of services needed to treat a particular diagnosis or the services provided for a particular procedure may be more costly than that assumed in the payment. If, on average, patients require more intensive services and, for hospitals, a longer length of stay than assumed in the prospective payment amount, the provider must bear the added costs.

Per diem reimbursement, whereby providers are paid a preset amount per patient day, is often used for hospitals and long-term care facilities. In addition to a single, all-inclusive per diem rate, *stratified per diems* are sometimes used whereby different rates are paid for dissimilar categories of care, such as general acute inpatient, obstetrical, and intensive care. Even under stratified per diems, where one rate usually covers a large number of diagnoses, providers bear case-mix risk along with intensity risk. In addition, providers bear the risk that the payer, through utilization reviews, will constrain lengths of stay, and hence increase intensity during the days that a patient is hospitalized. Thus, under per diem, the "compression" of services and shortened lengths of stay can put significant pressure on providers' profitability.

Under *global pricing*, payers pay a single prospective payment that covers all services delivered in a single episode, whether the services are rendered by a single or by multiple providers. For example, a global fee may be set for all obstetric services associated with a pregnancy provided by a single physician, including all prenatal and postnatal visits, as well as the delivery itself. Or, a global price may be paid for all physician and hospital services associated with a cardiac bypass operation.

From a payer's perspective, global pricing eliminates the potential for problems associated with unbundling and upcoding. *Unbundling* involves pricing the individual components of a service separately rather than as a package. For example, a physician's treatment of a fracture could be bundled, and hence billed as one episode, or it could be unbundled, with separate bills submitted for diagnosis, x-rays, setting the fracture, removing the cast, and so on. The rationale for unbundling usually is to provide more detailed records of treatments rendered, but often the result is higher total charges for the parts than would be charged for the entire package. *Upcoding* is the practice of billing for a procedure that yields a higher prospective payment than the one actually performed. Clearly, the more services that must be rendered for a single payment, the more providers are at risk for intensity of services.

Finally, under *capitation*, providers receive a fixed payment per member per month to provide all covered services to some defined population. Now, providers assume utilization and actuarial risks along with the risks assumed under the other reimbursement methods.

When the risks under different reimbursement systems are outlined in this descriptive fashion, it is easy to jump to the conclusion that capitation is by far the riskiest to providers, while fee-for-service is the least risky. However, before finalizing our conclusions regarding the risk to providers under capitation contracts, we need to examine the issue a little closer. We begin our more detailed examination with a discussion of the nature of financial risk.

The Nature of Financial Risk

As we discussed in Chapters 5 and 13, financial risk stems from uncertainties inherent in expected cash flows. If all forecasted cash flows were known with certainty, there would be no financial risk. However, because of uncertainties, there is some probability that a reimbursement contract will be less profitable than expected, and the greater the probability of a realized profitability far below that expected, the greater the financial risk.

Financial risk can be classified along several dimensions, but two dimensions are of particular relevance to our discussion of financial risk under capitation: (1) objective risk and (2) subjective risk. *Objective risk* occurs when the risk inherent in an uncertain outcome is known. For example, the flip of a coin has only objective risk. It is uncertain whether the flip will result in a head or a tail, so the flip is risky, but the probability of flipping a head or tail, 50 percent, is known. *Subjective risk* occurs when the probability distribution itself is uncertain. For example, a particular weather forecaster may predict that the chance of rain is 20 percent, but different forecasters may attach different probabilities to the event. Here, there are two dimensions to risk: (1) The risk inherent in the probability distribution (20 percent rain/80 percent no rain) and; (2) the risk that the probability distribution itself (the weather forecast) is wrong.[1]

We will see that the objective financial risk inherent in capitation contracts is not as high as many people suspect. However, their subjective financial risk is often very high, so the overall impact of capitation on the financial risk of most providers is much higher than indicated by an objective risk analysis because, by definition, subjective risk cannot be measured.

It is important to make one other point concerning financial risk. Under most types of reimbursement, rates can be set too low to cover costs. In such contracts, providers will lose money, but they do not necessarily bear a great deal of financial risk as defined here because such risk is a function of uncertainty, not profitability. If you loan $1,000 to your brother-in-law with every expectation that the loan will never be repaid, the loan is not very risky at all, even though its expected rate of return is -100 percent. Similarly, a hospital's reimbursement contract with a certain loss of, say, $100,000, has no financial risk because there is no uncertainty regarding the contract's profitability. The point here is that many payers that offer capitated contracts have a great deal of bargaining power that can be used to negotiate very tough terms with providers. These tough terms, and the resulting potential for losses on the contract, are not a result of the financial risk inherent in capitation contracts, but rather a result of the negotiating power of the payer. That same payer could negotiate a low-profitability contract regardless of the reimbursement method specified.

A Quantitative Analysis

The financial risk associated with provider contracts stems from uncertainty in profitability, so both revenues and costs must be considered. We will use hospitals to analyze the financial risk inherent in prospective payment and capitation contracts, but the results apply to physicians and other health-care providers.[2]

Under prospective payment, there is significant revenue risk because the amount of reimbursement depends on the number of admissions, with lower volume yielding reduced revenues. However, under capitation, and assuming a fixed number of enrollees, there is virtually no revenue risk. The hospital will receive the contractually fixed amount per member per month regardless of patient volume.

On the cost side, the financial risks are identical under the two contracts. There are fixed costs inherent in providing the service that must be met regardless of volume, and variable costs that are incurred for each patient admission. Thus, total costs, the sum of fixed and variable components, are dependent on volume. If we assume, at least initially, that the number and nature of admissions are unaffected by the reimbursement contract, then realized total costs are the same for a given population whether the payment method is prospective payment or capitation.

The financial risk facing hospitals is tied to uncertainty in profitability, and hence stems from both uncertainties in the revenue stream and uncertainties in total costs. To examine the impact of these uncertainties, we will consider two hospitals: (1) Hospital F, whose costs are all fixed; and (2) Hospital V, whose costs are all variable. Clearly, no real-world hospital has all fixed or all variable costs, but by looking at these extremes we can gain a better appreciation of the factors that influence financial risk under prospective payment and capitation.

To keep the analysis manageable, assume a hypothetical situation in which the contract involves 1,000 members; the annual capitation payment is $300 per member per year (PMPY); the expected number of inpatient stays is 0.1 PMPY, or 100 admissions per year; and the prospective payment per admission is $3,000. On the cost side, assume Hospital F has fixed costs of

TABLE 19.2
Annual Cash
Flows

	Hospital F		Hospital V	
	Prospective Payment	Capitation	Prospective Payment	Capitation
Total revenues	$300,000	$300,000	$300,000	$300,000
Fixed costs	300,000	300,000	0	0
Variable costs	0	0	300,000	300,000
Net income	$ 0	$ 0	$ 0	$ 0

$300,000 and no variable costs, to treat the population served; while Hospital V has variable costs of $3,000 per inpatient stay and no fixed costs.

Table 19.2 contains the annual cash flows to each hospital associated with the two contracts. Note that the initial values were chosen so that the revenues are the same under each contract type and that total costs are the same at both hospitals. Also, for ease, the values were chosen so that net income under both contracts is zero.

Now, let's introduce risk into the analysis. Again, to keep the example manageable, assume that the only uncertainty in the contracts is patient volume; that is, the capitation payment, prospective payment per admission, fixed costs, and variable costs per inpatient stay are known with certainty at the beginning of the year (beginning of the contract period). What would happen to profitability if realized volume differed from expected volume? Table 19.3 answers this question.

Uncertain volume has no effect on Hospital F under capitation or on Hospital V under prospective payment. In each instance, revenues and costs move in step with one another. Hospital F has all fixed costs, and under capitation its revenues are fixed, so changes in volume have no impact on

TABLE 19.3
Net Income at
Different
Volume Levels

Number of Inpatient Stays	Hospital F		Hospital V	
	Prospective Payment	Capitation	Prospective Payment	Capitation
80	($60,000)	$0	$0	$ 60,000
85	(45,000)	0	0	45,000
90	(30,000)	0	0	30,000
95	(15,000)	0	0	15,000
100	0	0	0	0
105	15,000	0	0	(15,000)
110	30,000	0	0	(30,000)
115	45,000	0	0	(45,000)
120	60,000	0	0	(60,000)

profitability. Under prospective payment, revenues vary with volume, while costs are fixed, so higher volume leads to higher profitability. Thus, with prospective payment contracts, Hospital F has a financial incentive to increase volume because increased volume leads to higher profits.

The situation is reversed at Hospital V. When all costs are variable, profits are constant under prospective payment but variable under capitation. Increased volume leads to increased revenue under prospective payment, but the revenue increase is offset exactly by higher costs. Hospital V receives $3,000 for each admission, but its variable costs also equal $3,000 per admission, so additional admissions add nothing to the bottom line. Lower volume means lower costs regardless of the reimbursement method, but under capitation, the revenue stream is fixed, so Hospital V has a financial incentive under capitation to decrease volume because lower volume leads to higher profits.

The analysis could be extended to include uncertainty in variable costs and prospective payment per admission, but the general results remain the same. If all costs are fixed, there is less objective financial risk to capitation contracts than to prospective payment contracts. If all costs are variable, there is less objective financial risk to prospective payment contracts than to capitation contracts.

When assessing the relative objective financial risk of capitation contracts, the key question to providers is: "Are the costs at my organization predominantly fixed or predominantly variable?" If the costs are mostly fixed, then objective financial risk is actually reduced when moving from prospective payment to capitation because the fixed revenue stream better matches the fixed cost structure. On the other hand, if the cost structure is predominantly variable, moving to capitation will increase objective financial risk because the fixed revenue stream is a poor match for a cost structure that is highly correlated to volume.

Most healthcare providers, and hospitals in particular, have relatively high fixed-to-total-cost ratios.[3] Thus, for most providers, capitation contracts actually have less objective financial risk than prospective payment contracts because financial risk is reduced by matching the uncertainties inherent in the revenue and cost streams. When organizations have a high percentage of fixed costs, a fixed revenue stream stabilizes profits, and hence reduces financial risk.

If objective financial risk is reduced under capitation contracts, why did our earlier descriptive analysis conclude that capitation is more risky than prospective payment? One reason, of course, is that the descriptive assessment did not consider in any systematic way the relationships between revenues and costs. More importantly, the numerical analysis ignored the subjective risk inherent in capitation contracts. The numerical analysis focused solely on objective financial risk—we assumed that providers know their cost structures and population characteristics well enough to be confident of the revenue and cost estimates. Under these conditions, capitation contracts are clearly less risky to providers with a high percentage of fixed costs.

However, to limit the overall financial risk of capitation contracts to objective risk, it is necessary that providers be able to accurately forecast costs and volumes for a large number of diagnoses for a given population. For example, assume that a hospital signs a capitation contract to provide all common inpatient services to a patient population of 100,000. If the hospital is to bear only objective financial risk, it must know with some confidence the expected volume by diagnosis, as well as the costs for treating those diagnoses. Thus, the hospital needs relatively sophisticated actuarial and cost data. In addition to the confidence in cost and utilization data, providers must have a sufficient number of capitated lives to make the law of large numbers work in their favor. With too few patients covered by capitation, just one or two adverse cases can easily push expected profitability into realized losses. Only with tens of thousands of members can providers take advantage of the risk reduction inherent in treating a "portfolio" of patients.

Even if a contract has substantial underlying financial risk, whether objective or subjective, its effective riskiness is lessened if management can take actions to counter unexpected adverse trends as they develop. Suppose a hospital enters into a capitation contract without good estimates of volume and costs. If six months into the contract managers realized that total costs exceed estimates and hence the contract will be less profitable than expected, they would try to take actions to increase the contract's profitability. The only two managerial actions available to turn a bad capitation contract into a good one is to decrease volume, lower costs, or both. In the past, hospitals with profitability problems solved such problems by raising charges and increasing volume. Under capitation, however, the prescription for increased profit requires actions—decreasing volume or lowering costs—with which providers have limited experience, and hence are more difficult to implement than previous prescriptions. Furthermore, when a high proportion of costs is fixed, cost-reduction efforts are extremely challenging because they can be achieved only by selling off plant and equipment and shrinking the labor force. Under capitation contracts, providers are less able to influence the profitability of a contract once it goes into force, so they are less able to cope with the given amount of financial risk faced.

Another risk that providers face under capitation is the impact of outliers. The costs associated with a single patient, especially to a hospital, can fall well beyond normal bounds, and hence one or just a few outliers can result in financial losses well beyond those estimated at the time a contract is signed. In general, prospective payment contracts have outlier provisions, so providers are somewhat protected against the risks associated with high-cost outliers. If capitation contracts do not contain such provisions, the risk of outliers increases the financial risk inherent in such contracts.[4] Furthermore, to increase the probability that realized volume, and hence cash flows, will be close to that forecasted, providers must have a relatively large number of covered lives under capitation contracts.

Our quantitative analysis leads to two primary conclusions about the relative risk of capitation contracts. First, the objective financial risk inherent in capitation contracts is not as high as most people think. Providers with a high percentage of fixed costs can actually stabilize earnings under capitation, and hence reduce financial risk. Second, the overall financial risk of capitation contracts, including both objective and subjective risk, can be very high if providers (1) do not have the actuarial and cost data available to make sound capitation pricing decisions; (2) do not have a sufficient number of capitated patients to take advantage of the law of large numbers; and (3) do not have the capability to reduce volume and cut costs, if necessary, to react to any adverse trends that might develop.

Taken together, these conclusions have several implications for healthcare providers. To prosper in a capitated environment, providers must be able to estimate accurately not only their own costs, but also the diagnoses and patient volumes that would result from a particular contract. This means that providers will need good costing systems and also that providers will need actuarial expertise, which is a domain historically left to insurers. Without these competencies, it will be impossible to enter into capitation contracts without bearing a high degree of subjective financial risk.

Also, providers will have to break with traditional paradigms. Financial problems can no longer be solved by raising charges and increasing volume. Under capitation, raising charges (having a high bid on a contract proposal) will mean fewer patients for the provider, which will have an adverse impact both on revenues and on achieving a capitated population sufficiently large to realize actuarial predictions. Furthermore, the key to success once the contract has been signed is to lower costs and utilization. This requires nontraditional strategies, so healthcare managers must exhibit flexibility and adaptability to successfully manage under capitation.

Finally, providers that are less efficient than their local counterparts confront very difficult issues when negotiating managed care contracts. Capitation contracts are usually set at rates that assume the efficient delivery of services to control unnecessary services and costs. Less-efficient providers will experience more challenges under capitation because they must choose between accepting rates, which, at least in the short run, may not cover costs, or lose market share that they may not be able to regain. The difficulties that inefficient providers face do not result from financial risk differentials, but rather from prior management practices that did not sufficiently stress the efficient delivery of services.

1. Briefly, describe the following reimbursement systems and, using the descriptive approach, analyze the risks to providers under each system:
    a. Fee-for-service
    b. Discounted fee-for-service
    c. Prospective payment

Self-Test Questions

d. Per diem
e. Global pricing
f. Capitation.
2. What is the basic source of financial risk?
3. Distinguish between objective and subjective financial risk.
4. What lessons can be learned from the quantitative risk assessment of prospective payment and capitation contracts?

Development of Premium Rates

One of the primary financial management functions within managed care plans and integrated delivery systems is the development of premium rates for healthcare buyers, which involves estimating the total costs of providing healthcare services. In this section, we discuss several methodologies for estimating provider payments, which are then aggregated to estimate total costs, the basis for the premium rate.

Allocation of Premium Dollars

HMOs and other managed care organizations collect premium dollars from employers and other purchasers of healthcare, and then use those dollars to pay providers, cover administrative expenses, and earn profits. To help better understand how HMOs set their premium rates, first consider Table 19.4, which illustrates how a typical premium dollar is spent. First, HMOs have the same types of management and marketing expenses as any other business, and the premium dollar must cover such costs. Also, it is necessary for HMOs to earn profits, both to create reserves for contingencies and for distribution to stockholders if investor-owned. About 16 percent of the premium dollar goes to administration and profit, while the remaining 84 percent is paid out to providers. The biggest provider expense typically is for physicians, with approximately 12 percent of the premium dollar going to primary care physicians and 32 percent to specialists that are part of the HMO's provider panel.

The next major item is payments for hospital and other institutional care provided within the system (within the HMO's provider panel), which totals 36 percent of the premium dollar. Finally, HMO members sometimes require services from providers that are out of the HMO's system, either because there are no in-system providers for that service or the services were required outside the geographic area served by the HMO. Payments to out-of-system providers, including both physicians and hospitals/institutions, average 4 percent of the premium dollar.

Note that the Table 19.4 percentages are averages, and there are wide variations among HMOs as to how the premium dollar is allocated. Healthcare purchasers want a high percentage of the premium dollar to go to providers to encourage them to provide needed services in a timely manner. Conversely,

Total premium dollar	<u>100%</u>	**TABLE 19.4**
		Typical
Administration and profit	16%	Allocation of
Paid to within-system physicians:		the HMO
Primary care	12%	Premium
Specialists	<u>32</u>	Dollar
Total to within-system physicians	<u>44%</u>	
Paid to within-system hospitals/institutions	36%	
Paid to out-of-system providers	<u>4%</u>	

Source: Jennings Ryan & Kolb, 1998.

HMOs have an incentive to lower the amount paid to providers, both to increase profits and to ensure competitive pricing to buyers in an increasingly hostile marketplace.

Developing Premium Rates: An Illustration

There are many ways to develop the premium rates that managed care plans charge to purchasers. In this section, we illustrate several methods that an HMO or integrated delivery system can use to estimate the payments it must make to its providers to cover a defined population, which it can then aggregate and combine with its own costs to estimate a premium rate.[5] Rates are developed as if all providers were capitated because the final premium rate will be quoted on a per member per month basis. However, actual reimbursement could be by capitation, discounted fee-for-service, or by any other method.

Assume that BetterCare, Inc., an aggressively managed HMO, must develop a premium bid to submit to Big Business, a major employer in BetterCare's service area. To keep the illustration manageable, assume that all medically necessary in-area services can be provided by a single hospital that offers both inpatient and outpatient services including emergency room services, a single nursing home, a panel of primary care physicians, and a panel of specialist physicians. In addition, BetterCare must budget for covered care to be delivered out of area when its members are traveling. Thus, to develop its bid, BetterCare has to estimate the amount of payments to this set of providers for the covered population, plus allow for administrative expenses and profits.

Hospital Inpatient Rate

The *fee-for-service equivalent method* is often used to set the within-system hospital inpatient capitation rate. This method is based on expected usage and negotiated charges, rather than underlying costs, although there clearly should be a link between charges and costs. To illustrate the concept, assume that BetterCare targets 350 inpatient days for each 1,000 members, or 0.350 inpatient days per member. Furthermore, BetterCare believes that a fair fee-for-service charge in a competitive environment would be $938 per inpatient day. Note that the values chosen both for utilization and payment are not based on conventional reimbursement experience. Rather, the number of inpatient days reflects a highly managed working-age population, and the fee-for-service charge is designed to cover all hospital costs, including profits, in an efficiently run hospital that operates in a highly competitive environment. The inpatient cost per member per month (PMPM) is found as follows:

$$\text{Inpatient cost PMPM} = \frac{\text{Per member utilization rate} \times \text{Fee-for-service rate}}{12}$$

$$= \frac{0.350 \times \$938}{12} = \$27.35 \text{ PMPM.}$$

Thus, using the fee-for-service method, BetterCare estimates inpatient costs for Big Business's HMO enrollees at $27.35 PMPM.

Other Institutional Rates

The rates for out-of-area hospital usage, hospital outpatient surgeries and emergency room visits, as well as for skilled nursing home stays, were developed using the fee-for-service equivalent method discussed above. Here is a summary of BetterCare's estimates for these services:

Service	Annual Utilization per 1,000 Members	Fee-for-Service Rate	Capitation Rate PMPM
Out-of-area inpatient days	25	$1,495	$ 3.11
Outpatient surgeries	50	1,082	4.51
Emergency room visits	125	138	1.44
Skilled nursing home days	5	150	0.06
			$9.12

Here, each PMPM capitation rate was calculated by multiplying annual utilization times the fee-for-service rate, and then dividing the resulting product first by 1,000 to obtain a per member amount and then by 12 to get the PMPM rate. The end result is a capitation estimate of $9.12 PMPM for the services listed above. Of course, actual payments to these providers typically would be made on a discounted fee-for-service basis.

Primary Care Rate

We will use the *budgetary*, or *cost*, *approach* to estimate primary physicians' costs for Big Business's enrollees. This method is the most common for setting physicians' payments, and it is based on utilization and underlying costs, as opposed to charges. The starting point is expected patient demand, by specialty, for physicians' services. This demand is then translated into the number of full-time equivalent (FTE) physicians required per 1,000 members (enrollees), which depends on physician productivity. Finally, the cost for physician services is estimated by multiplying staffing requirements by the average cost per FTE, including base compensation, fringe benefits, and malpractice premiums. In addition, an amount—usually some dollar amount per 1,000 members—is added for clinical and administrative support for physicians.

In developing its capitation rate for primary care physicians, BetterCare made the following assumptions:

- On average, each enrollee makes 3.0 visits to a primary care physician per year, so each 1,000 enrollees make 3,000 visits per year.
- Each primary care physician can handle 4,000 patient visits per year.
- Total compensation per primary care physician is $175,000 per year.

Under these assumptions, each 1,000 enrollees will require 3,000 / 4,000 = 0.75 primary care physicians, and hence each 1,000 enrollees will require 0.75 × $175,000 = $131,250 in primary care services. Finally, the annual cost per member is $131,250 / 1,000 = $131.25, and the cost PMPM = $131.25 / 12 = $10.94. Thus, the rate that BetterCare will propose to Big Business will include $10.94 PMPM for primary care physician compensation.

The capitation rate for specialists' care is developed using the cost approach in a similar manner to that for primary care. Here are BetterCare's assumptions: *Specialty Care Rate*

- On average, each enrollee is referred for 1.2 visits to specialty care physicians per year, so each 1,000 enrollees make 1,200 visits per year.
- Each specialty physician can handle 2,000 patient visits per year.
- Total compensation per specialist is $284,000 per year.

Under these assumptions, each 1,000 enrollees will require 1,200 / 2,000 = 0.60 specialists, and hence each 1,000 enrollees will require 0.60 × $284,000 = $170,400 in specialists' services. Finally, the annual cost per member is $170,400 / 1,000 = $170.40, so the cost PMPM = $170.40 / 12 = $14.20. Thus, the rate that BetterCare will propose to Big Business will include $14.20 PMPM for specialist physician compensation.

Thus far, we have estimated the capitation rate for physicians' compensation, but we have not accounted for other costs associated with physicians' practices. First, physicians require, on average, 1.7 FTEs for clinical and administrative support, and each supporting staff member receives an average of $35,000 per year in total compensation. Because the physician requirement to support 1,000 members is 0.75 primary care plus 0.60 specialists, for a total of 1.35 physicians, each 1,000 members will require 1.35 × 1.7 × $35,000 ≈ $80,000 of physician's support, or $80,000 / 1,000 / 12 = $6.67 PMPM. *Other Physician-Related Costs Rate*

Next, expenditures on supplies, including administrative, medical, and diagnostic supplies, average $10 per visit, and members are expected to make 4.2 visits per year to both primary and specialty care physicians. Thus, the annual cost per member is $42, and the cost PMPM is estimated to be $42 / 12 = $3.50 PMPM. Finally, overhead expenses, including depreciation, rent, utilities, and so on, are estimated at $6.00 PMPM.

Total Physician Rate   BetterCare has estimated numerous categories of costs related solely to physicians. For ease, assume now that BetterCare plans to contract with a single medical group practice to provide all physicians' service and to pay the group a capitated rate. Then, the total capitation rate for the medical group would be as follows:

Primary care	$ 10.94 PMPM
Specialist care	14.20
Support staff	6.67
Supplies	3.50
Overhead	6.00
Subtotal	$ 41.31 PMPM
Profit (10%)	4.13
In-area total	$45.44 PMPM
Outside referrals	3.40
Total	$48.84 PMPM

The $48.84 PMPM total capitation rate for the medical group is merely the aggregate of the rates previously developed for physicians' services, plus two additional elements. First, BetterCare believes that a fair profit margin on group practice businesses is 10 percent, so $4.13 PMPM is allowed for profit on the in-area physician subtotal of $41.31 PMPM. Second, $3.40 PMPM is allocated to cover referrals outside the group practice when needed either because a particular specialty is not available within the group or the member is outside the service area. Finally, note that the group might not capitate all its physicians even though it receives a capitated rate from BetterCare.

An Alternative Method for Physician's Rates   In general, the rates obtained from the first two methods would include adjustments for age and gender. An alternative method would be to start with utilization data already broken down by these categories. The *demographic-based approach* focuses on the age/gender distribution of the population being served, which is then coupled with cost or fee-for-service data to estimate the capitation rate. Table 19.5 illustrates the demographic-based approach by applying it to the population that would be served if BetterCare wins the contract to provide an HMO plan for Big Business.

The male/female costs were calculated by multiplying the population percentages for each gender times the applicable costs per member per month. The total cost for each service is merely the sum of the male and female costs. Note that the total cost for in-area physician services, $16.17 + $29.27 = $45.44 PMPM, is the same as BetterCare estimated using the budgetary approach. If the data are consistent, both methods should lead to the same capitation rate. Also, the hospital/other institutional capitation rate of $36.47 PMPM is the same as the rate obtained earlier for these services: $27.35 + $9.12 = $36.47. Clearly, we "fudged" the data so our results would be consistent. In most cases, capitation rates developed using different methodologies

TABLE 19.5
Demographic-Based Rates for the Medical Group

| Age Band | Demographics | | Cost per Member per Month | | | | | | | |
| | Male | Female | Primary Care | | Specialist/Referral | | Hospital/Other | |
			Male	Female	Male	Female	Male	Female
0–1	1.9%	1.9%	$47.00	$47.00	$31.42	$31.42	$29.93	$29.93
2–4	2.8	2.8	20.25	20.25	11.19	11.19	16.29	16.29
5–19	12.4	12.4	11.04	11.04	11.19	11.19	15.35	15.35
20–29	11.4	15.4	10.53	15.92	18.44	49.30	11.58	55.65
30–39	9.6	10.0	13.04	17.56	23.26	44.51	24.95	58.97
40–49	5.3	5.7	16.40	19.56	32.64	41.05	53.74	52.31
50–59	3.6	3.6	20.74	22.74	47.13	47.74	80.60	66.91
60+	0.7	0.5	24.93	25.60	73.43	58.91	121.54	87.60
Total	47.7%	52.3%						
Male/female cost			$ 7.07	$ 9.10	$10.58	$18.69	$13.24	$23.23
Total service cost			$16.17		$29.27		$36.47	

will be different, and hence a great deal of judgment will have to be applied in the rate-setting process.

**Setting the
Final Rate**
Remember that our goal here is to set a premium rate that BetterCare can use to make a bid to cover Big Business's employees. Thus far, we have estimated the PMPM rates required to pay all the providers needed to serve the population, both in area and out of area. In addition, we are assuming that pharmacy benefits will be handled separately, or *carved out*, and that the cost of these benefits would be $7.00 PMPM. After all costs have been considered, BetterCare concludes that it can submit a bid of $108.21 PMPM.[6]

Medical costs:	
Hospital inpatient	$27.35 PMPM
Other institutional	9.12
Outpatient prescription drugs	7.00
Physician care	48.84
Total medical costs	$92.31 PMPM
HMO costs:	
Administration	$13.85 PMPM
Contribution to reserves/profits	2.05
Total HMO costs	$15.90 PMPM
Total premium	$108.21 PMPM

Note that if BetterCare wins the contract from Big Business, the monthly revenue to providers will be somewhat higher (usually about 5 percent) than the embedded PMPM rates because enrollees will be required to make co-payments for selected services.

In closing, note that BetterCare's bid most likely will be subject to market forces—that is, there will be multiple bidders for Big Business's health contract. If BetterCare's bid is to be accepted, it must offer the right combination of price and quality. If BetterCare's costs, and hence bid, is too high or its quality too low, it will not get the contract and it must reassess its cost and quality structure to ensure that it is competitive on future bids.

**Self-Test
Questions**
1. Roughly, what is the allocation of an HMO premium dollar?
2. Briefly, describe the following three methods for developing capitation rates:
   a. Fee-for-service equivalent method
   b. Budgetary, or cost, approach
   c. Demographic-based approach
3. Of the three approaches, which one do you think would be the most accurate? The easiest to apply in practice?

Risk-Sharing Arrangements

In an integrated delivery system, or within the provider panel of a managed care plan, different providers are brought together in some type of formal or informal arrangement to provide healthcare services to a defined population. Often, system participants are paid under different reimbursement methods, and different reimbursement systems clearly create different incentives. To illustrate the concept, assume that an integrated delivery system uses capitation for primary care physicians, discounted fee-for-service for specialists, and per diem for institutional providers—hospitals and long-term care providers. In such a system, primary care physicians have the incentive to shift care to specialists and institutions because primary care physicians are capitated, and hence not rewarded for higher utilization. On the other hand, specialists and institutions would welcome the added volume because they are being paid on the basis of the amount of services provided. Overall, this differential in reimbursement creates incentives that increase total system costs, and hence costs to insurers and purchasers.

If both primary care and specialist physicians are capitated, primary care physicians would still have the incentive to make unnecessary referrals, but such referrals would no longer be welcome by specialists. If the institutions also are capitated, no provider wants increased volume, so conflicts are bound to occur between primary care physicians and specialists and between physicians and institutions.

In such situations, *risk-sharing* arrangements are often implemented to create incentives that encourage providers to act in the best interest of the system, rather than in their own self-interest. Generally, proper incentives are created within provider panels by establishing *withholds*, or *risk pools*, which are pools of money that are initially withheld and then distributed to panel members only if preestablished goals are met.

Risk-Sharing Basics

Risk pools can be used with any type of reimbursement system, such as the use of withholds in a per diem system, whereby the hospital is rewarded if utilization is less than expected and, in effect, penalized by not receiving some portion or all of the amount withheld if utilization exceeds the target. In effect, risk pools are designed to reward those providers that are most able to control costs through better utilization management, better cost control, or both. Risk-sharing arrangements can occur among physicians only, among physicians and institutions, or among all providers. Furthermore, risk pools can be established to promote only financial goals or some combination of financial and nonfinancial goals.

Note that if a system is fully integrated and all subsidiary providers are owned by, and hence directly responsible to, the same parent, there is only one bottom line and no need for risk-sharing arrangements, at least in theory. Proper incentives are created by managerial control. However, in most systems today, providers are loosely affiliated in some way rather than belonging to the same business entity, and hence risk-sharing arrangements are needed to align the incentives of the diverse parties involved.

Typically, risk-sharing arrangements allocate 10–20 percent of each reimbursement dollar to one or more risk pools, often for primary care, specialty (referral) care, and institutional. Then, throughout the year, expenses are charged against the applicable pools, and at year-end, each pool's expenses are reconciled—that is, compared with those budgeted. Any surpluses are distributed to the participating providers on the basis of a prearranged formula, while any deficits typically are funded from network reserves. (Reserves, which are risk management tools designed to help businesses cover system cost overruns, are discussed in Chapter 20.)

Primary Care Withhold: Single Risk Pool

The best way to grasp the basics of risk sharing is through examples. In this section, we illustrate a withhold system for primary care physicians only. In the next section, we will illustrate a risk-sharing system that encompasses primary care physicians, specialists, and a hospital.

Here is the risk pool arrangement for primary care physicians (PCPs) used by one HMO. The HMO pays its PCPs by capitation, but a percentage of the total capitated amount is held in reserve and distributed to individual physicians if certain financial goals are met. In general, PCP goals are based on specialty care and hospital costs. Of course, the goal is to lower the overall cost of providing care, but cost reduction goals should not reduce the quality of care afforded to patients.

Assume that the HMO's capitation payment to PCPs is $15 PMPM, but that 20 percent of this amount is placed into the PCP risk pool. The budgeted amount for specialty and hospital costs is $45 PMPM. Of course, the purpose of the pool is to encourage PCPs to take actions that result in realized specialty and hospital costs that are less than those budgeted. For simplicity, assume that there are only three PCPs in the plan: (1) Physician L (for low-cost), (2) Physician M (for medium-cost), and (3) Physician H (for high-cost). Furthermore, assume that each physician has 1,000 patients under the plan, so there are 3,000 patients in total.

Table 19.6 contains the risk pool distributions under two different outcome scenarios. Line 1 gives each PCP's initial annual capitation payment: $15 PMPM × 12 months × 1,000 members = $180,000. Thus, 3 × $180,000 = $540,000 in total is allocated for PCP payments. However, 20 percent of the capitated amount is placed into the risk pool, so each PCP's annual capitated payment is reduced by 0.20 × $180,000 = $36,000. This reduction and the resulting $144,000 initial allocation are shown on Lines 2 and 3. Note that each of the members served by the three PCPs is allocated $45 for specialty and hospital costs, so the budgeted goal for these costs is 1,000 × $45 × 12 = $540,000 per PCP, or $1,620,000 in total, as shown on Line 4. Also, note that the total amount in the PCP risk pool is 3 × $36,000 = $108,000.

Now, consider Scenario 1, contained in Lines 5, 6, 7, and 8. Here, the assumption is made that no PCP will receive any funds from the pool if it

TABLE 19.6
Primary Care
Physician
(PCP) Risk
Pool
(annual
amounts)

	Physician L	Physician M	Physician H
1. Allocated amount	$ 180,000	$ 180,000	$ 180,000
2. Withhold (20 percent)	(36,000)	(36,000)	(36,000)
3. Initial allocation	$ 144,000	$ 144,000	$ 144,000
4. Budgeted referral costs	$ 540,000	$ 540,000	$ 540,000
Scenario 1: Distribution Based on Aggregate PCP Performance			
5. Actual referral costs	500,000	560,000	680,000
6. Referral gain (loss)	40,000	(20,000)	(140,000)
7. Withhold returned	0	0	0
8. Total compensation	$ 144,000	$ 144,000	$ 144,000
Scenario 2: Distribution Based on Individual PCP Performance			
9. Actual referral costs	500,000	560,000	680,000
10. Referral gain (loss)	40,000	(20,000)	(140,000)
11. Withhold returned	36,000	16,000	0
12. Total compensation	$ 180,000	$ 160,000	$ 144,000

is empty at year-end. The actual referral costs for each PCP are the amounts shown on Line 5. The referral gain (loss) for each PCP is shown on Line 6, while the total gain (loss) for all three PCPs is $40,000 − $20,000 − $140,000 = −$120,000. This exceeds the $108,000 in the risk pool, so no funds remain for distribution. In fact, BetterCare will have to fund the $108,000 − $120,000 = $12,000 shortfall from its own reserves. Because no funds remain in the pool for distribution, each PCP's realized compensation would be his or her initial allocation, $144,000.

Clearly, there is a problem with the way that the risk pool is allocated. Because no funds remained in the pool, all three PCPs were equally penalized, even though Physician L did an excellent job of controlling costs and Physician M came in only $20,000 over budget. The real cause of the failure to meet the overall referral budget was Physician H, who was a whopping $140,000 over budget. Is it fair to penalize L and M because of H's actions? If, over time, it appears to Physicians L and M that the risk pool will always be exhausted as a result of actions beyond their control, they will have no motivation to continue to practice as efficiently as they do now. Also, it is important to know whether Physician H's failure to meet the risk pool budget was a result of practice patterns, or did H have an extraordinary number of high-cost patients? If the patient mix is not equal across PCPs, obvious problems will arise, so the HMO must be careful in assigning patients to ensure, to the extent possible, that the utilization and intensity mix is evenly spread across PCPs or that adjustments are made to account for such differences.

Scenario 2 in Table 19.6 is similar to Scenario 1, except that payments are made from the withhold to individual physicians regardless of the aggregate position of the pool. In this situation, the aggregate pool is really an artificiality. Because the HMO will reward individual PCPs that come in at or under budget regardless of aggregate performance, each PCP really has his or her own individual risk pool. Thus, as shown on Line 11, Physician L, because he or she came in below budget, received the entire withhold amount from his or her pool, which resulted in total compensation of $144,000 + $36,000 = $180,000. Physician M received $36,000 − $20,000 = $16,000 from his or her pool, for total compensation of $160,000; Physician H, on the other hand, received nothing from his or her pool, for a total compensation of $144,000. This type of arrangement creates better incentives for PCPs, but the HMO had to bear the total cost of the pool payments, $52,000, because the actions of Physician H depleted the pool. The key here is to modify the behavior of Physician H so that funds remain in the pool to make the incentive payments. Perhaps, after one year, Physician H will be motivated to follow lower-cost practice patterns because of the potential monetary rewards.

Note that there is an almost infinite number of ways in which a PCP risk pool can be distributed. Another alternative to Scenario 2 would be this: If the aggregate risk pool is depleted, payments to individual physicians will be cut in half. If this were the situation in Scenario 2 in Table 19.6, Physician L would get only $18,000 from the pool on Line 12, while Physician M would be paid $8,000. Now, the actions of Physician H have a direct bearing on the payments to L and M, so it is in the best interests of L, M, and the system to encourage H to lower costs. Also, with this distribution system, the HMO does not replace the full amount of the pool if it is depleted.

Primary Care and Referral Withholds: Two Risk Pools

The previous risk pool illustration placed only one set of providers at risk, the primary care physicians. In this section, we illustrate the use of two risk pools.

Assume that HealthyHMO, with 10,000 covered lives in a given service area, reimburses its primary care physicians under a capitated system, its specialty care physicians under a discounted fee-for-service system, and the hospital under a per diem system. To create proper incentives, HealthyHMO establishes two risk pools: (1) a professional services risk pool for the physicians only and (2) an inpatient services risk pool shared equally by the HMO, physicians, and hospital.

Professional Services Risk Pool (PSRP) Ten percent of the funds budgeted for specialty services are withheld in the professional services risk pool (PSRP). The total amount budgeted for professional services, including both primary and specialty care physicians, is $37 PMPM. With 10,000 members, the HMO's annual budget for professional services is $37 × 10,000 × 12 = $4,440,000.

The capitated payment for primary care physicians is $12 PMPM, for a total of $12 × 10,000 × 12 = $1,440,000. The difference between the total allocated for professional services and the capitated total for primary care services is $4,440,000 - $1,440,000 = $3,000,000$, which is the amount allocated for specialty services. Because 10 percent of the specialists' budget is placed in the PSRP, it is funded at a level of $300,000, and the budget for specialist payments, after withhold, is $2,700,000.

When the budget year is over, a year-end reconciliation process adjusts for under- and over-utilization, and allocates the pool among the primary care and specialist physicians. If actual costs exceed the $3,000,000 total specialty care budget, no distributions are made from the PSRP, and HealthyHMO must cover the shortfall. Table 19.7 illustrates end-of-year reconciliation under four different scenarios. In Scenario 1, actual payments for specialty services are assumed to be $3,000,000, as shown on Line 2. This results in a -$300,000 variance from the after-withhold budget, and the risk pool is depleted. Primary care physicians gain no additional income because the specialists have taken the entire amount in the pool in their fee-for-service payments.

Scenario 2 assumes specialist payments of $3,100,000, which results in a -$400,000 budget variance. Like Scenario 1, nothing is left for the primary care physicians. In fact, the specialists have not only exhausted the pool, but receive $100,000 in additional payments from HealthyHMO, which must bear all losses exceeding the amount placed into the pool.

Scenario 3, which begins on Line 13 in Table 19.7, presents a lower-cost situation, assuming specialty care payments of only $2,800,000. Now, the budget variance is -$100,000, which leaves $200,000 in the pool for distribution. There are many methodologies that could be used to make the distribution. The $200,000 could be evenly split among all physicians. Or, the pool could be distributed to physicians on a basis proportional to the amount of effort that they expend on HealthyHMO's patients, say, as measured by the number of patient visits or the dollar amount paid to each physician. Alternatively, the distribution could be based on the number of referrals made by primary care physicians and the number received by specialty physicians. In this situation, primary care physicians with fewer referrals would get a larger share of the pool, while specialists with a higher number of referrals would receive a larger share of the pool.

Scenario 4 is similar to Scenario 3, except that with only $2,600,000 paid to specialists over the year, the pool is left with $400,000. Now, $300,000 is available for distribution to physicians, and $100,000 is reclaimed by HealthyHMO.

HealthyHMO budgets for the inpatient services risk pool (ISRP) based on 350 **_Inpatient_** inpatient days per 1,000 members, which is the rate experienced by the HMO **_Services Risk_** last year for its entire membership. The negotiated per diem rate is $750. **_Pool (ISRP)_** Thus, its 10,000 members are expected to use $10 \times 350 = 3,500$ inpatient days, which gives a before-withhold amount of $3,500 \times \$750 = \$2,625,000$. HealthyHMO withholds 10 percent of the inpatient budget for the ISRP, or $262,500. Thus, the adjusted per diem rate is $0.90 \times \$750 = \$675$, which

TABLE 19.7

Professional Services Risk Pool (PSRP) (annual amounts)

Scenario 1: Specialty Payments of $3,000,000	
1. Budgeted payments for specialty services	$ 2,700,000
2. Actual payments for specialty services	3,000,000
3. Variance from budget	($ 300,000)
4. Risk pool starting amount	300,000
5. Remainder in pool	$ 0
6. Risk pool allocation	$ 0
Scenario 2: Specialty Payments of $3,100,000	
7. Budgeted payments for specialty services	$ 2,700,000
8. Actual payments for specialty services	3,100,000
9. Variance from budget	($ 400,000)
10. Risk pool starting amount	300,000
11. Remainder in pool	($ 100,000)
12. Risk pool allocation	$ 0
Scenario 3: Specialty Payments of $2,800,000	
13. Budgeted payments for specialty services	$ 2,700,000
14. Actual payments for specialty services	2,800,000
15. Variance from budget	($ 100,000)
16. Risk pool starting amount	300,000
17. Remainder in pool	$ 200,000
18. Risk pool allocation	$ 200,000
Scenario 4: Specialty Payments of $2,600,000	
19. Budgeted payments for specialty services	$ 2,700,000
20. Actual payments for specialty services	2,600,000
21. Variance from budget	$ 100,000
22. Risk pool starting amount	300,000
23. Remainder in pool	$ 400,000
24. Risk pool allocation	
a. Physicians	$ 300,000
b. HMO	100,000

results in a total budgeted payment for inpatient services of 3,500 × $675 = $2,362,500.

For reconciliation, suppose that actual utilization was 385 inpatient days versus the 350 forecast (10 percent variance higher than forecasted). The resulting ISRP distribution is contained in Table 19.8. With overutilization (as compared to the budget), realized payments total 3,850 × $675 = $2,598,750, as shown on Line 2, which results in a dollar variance of −$236,250, as shown on Line 3. Because the pool was initially funded with $262,500, the amount left in the pool after reconciliation is $262,500 − $236,250 = $26,250, which is shown on Line 5. This amount, according to distribution guidelines, is split evenly among primary care physicians, specialty care physicians, and the hospital, as shown on Lines 6a through 6c.

Note that the hospital's per diem payment before withhold was $750.

1. Budgeted payments for inpatient services	$ 2,362,500	**TABLE 19.8**
2. Actual payments for inpatient services	2,598,750	Inpatient
3. Variance from budget	($ 236,250)	Services Risk
4. Risk pool starting amount	262,500	Pool (ISRP)
5. Remainder in pool	$ 26,250	(annual
6. Risk pool allocation		amounts)
a. Hospital (1/3)	$ 8,750	
b. Primary care physicians (1/3)	8,750	
c. Specialty care physicians (1/3)	8,750	
7. Total allocated	$ 26,250	

After reconciliation, the hospital's total payment is $2,598,750 + $8,750 = $2,607,500. Because this total resulted from 3,850 inpatient days, the realized per diem payment was $2,607,500 / 3,850 = $677. This amount is less than the starting $750 amount because more than the budgeted amount was spent on inpatient care. However, because some funds remained in the pool, the final per diem amount is slightly more than the $675 after-withhold amount. Note that even if less than the budgeted amount is spent on inpatient care, the hospital will still receive less than the initial $750 per diem amount because any savings is split three ways.

The intent of the ISRP is to encourage the parties that have some control over hospital utilization to limit the number of inpatient days to those that are absolutely essential to patients' welfare. Of course, because the hospital is being reimbursed on a per diem basis, it has the incentive to maximize the number of inpatient days. Any gain from additional per diem payments will be three times as profitable as pool distributions because per diem payments are not shared with physicians. Therefore, the ISRP is really set up to motivate physicians, who actually control hospital admissions and discharges. Under per diem, the hospital does have the incentive to lower costs because lower costs lead to higher profits. However, the best way to motivate the hospital to control utilization would be to put it under capitation payments.

Performance-Based Pools

In our discussion of risk pools thus far, we have focused exclusively on risk pools designed to control utilization and costs, but such pools can be structured to influence other types of behavior. For example, primary care, as well as specialty physicians, may participate in a *performance-based pool*, wherein the pool is distributed on the basis of both financial and nonfinancial performance.

Here is how a performance-based pool might work for primary care physicians. As before, some percentage—say, 20—of the total capitation payment is withheld. At the end of the year, the pool is distributed to physicians based on performance in four areas: (1) quality of care, (2) quality of service, (3) cost control, and (4) organizational participation. Thirty percent of the pool is allocated to each of the first three areas, and 10 percent is allocated to organizational participation. Physicians are "graded" in each area. For example, quality of care could be based on chart reviews, continuing medical education hours, and number of liability claims; quality of service could be based on patient satisfaction surveys, as well as the ease with which patients can make appointments and visit waiting times; cost control could depend on the cost of referrals and other resource utilization; and organizational participation could be based on number of staff meetings attended and committee posts held.

At the end of the year, the pool distribution would reward those physicians that scored highest in each area and penalize those physicians that did worst. For example, assume that $10,000 remained in a pool for three physicians, so $0.30 \times \$10,000 = \$3,000$ is available for distribution based on quality of care performance. Furthermore, the physicians' quality of care performance scores are 55 for Physician X, 44 for Physician Y, and 33 for Physician Z. Note that these scores have no absolute meaning, but they do tell us how well the physicians have performed relative to one another on the quality-of-care dimension. Because the scores total 132, Physician X would receive $55 / 132 = 0.42$ of the $3,000 pool, or $1,260; Physician Y would receive $44 / 132 = 0.33$ of the pool, or $990; and Physician Z would receive the remaining $750. Of course, some minimum score could be established so that physicians would receive nothing from the pool if the minimum level of performance were not met. It is clear that the type of risk pool described in this section creates incentives for physicians to perform well along both financial and nonfinancial dimensions.

Self-Test Questions
1. What is the purpose of a risk pool?
2. Describe how a typical risk pool works.
3. Can a delivery system with multiple providers have more than one risk pool? Explain your answer.
4. What is a performance-based risk pool?

Key Concepts

Capitation and managed care have a profound influence on the risk and behavior of providers. In this chapter, some of the more important aspects of capitation and managed care are discussed. Here are its key concepts:

- *Capitation* is a flat periodic payment to a physician or other healthcare provider; it is the sole reimbursement for providing services to a defined population.
- Capitation payments are generally expressed as some dollar amount *per member per month (PMPM)*, where the word "member" typically means enrollee in some managed care plan—usually a *health maintenance organization (HMO)*.

- Although capitation payment is used mostly with *primary care physicians*, virtually any type of healthcare service can be reimbursed by capitation.
- Under *fee-for-service*, all volumes less than breakeven produce a loss for the provider, while all volumes greater than breakeven produce a profit. Under *capitation*, all volumes less than breakeven produce a profit, whereas all volumes greater than breakeven result in a loss. Thus, *provider incentives* under capitation are opposite those under conventional reimbursement.
- In markets where capitation and aggressive utilization management has made inroads, the trend is towards *fewer hospital beds* and a physician mix that contains a *greater proportion of primary care physicians*. Most importantly, as capitation and utilization management gain in importance, historical utilization rates based on conventional reimbursement methodologies are not good predictors of future utilization.
- *Objective risk* occurs when the risk inherent in an uncertain outcome can be specified with confidence. *Subjective risk* occurs when the probability distribution itself is uncertain. Although the objective risk in capitation contracts is no greater, and potentially less, than that under conventional reimbursement, the subjective risk can be high.
- Several methods are used to set capitation rates for providers including (1) the *fee-for-service equivalent method*, (2) the *budgetary*, or *cost, approach*, and (3) the *demographic-based approach*.
- In *integrated delivery systems*, it is important to establish incentives that encourage providers to act in the best interest of the system, rather than in their own self-interest. One way to create proper incentives is to establish *withholds*, or *risk pools*, which are pools of money that are initially withheld, and then distributed to providers only if pre-established goals are met.

This concludes our discussion of capitation, rate setting, and risk sharing. The next chapter, which is the final chapter of the book, covers financial risk management.

Selected References

Baker, Judith J. 1995. "Activity-Based Costing for Integrated Delivery Systems." *Journal of Health Care Finance* (Winter): 57–61.

Benoff, Marc and Daniel M. Grauman. 1997. "Risk Sharing in an Integrated Delivery System." *Healthcare Financial Management* (October): 42–48.

Boles, Keith E., and Steven T. Fleming. 1996. "Breakeven Under Capitation: Pure and Simple?" *Health Care Management Review* (Winter): 38–39.

Brown, Charles A., and John B. Reiss. 2000. "HMO Contracting Strategies: Protecting the Provider's Interests." *Healthcare Financial Management* (April): 36–42.

Brua, Kyle P. 1999. "Four Methods of Setting Group Premium Rates Require Different Insurer Resources." *Healthcare Financial Management* (December): 37–40.

Cave, Douglas G. 1995. "Vertical Integration Models to Prepare Health Systems for Capitation." *Health Care Management Review* (Winter): 26–39.

Coyne, Joseph S., and Stuart D. Simon. 1994. "Is Your Organization Ready to Share Financial Risk with HMOs?" *Healthcare Financial Management* (August): 30–34.

Davidson, Daniel M., and John Wester. 1995. "Addressing Integrated Systems' Tax-Exemption Problems." *Healthcare Financial Management* (January): 46–30.

Farley, Dean E. 2000. "Achieving a Balance Between Risk and Return." *Healthcare Financial Management* (June): 54–58.

Fine, Allan. 1998. "Preparing for Full-Risk Capitation." *Healthcare Financial Management* (March): 58–61.

Finkler, Steven A. 1995. "Capitated Hospital Contracts." *Health Care Management Review* (Summer): 88–91.

Frank, Cliff and Jon Brunsberg. 1999. "Using Contact Capitation to Align Payment Incentives Among Specialists." *Healthcare Financial Management* (October): 52–56.

Keegan, Arthur J. 1994. "Hospitals Become Cost Centers in Managed Care Scenario." *Healthcare Financial Management* (August): 36–39.

Kolb, Deborah S., and Judith L. Horowitz. 1995. "Managing the Transition to Capitation." *Healthcare Financial Management* (February): 65–69.

Herrle, Gregory N., and William M. Pollock. 1995. "Multispecialty Medical Groups: Adapting to Capitation." *Journal of Health Care Finance* (Spring): 37–43.

Pallarito, Karen. 1994. "Gatekeepers of Capitation." *Modern Healthcare* (June 27): 93–100.

Peregrine, Michael W., and D. Louis Glaser. 1995. "Choosing Medical Practice Acquisition Models." *Healthcare Financial Management* (March): 58–64.

Sauve, Marc. 1996. "Reassessing the Number and Mix of System Physicians Needed." *Healthcare Financial Management* (February): 56–60.

Seaver, Douglass J., and Stephen H. Kramer. 1994. "Direct Contracting: The Future of Managed Care." *Healthcare Financial Management* (August): 21–27.

Schultz, Donald V. 1995. "The Importance of Primary Care Providers in Integrated Systems." *Healthcare Financial Management* (January): 58–63.

Shortell, Stephen M. 1995. "The Future of Integrated Systems." *Healthcare Financial Management* (January): 24–30.

Teske, Jeffrey M. 1995. "Second-Generation Legal Issues in Integrated Delivery Systems." *Healthcare Financial Management* (January): 54–57.

Toso, Mark E., and Anne Farmer. 1994. "Using Cost Accounting Data to Develop Capitation Rates." *Topics in Health Care Financing* (Fall): 1–12.

Witek, J. Edward and Heather Davidson. 1994. "Assessing Organizational Readiness for Capitation and Risk Sharing." *Healthcare Financial Management* (August): 18–19.

Selected Web Sites

To learn more about the managed care industry, see the American Association of Health Plans site at *www.aahp.org.*

The InterStudy web site will give you some idea of the data available on managed care plans and capitation; see *www.hmodata.com*.

To obtain the current average insurance premiums for both HMO and indemnity plans, see *www.insure.com/health/ceridian200.html*.

Selected Cases

There is one case in *Cases in Healthcare Finance* that is applicable to this chapter: Case 26: Pinewood Health System PHO, which focuses on the premium setting process.

Notes

1. Decision scientists classify risk in a more rigorous fashion as follows: *Ignorance* is the condition when decision makers can't even estimate the probable outcomes, say, the cash flows associated with a research and development project; *uncertainty* is present when outcomes can be predicted, but no probabilities can be attached; and *risk* occurs when both outcomes and probabilities can be forecasted. These classifications are not commonly used by real-world decision makers, so we will stick to the simpler objective and subjective risk classifications discussed in this paragraph.

2. This section summarizes results reported in the following two articles by Louis C. Gapenski and Barbara Langland-Orban, "The Impact of Capitation Contracts on Financial Risk: A Monte Carlo Simulation," *Health Services Management Research*, August 1996, 181–191; and "The Financial Risk to Hospitals Inherent in DRG, Per Diem, and Capitation Reimbursement Methodologies," *Journal of Healthcare Management*, July/August 1998, 323–338.

3. According to the American Hospital Association, the average general acute care hospital has a cost structure of 75 percent fixed costs and 25 percent variable costs.

4. Providers that have capitation contracts can limit outlier risk by purchasing *stop-loss* insurance. However, such insurance reduces the profitability of the capitation contract. Stop-loss insurance is discussed in detail in Chapter 20.

5. Note that the utilization, charge, and cost data used in this section to develop capitation rates are for illustration only and do not necessarily reflect actual values being used today.

6. In early 2000, the average HMO single coverage premium was about $190 PMPM, which is much higher than the amount in our example. However, the average includes Medicare HMOs, which have much higher healthcare costs than do commercial HMOs. Still, it would require a very healthy population to justify the low premium in the example.

FINANCIAL RISK MANAGEMENT

Learning Objectives

After studying this chapter, readers should be able to:

- Discuss the fundamentals of risk management, including some types of risk and the general approach that businesses take to manage risk.
- Explain how reserves and reinsurance can be used to manage the risk inherent in capitation contracts.
- Describe the features of options as well as the factors that influence a call option's value.
- Describe futures contracts and explain how they can be used within health services organizations to reduce the riskiness of financial transactions.

Introduction

In this chapter, we discuss financial risk management—a topic of increasing importance to healthcare managers. The term *risk management* can mean many things, but in a financial context it involves identifying events that could have adverse financial consequences and then taking actions to prevent and/or minimize the damage caused by these events. Years ago, financial risk management dealt primarily with insurance—managers made sure a provider was adequately insured against fire, theft, and other casualties, and that it had adequate medical liability coverage. More recently, the scope of financial risk management has been broadened to include such things as protecting against adverse changes in interest rates or ensuring that greater-than-expected utilization or illness severity will not have a catastrophic negative impact on the business's financial condition.

As the healthcare environment increases in complexity, it is becoming more and more difficult for managers to know what financial pitfalls might lie in wait. Therefore, providers need to have someone systematically look for potential problems and design safeguards to minimize potential damage. With this fact in mind, most large businesses have designated *risk managers* who report to the CFO, while the CFOs of medium-sized firms or the owners of small businesses personally assume risk-management responsibilities. In any event, financial risk management is becoming increasingly important, and it is something health administration students should understand. In this chapter, we present a diverse collection of financial risk management topics of relevance to healthcare providers.

Fundamentals of Financial Risk Management

Risks can be categorized along several dimensions. In addition, there are multiple approaches to financial risk management within businesses. In this section, we introduce some fundamental concepts.

Risk Terminology

We begin by defining some commonly used risk terminology.

- **Pure risks** are risks that offer only the prospect of a loss. Examples include the risk that a facility will be destroyed by fire or that a medical liability suit will result in a large judgment against the business.
- **Speculative risks** are situations that offer the chance of a gain, but might result in a loss. Thus, investments in new service lines and securities involve speculative risks.
- **Utilization risks** are associated with the demand for a provider's services. Because the provision of services at appropriate volumes is essential to the survival of all health services organizations, utilization risk is one of the most significant risks that providers face.
- **Severity risks** stem from the fact that costs may be higher than expected because the realized severity of patients' illnesses is greater than that expected. For example, if a provider accepts a capitated contract with the expectation of a given average level of severity, and it turns out to be much higher, costs will be higher than expected with no matching increase in revenues.
- **Input risks** are associated with input costs, including both labor and supplies. For example, a provider faces the risk that its nursing costs will increase and that it will not be able to pass this increase on to its payers because of prospective payment or capitation contracts.
- **Financial risks** are risks that result from financial transactions. For example, if a hospital plans to issue new bonds, it faces the risk that interest rates will rise before the bonds can be brought to market. As we will explain in a later section, this type of risk can be mitigated by taking a position in the futures market.
- **Property risks** are associated with destruction of productive assets. Thus, the threat of fire, floods, and riots imposes property risks on a business.
- **Personnel risks** are risks that result from employees' action. Examples include the risks associated with employee fraud or embezzlement, or suits against a business on the basis of age or sex discrimination.
- **Environmental risks** include risks associated with polluting the environment. Public awareness in recent years, coupled with the huge costs of environmental cleanup, has increased the importance of this risk.
- **Liability risks** are associated with product, service, or employee actions. For providers, the risk of very large judgments for medical mistakes is especially severe.

- **Insurable risks** are risks that can be covered by insurance. In general, property, personnel, environmental, liability, and even severity risks can be transferred to insurance companies. Note, though, that the ability to insure a risk does not necessarily mean that the risk should be insured. Indeed, a major function of risk management involves evaluating all alternatives for managing a particular risk, including self-insurance, and then choosing the optimal alternative.

Note that the risk classifications given above are somewhat arbitrary, and different classifications are commonly used in specific situations—for example, when defining the risks associated with capitation contracts. Still, the list does give an idea of the wide variety of risks to which a provider can be exposed.

An Approach to Risk Management

Although there are several alternative approaches to risk management, most businesses use the following process for managing risks.

- **Identify the risks faced by the business.** Here, the risk manager identifies the potential risks faced by his or her firm. Unfortunately, this process is neither glamorous or exciting. Nevertheless, it is critical to the risk management function. Generally, data collection from previous incidents, surveys, and annual reviews are used for this purpose.
- **Estimate the potential impact of each risk.** Some risks are so small that they are immaterial, whereas others are so severe that they have the potential to doom the business. Furthermore, some risks are extremely remote, while others may occur with relatively high frequency. It is useful to segregate risks by potential frequency and severity—often by use of a *frequency/severity matrix*—and then focus most risk management attention on those risks with both high frequency and high severity.
- **Decide how each relevant risk should be handled.** In most situations, risk exposure can be reduced through one of the following techniques:
  1. Transfer the risk to an insurance company. Often, it is advantageous to insure against, and hence transfer, a risk. However, the fact that a risk is insurable does not necessarily mean that it should be covered by insurance. In many instances, it might be better for the company to *self-insure*, which means bearing the risk directly rather than paying another party to bear it.
  2. Transfer the function that produces the risk to a third party. Sometimes it is best, if possible, to transfer the entire function, and hence risk, to another party. For example, suppose a hospital is concerned about potential liabilities arising from its in-house disposal of medical wastes. One way to eliminate this risk would be to contract with another company to do the disposal, thus passing the risk to a third party.

3. Purchase derivative contracts to reduce risk. As we will discuss in more detail in later sections, businesses can use derivatives to hedge some types of risk. For companies using commodities as inputs, commodity derivatives can be used to reduce input risks. For example, a surgical equipment manufacturer may use metal futures to hedge against increases in raw material prices. Similarly, financial derivatives can be used to reduce risks that arise from changes in interest rates and exchange rates.

4. Reduce the probability of occurrence of an adverse event. The expected loss arising from any risk is a function of both the expected frequency of occurrence and the expected dollar loss if the adverse event occurs. In some instances, it is possible to reduce the probability that an adverse event will occur. For example, the probability that a fire will occur can be reduced by instituting a fire-prevention program, by replacing old electrical wiring, and by using fire-resistant materials in areas with the greatest fire potential.

5. Reduce the magnitude of the loss associated with an adverse event. Continuing with the fire risk example, the dollar cost associated with a fire can be reduced by such actions as installing sprinkler systems, designing facilities with self-contained fire zones, and locating facilities close to a fire station.

6. Totally avoid the activity that gives rise to the risk. A business might discontinue a product or service line because the risks outweigh the rewards. For example, a hospital might decline an offer to participate in a medical device clinical trial because the liability risk is too great.

Note that risk-management decisions, like all corporate decisions, should be supported by a cost/benefit analysis of each feasible management alternative. For example, suppose it would cost a clinic $50,000 per year to purchase a first-dollar coverage medical liability policy. An alternative might be to purchase a lower-cost policy without first-dollar coverage, and to use the money saved to establish a liability reserve. Both alternatives involve expected cash flows, and from an economic standpoint the choice should be made on the basis of the lowest present value of future costs. Thus, the same financial management techniques applied to other business decisions can also, at least in theory, be applied to risk-management decisions.

Self-Test Questions

1. Define the following terms:
   a. Pure risks
   b. Speculative risks
   c. Demand risks
   d. Input risks
   e. Financial risks
   f. Property risks
   g. Personnel risks

h. Environmental risks
i. Liability risks
j. Insurable risks
k. Self-insurance
2. Briefly, describe one common approach to risk management.
3. Should a business insure itself against all of the insurable risks it faces? Explain your answer.

Risk Management of Capitated Contracts

As discussed in previous chapters, capitated payments expose providers to financial risks that differ from those associated with conventional reimbursement systems. As with all financial risks, there are actions that can be taken to reduce the impact of capitation-induced risks. We discuss two in this section: (1) the establishment of reserves and (2) stop-loss provisions (reinsurance).

Reserves

The first line of defense against financial risk by any organization is the maintenance of adequate *reserves*. Any provider—including medical practices and hospitals—that assumes the financial risk for covered lives without having adequate reserves could easily end up, so to speak, as "roadkill along the capitation highway." When healthcare providers accept capitated rates, they agree to provide whatever services are required for a fixed monthly fee. If all goes well—that is, if utilization and costs are controlled—the provider will end the year with a profit. But, if realized utilization, and hence costs, exceed estimates, or if costs are higher than expected, on average, for each patient encounter, any losses that arise have to be covered. In such situations, the need for reserves becomes apparent. There are several classifications of reserves. We will cover the two most important types: (1) required reserves and (2) reserves for incurred but not reported costs.

Required reserves are those reserves specifically designed to cover random periods when costs exceed capitation revenues. The term "required reserves" stems from the fact that insurance companies are required by state regulators to maintain reserves. Typically, such regulations specify a minimum fixed dollar amount of reserves, some percentage of premium income, or even some dollar amount per individual insured. It is interesting to note that some state insurance regulators are now examining the risk positions of providers that accept capitation contracts, and hence assume the insurance function, to ascertain whether or not requiring licensure and mandatory reserves for these businesses is appropriate. **Required Reserves**

At the provider level, where reserves are not currently required by law, it makes good business sense to have sufficient cash and marketable securities on hand (in reserve) to cover losses that have a reasonable likelihood of occurring. One approach to setting reserve requirements within businesses is to use *Monte Carlo simulation*, which we discussed in Chapter 13 in regards to project risk assessment, to estimate the extent of the risk. Think in terms of a business's cash budget, which was discussed in Chapter 15. Here, we noted that a business's cash inflows and outflows are not known with certainty, so in any period—say, a month—cash outflows could exceed inflows. Most firms set their target cash balances high enough to cover routine shortfalls. The concept is exactly the same for capitation reserves, but here it is applied to a particular contract. By applying Monte Carlo simulation to utilization and costs, it is possible to estimate the sizes and probabilities of occurrence of potential contract losses. Then, based on the risk aversion of the organization's managers, a reserve can be established to cover all, but the most unlikely, loss scenarios.

To illustrate the concept, consider a capitation contract that Westside Memorial Hospital has with a local HMO to serve 50,000 enrollees. The capitation rate is $27.50 PMPM, resulting in $16.50 million in total revenue. Table 20.1 contains Westside's best estimate for the cost distribution of enrollees, along with the resulting profit distribution. These distributions were developed on the basis of estimates of enrollee's admission rates, average length of stay, and average per diem cost. The expected total contract cost is $15.78 million, resulting in an expected profit of $720,000, which gives Westside a profit margin on the contract of 4.4 percent.

Focusing solely on this one contract, it is clear that Westside's profit is not guaranteed. There is a $10 + 20 + 30 = 60$ percent chance that the profit realized will be greater than the $720,000 estimate. That's the good news! The bad news is that there is a 40 percent chance that the profit will be less than expected, and a $5 + 3 + 2 = 10$ percent chance that the contract will lose money. How can Westside protect itself against the possibility that losses on this contract will push the hospital into financial distress? Of course, one answer

TABLE 20.1
Westside Memorial Hospital: Contract Cost and Profit Distribution (millions of dollars)

Probability	Contract Cost	Contract Profit (Loss)
0.10	$14.00	$ 2.50
0.20	15.00	1.50
0.30	15.50	1.00
0.20	16.00	0.50
0.10	16.50	0.00
0.05	17.50	(1.00)
0.03	19.00	(2.50)
0.02	21.50	(5.00)
1.00		
	Expected value = $15.78	$0.72

Note: Contract revenues are expected to total $16.50 million.

is to have sufficient reserves. On the basis of the Table 20.1 distributions, Westside could fund a $5 million reserve that would totally protect it against losses on this contract, assuming that the probability distribution itself is correct. But this very conservative approach to reserves would, assuming a opportunity cost rate of 10 percent, cost Westside $500,000 in carrying costs, and hence almost wipe out the contract's expected profit.

As an alternative, Westside might conclude that a 2 percent probability of occurrence represents a very unlikely event, and hence does not warrant reserve protection. If this were the case, Westside would set a reserve for the contract of less than $5 million—say, $1 million or $2.5 million. The choice is a risk/return trade-off, with more risk protection requiring a larger reserve, which in turn leads to lower contract profits. In general, the larger the contract, and the greater the uncertainty in contract costs, and hence profits, the higher the reserve must be to offer realistic protection against negative outcomes.

Unfortunately, in most situations the reserve requirement is not as clear-cut as discussed here. First, it is not easy to estimate utilization and cost distributions, so it is very difficult to have much confidence in the Table 20.1 values. Second, most providers have a large number of contracts with numerous payers, and what is most relevant is the chance of an overall loss rather than the probability of a loss on a particular contract. If the loss distributions on the individual contracts are not perfectly positively correlated, then portfolio effects will somewhat mitigate the risks inherent in each contract.

Note that financial withholds, as discussed in Chapter 19, are, in effect, a type of reserve. If certain financial goals are met, the withhold is distributed to providers. However, if goals are not met, the withhold is used to cover the excess costs incurred. Also, note that of all the providers, physicians are particularly vulnerable when entering capitation contracts because historically they have not used reserves. In most cases, physician practices distribute most, if not all, of their profits each year, reinvesting only those amounts absolutely necessary to fund new equipment. With this type of behavior as the norm, it is especially difficult to think in terms of establishing reserves.

Reserves for Incurred But Not Reported (IBNR) Costs

Consider the situation facing HealthyHMO. At the end of every accounting period—for purposes here, assume a year—HealthyHMO must close its books and reconcile its established risk pools. HealthyHMO uses capitation to pay for primary care services, but it uses fee-for-service reimbursement to pay for specialist services. When it closes its books at the end of the year, HealthyHMO might not realize that there are specialist referrals that have been made by its primary care physicians that have not yet been billed. Indeed, some required specialist services may not have even been performed. The costs associated with referrals that have been made but which, for one reason or another, have not yet been reported in the organization's managerial accounting system are called *incurred but not reported (IBNR) costs*.

If a provider is capitated, yet has referral responsibility for services that it does not provide, there is a strong likelihood that at the end of the year there will be payment obligations for costs that have been incurred but not reported. Obviously, such costs must be planned for and covered, and the impact of such costs on risk-pool distributions must be taken into account. There are relatively sophisticated methods available for establishing IBNR reserves, as well as some rather ad hoc methods such as setting two or three months worth of historical IBNR dollar claims aside as a reserve. It is not important for you to know the details of setting up IBNR reserves, we will leave that to the accountants, but it is important for you to recognize that providers bear extra risk whenever they are responsible for payments for services that they do not provide.[1]

Stop-Loss Provisions (Reinsurance)

Rather than establish reserves to cover every conceivable cost situation, many providers elect to "reinsure" the risk. Such insurance, which is now offered by dozens of insurance companies, is called *reinsurance* or medical *stop-loss insurance*.[2] Providers have several alternatives for handling stop-loss insurance. One alternative is to have the HMO withhold a portion of the capitation rate for the sole purpose of buying insurance. However, if the HMO elects to self-insure, and then fails to establish adequate reserves, the provider remains at risk. Another alternative is for the provider to receive the full capitation payment, and then purchase stop-loss insurance directly from a company that specializes in such insurance. Of course, the alternative always exists for the provider to self-insure.

Typically, stop-loss insurance is written to protect providers from losses on individual patients, rather than from aggregate losses on a contract. The idea is to insure the provider against catastrophic "budget-buster" patients, not to guarantee a certain level of overall profitability. For example, a hospital might purchase stop-loss insurance with a deductible, or *threshold*, of $100,000. For any patient with charges over $100,000, the insurer might agree to pay 80 percent of billed charges in excess of this threshold amount. Of course, the lower the threshold and the higher the percentage of any excess paid by the insurer, the higher the stop-loss insurance premium.

Self-Test Questions
1. Why is it important that capitated providers establish reserves?
2. What are the two primary types of reserves?
3. What is stop-loss insurance, and when should it be taken?

Debt Portfolio Immunization

Healthcare providers, especially not-for-profit hospitals, often maintain large portfolios of debt securities to either fund future capital investments or maintain endowments. As we discussed in Chapter 8, debt securities carry interest rate risk, which is composed of price risk and reinvestment rate risk. *Price risk* occurs because rising interest rates lower the values of existing securities, and *reinvestment rate risk* occurs because falling rates mean that reinvested principal and interest will earn less in the future.

To illustrate these risks, assume that a hospital is planning to add a new wing in ten years and is creating a portfolio of Treasury securities to pay for the required construction and equipment. Furthermore, assume that the yield curve is flat and the interest rate on such securities, regardless of maturity, is 6 percent. Finally, assume that the hospital will buy securities in $10,000 increments and the bonds have annual coupons. Here are some possible interest rate scenarios and final values, assuming the bonds have a **ten-year maturity**:

- **Interest rates remain at 6 percent.** If interest rates remain at 6 percent, the value of one increment would be the initial $10,000 plus $7,908 future value of interest payments at the end of ten years for a total amount of $17,908. This constant interest rate scenario is the base case, so the hospital is expecting each increment of bonds to be worth $17,908 in ten years when needed to pay for the new wing.
- **Interest rates drop to 4 percent immediately after purchase.** If interest rates fall, and remain at the new level, the value of one increment will be only $10,000 + $7,204 = $17,204. Here, the lower interest rate means that the reinvested coupon payments will earn less than in the base case.
- **Interest rates rise to 8 percent immediately after purchase.** If interest rates rise, and remain at the new level, the value of one increment will be $10,000 + $8,692 = $18,692. As opposed to the previous scenario, the reinvested coupon payments will now earn more than in the base case.

Because of interest rate risk, the hospital might find itself after ten years in a position with less money saved than it had expected. The shortfall would be realized if interest rates fall because the bonds have reinvestment rate risk. However, because the bonds have a ten-year maturity, the hospital is not bearing any price risk—the bonds will be worth $10,000 per increment at the end of ten years regardless of the level of interest rates.

Now, assume that the hospital invests in 30-year, rather than ten-year, Treasury securities. Here are the results, assuming a **30-year maturity**:

- **Interest rates remain at 6 percent.** If interest rates remain at 6 percent, the value of one increment would be the initial $10,000 plus $7,908 future value of interest payments at the end of ten years for a total amount of $17,908. These results are the same as with ten-year bonds because the constant interest rate holds the value of the 30-year bonds at $10,000 per increment over their entire maturity.
- **Interest rates drop to 4 percent immediately after purchase.** If interest rates fall, and remain at the new level, the value of one increment will be $12,718 + $7,204 = $19,922. Note that the $12,718 value per $10,000

increment is the value of the bonds with only 20 years remaining to maturity, which is the time remaining at the end of the ten-year holding period. In this scenario, the future value of the interest payments declines, but the bond is worth more when it would be sold. The net effect is an amount that is higher than the expected $17,908.

- **Interest rates rise to 8 percent immediately after purchase.** If interest rates rise, and remain at the new level, the value of one increment will be $8,036 + $8,692 = $16,728. Although the interest payments are worth more, the value of the bonds has dropped by an even greater amount, so the total value of one increment is now less than the amount expected.

With a 30-year bond, the hospital is bearing both price risk and reinvestment rate risk. Thus, the possible shortfall is greater than it was in the case of ten-year bonds. Because the price risk is much greater than the reinvestment rate risk, the shortfall occurs when interest rates rise.

There are two ways for the hospital to create a portfolio that is riskless, or close to it, in the sense that the ending amount is known with relative certainty today. The first way is to buy *zero-coupon bonds* with a ten-year maturity. If this way is followed, there is no reinvestment rate risk because there are no coupon payments and there is no price risk because the maturity of the bond matches the hospital's ten-year holding period.

The second way is to *immunize* the portfolio. The term "immunize" is used because it allows the portfolio to be free of interest rate risk just as a vaccination allows an individual to be free of the risk of getting some disease. The key to immunizing a portfolio is to buy bonds that have a *duration* equal to the holding period. Duration cannot be as easily defined as maturity, but it can be thought of as the weighted average maturity of a bond when all of its cash flows are considered, including both interest payments and return of principal. For zero-coupon bonds, the duration is the same as the bond's maturity. Thus, when we said that interest rate risk could be eliminated by investing in ten-year zero-coupon bonds, we were actually choosing bonds with a duration that matched the hospital's ten-year holding period. However, when bonds have coupon payments, duration is shorter than maturity, and the higher the coupon payment, the shorter the duration. (Higher coupon payments mean that the cash flows from the bond, on average, occur earlier in the bond's life.)

Duration is calculated in the following way:

1. Lay out the cash flows expected from the bond in each Year t.
2. Find the present value of each cash flow when discounted at the required rate of return on the bond.
3. Divide each present value by the bond's current value.
4. Multiply each amount from the previous step by the year in which it occurs.
5. Sum the resulting products. This sum is the bond's duration.

To illustrate the calculation of duration, consider the ten-year, 6 percent annual coupon bonds described previously. Assume that the par value is $10,000 and the current required rate of return on the bond is 6 percent. Because the required rate of return equals the coupon rate, the bond's par value is also its current value. Table 20.2 contains the duration calculation. As we stated previously, when a bond has coupon payments, its duration is shorter than its maturity. In this case, the duration is 7.8 years versus a maturity of ten years.

In addition to being used for immunization, duration can be used to estimate the sensitivity of a bond to changes in interest rates. For each 1-percent change in interest rates, the value of a bond will roughly change by a percentage amount equal to its duration. Thus, if interest rates rose by 1 percentage point, the bond in Table 20.2 would lose about 7.8 percent of its value, or fall to about $9,220. The precise value is $9,298, so using duration to determine the impact of interest rate changes is only an approximation, but it demonstrates that price risk is more closely related to duration than it is to maturity.[3]

Healthcare managers immunize a bond portfolio—protect it against interest rate risk—by creating a portfolio with a duration that equals the holding period. Thus, in our example, the hospital would want to create a bond portfolio with a ten-year duration. To illustrate the effects of immunization, consider a 14-year bond with a 6 percent coupon when the required rate of return is 6 percent. Its duration is 9.85 years, so it closely matches the ten-year holding period. When we change the interest rate environment as before, here are the results:

TABLE 20.2
Duration
Calculation

Year (t)	Cash Flow	Present Value	Present Value / Current Value	t × (Present Value / Current Value)
1	$ 600	$ 566.04	0.0566	0.0566
2	600	534.00	0.0534	0.1068
3	600	503.77	0.0504	0.1511
4	600	475.26	0.0475	0.1901
5	600	448.35	0.0448	0.2242
6	600	422.89	0.0423	0.2538
7	600	399.03	0.0399	0.2793
8	600	376.45	0.0376	0.3102
9	600	355.14	0.0355	0.3196
10	10,600	5,918.98	0.5919	5.9190
				7.8017

Notes: (1) The present value is found by discounting each cash flow back to Year 0 at the 6 percent required rate of return.

(2) The fourth column contains the present values divided by the $10,000 current value.

(3) Values in the final column are found by multiplying each value in the fourth column by the corresponding value of t in the first column.

- **Interest rates remain at 6 percent.** If interest rates remain at 6 percent, we again have the base case situation of $10,000 in principal amount plus $7,908 future value of interest payments for a total amount of $17,908.
- **Interest rates drop to 4 percent immediately after purchase.** If interest rates fall, and remain at the new level, the value of one increment will be $10,726 + $7,204 = $17,930. Here, the future value of the interest payments declines, but the bond is worth more when it would be sold, and the two value changes just about cancel each other out.
- **Interest rates rise to 8 percent immediately after purchase.** If interest rates rise, and remain at the new level, the value of one increment will be $9,338 + $8,692 = $18,030. Although the interest payments are worth more, the value of the bond has dropped, and again the two changes come close to offsetting one other.

With a duration roughly equal to the holding period, any gains from coupon reinvestment at a higher rate are offset by a loss of principal value, and vice versa. In effect, price risk and reinvestment rate risk are played off against one another, with the resulting value at the end of ten years being close to $18,000 regardless of interest rate changes.

Unfortunately, life is not as easy as textbook examples. Although our example illustrates the basic concept of using duration to immunize bond portfolios, it oversimplifies the situation by assuming only one interest rate change during the hospital's ten-year holding period. In reality, interest rates change on a daily basis, which causes bonds' durations to change. This change in duration, in turn, means that real-world portfolios must be periodically *rebalanced* to remain immunized. Still, with the right software, rebalancing is not an overwhelming task, and it is done by thousands of businesses as part of their financial risk-management programs.

Self-Test Questions

1. What are the two components of interest rate risk?
2. Why do zero-coupon bonds that match the holding period eliminate interest rate risk?
3. What is duration?
4. How is duration used to immunize debt portfolios?

An Overview of Derivatives

Derivatives are a type of security whose value stems from the value of a commodity item or other security, so its value is "derived" from the value of some other "instrument." Because their values are derived from other instruments, or claims, derivatives are also called *indirect claims*. In contrast, stocks and bonds are *direct claims* because they have claims tied directly to the cash flows of a business. Because derivatives play an important role in financial risk management, an overview of these securities will help you understand the material to follow.

One of the first formal markets for derivatives was the *futures market* for wheat. Farmers were concerned about the price they would receive for their wheat when they sold it in the fall, and millers were concerned about the price they would have to pay. The risks faced by both parties could be reduced, or *hedged*, if they could establish a price earlier in the year. Accordingly, mill agents would go out to the wheat belt and make contracts with farmers that called for the farmers to deliver grain at a predetermined price. Both parties benefited from the transaction in the sense that their risks were reduced. The farmers could concentrate on growing their crop without worrying about the price of grain, and the millers could concentrate on their milling operations. Thus, in this case, hedging in the futures market reduced the price uncertainty to both parties, and hence lowered aggregate risk in the economy.

These early futures dealings were between two parties who arranged the transactions themselves. Furthermore, the *underlying asset*, which was wheat in the illustration, was actually delivered when the contract expired. Such a contract is called a *forward contract,* and the two parties that establish the contract are called *counterparties.* Because forward contracts require delivery, they are most useful when one counterparty actually owns the underlying asset and the other needs that asset. A *futures contract* is similar to a forward contract, but with three key differences:

1. Futures contracts are generally standardized instruments that are traded on exchanges, whereas forward contracts are generally tailor made, are negotiated between two counterparties, and are not traded after they have been signed.
2. Futures contracts are "marked to market" on a daily basis, which means that gains and losses are noted by the exchange and money must be put up by buyers to cover losses. This process greatly reduces the risk of default that exists with forward contracts.
3. With futures, physical delivery of the underlying assets is virtually never taken—the two counterparties simply settle up with cash for the difference between the contracted price and the actual price on the expiration date.

The formation of futures markets allowed the contracts to be easily traded. The Chicago Board of Trade was an early marketplace for this dealing, and *futures dealers* helped make a market in futures contracts. Farmers could sell futures on the exchange, and millers could buy them there, rather than contract directly. Thus, millers could buy wheat from any supplier at the prevailing harvest price, yet still lock in an effective price much earlier through futures contracts. Similarly, farmers could sell their crops to anyone at harvest and use the futures market to offset any adverse price trends that occurred during the growing season. The advent of a dealer system improved the efficiency and lowered the cost of hedging operations.

Quickly, a third group—*speculators*—entered the scene. Most derivatives, including futures, are highly leveraged, which means that a small change in the value of the underlying asset will produce a large change in the price of the derivative. This leverage appealed to speculators. At first blush, one might think that the appearance of speculators would increase risk, but this is not true. Speculators add capital and players (counterparties) to the market, and this tends to create more liquidity and stabilize the market. Of course, derivatives markets are inherently volatile because of the amount of leverage involved, and hence risk to the speculators is high. Still, their willingness to bear that risk makes the derivatives markets more efficient for hedging.

Natural hedges—defined as situations in which aggregate risk can be reduced by derivatives transactions between the counterparties—exist for many commodities, for foreign currencies, for interest rates on securities with different maturities, and even for common stocks where portfolio managers want to "hedge their bets." Natural hedges occur when futures are traded between cotton farmers and cotton mills, copper mines and copper fabricators, importers and foreign manufacturers (which hedge currency exchange rates), electric utilities and coal miners, and oil producers and oil users. In all such situations, hedging reduces aggregate risk and, thus, benefits the economy.

Hedging can also be done in situations where no natural hedge exists. Here, one party wants to reduce some type of risk, and another party agrees to sell a contract that protects the first party from that specific event or situation. Insurance is an obvious example of this type of hedge. Note, though, that with nonsymmetric hedges, risks are generally *transferred* rather than *eliminated*. Even here, though, insurance companies can reduce certain types of risk through diversification.

The derivatives markets have grown more rapidly than any other major market in recent years for a number of reasons. First, analytical techniques have been developed to help establish "fair" prices, and having a better basis for pricing contracts makes the counterparties more comfortable with deals. Second, computers and electronic communications make it much easier for counterparties to deal with one another. Third, globalization has greatly increased the importance of currency markets and the need for reducing the exchange rate risks brought on by global trade. Recent trends and developments are sure to continue if not accelerate, so the use of derivatives for risk management is bound to grow.

Note, though, that derivatives do have a potential downside. Because these instruments are highly leveraged, small miscalculations can lead to huge losses. Also, they are complicated, and hence not well understood by most people. This complexity makes mistakes more likely than with less complex instruments, and it makes it harder for a firm's top management to exercise proper control over derivative transactions. One 28-year-old, relatively low-level employee, who operated in the Far East, entered into transactions that led to the bankruptcy of Britain's oldest bank—Barings —which held the accounts of the Queen of England. Hundreds of other horror stories could be told.

Still, derivatives are used far more often to hedge risks than in harmful speculations, but these beneficial transactions never make the headlines. Therefore, while the horror stories point out the need for top managers to exercise control over the personnel who deal with derivatives, they certainly do not justify the elimination of derivatives. In the balance of this chapter, we discuss some specific types of derivative securities and how healthcare businesses can use them for risk management.

1. What is the difference between direct and indirect claims?
2. How did derivatives begin?
3. What is a natural hedge? Give some examples of natural hedges.
4. What is the difference between using derivatives for hedging as opposed to speculation?
5. Why are derivatives better than direct claims for speculation?

Options

An *option* is a particular type of derivative that gives its holder the right to buy, or sell, an *underlying asset* at some predetermined price within a specified period of time. Healthcare managers should have some understanding of options both for risk management and also because of the impact of real options on the value of capital projects under consideration.

Option Types and Markets

There are many types of options and option markets.[4] To illustrate how options work, suppose you owned 100 shares of Tenet Healthcare, which on Monday, July 10, 2000, sold for $28.50 per share. You might sell to someone else the right to buy your 100 shares at any time during the next four months at a price of, say, $30 per share. The $30 is called the *strike*, or *exercise, price*. Such options exist, and they are traded on a number of exchanges, with the Chicago Board Options Exchange (CBOE) being the oldest and the largest. This type of option is a *call option* because the purchaser has a "call" on 100 shares of stock. The seller of an option is called the option *writer*. An investor who "writes" call options against stock held in his or her portfolio is said to be selling *covered options*. Options sold without the stock to back them up are called *naked options*. When the exercise price exceeds the current stock price, a call option is said to be *out-of-the-money*. When the exercise price is below the current price of the stock, the option is *in-the-money*.

Suppose that the call options described above were selling for $2.70. Thus, for $270 an individual or business could buy the right to purchase 100 shares of Tenet Healthcare stock at a price of $30 per share at any time over the next four months.[5] If the stock price stayed below $30 during that period, the buyer would lose $270, but if it rose to $40, the $270 investment would increase in value to ($40 − $30) × 100 = $1,000 in less than 120 days, which translates into a very healthy annual rate of return. Incidentally, if the stock price did go up, the holder would not actually exercise the options, buy the stock, and then resell it at a higher price. Rather, the holder would merely sell the options, which would then have a value of somewhat more than $1,000 versus the $270 purchase price, to another option buyer or back to the original seller.

An individual or business can also buy an option that gives the holder the right to sell a stock at a specified price within some future period—this is called a *put option*. For example, suppose someone believes Tenet Healthcare's stock price is likely to decline from its current level of $28.50 sometime during the next four months. This individual might buy a four-month put option for, say, $150 that would give the buyer the right to sell 100 shares (which the option buyer would not necessarily own) at a price of $25 per share ($25 is the strike price). If the individual bought this 100-share contract and then Tenet's stock price fell to $20, the holder could, in theory, buy a share of stock for $20 and exercise the put option by selling it for $25. The profit from exercising the option would be ($25 − $20) × 100 = $500. After subtracting the $150 you paid for the option, the profit (before taxes and commissions) would be $350. As with call options, the holder would not actually exercise the put option. Rather, he or she would sell the put option, which would have a value of over $500.

In addition to options on individual stocks, options are also available on several stock indexes such as the NYSE Index and the S&P 500 Index. Index options permit someone to hedge, or bet, on a rise or fall in the general market as well as on individual stocks. Option trading is one of the hottest financial activities in the United States. The leverage involved makes it possible for speculators with just a few dollars to make a fortune almost overnight. Also, investors with sizable portfolios can sell options against their stocks and earn the value of the option (less brokerage commissions), even if the stock's price remains constant. Most importantly, though, options can be used to create *hedges* that protect the value of an individual stock or portfolio.

Corporations on whose stocks options are written have nothing to do with the options markets. Corporations do not raise money in the options markets, nor do they have any direct transactions in it. Moreover, option holders do not vote for corporate directors or receive dividends. There have been numerous studies conducted to ascertain whether option trading stabilizes or destabilizes the stock market, and whether this activity helps or hinders corporations that seek to raise new capital. The studies have not been conclusive, but option trading is here to stay, and many regard it as the most exciting game in town.

Factors That Affect the Value of a Call Option

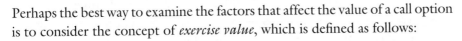

Perhaps the best way to examine the factors that affect the value of a call option is to consider the concept of *exercise value*, which is defined as follows:

Exercise value = Current price of the stock − Exercise (strike) price.

In other words, the exercise value is what the option would be worth if it were exercised immediately. For example, if a stock sells for $50 and its option has an exercise price of $20, then you could buy the stock for $20 by exercising the option. You would own a stock worth $50, but you would have to pay only $20. Therefore, the option would be worth $30 if you had to exercise it immediately. Note that the calculated exercise value of a call option could be negative, but realistically the minimum "true" value of an option is zero because no one would exercise an out-of-the-money option. Note also that an option's exercise value is only a first approximation value—it merely provides a starting point for finding the actual value of the option.

Now, consider Figure 20.1, which contains some call option data on West Coast Genetics, Inc. (WCG)—a company that recently went public and whose stock price has fluctuated widely during its short history. Column 1 in the tabular data section contains a list of selected recent stock prices, while Column 2 shows the constant $20 strike price. Column 3 shows the exercise values for WCG's call option when the stock was selling at the listed prices; Column 4 gives the actual market prices for the option; and Column 5 shows the premium of the actual call option price over its exercise value. At any stock price below $20, the exercise value is set at zero, but above $20; each $1 increase in the price of the stock brings with it a $1 increase in the option's exercise value. Note, however, that the actual market price of the option lies above the exercise value at each stock price, although the premium declines as the price of the stock increases. For example, when the stock sold for $20 and the option had a zero exercise value, its actual price, and the premium, was $9. Then, as the price of the stock rose, the exercise value's increase matched the stock's increase dollar for dollar, but the market price of the option climbed less rapidly, causing the premium to decline. The premium was $9 when the stock sold for $20 a share, but it had declined to $1 by the time the stock price had risen to $73 a share. Beyond that point, the premium virtually disappeared.

Why does this pattern exist? Why should a call option ever sell for more than its exercise value, and why does the premium decline as the price of the stock increases? The answer lies in part in the speculative appeal of options—they enable buyers to gain a high degree of personal leverage when buying securities. To illustrate the concept, suppose WCG's option **sold for exactly its exercise value**. Now, suppose you were thinking of investing in the company's common stock at a time when it was selling for $21 a share. If you bought a share and the price rose to $42, you would have made a 100 percent capital gain. However, had you bought the option at its exercise value—$1 when the stock was selling for $21—your capital gain would have been $22 − $1 = $21 on a $1 investment, or 2,100 percent! At the same time, your total loss potential with the option would be only $1 versus a potential loss of $21 if you purchased the stock. The huge capital gains potential, combined with the loss limitation, is clearly worth something—the exact amount it is worth to investors is the amount of the premium. Note, however, that buying the option is riskier than buying WCG's stock because there is a higher probability of losing money on the option. If WCG's stock price fell to $20, you would have a 4.76 percent loss if you bought the stock (ignoring transaction costs), but you would have a 100 percent loss on the option investment.

Why does the premium decline as the price of the stock rises? Part of the answer is that both the leverage effect and the loss protection feature decline as the stock price rises. For example, if you were thinking of buying WCG's stock when its price was $73 a share, the exercise value of the option would be $53. If the stock price doubled to $146, you would have a 100 percent gain on the stock. But, the exercise value of the option would go from $53 to $126, for a percentage gain of only 138 percent versus 2,100 percent in the earlier case. Note also that the potential loss per dollar of potential gain on the option is much greater when the option is selling at high prices. These two factors, the declining leverage impact and the increasing danger of large losses, help explain why the premium diminishes as the price of the common stock rises.

Option pricing models can be used to precisely identify the factors that affect the value of a call option, but these factors can also be discussed in a more intuitive way.[6]

- The higher the stock's market price in relation to the exercise price, the higher will be the exercise value and, hence, the option's value.
- The lower the exercise price, the higher the call option value. Again, call option value stems from the spread between the stock price and the exercise price (the exercise value), so a higher strike price reduces call option value.
- The longer the option period, the higher the option value. This occurs because the longer the time before expiration, the greater the chance that the stock price will climb substantially above the exercise price. Thus, option premiums and, hence, values increase as the expiration date is lengthened.
- An option on an extremely volatile stock is worth more than one on a very stable stock. If the stock price rarely moves, then there is only a small chance of a large gain. However, if the stock price is highly volatile, the option could easily become very valuable. At the same time, losses on options are limited—you can make an unlimited amount, but you can lose only what you paid for the option. Therefore, a large decline in a stock's price does not have a corresponding bad effect on option holders. As a result of the unlimited upside but limited downside, the more volatile the

stock price, the higher the premium and, hence, value of the
call option.

• The payoff on an option will occur sometime in the future, so the value of
the option is, in a sense, the present value of an expected future payoff.
Because of the time value of money, the higher the current level of interest
rates, the higher the future payoff, and hence the higher the premium and
value of the option.

1. What is an option? A call option? A put option?
2. Define a call option's exercise value. Why is the actual market price of a
call option usually above its exercise value?
3. What are some factors that affect a call option's value?

**Self-Test
Questions**

Futures

One of the most useful tools for reducing interest rate, exchange rate, and
input risk is to hedge in the futures markets. Most financial and real-asset
transactions occur in what is known as the *spot*, or *cash, market*, where the
asset is delivered immediately or within a few days. *Futures markets* involve
the purchase or sale of an asset at some future date, but at a price which is
fixed today.

Types of Contracts

Futures contracts are available on more than 30 real and financial assets traded
on 14 U. S. exchanges, the largest of which are the Chicago Board of Trade
(CBOT) and the Chicago Mercantile Exchange (CME). Futures contracts
are divided into two classes: (1) *commodity futures* and (2) *financial futures*.
Commodity futures, which cover oil, various grains, oilseeds, livestock, meats,
fibers, metals, and wood, were first traded in the United States in the mid-
1800s. Financial futures, which were first traded in 1975, include Treasury
bills, notes, bonds, certificates of deposit, Eurodollar deposits, foreign currencies, and stock indexes. Although commodity contracts are still very important,
today more trading is done in foreign exchange and interest rate futures.

When futures contracts are purchased, the buyer does not have to put
up the full amount of the purchase price; rather, the purchaser is required to
post an *initial margin*, which for CBOT Treasury bond contracts is $3,000 per
$100,000 contract. The fact that the full value of the contract is not required
from the counterparties to initiate the contract creates significant leverage.
However, investors are required to maintain a certain value in the margin
account, called a *maintenance margin*. If the value of the contract declines,
then the owner may be required to add additional funds to the margin account,
and the more the contract value falls, the more money must be added. The
value of the contract is checked at the end of every working day, and margin
account adjustments are made at that time. This process is called *marking
to market*.

Futures contracts and options are similar to one another—so similar that people often confuse the two. Therefore, it is useful to compare the two instruments. A *futures contract* is a definite agreement on the part of one party to buy the underlying asset on a specific date and at a specific price, and the other party agrees to sell on the same terms. No matter how low or how high the price goes, the two parties must settle the contract at the agreed-upon price. An *option*, on the other hand, gives someone the right to buy (call) or sell (put) an asset, but the holder of the option does not have to complete the transaction. The two types of instruments can be used for the same purposes. One is not necessarily better or worse than another—they are simply different.

Using Futures to Hedge Interest Rate Risk

To illustrate the use of interest rate futures to hedge (manage) risk, assume that HCA decides to build a new hospital at a cost of $100 million. It plans to finance the project with 20-year bonds that would carry a 10 percent interest rate if they were issued today. However, the company will not need the money for about six months. HCA could go ahead and sell 20-year bonds now, locking in the 10 percent rate, but it would have the money before it was needed, so it would have to invest the $100 million in short-term securities that would yield significantly less than 10 percent. However, if HCA waits six months to sell the bond issue, interest rates might be higher than they are today, in which case the cost of financing would increase, perhaps to the point of making the hospital unprofitable. One solution to HCA's dilemma is to hedge the bond issue transaction with *interest rate futures*, which are based on a hypothetical 20-year Treasury bond with a 6 percent semiannual coupon. If interest rates in the economy go up, the value of the hypothetical T-bond will go down, and vice versa.

Hedging involves protecting some underlying asset against adverse price trends. Because prices can go up or down, there are two basic types of futures hedges: (1) *long hedges*, in which a contract is purchased to guard against price increases, and (2) *short hedges*, in which a contract is sold to guard against price declines. In our example, HCA is worried about an increase in interest rates, which is actually a fall in bond prices. Thus, HCA should use a short hedge; that is, it should sell T-bond futures for delivery in six months. Then, if interest rates rise, HCA will have to pay more when it issues its own bonds. However, it will make a profit on its futures position because it will have pre-sold the hypothetical bonds at a higher price than it will have to pay to cover (repurchase) them. Of course, if interest rates decline, HCA will lose on its futures position, but this will be offset by the fact that HCA will pay a lower interest rate when it issues its bonds.

If futures contracts existed on HCA's own debt, and interest rates moved identically in the spot (current) and futures markets, HCA could construct a *perfect hedge*, in which gains on the futures contract would exactly offset losses on the bonds. In reality, it is virtually impossible to construct perfect hedges because in most cases the underlying asset is not identical to the futures asset, and even when they are, prices, and interest rates, may not move exactly together in the spot and futures markets.

Note that if HCA had been planning an equity offering, and if its stock tended to move fairly closely with one of the stock indexes, the company could have hedged against falling stock prices by selling short the index future. Even better, because options on HCA's stock are traded in the options markets, it could use options, rather than futures, to hedge against falling stock prices. The general approach would be the same as that just described using the futures market.

The futures and options markets permit flexibility in the timing of financial transactions because the firm can be protected, at least partially, against changes that occur between the time a decision is reached and the time when the transaction will be completed. However, this protection has a cost—the firm must pay commissions. Whether or not the protection is worth the cost is a matter of judgment. The decision to hedge also depends on management's risk aversion as well as the company's strength and ability to assume the risk in question. In theory, the reduction in risk that results from a hedge transaction should have a value exactly equal to the cost of the hedge. Thus, a firm should be indifferent to hedging. However, many firms believe that the peace of mind is worth the cost.

Using Futures to Hedge Input Risk

As we noted earlier, futures markets were established for many commodities long before they began to be used for financial instruments. We can use American Dental Products (ADP), which uses large quantities of palladium for dental alloys, to illustrate input risk hedging. Suppose that in July 2000, ADP became especially concerned about the market price of palladium. Russia supplies about 60 percent of the world supply, and the increasing political instability there has created concern among ADP's managers. Because ADP has many long-term fixed price contracts with buyers of dental alloys, a spike in palladium costs could easily result in significant damage to its bottom line.

ADP could, of course, go ahead and buy palladium today to meet its needs over, say, the next year, but if it does it will incur substantial carrying costs. As an alternative, the company could hedge against increasing palladium prices in the futures market. The New York Mercantile Exchange trades standard palladium futures contracts of 100 troy ounces each.[7] Thus, ADP could buy 100 contracts (go long) for delivery in, say, December, which would lock in a price of $637 per ounce. If palladium prices do rise appreciably over the next five months, the value of ADP's long position in palladium futures would increase; thus offsetting some of the price increase in the commodity itself. Of course, if palladium prices fall, ADP would lose money on its futures contract, but the company would be buying the metal on the spot market at a cheaper price, so it would make a higher-than-anticipated profit on its dental alloy sales. Thus, hedging in the futures market locks in the cost of ADP's raw materials and removes some risk to which the firm would otherwise be exposed.

1. Briefly, describe the features of a futures contract.
2. How do options and futures differ?
3. How can futures contracts be used to hedge interest rate risk?
4. How can futures contracts be used to hedge input risk?

Swaps

A *swap* is just what the name implies. Two parties agree to swap something—generally obligations to make specified payment streams. Most swaps today involve either interest payments or currencies. To illustrate an interest rate swap, suppose Company S has a 20-year, $100 million floating bond outstanding, while Company F has a $100 million, 20-year, fixed rate issue outstanding. Thus, each company has an obligation to make a stream of interest payments, but one payment stream is fixed while the other will vary as interest rates change in the future.

Now, suppose Company S has stable cash flows, and it wants to lock in its cost of debt. Company F has cash flows that fluctuate with the economy, rising when the economy is strong and falling when it is weak. Recognizing that interest rates also move up and down with the economy, Company F has concluded that it would be better off with variable rate debt. If the companies swapped their payment obligations, an *interest rate swap* would occur. Company S would now have to make fixed payments, which is consistent with its stable cash inflows, and Company F would have a floating stream, which for it is less risky.

Our example illustrates how swaps can reduce risk by allowing each company to match the variability of its interest payments with that of its cash flows. However, there are also situations where swaps can reduce both the riskiness and the amount of interest payments. For example, Antron Pharmaceuticals, which has a high credit rating, can issue either floating rate debt at LIBOR + 1 percent or fixed rate debt at 10 percent.[8] Bosworth Medical Instruments is less creditworthy, and its cost for floating rate debt would be LIBOR + 1.5 percent, and its fixed rate cost would be 10.4 percent. Because of the nature of its operations, Antron's managers have decided that it would be better off with fixed rate debt, while Bosworth's managers would prefer floating rate debt. Paradoxically, both firms can benefit by issuing the type of debt they do not want, but then swapping their payment obligations.

First, each company would issue an identical amount of debt, which is called the *notional principal*. Even though Antron wants fixed rate debt, it issues floating rate debt at LIBOR + 1 percent, and Bosworth issues fixed rate debt at 10.4 percent. Next, the two companies swap their interest payments:

Antron will make 10.4 percent fixed rate payments to Bosworth, and Bosworth will make LIBOR + 1 percent payments to Antron.[9]

In addition, Bosworth must make an additional fixed payment of 0.45 percent to Antron. Antron ends up making fixed payments, which it desires, but because of the swap, the rate paid is 9.95 percent versus the 10 percent rate it would have paid had it issued fixed rate debt directly. At the same time, the swap leaves Bosworth with floating rate debt, which it wanted, but at a rate of LIBOR + 0.45 percent versus the LIBOR + 0.50 percent it would have paid on directly issued floating rate debt. As this example illustrates, swaps can sometimes lower the interest rate paid by each party.

As in the illustration, swap arrangements often involve *side payments*. For example, if interest rates had fallen sharply since Company F issued its bonds, then its old payment obligations would be relatively high, and it would have to make a side payment to get S to agree to the swap. Similarly, if the credit risk of one company were higher than that of the other, the stronger company would be concerned about the ability of the weaker counterparty to make the required payments. This high credit risk would also lead to the need for a side payment.

Major changes have occurred over time in the swaps market. First, standardized contracts have been developed for the most common types of swaps, and this has had two effects: (1) Standardized contracts lower the time and effort involved in arranging swaps, and thus lower transactions costs; and (2) the development of standardized contracts has led to a secondary market for swaps, which has increased the liquidity and efficiency of the swaps market. A number of international banks now make markets in swaps and offer quotes on several standard types. Also, banks now take counterparty positions in swaps, so it is not necessary to find another firm with mirror-image needs before a swap transaction can be completed. The bank would generally find a final counterparty for the swap at a later date, so its positioning helps make the swap market more operationally efficient.

Currency swaps, which are similar to interest rate swaps, are of significant value to businesses with overseas operations. They are structured in a manner similar to that described for interest rate swaps, except that the counterparties are exchanging currency types rather than interest rate types. Because few healthcare providers operate in foreign countries, we will not provide an illustration here.

Self-Test Questions

1. What are swaps?
2. How can swaps be used to reduce risk? To lower borrowing costs?

The Use and Misuse of Derivatives

Most of the news stories about derivatives are related to financial disasters. Much less is heard about the benefits of derivatives. However, because of these benefits, more than 90 percent of large U. S. companies use derivatives on a regular basis. These data lead to one conclusion: If a company can safely and inexpensively hedge its financial risks, it should do so.

There can, however, be a downside to the use of derivatives. Hedging is invariably cited by authorities as a "good" use of derivatives, whereas speculating with derivatives is often cited as a "bad" use. Some people and organizations can afford to bear the risks involved in speculating with derivatives, but others are either not sufficiently knowledgeable about the risks they are taking or else should not be taking those risks in the first place. Most would agree that the typical corporation should use derivatives only to hedge risks, not to speculate in an effort to increase profits. Hedging allows managers to concentrate on running their core businesses without having to worry about interest rate, currency, and commodity price variability. However, problems can arise quickly when hedges are improperly constructed or when managers, who are eager to report high returns, uses derivatives for speculative purposes.

Our position is that derivatives can and should be used to hedge against certain risks, but that the leverage inherent in derivative contracts makes them potentially dangerous instruments. Also, healthcare managers should be reasonably knowledgeable about the derivatives their firms use, should establish policies regarding when they can and cannot be used, and should establish audit procedures to ensure that the policies are actually carried out. Moreover, a firm's derivative position should be known by the board and reported to stockholders because stockholders have a right to know the extent to which companies are using derivatives.

Not surprisingly, the Financial Accounting Standards Board (FASB) recently issued new guidelines regarding the disclosure of derivative transactions. The rules, which became effective on July 1, 2000, require that nearly all derivative contracts be marked to market every quarter. This means that a derivative position that has lost value will have to be charged against earnings even though the contract has not expired and may well rise in price later. Before these guidelines were issued, the values of derivative transactions were commonly deferred or shown only in footnotes. Critics of the guidelines contend that they cause reported earnings to fluctuate unnecessarily, and hence force managers to rethink their use of hedging strategies. Proponents contend that the new guidelines allow investors to see what derivative strategies are being used and how well they are working.

Self-Test Questions

1. What is a futures contract?
2. Explain how a company can use the futures market to hedge against rising interest rates.
3. What is a swap? Describe the mechanics of a fixed rate to floating rate swap.
4. Explain how a company can use the futures market to hedge against rising raw materials prices.

5. How should derivatives be used in financial risk management? What problems can occur?

Key Concepts

This chapter provided an introduction to financial risk management. Here are its key concepts:

- In general, *financial risk management* involves the management of unpredictable events that have adverse financial consequences for the business.
- The three steps in risk management are as follows: (1) *identify* the risks faced by the company, (2) *measure* the potential impacts of these risks, and (3) *decide* how each relevant risk should be handled.
- In most situations, risk exposure can be mitigated by one or more of the following techniques: (1) *transfer the risk* to an insurance company, (2) *transfer the function* that produces the risk to a third party, (3) *purchase derivative contracts*, (4) *reduce the probability* of occurrence of an adverse event, (5) *reduce the magnitude* of the loss associated with an adverse event, and (6) totally *avoid* the activity that gives rise to the risk.
- *Derivatives* are securities whose values are determined by the market price of a commodity item or other security.
- A *hedge* is a transaction that lowers risk. A *natural hedge* is a transaction between two *counterparties* where both parties' risks are reduced.
- *Options* are financial instruments that (1) are created by exchanges rather than firms, (2) are bought and sold primarily by investors, and (3) are of importance to both investors and managers.
- The two primary types of options are (1) *call options*, which give the holder the right to purchase a specified asset at a given price (the *exercise,* or *strike, price*) for a given period of time; and (2) *put options*, which give the holder the right to sell an asset at a given price for a given period of time.
- A call option's *exercise value* is defined as the current price of the stock less the strike price.
- Under a *forward contract*, one party agrees to buy a commodity at a specific price on a specific future date and the other party agrees to make the sale. With a forward contract, delivery does occur.
- A *futures contract* is a standardized contract that is traded on an exchange and is "marked to market" daily, but where physical delivery of the underlying asset usually does not occur.
- *Financial futures* permit businesses to create hedge positions to protect themselves against fluctuating interest rates, stock prices, and exchange rates.
- *Commodity futures* can be used to hedge against input price increases.
- *Long hedges* involve buying futures contracts to guard against price increases.

- *Short hedges* involve selling futures contracts to guard against price declines.
- A *perfect hedge* occurs when the gain or loss on the hedged transaction exactly offsets the loss or gain on the underlying asset. Unfortunately, it is difficult to create perfect hedges in the real world because of inherent differences in spot and future markets.
- A *swap* is an exchange of cash payment obligations. Swaps occur because the counterparties involved prefer the other party's payment stream.
- Derivatives can and should be used to hedge against certain risks, but the leverage inherent in derivative contracts makes them potentially dangerous instruments.

This chapter ends our discussion of financial risk management as well as concludes the text. We sincerely hope that you have found this text useful to you as you develop your healthcare financial management skills.

Selected References

Aderholdt, John M., and Robert H. Rasmussen. 1996. "Using Derivatives to Hedge Against the Unexpected." *Healthcare Financial Management* (February): 62–69.

Bond, Michael T., and Brenda Stevenson Marshall. 1994. "Offsetting Unexpected Healthcare Costs with Futures Contracts." *Healthcare Financial Management* (December): 54–58.

———. 1995. "Managing Financial Risk with Options on Futures." *Healthcare Financial Management* (May): 50–56.

Elrod, James L., Jr. 1986. "Can Municipal Bond Futures Contracts Minimize Financial Risk?" *Healthcare Financial Management* (April): 40–44.

LeBuhn, James. 1994. "Primary Market Derivatives: Satisfying Investor Appetites." *Journal of Health Care Finance* (Winter): 11–21.

Patterson, Mary A., and Jeanne Wendel. 1996. "Managing Risk in a Changing Health Care System." *Journal of Health Care Finance* (Spring): 15–22.

Ryan, J. Bruce and Scott B. Clay. 1995. "How to Determine Financial Reserves for Capitated Contracts." *Healthcare Financial Management* (March): 18.

Ryan, J. Bruce and Anne C. Desonier. 1996. "Cost Effective Choices for Provider Stop Loss Insurance." *Healthcare Financial Management* (February): 20–21.

Smith, Scott D. 1994. "The Use of Interest Rate Swaps in Hospital Capital Finance." *Journal of Health Care Finance* (Winter): 35–44.

Woodward, Mark A. 1993. "Interest Rate Swaps: Financial Tool of the '90s." *Healthcare Financial Management* (November): 56–64.

Selected Web Sites

To learn more about the risk-management function in the health services industry, see the web site of the American Society of Healthcare Risk Management at *www.ashrm.org*.

For more information on options and futures markets, see the following:

- *www.cbot.com* for the Chicago Board of Trade;
- *www.cme.com* for the Chicago Mercantile Exchange;
- *www.cboe.com* for the Chicago Board Options Exchange; and
- *www.nymex.com* for the New York Mercantile Exchange.

All of the above web sites contain a large amount of general information as well as specific information regarding the contracts offered.

Notes

1. For more information on IBNR reserves, see J. Bruce Ryan and Scott B. Clay, "How to Determine Financial Reserves for Capitated Contracts," *Healthcare Financial Management*, March 1995, 18.
2. The term "reinsurance" has traditionally been used to mean insurance bought by insurance companies from other insurance companies to limit the risk assumed by the first insurer in covering a potential loss. However, the term is also used in the health services industry when a provider seeks insurance to limit capitation risk.
3. There is a way to modify the duration of a bond to make it a more exact predictor of price risk. See Robert C. Radcliffe, *Investment: Concept, Analysis, and Strategy* (Reading, MA: Addison-Wesley, 1997), 430–431.
4. For an in-depth treatment of options, see Don M. Chance, *An Introduction to Derivatives* (Fort Worth, TX: Dryden Press, 1998).
5. Actually, the *expiration date*, which is the last date that the option can be exercised, is the Friday before the third Saturday of the exercise month. Also, note that option contracts are generally written in 100-share multiples.
6. For purposes of our discussion of healthcare finance, it is not necessary to discuss option pricing models. For a discussion of such models, see the text referenced in Note 4.
7. A *troy ounce* is a unit of weight commonly used in metals. It is equal to 1.0977 avoirdupois (regular) ounces.
8. LIBOR stands for London Interbank Offer Rate, which is the rate charged on dollar loans between banks in the Eurodollar market (the market for U.S. dollars traded overseas).
9. Actually, such transactions generally are arranged by large money-center banks, and payments are made to the bank, which in turn pays the interest on the original loans. The bank would assume the credit risk and guarantee the payments should one of the parties default. For its services, the bank would receive a percentage of the payments as its fee.

Index

ABOUT THE AUTHOR

Louis C. Gapenski, Ph.D., is a professor in both health services administration and finance at the University of Florida. He is the author or coauthor of over twenty textbooks on corporate and healthcare finance. Dr. Gapenski's books are used world wide, with Canadian and international editions, as well as translations into Russian, Bulgarian, Chinese, Indonesian, and Spanish. In addition, he has published numerous journal articles related to corporate and healthcare finance.

Dr. Gapenski received a B.S. degree from the Virginia Military Institute, a M.S. degree from the U.S. Naval Postgraduate School, and M.B.A. and Ph.D. degrees from the University of Florida.

Dr. Gapenski is an active member of the Association of University Programs in Health Administration, the American College of Healthcare Executives, and the Healthcare Financial Management Association. He has acted as academic advisor, chaired sessions, and presented papers at numerous national meetings. Additionally, Dr. Gapenski has acted as a reviewer for eleven academic and professional journals.